Neuropsychology and Substance Use

STUDIES ON NEUROPSYCHOLOGY, NEUROLOGY AND COGNITION

Series Editor:

Linas Bieliauskas, Ph.D.
University of Michigan, Ann Arbor, MI, USA

Other titles in this series:

Fundamentals of Functional Brain Imaging: A Guide to the Methods and their Applications to Psychology and Behavioral Neuroscience. A. C. Papanicolaou

Forensic Neuropsychology: Fundamentals and Practice. Edited by J. J. Sweet

Neuropsychological Differential Diagnosis. K. K. Zakzanis, L. Leach, & E. Kaplan

Minority and Cross-Cultural Aspects of Neuropsychological Assessment. Edited by F. R. Ferraro

Ethical Issues in Clinical Neuropsychology. Edited by S. S. Bush & M. L. Drexler

Practice of Child-Clinical Neuropsychology: An Introduction. B. P. Rourke, H. van der Vlugt, & S. B. Rourke

The Practice of Clinical Neuropsychology. A Survey of Practice and Settings. Edited by G. J. Lamberty, J. C. Courtney, & R. L. Heilbronner

Neuropsychological Rehabilitation: Theory and Practice. Edited by B. E. Wilson

Traumatic Brain Injury in Sports: An International Neuropsychological Perspective. Edited by M. R. Lovell, R. J. Echemendia, J. T. Barth, & M. W. Collins

Methodological and Biostatistical Foundations of Clinical Neuropsychology and Medical and Health Disciplines. Edited by D. V. Cicchetti & B. P. Rourke

A Casebook of Ethical Challenges in Neuropsychology. Edited by S. S. Bush

Neurobehavioral Toxicology: Neurological and Neuropsychological Perspectives. Volume I Foundations and Methods. S. Berent & J. W. Albers

Neurobehavioral Toxicology: Neurological and Neuropsychological Perspectives. Volume II Peripheral Nervous System. J. W. Albers & S. Berent

Geriatric Neuropsychology: Practice Essentials. Edited by S. S. Bush & T. A. Martin

Brain Injury Treatment: Theories and Practices. J. Leon-Carrion, K. R. H. Von Wild, & G. Zitnay

The Quantified Process Approach to Neuropsychological Assessment. Edited by A. Poreh

Mild Cognitive Impairment: International Perspectives. Edited by H. A. Tuokko & D. F. Hultsch

Cognitive Reserve: Theory and Applications. Edited by Y. Stern

Forthcoming titles:

Geriatric Neuropsychology Casebook. J. J. Dunkin

Neuropsychology of Malingering Casebook. J. E. Morgan & J. J. Sweet

For continually updated information about the *Studies on Neuropsychology, Neurology and Cognition* series, please visit: **www.psypress.co.uk/nnc/**

Neuropsychology and Substance Use
State-of-the-Art and Future Directions

Edited by
Ari Kalechstein and Wilfred G. van Gorp

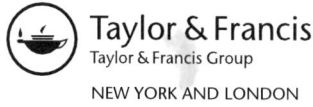
Taylor & Francis Group
NEW YORK AND LONDON

Published 2007
by Taylor & Francis, an informa business
270 Madison Avenue
New York, NY 10016
www.taylorandfrancis.com

Published in Great Britain
by Taylor & Francis Group, an informa business
27 Church Road
Hove, East Sussex BN3 2FA
www.tandf.co.uk

Copyright © 2007 by Taylor & Francis

Typeset in Times by RefineCatch Limited, Bungay, Suffolk, UK
Printed and bound in the USA by Edwards Brothers, Inc. on acid-free paper
Cover design by Hybert Design

All rights reserved. No part of this book may be reprinted or reproduced or utilized in any form or by any electronic, mechanical, or other means, now known or hereafter invented, including photocopying and recording, or in any information storage or retrieval system, without permission in writing from the publishers.

10 9 8 7 6 5 4 3 2 1

Library of Congress Cataloging in Publication Data
Neuropsychology and substance use : state-of-the-art and future directions / edited by Ari Kalechstein, Wilfred Van Gorp.
    p. ; cm. – (Studies on neuropsychology, neurology, and cognition)
  Includes bibliographical references and indexes.
  ISBN 978-1-84169-457-3 (hardcover : alk. paper) 1. Brain – Effect of drugs on. 2. Substance abuse – Physiological aspects. 3. Neuropsychology. I. Kalechstein, Ari. II. Van Gorp, W. G. (Wilfred G.) III. Series.
  [DNLM: 1. Substance-Related Disorders – physiopathology. 2. Comorbidity. 3. Neuropsychology. WM 270 N49457 2007]
  RC564.N477 2007
  362.29 – dc22
                                                  2006100609

ISBN: 978-1-84169-457-3 (hbk)

Contents

About the editors vii
List of contributors ix
From the series editor xi
Preface xiii

1 **Substance abuse epidemiology in the United States: A review of the indicator data** 1
JANE C. MAXWELL, BETH A. RUTOWSKI, AND RICHARD A. RAWSON

Part I
Popular Drugs of Misuse 41

2 **Alcohol** 43
MARLENE OSCAR-BERMAN AND KSENIJA MARINKOVIĆ

3 **Benzodiazepines** 75
SIMON F. CROWE AND MELINDA J. BARKER

4 **Cocaine** 111
KAREN I. BOLLA AND JEAN L. CADET

5 **Marijuana** 139
RAUL GONZALEZ, EILEEN M. MARTIN, AND IGOR GRANT

6 **MDMA** 171
ARI KALECHSTEIN, WILLIAM E. FANTEGROSSI, RONALD L. COWAN, AND JAMES J. MAHONEY

7 **Methamphetamine** 207
ARI KALECHSTEIN AND THOMAS F. NEWTON

8	**Nicotine**	227
	HEATHER G. BELANGER, VANI SIMMONS, AND JOHN SCHINKA	
9	**Opioids**	263
	MIRIAM Z. MINTZER AND MATTHEW W. JOHNSON	

Part II
Populations of Interest   321

10	Substance use and neuropsychological disorders in aging	323
	DYLAN G. HARWOOD, ARI KALECHSTEIN, AND DAVID L. SULTZER	
11	Neurobehavioral consequences of substance abuse and HIV infection	349
	MICHAEL R. BASSO, ROBERT A. BORNSTEIN, AND TAEH WARD	
12	The neurocognitive consequences of substance use in schizophrenia: Are there additive effects?	375
	KARI TERVO	

Part III
Future Directions   405

13	If only the hangover preceded intoxication: An integration of behavioral economic and neuropsychological approaches to impulsive choice	407
	JOHN R. MONTEROSSO, ARI KALECHSTEIN, AND XOCHITL CORDOVA	
14	The influence of environmental context on the effects of drugs of abuse	435
	JASON M. USLANER, HANS S. CROMBAG, AND TERRY E. ROBINSON	

Author index	457
Subject index	487

About the editors

Ari Kalechstein is a senior faculty member at the Semel Institute for Neuroscience and Human Behavior at the David Geffen School of Medicine at UCLA. The primary focus of Dr. Kalechstein's research is the neuropsychological consequences of substance, the identification of compounds that remedy these impairments, and the relationship between neuropsychological impairment and day-to-day functioning.

Wilfred G. van Gorp is Professor of Clinical Psychology and Director of Neuropsychology in the Department of Psychiatry at Columbia University, College of Physicians and Surgeons. He is Editor of *Journal of Clinical and Experimental Neuropsychology* and Past President of the American Academy of Clinical Neuropsychology. Dr. van Gorp has served for many years on the Executive Committee of Division 40 (Clinical Neuropsychology) of the American Psychological Association, and has also served on the APA's Council of Representatives.

List of contributors

Melinda J. Barker, Ph.D., Centre for Community Child Health, Royal Children's Hospital, Victoria, BC, Australia

Michael R. Basso, Ph.D., University of Tulsa, Tulsa, OK

Heather G. Belanger, Ph.D., James A. Haley Veterans' Hospital, University of South Florida, Tampa, FL

Karen I. Bolla, Ph.D., Johns Hopkins Bayview Medical Center, Johns Hopkins University School of Medicine, Baltimore, MD

Robert A. Bornstein, Ph.D., The Ohio State University Medical Center, Columbus, OH

Jean L. Cadet, M.D., National Institute on Drug Abuse (NIDA), Baltimore, MD

Xochitl Cordova, Department of Psychiatry and Biobehavioral Sciences, University of California, Los Angeles, CA

Ronald L. Cowan, M.D., Ph.D., Vanderbilt University Medical Center, Nashville, TN

Hans S. Crombag, Ph.D., Biopsychology and Neuroscience Departments, Johns Hopkins University, Baltimore, MD

Simon F. Crowe, Ph.D., US Department of Veterans Affairs Healthcare System, Jamaica Plain Division, La Trobe University, Victoria, BC, Australia

William E. Fantegrossi, Ph.D., University of Michigan Medical School, Ann Arbor, MI

Raul Gonzalez, Ph.D., University of Illinois, Chicago, IL

Igor Grant, M.D., University of California, San Diego School of Medicine, HIV Neurobehavioral Research Center, California NeuroAIDS Tissue Network, University of California Center for Medicinal Cannabis Research, San Diego, CA

Dylan G. Harwood, Ph.D., UCLA David Geffen School of Medicine, VA Greater Los Angeles Healthcare System, Los Angeles, CA

Matthew W. Johnson, Ph.D., Johns Hopkins University School of Medicine, Baltimore, MD

Ari Kalechstein, David Geffen School of Medicine, University of California, Los Angeles, CA

James J. Mahoney, Ph.D., David Geffen School of Medicine and Semel Institute for Neuroscience and Human Behavior, University of California, Los Angeles, CA

Ksenija Marinković, Ph.D., Athinoula A. Martinos Center for Biomedical Imaging, Harvard Medical School, Massachusetts General Hospital, Boston, MA

Eileen M. Martin, Ph.D., University of Illinois, Chicago, IL

Jane C. Maxwell, Ph.D., University of Texas, Austin, TX

Miriam Z. Mintzer, Ph.D., Johns Hopkins Bayview Medical Center, Johns Hopkins University School of Medicine, Baltimore, MD

John R. Monterosso, Ph.D., Neuropsychiatric Institute, University of California, Los Angeles, CA

Thomas F. Newton, M.D., University of California, Los Angeles, CA

Marlene Oscar-Berman, Ph.D., Boston University School of Medicine, Boston, MA

Richard A. Rawson, Ph.D., UCLA Integrated Substance Abuse Programs, Los Angeles, CA

Terry E. Robinson, Ph.D., Biopsychology and Neuroscience Departments, University of Michigan, Ann Arbor, MI

Beth A. Rutowski, MPH, UCLA Integrated Substance Abuse Programs, Los Angeles, CA

John Schinka, Ph.D., James A. Haley VA Medical Center, University of South Florida, Tampa, FL

Vani Simmons, Ph.D., James A. Haley Veterans' Hospital, University of South Florida, Tampa, FL

David L. Sultzer, M.D., UCLA David Geffen School of Medicine, VA Greater Los Angeles Healthcare System, Los Angeles, CA

Kari Tervo, Ph.D., Department of Psychiatry, Neuropsychiatry Section, University of Pennsylvania School of Medicine, Philadelphia, PA

Jason M. Uslaner, Ph.D., Sleep and Schizophrenia Departments, Merck, West Point, PA

Wilfred G. van Gorp, Ph.D., Columbia University College of Physicians and Surgeons, New York, NY

Taeh Ward, University of Tulsa, Tulsa, OK

From the series editor

Though the neuropsychology of substance use is a topic that has been the subject of multiple research studies over the past 30 years, the literature has varied in terms of quality and quantity and is spread over widely varied journals and presentations.

In *Neuropsychology and Substance Use: State-of-the-Art and Future Directions*, Drs. Kalechstein and van Gorp have collected contemporary, yet practical, reviews of the cognitive implications of the misuse of a variety of commonly encountered substances. While the agents addressed range from alcohol to opioids, sections of the text explore implications of substance use in varying populations of interest and environmental, social, and economic aspects of abuse.

The text is a stellar example of the integration of science and practical implications for which we strive in our book series. I commend this volume as a centralized, ready reference for all who are interested in a centralized summary of the cognitive and social consequences of using and misusing commonly encountered substances with psychoactive effects.

Linas A. Bieliauskas
Ann Arbor
January, 2007

Preface

Ari Kalechstein and Wilfred G. van Gorp

Substance misuse continues to be a major public health problem, and the ramifications of this are manifold. For instance, at present, on a yearly basis, the total economic cost of substance misuse is literally hundreds of billions of dollars. These costs are related to a number of factors, including, but not limited to, treatment and prevention, reduced job productivity and/or absenteeism, interdiction by the criminal justice system, and incarceration.

The adverse effects of substance misuse can also be measured by calculating the number of treatment admissions for substance misuse. For example, in 2003 there were 1.7 million admissions to publicly funded substance abuse treatment programs. This does not take into account the number of admissions into private facilities. While the substance most likely to be misused was alcohol, there was marked misuse of other drugs, such as marijuana, opioids, cocaine, and amphetamine/methamphetamine. Thus, the issue does not appear to be specific to any particular substance.

There are many more psychosocial consequences of substance misuse, and these have been well documented over the past four to five decades; in contrast, with the exception of alcohol, the cognitive effects of substance misuse on the brain have received attention only in the past 10–15 years. An emerging body of literature has reported on the effects of various drugs on neuropsychological functioning, including benzodiazepines, cocaine, marijuana, MDMA, methamphetamine, nicotine, and opioids. Notably, there has been debate of whether certain drugs, such as MDMA, actually cause residual neuropsychological impairment. Furthermore, the co-occurrence of substance misuse and various medical and mental health disorders, such as schizophrenia and HIV, has received increased attention. Moreover, innovative researchers have sought to clarify the associations between these neuropsychological abnormalities and other indices of brain function, such as neuroimaging. Additionally, within the last two to three years, researchers have begun to document the relationship between neuropsychological profile and important functional outcomes, such as relapse to dependence.

Despite the fact that the neuropsychological consequences of many drugs of abuse are well documented, to our knowledge, no one has previously published an edited volume that focused exclusively on this issue involving multiple substances of misuse. Based on this fact, we decided to create a volume that would review the available literature regarding this topic. For example, in order to highlight the incidence and prevalence of substance misuse, the first chapter of the volume focuses exclusively on epidemiology. The next eight chapters discuss the neuropsychological consequences of substances that are most likely to be misused. Three additional chapters focus on the co-occurrence of substance misuse in at-risk populations.

Astute readers may note that the neuropsychological consequences of certain drugs, such as PCP and LSD, were not reviewed. There are a number of reasons for this. First, and to our surprise, there were very few studies that examined the neuropsychological consequences of these drugs. Moreover, the prevalence rate of misuse of these substances was relatively low in comparison to that of other drugs. Because one of our goals was to maximize the relevance of this volume, it seemed most appropriate to include reviews on substances that are currently misused rather than those that might have been abused in decades past.

While we recognized the need to include thorough reviews of the literature for each topic, it was our intent to have chapters that were innovative and/or challenged current thinking in the field. For instance, one of the chapters focuses on an exciting new field, neuroeconomics, which addresses the link between neuropsychological functioning and cost/benefit analyses. Another chapter examines the manner in which context can influence brain structure and function, as well as behavior. These are exciting new fields of scientific endeavor.

Finally, to the extent that it was feasible, we asked authors to address ecologically valid questions related to the use of various drugs. For example, with respect to the use of benzodiazepines, it is clear that these medications are an effective treatment for various types of anxiety disorder; however, if individuals who take benzodiazepines are at risk to experience neuropsychological impairment, then what does that mean for the ability of these individuals to perform various day-to-day activities? Similarly, it has been demonstrated that marijuana can be used effectively as an analgesic and to counteract the anorectic effects of various medical disorders (e.g., HIV, cancer). Nonetheless, it is important to consider if there are potentially detrimental effects of controlled marijuana use that outweigh these benefits.

Before proceeding to the body of the volume, we wish to express our profound gratitude to each of the authors who contributed to this volume. Their dedication and hard work made this volume possible.

1 Substance abuse epidemiology in the United States: A review of the indicator data

Jane C. Maxwell, Beth A. Rutowski, and Richard A. Rawson

Ask any seven people in the United States "What is the worst drug problem in America in 2004?" and you are likely to get seven different answers. For the high school teacher in Pennsylvania, it might appear that marijuana use is rampant among his/her students; for the emergency room doctor in Hawaii, it most certainly is methamphetamine; for the policeman in Washington, DC, "crack" is king; for the parent on an Indian reservation in Arizona, the big concern may be gasoline sniffing; for the primary care physician in Kentucky, OxyContin appears to be an overnight epidemic; the coroner in Baltimore will certainly maintain that heroin is the biggest killer in that city; and, of course, as any highway patrol officer will report across the USA, alcohol is the drug that creates the most problems and costs the most lives.

If you were the Director of the White House Office of National Drug Control Policy, how would you decide which of these problems represented the top priority for spending the limited resources available to prevent and treat substance abuse problems in the USA? In an attempt to answer this question, a set of data collection systems has been established to quantify shifts in drug use patterns in the USA. While the use of multiple data collection systems leads to some inconsistencies in trend information due to the fact that each data system sees the problem from a different point of view, an overview of drug use trends can be constructed by considering a number of different indicators, including both quantitative and qualitative sources.

This chapter evaluates the data from a number of sources to identify trends and patterns of use of alcohol and illicit drugs. The data are arrayed to put together a somewhat cohesive picture of who tends to use which drugs, the trends in use, and the medical and psychological (including neuropsychological) consequences of substance use. The following data sources are discussed in detail in each drug section, and will be referred to hereafter by their abbreviated acronyms.

The Monitoring the Future Survey (MTF) is conducted by the University of Michigan's Institute for Social Research and is funded by the National Institute on Drug Abuse (NIDA). It tracks illicit drug use and attitudes toward drugs by eighth, tenth, and twelfth graders, as well as college students, their age peers not in college, young adult high school graduates through to age 30, and high school graduates aged 35, 40, and 45. The data presented in this chapter cover eighth, tenth, and twelfth graders, college students, and young adults aged 19–28. The MTF reports can be accessed at http://monitoringthefuture.org.

The National Survey on Drug Use and Health (NSDUH), formerly called the National Household Survey on Drug Abuse (NHSDA), is conducted by the Office of Applied Studies of the Substance Abuse and Mental Health Services Administration. It collects information on the prevalence, patterns, and consequences of alcohol, tobacco, and illegal drug use and abuse in the US civilian non-institutionalized population, ages 12 and older. In 2003, a total of 67,784 individuals were sampled in this survey, which is representative of the US general population. The survey reports can be found at http://oas.samhsa.gov/nhsda.htm.

The Drug Abuse Warning Network (DAWN) comprises two components: emergency department (ED) data and mortality data from medical examiners (ME). The ED component provides statistical estimates of drug-related visits to emergency departments for 21 metropolitan areas as well as for the nation. Reasons for visits can include drug abuse and misuse, adverse reactions, accidental ingestion, overmedication, malicious poisoning, suicide attempts, underage drinking, and patients seeking detoxification or drug abuse treatment. The ME component collects data on deaths involving drug abuse (drug-induced or drug-related) that were identified and submitted by participating medical examiners in approximately 40 metropolitan areas across the United States. Unlike the ED component, the ME component is not a sample and it does not provide statistical estimates for the nation as a whole; it simply collects data voluntarily reported by interested medical examiners. DAWN is conducted by the Office of Applied Studies of the Substance Abuse and Mental Health Services Administration. The reports can be found at http://dawninfo.samhsa.gov.

The Treatment Episode Data Set (TEDS) collects information on individuals admitted to substance abuse treatment facilities that are licensed or certified by the 50 state substance abuse agencies. Reporting facilities tend to be those that receive state alcohol and/or drug agency funds, including Federal Block Grant funds. In 2002, over 1.9 million treatment admissions were reported. TEDS is conducted by the Office of Applied Studies of the Substance Abuse and Mental Health Services Administration. The reports can be found at http://oas.samhsa.gov/dasis.htm#teds2.

The Arrestee Drug Abuse Monitoring Program (ADAM) measures the extent of drug use in the high-risk population of people who have been arrested and booked or detained. The 2003 data were collected through probability-based sampling of male arrestees in adult facilities in 39 participating counties (weighted sample of 180,455) and purposive sampling of female arrestees in 25 counties (sample of 3664 females). Information comes from interviews and urine analyses obtained voluntarily and recorded confidentially in booking facilities, usually on the day of arrest and always within

48 hours of arrest. In addition to testing for several drugs, in 2003 data were included for arrestees testing positive for recent alcohol consumption. ADAM was funded by the National Institute of Justice but was discontinued after 2003. The reports are available at http://www.ojp.usdoj.gov/nij/adam/welcome.html.

The National Forensic Laboratory Information System (NFLIS), sponsored by the Drug Enforcement Administration (DEA), is a program that systematically collects results from toxicological analyses conducted by state and local forensic laboratories on substances seized in law enforcement operations. The NFLIS, which was begun in 1997, now collects data from nearly 200 laboratories in 35 states and 55 localities. In 2003, a total of 1,596,780 items were reported (Drug Enforcement Administration, 2004b). The NFLIS reports are available at http://www.deadiversion.usdoj.gov/nflis/index.html. The authors downloaded most of the data in this chapter from the NFLIS online system.

The Community Epidemiology Work Group (CEWG) is sponsored by the National Institute on Drug Abuse (NIDA). The CEWG is composed of 21 researchers from across the nation. They meet twice per year to report on drug abuse patterns and trends and emerging problems in their local areas. Members use quantitative statistics and qualitative techniques such as focus groups and key informant interviews to monitor drug trends. The full reports of the CEWG can be accessed at http://www.nida.nih.gov/about/organization/cewg/Reports.html.

The Drug Enforcement Administration (DEA) reports the price and purity of drugs in various geographic regions of the country. The reports are available at http://www.usdoj.gov/dea/statistics.html.

Alcohol

Alcohol is the most widely used drug, with an economic cost in terms of health care, lost productivity, and criminal justice costs of $166.5 billion to American society in 1995, as compared to an economic cost of $109.8 billion for drug abuse (Harwood et al., 1998). Binge and heavy drinking remains a problem, and alcohol is often misused in combination with other drugs.

According to results from the 2003 MTF, there was little change in alcohol use among survey participants in the 12 months since the last survey was administered (Exhibit 1.1). Twelfth graders were the only group of students who showed further decline in 30-day prevalence of drinking (from 48.6% in 2002 to 47.5% in 2003). Occurrences of heavy drinking (which is defined as consumption of five or more drinks in a row in the past two weeks) continued to decrease slightly (although not significantly) in all three grades, and the prevalence of daily alcohol use remained low in all three grades, decreasing slightly among tenth graders (1.8% to 1.5%) and twelfth graders (3.5% to 3.2%). In terms of long-term trends in lifetime alcohol use, 70.1% of eighth graders, 83.8% of tenth graders, 88.0% of twelfth graders, 93.6% of college

Exhibit 1.1 Lifetime prevalence of drugs from the Monitoring the Future Surveys: 1991–2003

Percent of All Respondents, By Grade/Age Group

	1991	1992	1993	1994	1995	1996	1997	1998	1999	2000	2001	2002	2003	Change
Alcohol														
8th grade	70.1	69.3	55.7	55.8	54.5	55.3	53.8	52.5	52.1	51.7	50.5	47	45.6	
10th grade	83.8	82.3	71.6	71.1	70.5	71.8	72	69.8	70.6	71.4	70.1	66.9	66	
12th grade	88	87.5	80	80.4	80.7	79.2	81.7	81.4	80	80.3	79.7	78.4	76.6	
College Students	93.6	91.8	89.3	88.2	88.5	88.4	87.3	88.5	88	86.6	86.1	86	86.2	
Young Adults	94.1	93.4	92.1	91.2	91.6	91.2	90.7	90.6	90.2	90.7	89.9	90.2	89.3	
Inhalants														
8th grade	17.6	17.4	19.4	19.9	21.6	21.2	21	20.5	19.7	17.9	17.1	15.2	15.8	
10th grade	15.7	16.6	17.5	18	19	19.3	18.3	18.3	17	16.6	15.2	13.5	12.7	
12th grade	17.6	16.6	17.4	17.7	17.4	16.6	16.1	15.2	15.4	14.2	13	11.7	11.2	
College Students	14.4	14.2	14.8	12	13.8	11.4	12.4	12.8	12.4	12.9	9.6	7.7	9.7	
Young Adults	13.4	13.5	14.1	13.2	14.5	14.1	14.1	14.2	14.2	14.3	12.8	12.4	12.2	
Powder Cocaine														
8th grade	2.3	2.9	2.9	3.6	4.2	4.5	4.4	4.6	4.7	4.5	4.3	3.6	3.6	
10th grade	4.1	3.3	3.6	4.3	5	6.5	7.1	7.2	7.7	6.9	5.7	6.1	5.1	
12th grade	7.8	6.1	6.1	5.9	6	7.1	8.7	9.3	9.8	8.6	8.2	7.8	7.7	
College Students	9.4	7.9	6.3	5	5.5	5	5.6	8.1	8.4	9.1	8.6	8.2	9.2	
Young Adults	21	19.5	16.9	15.2	13.7	12.9	12.1	12.3	12.8	12.7	13.1	13.5	14.7	
Crack Cocaine														
8th grade	1.3	1.6	1.7	2.4	2.7	2.9	2.7	3.2	3.1	3.1	3	2.5	2.5	
10th grade	1.7	1.5	1.8	2.1	2.8	3.3	3.6	3.9	4	3.7	3.1	3.6	2.7	**

12th grade	3.1	2.6	2.6	3	3	3.3	3.9	4.4	4.6	3.9	3.7	3.8	3.6
College Students	1.5	1.7	1.3	1	1.8	1.2	1.4	2.2	2.4	2.5	2	1.9	3.1
Young Adults	4.8	5.1	4.3	4.4	3.8	3.9	3.6	3.8	4.3	4.6	4.7	4.3	4.7
Methamphetamine													
8th grade	…	…	…	…	…	…	…	…	4.5	4.2	4.4	3.5	3.9
10th grade	…	…	…	…	…	…	…	…	7.3	6.9	6.4	6.1	5.2
12th grade	…	…	…	…	…	…	…	…	8.2	7.9	6.9	6.7	6.2
College Students	…	…	…	…	…	…	…	…	7.1	5.1	5.3	5	5.8
Young Adults	…	…	…	…	…	…	…	…	8.8	9.3	9	9.1	8.9
Ice													
12th grade	3.3	2.9	3.1	3.4	3.9	4.4	4.4	5.3	4.8	4	4.1	4.7	3.9
College Students	1.3	0.6	1.6	1.3	1	0.8	1.6	2.2	2.8	1.3	2.3	2	2.9
Young Adults	2.9	2.2	2.7	2.5	2.1	3.1	2.5	3.4	3.3	3.9	4	4.1	4.7
Marijuana													
8th grade	10.2	11.2	12.6	16.7	19.9	23.1	22.6	22.2	22	20.3	20.4	19.2	17.5
10th grade	23.4	21.4	24.4	30.4	34.1	39.8	42.3	39.6	40.9	40.3	40.1	38.7	36.4
12th grade	36.7	32.6	35.3	38.2	41.7	44.9	49.6	49.1	49.7	48.8	49	47.8	46.1
College Students	46.3	44.1	42	42.2	41.7	45.1	46.1	49.9	50.8	51.2	51	49.5	50.7
Young Adults	58.6	56.4	55.9	53.7	53.6	53.4	53.8	54.4	54.6	55.1	55.7	56.8	57.2
Heroin													
8th grade	1.2	1.4	1.4	2	2.3	2.4	2.1	2.3	2.3	1.9	1.7	1.6	1.6
10th grade	1.2	1.2	1.3	1.5	1.7	2.1	2.1	2.3	2.3	2.2	1.7	1.8	1.5
12th grade	0.9	1.2	1.1	1.2	1.6	1.8	2.1	2	2	2.4	1.8	1.7	1.5
College Students	0.5	0.5	0.6	0.1	0.6	0.7	0.9	1.7	0.9	1.7	1.2	1	1
Young Adults	0.9	0.9	0.9	0.8	1.1	1.3	1.3	1.6	1.7	1.8	2	1.8	1.9

(Continued Overleaf)

Exhibit 1.1 (Continued)

Percent of All Respondents, By Grade/Age Group

	1991	1992	1993	1994	1995	1996	1997	1998	1999	2000	2001	2002	2003	Change
LSD														
8th grade	2.7	3.2	3.5	3.7	4.4	5.1	4.7	4.1	4.1	3.9	3.4	2.5	2.1	
10th grade	5.6	5.8	6.2	7.2	8.4	9.4	9.5	8.5	8.5	7.6	6.3	5	3.5	**
12th grade	8.8	8.6	10.3	10.5	11.7	12.6	13.6	12.6	12.2	11.1	10.9	8.4	5.9	***
College Students	9.6	10.6	10.6	9.2	11.5	10.8	11.7	13.1	12.7	11.8	12.2	8.6	8.7	
Young Adults	13.5	13.8	13.6	13.8	14.5	15	15	15.7	16.2	16.4	16	15.1	14.6	
PCP														
12th grade	2.9	2.4	2.9	2.8	2.7	4	3.9	3.9	3.4	3.4	3.5	3.1	2.5	
Young Adults	3.1	2	1.9	2	2.2	1.9	2.4	2.7	2.3	2.3	3.1	2.5	3	
MDMA (Ecstasy)														
8th grade	...	...	...	...	...	3.4	3.2	2.7	2.7	4.3	5.2	4.3	3.2	*
10th grade	...	...	...	...	...	5.6	5.7	5.1	6	7.3	8	6.6	5.4	
12th grade	...	...	...	...	...	6.1	6.9	5.8	8	11	11.7	10.5	8.3	*
College Students	2	2.9	2.3	2.1	3.1	4.3	4.7	6.8	8.4	13.1	14.7	12.7	12.9	
Young Adults	3.2	3.9	3.8	3.8	4.5	5.2	5.1	7.2	7.1	11.6	13	14.6	15.3	

Levels of significance of difference between the two most recent years: * = 0.05; ** = 0.01, *** = 0.001.
Young Adult category includes individuals aged 19–28.
(...) Data not available.
Source: Monitoring the Future Survey, NIDA.

students, and 94.1% of young adults reported any alcohol use in 1991. Twelve years later, in 2003, these rates had fallen to 45.6% among eighth graders, 66.0% among tenth graders, 76.6% among twelfth graders, 86.2% among college students, and 89.3% among young adults. Lifetime, past year, and past month use by girls aged 12–17 now equals or surpasses that of boys (Johnston et al., 2004a, 2004b).

The 2003 NSDUH reported that 50% or an estimated 119 million Americans aged 12 or older consumed alcohol in the 30 days preceding their survey. Approximately 54 million (22.6%) individuals binged (defined as consumption of five or more drinks on the same occasion at least once in the past 30 days) at least once in the 30 days prior to the survey, and 16 million (6.8%) drank heavily (defined as consumption of five or more drinks on the same occasion on at least five different days in the past 30 days). Young adults aged 18–25 were most likely to report patterns of both binge and heavy drinking in 2003. Binge and heavy alcohol use rates decreased faster with increasing age than did rates of past month alcohol use.

Of all racial/ethnic groups, Whites were most likely to report current use of alcohol in 2003 (54.4%), followed by American Indians/Alaska Natives (42.0%) and Hispanics (41.5%), and then Blacks (37.9%). In terms of geographic differences in self-reported alcohol use, the rate of past month alcohol use among persons aged 12 and older was highest in large metropolitan areas (53.3%), as compared to small metropolitan areas (48.9%) and nonmetropolitan areas (42.1%).

With regard to underage alcohol use, nearly 11 million persons aged 12–20 consumed alcohol in the 30 days prior to their survey, which represented 29% of the age group. Of these individuals, 7.2 million (19.2%) binge drank and 2.3 million (6.1%) drank heavily. The prevalence of current alcohol use among adolescents increased with increasing age, from 2.9% of 12-year-olds to 59.6% of 20-year-olds.

Girls aged 12–17 reported higher rates of lifetime, past year, and past month use of alcohol (43.9%, 36.5%, 18.3%) than their male peers (41.9%, 32.1%, 17.1%), although boys reported higher rates of binge and heavy alcohol use. Among those aged 18–25, males reported higher lifetime, past year, and past month use than females, as well as higher rates of binge and heavy alcohol use.

In 2003, current self-reported alcohol use was strongly associated with other substance use, including tobacco and illicit drugs. Among the 16.1 million heavy drinkers aged 12 and older, 32.5% were also current illicit drug users. Moreover, 61.7% of heavy drinkers smoked cigarettes in the past month. Smokeless tobacco and cigar use were higher among heavy drinkers than among nonbinge drinkers and nondrinkers.

The number of new alcohol users rose steadily during the 1990s, from 2.9 million new alcohol users in 1990 to 5.3 million in 2001. Much of this increase can be accounted for by initiation of use among young persons under the age of 21. The number of new adolescent users nearly doubled in the past decade, from 2.0 million in 1990 to 3.8 million in 2001. Of the estimated 21.6 million Americans aged 12 or older who were classified with substance dependence or abuse in 2003 (9.1% of the total population aged 12 or older), 14.8 million were dependent upon or abused alcohol, but not illicit drugs. In 2003, 1.1 million individuals received alcohol treatment (SAMHSA, 2004d, 2004e).

The DAWN ED system reported that the rate of mentions of alcohol in combination with other drugs had increased significantly from 71.7 per 100,000 in 1995 to 80.8 per 100,000 in 2002. The increase was significant for males, for all persons aged 18–25, and for those aged 35 and older. Of the 207,395 cases seen, 61% were male, 55% White, 26% Black, and 10% Hispanic. Fifty-five percent were aged 35 or older. Forty-one of the cases reported their motive for seeking emergency department care was dependence, while 25% reported a suicide attempt, and 21% reported psychic effects. The reason for the contact for 35% was an overdose, with 23% seeking detoxification. Fifty-five percent of the cases were admitted to hospital for further care (SAMHSA, 2003).

The proportion of TEDS treatment admissions with a primary problem of alcohol dropped from 59% in 1992 to 43% in 2002 (Exhibit 1.2). In 2002, there were 807,939 alcohol admissions. Of these admissions, 45% reported that they also had secondary problems with other drugs. Clients who were alcohol-only admissions in 2002 were likely to be male (76%), White (71%), and with an average age of 39 years. Those with a primary alcohol problem and a secondary drug problem were also more likely to be male (74%), less likely than alcohol-only clients to be White (59%), and to be younger (average age 34 years). Forty percent of alcohol-only admissions and 34% of alcohol and drug admissions were referred to treatment from criminal justice agencies (SAMHSA, 2004a). Marijuana was the most frequently reported second problem drug (24%), followed by cocaine (19%; SAMHSA, 2004b).

The DAWN ME component includes data on two categories of deaths: drug-induced and drug-related. One to six drugs can be mentioned in conjunction with a reportable case. To facilitate the interpretation of DAWN ME findings for each participating metropolitan area, deaths involving only one drug ("single-drug" deaths) are differentiated from those involving more ("multiple-drug" deaths). Alcohol is frequently mentioned in combination with other commonly reported drugs, such as cocaine, heroin/morphine, and narcotic analgesics. It is important to note that the number of cases involving these combinations varies across participating metropolitan areas, and many other drug combinations are reported. In 19 of the 31 metropolitan areas in 2002, alcohol (in combination with at least one other drug) was one of the three most frequently mentioned drugs in reported cases (SAMHSA, 2004c).

According to ADAM data collected in 2003, 10% of adult male and 86% of adult female arrestees tested positive for recent alcohol consumption. Median past 30-day binge and heavy alcohol use was higher among males than females (48% and 26% respectively for males, compared with 35% and 16% respectively for females; Zhang, 2004).

Exhibit 1.2 US admissions to treatment by primary drug of abuse: 1992–2002

	Percent of All Admissions										
	1992	1993	1994	1995	1996	1997	1998	1999	2000	2001	2002
Alcohol	58.8	56.5	52.5	50.5	50.2	49.5	48.4	47.7	46.3	44.2	42.9
Heroin	11	12.2	13	13.5	13.5	14.6	14.4	14.8	15.5	15.8	15.2
Other Opiates	0.9	0.9	0.9	1	1	1	1.2	1.3	1.6	2.1	2.4
Cocaine											
Crack	12	12.7	13.3	12.4	11.9	10.9	10.9	10.4	9.9	9.4	9.3
Powder	5.5	4.8	4.6	4.2	4.2	3.8	3.9	3.8	3.7	3.5	3.5
Marijuana	6	7	8.7	10.5	12	12.3	12.9	13.5	14.1	14.7	15.1
Stimulants*	1.4	1.8	2.8	3.9	3.3	4.2	4.2	4.3	4.7	5.6	6.7
Tranquilizers	0.3	0.3	0.3	0.3	0.3	0.3	0.3	0.3	0.4	0.4	0.4
Sedatives/ Hypnotics	0.2	0.2	0.2	0.2	0.2	0.2	0.2	0.2	0.2	0.2	0.2
Hallucinogens	0.2	0.2	0.2	0.2	0.2	0.2	0.1	0.2	0.2	0.2	0.1
PCP	0.2	0.2	0.2	0.2	0.2	0.1	0.1	0.1	0.2	0.2	0.2
Inhalants	0.2	0.2	0.2	0.1	0.1	0.1	0.1	0.1	0.1	0.1	0.1

*Includes methamphetamine, other amphetamines, and other stimulants.
Source: Treatment Episode Data Set, SAMHSA.

Inhalants

Inhalants are breathable chemical vapors or gases that produce psychoactive (mind-altering) effects when abused or misused. They include a broad range of volatile solvents and gas products (e.g., model airplane glue, paint thinner, gasoline, and nail polish remover), aerosols (e.g., nonstick cooking spray and hair spray), anesthetics (e.g., nitrous oxide, or "laughing gas," and ether), and nitrites (e.g., amyl, butyl, and isobutyl nitrites, often marketed as "poppers" or room odorizers).

Inhalant abuse is often a hidden problem. While surveys show that inhalant use is highest among the young, its use is still relatively low compared to the prevalence of marijuana and alcohol use. In the 2003 MTF, lifetime use of inhalants was 15.8% for eighth graders, 12.7% for tenth graders, and 11.2% for seniors. One of the most remarkable and consistent findings of school surveys is the decline in students reporting lifetime and recent prevalence of inhalant usage between eighth and twelfth grades (Johnston et al., 2004a), a pattern that contrasts with the increase in lifetime and current use of all other substances with age. The decrease in prevalence rates is best understood in the context of other research showing that inhalant-using students are more likely to drop out of school before graduation (National Institute on Drug Abuse, 2000). Ongoing inhalant abuse has been associated with failure in school, delinquency, and an inability to achieve societal adjustment (Chadwick & Anderson, 1989; Chadwick et al., 1990).

In the 2003 MTF, the pattern of decline as students age was evident among students of all ethnicities, although slightly less steep for White students (from 16% lifetime in eighth grade to 13% in twelfth grade) than for African American students (12% in eighth grade and 5% in twelfth grade) and Hispanic students (19% in eighth grade to 10% in twelfth grade). In addition, after a lengthy and marked decrease over the years in the use of inhalants by eighth, tenth, and twelfth graders, past-year use by eighth graders increased significantly, from 7.7% to 8.7%, in 2003 (Johnson et al., 2004a).

The NSDUH shows a lifetime prevalence of inhalant use in 2003 at approximately 9.7% of the population aged 12 and older. Lifetime use was 10.7% for ages 12–17, 14.9% for ages 18–25, and 8.6% for ages 26 and older. Further, lifetime use was 12.9% for males and 6.6% for females; 11.5% for Whites, 6.4% for Hispanics, and 3.9% for Blacks. For all ages combined, lifetime use of inhalants was higher than the use of stimulants, methamphetamines, MDMA (ecstasy), crack cocaine, heroin, PCP, tranquilizers, or sedatives, and past month use of inhalants was higher than the use of LSD, heroin, crack cocaine, PCP, methamphetamines, or sedatives.

The inhalants that were most commonly reported as having ever been used included nitrous oxide or "whippets" (4.9%), amyl nitrite ("poppers," "locker room," or "rush") (3.8%), glue, shoe polish, or toluene (1.8%), gasoline or lighter fluid (1.6%), correction fluid, degreaser, or cleaning fluid (1.0%), lacquer thinner or other paint solvents (0.8%), spray paints (0.9%), and other aerosol sprays (0.9%). Reported lifetime use varied by age group and substance. Those aged 26 and older reported the highest lifetime use of amyl nitrite, those aged 18–25 reported the highest use of nitrous oxide or "whippets," and gases such as halothane, ether, or other anesthetics, while those aged 12–17 reported highest lifetime use of glue, shoe polish, or toluene, gasoline or lighter fluid, correction fluid, degreaser or cleaning fluid, other aerosol sprays, lacquer thinner or other paint solvents, lighter gases (butane, propane), spray paints, and other aerosol sprays.

The number of new initiates of inhalant use has risen from 472,000 in 1990 to 1.1 million in 2001, before dropping to 1.0 million in 2002. Average age of new users has dropped from 19.0 in 1985 to 15.6 in 2002 (SAMHSA, 2004d, 2004e).

Exhibit 1.3 shows the number of confirmed intentional misuse and abuse calls to Texas Poison Control Centers. While the numbers of cases are not large, they demonstrate the variations in substances used and different age groups. The youngest inhalers misused typewriter correction fluid, aerosol air

Exhibit 1.3 Exposures involving misuse or abuse of inhalants reported to the Texas Poison Center Network, by year: 1998–2003

Product	Total Number of Calls 1998–2003	Average Age 1998–2003
Air Freshener: Aerosol	33	14.6
Amyl/Butyl Nitrite	13	27.6
Automotive Product: Hydrocarbon	78	20.2
Automotive Product: Methanol	74	25.3
Formaldehyde/Formalin	49	22.1
Freon/Other Propellant	126	17.6
Gasoline	101	14.8
Lighter Fluid/Naphtha	6	24.3
Mineral Spirits/Varsol/Stoddard	26	23.5
Nitrous Oxide	21	23.4
Paint: Oil-Base	114	23.6
Propane & Other Simple	63	15.5
Toluene/Xylene (excluding adhesives)	67	24.3
Typewriter Correction Fluid	15	12.9
Unknown Paint, Varnish, or Lacquer	62	23.8
Varnish & Lacquer	10	20.2

Source: Texas Poison Center Network.

freshener, and gasoline, while the oldest group of misusers inhaled amyl or butyl nitrite (poppers), and another group in their mid-20s used automotive products, lighter fluid, or paint products (Maxwell, 2004). An earlier study found that the average age of Texas decedents where inhalants were mentioned on the death certificates was 25.6 years and the ages ranged from 8 to 62 years; approximately 81% were White. The relationship between the specific inhalant substance used and occupation of the decedent was statistically significant (e.g., mechanics, installers, and repairers used Freon, and other blue-collar workers used toluene; Maxwell, 2001).

The 2002 DAWN ED data showed that of the 1496 persons seen in emergency departments with problems with inhalant use, 19% were under 18, 22% were 18–25, 32% were 26–34, and 27% were 35 or older. Some 63% were male; 45% were White and 17% were Black (the percentage of Hispanics was not reported). The motives for using inhalants included suicide (36%), psychic effects (27%), and dependence (21%; SAMHSA, 2003a).

Nationally, inhalant abusers constituted only 0.1% (1199) of the TEDS treatment admissions in 2002 (Exhibit 1.2). Of these admissions, 72% were male; 70% were White and 18% were Hispanic. The average age was 24 years. Some 33% were referred by the criminal justice system (SAMHSA, 2004a). Secondary drugs of abuse were alcohol (29%) and marijuana (28%; SAMHSA, 2004b).

Cocaine

Powder cocaine is normally either inhaled or injected, while crack cocaine is smoked. Crack cocaine is made by adding baking soda and water to powder cocaine and then cooking the mixture until it forms a hard substance that can be broken into pieces, known as "rocks," for smoking. Use of cocaine remains at a high endemic level. Crack cocaine has spread out of the Black community into White and Hispanic user groups, and females are more likely to use crack rather than powder cocaine, according to TEDS and ADAM data, although this trend is not seen in the NSDUH.

The 2003 MTF findings indicate that lifetime prevalence of powder and crack cocaine use has remained stable among eighth graders (at 3.6% and 2.5%, respectively), but has continued to decline among tenth (5.1% and 2.7%, respectively) and twelfth graders (7.7% and 3.6% respectively; Exhibit 1.1). Furthermore, the decline in crack cocaine use among tenth graders was significant. Annual and past 30-day use of cocaine and crack remained low, decreasing slightly among students in all three grade levels. Current crack use declined significantly among tenth graders (from 1% to 0.7%; Johnston et al., 2004a). Among college students, lifetime use of cocaine was stable at 9.4% in 1991 and 9.2% in 2003, but use of crack cocaine doubled from 1.5% to 3.1% in the same time period. Among young adults, lifetime use of powder cocaine decreased from 21.0% in 1991 to 14.7% in 2003, while lifetime use of crack cocaine was steady at 4.8% in 1991 and 4.7% in 2003 (Johnston et al., 2004a, 2004b).

According to findings from the 2003 NSDUH, an estimated 34.9 million Americans aged 12 or older (14.7%) reported cocaine use at least once in their lifetime, and 7.9 million (3.3%) of these individuals reported lifetime use of crack cocaine. Approximately 2.3 million (1.0%) reported past-month use of cocaine, and 604,000 (0.3%) used crack cocaine in the past month. Rates of current cocaine use were highest among young adults aged 18–25 (2.2%), followed by adults aged 26 and older (0.8%), and youths aged 12–17 (0.6%).

Following a steady decline in the number of new cocaine users from 1980 to 1993, the incidence of cocaine use increased during the 1990s to 1.1 million new users in 2002. The average age of new cocaine initiates dropped from 24.5 in 1992 to 20.3 in 2002. New crack users are older, but the average age has dropped from 28.8 in 1993 to 22.9 in 2002. Males are more likely than females to initiate cocaine use. In 2002, nearly 0.6 million new cocaine users were male, compared to less than 0.5 million female users (SAMHSA, 2004d, 2004e).

DAWN ED mentions of cocaine (199,198 in 2002) have increased from 58.3 per 100,000 in 1995 to 77.6 per 100,000 in 2002, a 33% change that was statistically significant. Significant increases were observed between 1995 and 2002 for males and females and all age groups except those aged 26–34. Of the patients in 2002, 64% were male, 40% were White, 40% were Black, and 12% were Hispanic. Fifty-six percent were aged 35 and older. Fifty-four percent of the cases reported that their motive for using cocaine was dependence, and 28% came to the emergency department because of an unexpected reaction to the cocaine. Fifty percent were subsequently admitted to hospital (SAMHSA, 2003a).

The proportion of TEDS treatment admissions for primary cocaine abuse has declined from 18% in 1992 to 13% in 2002 (Exhibit 1.2). Crack cocaine smokers (176,014 in 2002) represented 73% of the cocaine admissions in 2002, which is an increase from 69% in 1992. Of the powder cocaine users (65,685 in 2002), 73% inhaled and 14% injected. Males constituted 59% of the crack cocaine admissions and 67% of the powder cocaine admissions. Crack users were older, with an average age of 37, as compared to powder cocaine users, whose average age was 34. The racial distribution of crack admissions has changed: in 1992, 26% were White, 69% Black, and 5% Hispanic; in 2002, 34% were White, 57% Black, and 7% Hispanic. Among powder cocaine admissions, the proportion who were White was 47% in 1992 and 2002, while the proportion who were Black has declined from 40% to 33%, and the proportion who were Hispanic increased from 13% to 17% (SAMHSA, 2004a).

Forty-seven percent of crack smokers, 30% of the cocaine injectors, and 43% of the cocaine inhalers reported that they also had problems with alcohol, while 20% of crack smokers, 14% of injectors, and 25% of inhalers reported problems with marijuana. Twenty-five percent of crack smokers and 34% of powder cocaine users were referred to treatment by the criminal justice system. Twenty-two percent of cocaine injectors reported problems with heroin, which shows the preference for "speedballing" (the combining of cocaine and heroin) among some users (SAMHSA, 2004b).

Twenty-eight of the 31 metropolitan areas that reported drug death data to the DAWN ME system in 2002 had heroin/morphine, cocaine, and alcohol in combination listed as the most frequently mentioned substances among drug deaths. In addition to being frequently reported in combination, cocaine was also one of the drugs commonly reported singly. In terms of the most commonly reported drug combinations, cocaine was frequently mentioned in combination with alcohol or heroin/morphine. In 19 of the 31 participating metropolitan areas, cocaine was one of the three most frequently mentioned drugs in reported cases. According to trend data, which were available for 29 metropolitan areas, 15 areas reported a decrease in the frequency of cocaine involvement in drug abuse deaths, whereas the remaining 14 areas saw an overall increase in cocaine relative to 2001 (SAMHSA, 2004c).

According to ADAM data collected in 2003, 30% of adult male and 35% of adult female arrestees tested positive for recent crack or powder cocaine use. The rate of recent use among adult males ranged from a low of 2.6% in Woodbury, IA, to a high of 49.84% in Atlanta, GA. The rate of recent use among adult females ranged from a low of 8.5% in Honolulu, HI, to a high of 55.7% in Indianapolis, IN.

In addition to testing for recent cocaine use using urine analysis, adult male and female arrestees were asked to self-report past year and past 30-day use of crack and powder cocaine. A higher percentage of adult females than males reported past year (24.5% vs. 17.2%) and past 30-day crack cocaine use (20.5% vs. 13.8%). Past year and past 30-day powder cocaine use, on the other hand, was slightly higher among males (13.6% and 9.6%, respectively) and females (12.9% and 7.6%, respectively; Zhang, 2004).

Between 1997 and 2003, cocaine was the second most commonly identified drug by law enforcement laboratories reporting to the NFLIS, although the proportion has dropped from 35.0% in 1997 to 30.8% in 2003 (Exhibit 1.4; National Forensic Laboratory Information System, 2004). During the December 2003 CEWG meeting, many members reported that cocaine, crack cocaine in particular, continued to be widely available, dominating many of the major indicator systems in cities such as Chicago, New Orleans, Philadelphia, and Washington, DC. In Chicago, for example, many cocaine indicators, such as treatment admissions and use among Chicago school students, increased in 2002. In Washington, DC, where "cocaine is king," crack cocaine accounted for more emergency department episodes, admissions to publicly funded treatment programs, and drug-related deaths than any other drug.

Exhibit 1.4 Substances identified by laboratories participating in the National Forensic Laboratory Identification System: 2003

	1997	1998	1999	2000	2001	2002	2003
Cannabis	47.1%	46.3%	37.8%	38.5%	35.7%	35.0%	36.1%
Cocaine	34.6%	33.8%	34.2%	32.1%	31.0%	32.1%	30.8%
Methamphetamine	3.7%	2.7%	7.9%	8.8%	12.2%	12.8%	11.9%
Heroin	0.5%	5.2%	8.5%	7.5%	6.8%	6.3%	6.1%
MDMA	0.0%	0.0%	0.5%	1.2%	1.5%	1.1%	0.6%

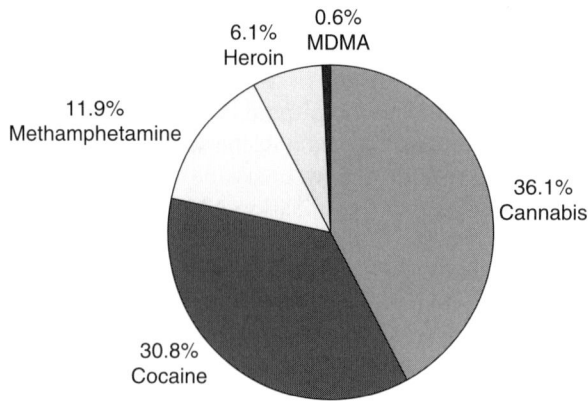

Source: National Forensic Laboratory Identification System.

In addition to reports of increased use in general, reemergence of powder cocaine (or a shift from crack to powder) and new populations of cocaine users were discussed. In Denver, a shift in how and to whom powder cocaine is marketed was reported. Drug markets have shifted as distributors have moved the supply to sell to new customers or new communities. Use among Hispanic communities has increased. In Texas, the proportion of treatment admissions reporting powder cocaine use who were Hispanic increased from 23% to 46%, whereas the percentage of powder cocaine admissions who were White decreased from 48% to 42%, and the percentage of powder cocaine admissions who were African American dropped from 28% to 10%. Other demographic changes included a shift in the age of cocaine users, as well as a shift in socioeconomic status. In New York, cocaine-using treatment admissions were reported as an "aging population," with crack smokers tending to be older than intranasal cocaine users. There was also an influx of white-collar professional powder cocaine users. Finally, several CEWG members, especially those who represent Western US cities, echoed reports that cocaine use and availability is becoming overshadowed by another stimulant, methamphetamine (National Institute on Drug Abuse, 2004).

Methamphetamine

In the United States, the use and abuse of methamphetamine has been described as a series of epidemics, with use stabilized at high endemic levels in the West, where, other than marijuana, it is the major illicit drug of abuse. At the same time its use is growing in the Midwest and only beginning to emerge on the East Coast, except in the gay male bar scene, where it has become a significant problem. To provide more insight into the different levels of use, this section will look at reports from CEWG members in detail.

One of the problems in monitoring patterns of use is that in the United States the distinctions between amphetamine and methamphetamine are not well defined. Although they are different substances, the terms are often interchanged or reported in a combination "amphetamine/methamphetamine" or "stimulant" category. Methamphetamine comes in different forms and with different names. "Speed" is often powdered and ranges in color from white to yellow, orange, brown, or pink. It is usually of relatively low purity. "Pills" can be pharmaceutical grade amphetamine, such as Adderall, Ritalin, or Phenteramine, or the pills can be methamphetamine powder that has been pressed into tablets that are sold as amphetamine or ecstasy. "Ice," also known as "shard," "shabu," "tweak," "crystal," or "crystal meth," is methamphetamine that has been "washed" in a solvent, such as denatured alcohol, to remove impurities. Evaporation of the solvent yields crystals that resemble glass shards or ice shavings. It is usually smoked and has longer-lasting physical effects and purity levels above 80%, although low-quality methamphetamine may also be marketed as Ice.

According to the 2003 MTF, lifetime use of methamphetamine was down for twelfth graders, tenth graders, and young adults, while use was up for eighth graders and college students (Exhibit 1.1). The MTF also queried twelfth graders, college students, and young adults about their past year use of Ice. Use by twelfth graders decreased between 2002 and 2003, while use by college students and young adults increased. Among twelfth graders, the percentage who thought it harmful to try crystal meth or Ice once or twice dropped from an all-time high of 53.8% in 2002 to 51.2% in 2003, and perceived availability of crystal meth dropped from a high of 29.8% in 1998 to 26.1% in 2003 (Johnston et al., 2004a, 2004b).

The NSDUH in 2003 reported that 5.2% of the US population aged 12 and over (12.3 million individuals) had ever used methamphetamine (defined as crank, crystal, ice, speed, Desoxyn, or methedrine), 0.6% (1.3 million) had used in the past year, and 0.3% (607,000) had used in the past month. Some 1.6% of those aged 18–25 had used methamphetamine in the past year, as compared to 0.4% of those aged 26 or older. Lifetime use was 1.3% for those aged 12–17, 5.2% for those aged 18–25, and 5.7% for those aged 26 and older.

Incidence of methamphetamine use had remained fairly level since the early 1980s, but increased to a high of 372,000 new users in 1998. In 2002, there were approximately 323,000 new methamphetamine users. Average age of new initiates dropped from a high of 22.1 in 1991 to 18.8 in 2001 and then increased to 20.2 in 2002. In addition, the NSDUH found that 3.6% reported lifetime use of prescription diet pills and 1.8% reported lifetime use of Ritalin or methylphenidate. Persons aged 26 and older reported the highest lifetime use of prescription diet pills (4.2%), and those aged 18–25 reported the highest usage of Ritalin or methylphenidate (5.7%) (SAMHSA, 2004d, 2004e).

The rate of DAWN ED mentions of methamphetamine/amphetamine has increased from 11 per 100,000 in 1995 to 15 per 100,000 in 2002, which is a 39.9% increase. In 2002, 59% of the patients were male, but visits by females have risen from 37% in 1995 to 40% in 2002. Some 65% were White, 6% were Black, and 11% were Hispanic. Thirty-three percent were age 35 and older and 56% were between 18 and 34. The motives for using the drug included dependence (39%) or psychic effects (24%), and the reasons for seeking emergency department treatment included overdose (30%) or unexpected reaction (24%). Sixty-two percent also used other drugs: marijuana, alcohol, cocaine, benzodiazepines, opioid pain relievers, and heroin (SAMHSA, 2003a).

Geographically, the areas with the highest rates per 100,000 were San Francisco (91), San Diego (68), Phoenix (65), Seattle (46), and Los Angeles (39). But use of the drug is spreading eastward. Compared to 1995, the 2002 rates had more than doubled in Atlanta (23 in 2002), Baltimore (10), Chicago (8), Miami (4), Minneapolis (19), New Orleans (16), Newark (9), and St. Louis (24) (Office of Applied Studies, 2004a).

The TEDS reports a combined category of "methamphetamine/amphetamine" admissions. The proportion of these admissions in the TEDS treatment database increased from 1.4% in 1994 to 6.7% in 2002 (Exhibit 1.2). During that time, the proportion who were Hispanic doubled from 6% to 12%, while the proportion who were White dropped from 83% to 74%. The proportion who were Black remained less than 3%. Use of Ice (a street name for crystal methamphetamine hydrochloride, which is more pure than the powder form of methamphetamine) has increased, as shown by the fact that smoking methamphetamine (Ice) increased from 12% to 50%, while the proportion who were inhaling has dropped from 39% to 17% and the proportion who were injecting has dropped from 32% to 23%. Approximately 52% of the clients were referred to treatment by the criminal justice system. In 2002, another 9% took amphetamine-type pills by mouth (SAMHSA, 2004a). Secondary problem drugs were marijuana for 35% of the clients and alcohol for 27% (SAMHSA, 2004b).

Exhibit 1.5 illustrates the increases in the rate of methamphetamine/amphetamine treatment admissions over the ten-year period of 1992–2002. Nationally, the rate rose from 10.4 admissions per 100,000 in 1992 to 52.1 per 100,000 in 2002. The impact on the individual states is shown by the fact that in 1992 only one state had a rate higher than 50 per 100,000. By 2002, 19 states had rates of 50 or more per 100,000 and 13 of those 19 states reported rates of 100 or more per 100,000. The magnitude of the problem varies from region to region. Use has stabilized at endemic levels in the West while it is still a growing epidemic in the Midwest and is just beginning in the East, although its use has been well-documented in the gay club scene.

According to 2002 DAWN ME data, methamphetamine-induced and methamphetamine-related deaths continued to be geographically concentrated in the Midwest and West. In 11 of the 31 areas, including Dallas, Denver, Salt Lake City, and San Francisco, methamphetamine was listed among the top 10 most common drugs mentioned in drug data reported to DAWN. San Francisco, Dallas, Las Vegas, San Diego, and Phoenix were the five metropolitan areas reporting the highest number of methamphetamine mentions (38, 46, 72, 81, and 132 mentions, respectively). Alternatively, only one Eastern metropolitan area, Philadelphia, reported more than five methamphetamine mentions. Among the 23 metropolitan areas reporting any methamphetamine mentions, the drug was reported in combination with at least one additional drug in 88% of the cases, on average. San Diego and Dallas had the highest number of methamphetamine-only deaths (10 and 13, respectively) of the 13 metropolitan areas that reported any single-drug methamphetamine deaths (SAMHSA, 2004c).

ADAM data in 2003 showed, on average, that females were nearly twice as likely as males to test positive for recent methamphetamine use (8.8% vs. 4.7%). The highest percentage of adult males and females testing positive was in Honolulu, HI (40.3% of males and 57.4% of females). Twelve of 29 sites, concentrated in the Western United States, had more than 20% of adult males test positive for methamphetamine, and nine of 25 sites, again concentrated

Exhibit 1.5 Methamphetamine/amphetamine admission rates per 100,000 population aged 12 and older, by state: 1992 vs. 2002

	Rate per 100,000 Population			Rate per 100,000 Population	
	1992	2002		1992	2002
Total USA	10.4	52.1	Montana	33.5	118.6
Alaska	4.2	15	North	1.1	3.2
Alabama	1.3	35.9	North Dakota	2.3	65.4
Arkansas	7.2	124.9	Nebraska	6.8	102.2
Arizona	*	27.7	New	0.3	7
California	48.6	200.1	New Jersey	2.6	1.9
Colorado	14	67.7	New Mexico	4.9	4.5
Connecticut	1	3.8	Nevada	34.6	156.8
Delaware	2.1	1.8	New York	1.8	3.4
Florida	1.5	5.3	Ohio	5.3	1.9
Georgia	1.9	22.2	Oklahoma	15.5	118.8
Hawaii	32.8	217.2	Oregon	72.4	323.6
Iowa	9.2	198.1	Pennsylvania	2.5	2.3
Idaho	9.7	116.2	Rhode Island	2.1	2.4
Illinois	2	13.4	South	1.3	6.7
Indiana	1.6	22.8	South Dakota	4	68.9
Kansas	9.8	61.3	Tennessee	0.1	9.3
Kentucky	*	13.3	Texas	7.2	13
Louisiana	3.9	18.4	Utah	10	115.2
Massachusetts	1.1	1.3	Virginia	0.9	3.2
Maryland	1.5	2.6	Vermont	4.7	4.3
Maine	1.5	3.5	Washington	11.4	150.4
Michigan	2.1	5.1	Washington	*	3.6
Minnesota	4.6	77.6	Wisconsin	0.4	3.5
Missouri	5.2	86.2	West Virginia	1.4	0.5
Mississippi	*	17.5	Wyoming	15.2	166.9

* Indicates states with incomplete data.
Source: Treatment Episode Data Set, SAMHSA.

in the Western United States, had more than 20% of adult females test positive for methamphetamine. In almost every case, a higher percentage of adult females tested positive for recent methamphetamine use. In terms of self-reported use of methamphetamine, a higher percentage of adult females than males reported past year (15.3% vs. 7.7%) and past 30-day use (11.3% vs. 4.7%; Zhang, 2004).

The proportion of substances identified in the NFLIS as being methamphetamine rose from 4.0% in 1997 to 11.9% in 2003 (Exhibit 1.4). In the Western region, 37.0% of the items were methamphetamine, as compared to 7.5% in the Midwest, 6.4% in the South, and 0.3% in the Northeast (National Forensic Laboratory Information System, 2004).

Ice is predominately available in Hawaii and on the West Coast, but it is becoming more available elsewhere in the United States. A gram on the West Coast sells for $140, an ounce from $1200 to $1500, and a pound from $10,000 to $18,000. In Hawaii, a gram costs between $200 and $400, an ounce costs $2300, and a pound can cost as much as $30,000.

During the June and December 2003 meetings, CEWG members reported that in Hawaii the use of Ice was increasing. There were more deaths due to methamphetamine than due to alcohol in 2002. The suicide rate involving methamphetamine was high, and treatment admissions were increasing. In San Diego, methamphetamine use was increasing and it was primarily imported from Mexico. Ice use was also prevalent in San Diego. In Los Angeles, the numbers of methamphetamine treatment admissions and arrestees testing positive for methamphetamine were increasing, drug purity was stable, and the price was increasing. In San Francisco, emergency department mentions and treatment admissions were increasing. Use was widespread, with increased dealing and usage, especially among "fast lane" gay and bisexual males. In Seattle, treatment admissions were level and emergency department admissions were down from earlier years. While the number of laboratories seized in Washington State was down, there were still many small "mom and pop" operations.

In Phoenix, Ice was a problem and the quality was high, with most of the drug coming from "superlabs" in California or Mexico. The price was up due to the demand. In Colorado, methamphetamine was the "big story," with indicators such as poison control center calls, overdose deaths, and hospital discharges increasing. It was a major problem in the rural areas. The proportions of Hispanic treatment admissions and admissions over age 35 were increasing and crack cocaine users were reported to be switching to methamphetamine. Most new users were smoking rather than injecting the drug.

In Texas, treatment admissions had increased, overdose deaths were up, and drug seizures were increasing. Methamphetamine and amphetamines were greater problems in the northern half of the state, as documented by the Texas NFLIS data. Methamphetamine was both imported from Mexico and also manufactured in small laboratories in the more rural areas of the state. Ice was a growing problem in the state, with more treatment admissions for smoking than inhaling or "snorting" the drug.

In Minneapolis and St. Paul, methamphetamine use was increasing, especially in the rural areas. In Missouri, methamphetamine was the primary illicit drug of abuse in rural areas, and treatment admissions were increasing. Use was increasing among African American users in Kansas City. In

Michigan, laboratory seizures were increasing, smoking was the primary route of administration, and treatment admissions were increasing for both methamphetamine and prescription amphetamines. In Chicago, use had remained low but was more prevalent in the downstate rural counties. "Tweak," which has a crystal-like appearance, was seen in Chicago clubs and it was more commonly smoked than injected.

In Atlanta, methamphetamine had increased, with more local laboratories seized. Mexican methamphetamine was also available. Use among African Americans was increasing, as well as use among teenagers. Among rural users, some 60% were female and smoking was the most popular route of administration. Ice and "shards" were the choices. In Miami, "Tina" was popular in the gay bathhouse scene and methamphetamine abuse was described as an emerging drug epidemic. In New York City there had been a slight increase in availability of methamphetamine, and some crystal meth was being sold. Recent seizures of laboratories in rural areas in New York indicated the continuing spread of methamphetamine eastward. In Boston, methamphetamine was emerging as the drug in the club scene.

Marijuana

Marijuana is the most frequently used illicit drug. Survey data, emergency department reports, and treatment admissions are now documenting an increase in marijuana users who are reporting adverse events or meeting the criteria for dependence, although use by adolescents has decreased recently (Exhibit 1.6).

Marijuana is the most widely used illicit drug, according to findings from the MTF. In 2003, 12.8% of eighth graders, 28.2% of tenth graders, 34.9% of twelfth graders, 33.7% of college students, and 29% of young adults smoked marijuana in the previous year. One percent of eighth graders, 3.6% of tenth graders, 6% of twelfth graders, 4.7% of college students, and 5.3% of young adults reported daily use of marijuana. In a reversal of trends, a significantly higher proportion of students in all three grades thought that it was a great risk to smoke marijuana occasionally or to smoke marijuana regularly. These findings may relate to the recent declines in marijuana use (Johnston et al., 2004a, 2004b).

Marijuana is also the most commonly used illicit drug among persons aged 12 and older (6.2% used marijuana in the past 30 days), according to findings from the 2003 NSDUH. Some 96.6 million Americans aged 12 and older (or approximately 41% of the general population) reported trying marijuana/hashish at least once in their lifetime. Seventy-five percent of the current illicit drug users reported marijuana use either alone (55%) or with at least one other illicit drug (21%). The rate of current marijuana use was highest among 18–25-year-olds (17.0%), followed by youths aged 12–17 (7.9%), and adults aged 26 or older (4.0%). When asked to report the frequency with which they used marijuana, 12.2% of past year marijuana users

Exhibit 1.6 Marijuana indicators: 1995–2002

	1995	1996	1997	1998	1999	2000	2001	2002
Marijuana Admissions of All Illicit Drug Admissions (TEDS)	10.5	12	12.3	12.9	13.5	14.1	14.7	15.1
ED Mentions/ 100,000 (DAWN)	19.5	22.9	27.2	31.9	35.8	39	43.6	46.5
Lifetime Use by 18–25 (NSDUH)	44.1	44.3	45.7	47	50.3	51.8	53	53.8
Past Month Use by 12th Graders (MTF)	21.2	21.9	23.7	22.8	23.1	21.6	22.4	21.5

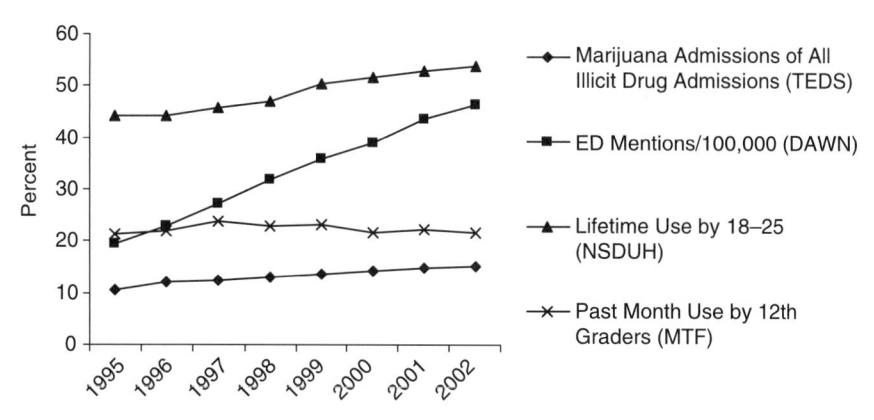

Source: Treatment Episode Data Set, Drug Abuse Warning Network, and National Survey on Drug Use and Health, SAMHSA; Monitoring the Future, NIDA.

used the drug on 300 or more days. This rate translates into 3.1 million persons using marijuana on a daily or almost daily basis.

The NSDUH includes questions about how marijuana is obtained. In 2003, more than half of all marijuana users (57%) obtained the drug for free or smoked marijuana that was obtained by another individual, while 40% bought their marijuana.

In 1990, 1.5 million individuals tried marijuana for the first time. The number of new marijuana users increased over the next few years to a high of nearly 2.9 million in 2000, before dropping to an estimated 2.6 million individuals initiating marijuana use in 2002. Average age of the new initiates has decreased from 19.4 in 1982 to 17.2 in 2002, and over half (53%) of marijuana initiates were female. Lastly, of the 6.8 million Americans classified as being dependent on or abusing illicit drugs, over half (4.2 million) were dependent on or abused marijuana. This translates into 1.8% of the total US population aged 12 and older (SAMHSA, 2004d, 2004e).

Analysis of the 1991–1992 National Longitudinal Alcohol Epidemiologic Survey (NLAES) and the 2001–2002 National Epidemiologic Survey on Alcohol and Related Conditions (NESARC) found that, although the prevalence of marijuana use remained stable at about 4.0% over the past decade among the adult US population, the prevalence of DSM-IV marijuana abuse or dependence increased significantly from 1.2% to 1.5%. The greatest increases were among young Black men and women and young Hispanic men. Further, the reports of marijuana use disorders significantly increased, although the frequency and quantity of use did not increase, which suggests that the increase in potency of delta-9-tetrahydrocannabinol may have contributed to the rising rates. The average potency of confiscated marijuana increased by 66%, from 3.1% in 1992 to 5.1% in 2002 (Compton et al., 2004).

The rate of mentions of marijuana in DAWN ED admissions increased from 19.5 in 1995 to 46.5 per 100,000 in 2002, a 139% increase that was statistically significant. The increases were also significant for both males and females and for all age groups. Of the patients mentioning marijuana, 64% were male, 55% White, 26% Black, and 11% Hispanic. With respect to age, 32% were aged 35 and older, 21% were aged 26–34, 31% were aged 18–25, and 16% were aged 12–17. Thirty-three percent reported that they used marijuana for psychic effects, and 29% said they used it because they were dependent. The reason for seeking emergency department assistance included unexpected reaction (38%), overdose (19%), and seeking detoxification (12%; SAMHSA, 2003a).

Admissions to treatment with a primary marijuana problem increased from 6% in 1992 to 15% in 2002 (Exhibit 1.2). Marijuana admissions tend to be male (76%), White (55%), and young (23 years). Some 57% of marijuana admissions were referred to treatment through the criminal justice system (SAMHSA, 2004a). Two-thirds reported abuse of additional substances, with 53% reporting also having problems with alcohol (SAMHSA, 2004b).

In terms of 2002 DAWN ME data, marijuana is reported in a number of cases, but to a much lower extent than alcohol, cocaine, or heroin/morphine. Marijuana is listed among the 10 most commonly mentioned drugs in 14 participating metropolitan areas, such as Detroit (111 mentions), New Orleans (56 mentions), and New York (55 mentions). Further, marijuana was one of the three most frequently mentioned drugs in three areas: Kansas City, MO, Louisville, KY, and Omaha, NB. Because many participating jurisdictions do not test for the presence of marijuana among decedents, it is hard to quantify the full extent of marijuana involvement in the DAWN ME system.

According to ADAM data collected in 2003, males were more likely than females to test positive for recent marijuana use (44.1% vs. 31.6%). In 9 of 39 sites, more than 50% of adult male arrestees tested positive for recent marijuana use. For adult females, the percentage of positive tests ranged from 24.5% in Anchorage, AK, to 43.3% in Oklahoma City, OK. In terms of self-reported use of marijuana, a slightly higher percentage of adult males than females reported past year (51.9% vs. 44.4%) and past 30-day (44.9% vs. 36.0%) marijuana use (Zhang, 2004). Marijuana is also the substance most often identified in state and local laboratories reporting to the NFLIS, although the proportion of items identified has dropped from 49% in 1997 to 36% in 2003 (Exhibit 1.4; National Forensic Laboratory Information System, 2004).

Much discussion ensued during the December 2003 CEWG meeting with regard to the high levels of marijuana use, especially among youths. Overall, indicators of marijuana use remained very high throughout 2002 and into early 2003, and even increased in some cities. High proportions of treatment resources were devoted to marijuana abusers, large percentages of adult arrestees tested positive for recent marijuana use, and rates of emergency department mentions of marijuana remained high. Some CEWG members raised a concern about the availability of higher-potency marijuana, the use of marijuana in combination with other drugs, and both younger and older cohorts of marijuana users seeking treatment for their marijuana use. In addition, young marijuana users (especially under the age of 18) continued to enter treatment because of referrals from the criminal justice system. In Texas, clients entering treatment as a result of criminal justice referrals were less impaired on the Addiction Severity Index than those who were not criminal justice referrals, and the criminal justice referrals reported using marijuana and other drugs on fewer days in the month prior to admission.

In New Orleans, marijuana remained a major problem, especially among youths. And because of an abundance of Mexican marijuana, prices decreased in some areas of Louisiana. Increases in both marijuana-related arrests and seizures were reported for Los Angeles. In Phoenix, marijuana remained readily available in large quantities, despite recent seizures by the US Border Patrol. The average size of a seized marijuana load ranged from 200 to 500 pounds. In San Diego, increases in emergency department mentions, treatment admissions, and positive drug screens among arrestees were reported in a discussion of recent marijuana-specific trends (National Institute on Drug Abuse, 2004).

Heroin

There are four types of heroin in the United States. East of the Mississippi River, 93% of heroin samples were from South America. That type of heroin is powdered, with an average street-level purity of 42% and a cost of $0.89 per milligram pure. West of the Mississippi River, 95% of the samples in 2003 were Mexican heroin (black tar and, to a lesser extent, brown powder), with an average purity of 26% and a cost of $0.75 per milligram pure in 2003. Mexican black tar may be sticky like roofing tar or hard like coal. Mexican brown powder may be either a powdered heroin produced in Mexico, or it may be black tar that has been turned into a powder by local dealers or users by adding a diluent such as lactose. Smaller quantities of Southeast and Southwest Asian heroin are found throughout the USA. Southeast Asian heroin was 38% pure at a cost of $0.44 per milligram pure, and Southwest Asian was 26% pure and cost $0.97 per milligram pure (Drug Enforcement Administration, 2003, 2004a).

While South American and Asian powdered heroin can be inhaled, smoked, or injected, the most common route of administration of black tar is injection. Because of its oily, gummy consistency, special steps are required to convert the heroin into a powder that can be snorted. Because brown powder is diluted, it is preferred by novices and users who fear overdoses. Diluents ("cuts") can include lactose, Benedryl, Nytol, baby laxative, vitamin B, and coffee creamer. Tar heroin can be frozen, the "cut" added, and then pulverized or ground into a powder in a coffee grinder or with a mortar and pestle. It can also be dried out on a plate over the stove or under a heat lamp prior to pulverizing.

Lifetime prevalence of heroin use as reported in the MTF was nearly identical across grade levels in 2003: 1.6% of eighth graders and 1.5% of both tenth and twelfth graders, 1.0% of college students and 1.9% of young adults reported using heroin at least once in their lives (Exhibit 1.1; Johnston et al., 2004a, 2004b). According to results from the 2003 NSDUH, 3.7 million Americans aged 12 or older reported lifetime heroin use, which translates to 1.6% of the general population. Some 314,000 individuals reported past year use of heroin, and 119,000 persons were current heroin users. The number of new initiates increased from 32,000 in 1985 to 162,000 in 2001 and then dropped to 122,000 in 2002. Average age of the new initiates has dropped from 27.2 in 1992 to 21.4 in 2002. In 2003, 1.1% reported that they had sniffed or snorted heroin at least once in their lifetimes, while 0.5% reported having smoked heroin, and 0.7% reported injecting heroin (SAMHSA, 2004d, 2004e).

The rate of mentions of heroin in DAWN emergency departments has increased from 29.9 per 100,000 in 1995 to 36.4 in 2002 (265,667 mentions), a statistically significant increase of 21.9%. The rates of increase for males and females and for those aged 18–25 and 35 and older were also significant for this time period. Some 66% of the patients in 2002 were male; 43% White, 31% Black, and 14% Hispanic. The patients tended to be older: 56% were 35 and older. Eighty-one percent said their motive for use was dependence, and 37% came to the emergency department seeking detoxification (SAMHSA, 2003a),

Treatment admissions with a primary problem with heroin increased from 11% in 1992 to 15.2 in 2002 (Exhibit 1.2). Of the 2002 admissions, 48% were White, 25% Hispanic, and 24% Black; 69% were male. The average age was 36. The preferred route of admission changed over the ten-year period. In 1992, 77% were injectors, as compared to 62% in 2002; in contrast, inhaling of heroin has increased from 20% in 1992 to 33% in 2002, while smoking heroin has gone from 1% to 3% in the same time period. Clients with problems with opiates were much less likely than users of other drugs to be referred by the criminal justice system, i.e., only 13% of heroin users were referred by the criminal justice system (SAMHSA, 2004a). Other drugs of abuse include alcohol for 35% of the heroin admissions and powder cocaine for 21%, which shows the pattern of "speedballing" heroin and cocaine (SAMHSA, 2004b).

Like cocaine, heroin/morphine was one of the drugs commonly reported by itself, according to DAWN ME data in 2002. In terms of the most commonly reported drug combinations, heroin/morphine was frequently mentioned in combination with alcohol, cocaine, or other narcotic analgesics. In 19 of the 31 metropolitan areas, heroin/morphine was one of the three most frequently mentioned drugs in reported cases. In 2002, 15 metropolitan areas reported a lesser number of heroin/morphine mentions than in 2001, whereas the remaining 12 reported a higher number of heroin/morphine mentions than the previous year (SAMHSA, 2004c). In 2003, heroin ranked fourth in terms of the drugs most commonly identified by NFLIS laboratories. It constituted 6% of all items identified (Exhibit 1.4; National Forensic Laboratory Information System, 2004).

An average of 5.8% of adult males and 6.6% of adult females tested positive for recent opiate use, according to 2003 ADAM data. Among adult males, the percentage of positive opiate urine analyses ranged from a low of 1.6% in Woodbury, IA, to a high of 28.4% in Rio Arriba, NM. Among females, the percentage of positive opiate urine analyses ranged from 0% in Los Angeles and Omaha, NE, to a high of 23.2% in New York City. In terms of self-reported use of heroin, 5.1% of males and 7.1% of females reported past year use and 3.9% of males and 4.4% of females reported past 30-day heroin use (Zhang, 2004).

Despite discussion of increased use of several drugs by attendees at the December 2003 CEWG meeting, heroin indicators remained relatively stable in most CEWG areas. Northeastern/mid-Atlantic areas (where high-purity South American powder heroin is marketed) tended to report high levels of heroin use, but indicators of use were also high in San Francisco and Seattle, two cities where Mexican black tar heroin is the predominant form available for use. Increases were also reported in Boston, Chicago, Los Angeles, and Minneapolis/St. Paul. CEWG members from Denver and Detroit reported changes in user demographics, including a shift away from injection use toward smoking or inhaling, and a shift toward White suburban user groups. The Detroit members mentioned continued reports of oxycodone users shifting to heroin because of the reduced availability of oxycodone.

Other opiates

This group excludes heroin but includes opiates such as methadone, codeine, hydrocodone (Vicodin, Tussionex), oxycodone (OxyContin, Percodan,

Percocet-5, Tylox), *d*-propoxyphene (Darvon), hydromorphone (Dilaudid), morphine, meperidine (Demerol), and opium. In recent years, data have documented increasing sales (and diversion) of some of these drugs and increasing numbers of adverse events, as well as patterns of misuse by young adults and by persons in rural areas.

The 2003 MTF showed that lifetime and past month use of "narcotic drugs other than heroin" peaked among twelfth graders in 2002, while past month use continued to rise into 2003. Starting in 2002, the MTF queried the five age groups about past year use of OxyContin and Vicodin. The annual prevalence rates for OxyContin in 2003 were 1.7% among eighth graders, 3.6% among tenth graders, 4.5% among twelfth graders, 2.2% for college and 2.6% for young adults. Students were more likely to report annual use of Vicodin than OxyContin: the 2003 annual prevalence rates for Vicodin were 2.8% among eighth graders, 7.2% among tenth graders, 10.5% among twelfth graders, 7.5% for college students, and 8.6% for young adults. Both of these narcotic drugs showed gradually but not statistically significant increases in all five populations in 2003 (Johnston et al., 2004a, 2004b).

The 2003 NSDUH findings showed that an estimated 4.7 million persons, corresponding to about 2.0% of the population aged 12 or older, were current users of pain relievers taken nonmedically. The lifetime prevalence rate for nonmedical use of other opiates was 8.3% for Darvocet, Darvon, or Tylenol with codeine; 6.6% for Vicodin, Lortab, or Lorcet; 4.5% for Percocet, Percodan, or Tylox; 2.9% for codeine; 2.4% for hydrocodone; 1.3% for Demerol; 0.9% for morphine; and 1.2% for OxyContin. Young adults aged 18–25 reported the highest rates of use for each of these drugs.

The number of new initiates of pain relievers has increased annually, rising from 41,000 in 1966 to 2.5 million in 2002. Average age has decreased from 24.9 in 1987 to 22.2 in 2002 (SAMHSA, 2004d, 2004e).

DAWN ED mentions of hydrocodone alone or in combination with substances such as aspirin or acetaminophen have increased from 9686 mentions in 1995 to 25,197 in 2002, which is a 160% increase (Exhibit 1.7). Mentions of oxycodone, by itself or in combination with other substances, increased from 3393 mentions in 1995 to 22,397 in 2002, which is an increase of 560%. This increase in oxycodone mentions is primarily due to the introduction of OxyContin, a slow-release oxycodone. In 1997, there were four DAWN ED mentions of slow-release oxycodone; in 2002, there were 14,087 (SAMHSA, 2003a). Polydrug use was prevalent among users of other opiates. In 2002, 71% of oxycodone-related emergency department visits and 78% of hydrocodone-related visits involved multiple drugs. Alcohol was the substance most frequently mentioned, followed by cocaine, heroin, marijuana, and alprazolam (Office of Applied Studies, 2004d).

The proportion of treatment admissions with a primary problem with opiates other than heroin has increased from 0.9% in 1992 to 2.4% in 2002 (Exhibit 1.2). Unlike users of many other drugs, clients with problems with these opiates were not as likely to be male: 46% were female. In addition, 88%

Exhibit 1.7 DAWN ED mentions of selected opiates

	1995	1996	1997	1998	1999	2000	2001	2002
Hydrocodone/combinations	9686	11,419	11,570	13,611	15,252	20,098	21,567	25,197
Oxycodone/combinations	3393	3190	5012	5211	6429	10,825	18,409	22,397

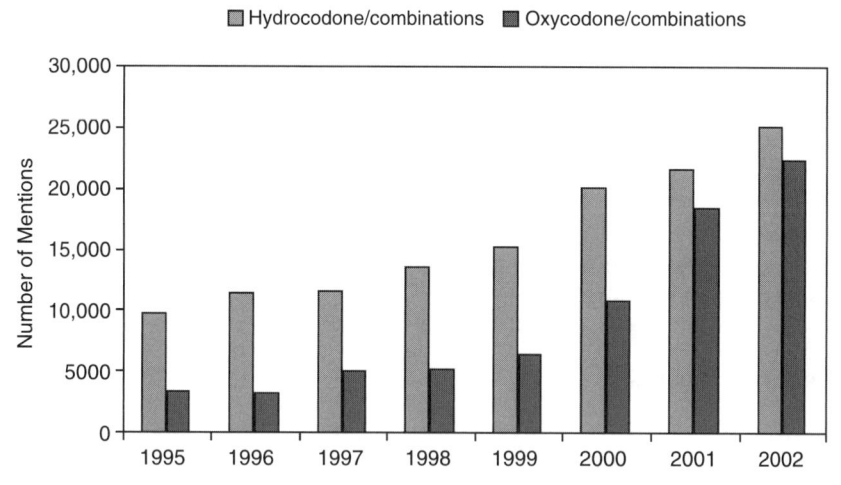

Source: Drug Abuse Warning Network, SAMHSA.

were White and their average age was 35 years. Fifteen percent were referred by the criminal justice system (SAMHSA, 2004a). In comparison to heroin users, patients who used other opiates also had problems with other drugs: alcohol (18%), marijuana (11%), crack cocaine (10%), benzodiazepines (8%), and heroin (8%; SAMHSA, 2004b).

The major change between 1997 and 2002 was the increase in the proportion of new users (those who entered treatment within three years of beginning use). The proportion of new users increased from 26% in 1997 to 39% in 2002 and the largest increase was in the number of admissions among persons aged 20–30 (Office of Applied Studies, 2004e). In addition, the increase was greatest (269%) in the most rural areas (nonmetropolitan areas with a city), and the smallest in large central metropolitan areas (58%; Office of Applied Studies, 2004f).

A wide variety of prescription and over-the-counter drugs are reported to the DAWN ME system as playing a role in drug deaths; the most frequently mentioned include benzodiazepines and narcotic analgesics. In 2002, hydrocodone ranked among the 10 most commonly mentioned drugs in deaths in 14 metropolitan areas, including Detroit (80 mentions), New Orleans (80), Las Vegas (60), Dallas (50), and San Diego (31). Methadone ranked in the top 10 in 24 areas, including New York (169 mentions), New Orleans (95),

Philadelphia (80), Baltimore (74), Detroit and Las Vegas (each with 61), and Chicago (53). Oxycodone ranked among the 10 most commonly mentioned drugs in deaths in 17 areas, including Philadelphia (93 mentions), Boston (49), Las Vegas (42), Baltimore (33), and Seattle (29). Lastly, codeine ranked in the top 10 drugs mentioned in 19 areas, including Detroit (149 mentions), Philadelphia (120), Baltimore (89), Phoenix (80), and Newark (68; SAMHSA, 2004c). Of all the items examined by the NFLIS, hydrocodone and oxycodone each made up no more than 1% (National Forensic Laboratory Information System, 2004).

At the December 2003 CEWG meeting, OxyContin use generally increased. In Detroit, OxyContin users were transitioning to heroin use. In New York City, OxyContin was being mixed with heroin to enhance the "high." In Boston, there were increased calls to local authorities on problems related to OxyContin use. In San Francisco, hydrocodone and oxycodone use had increased. In Phoenix, use of narcotic analgesics had increased. The use of Vicodin and OxyContin was increasing in Denver. In Texas, Vicodin use was more prevalent than OxyContin use.

Sedatives/tranquilizers

This category includes sedatives such as phenobarbital and secobarbital (Seconal), nonbarbiturate sedatives such as methaqualone, over-the-counter sleeping aids, and chloral hydrate, and tranquilizers and benzodiazepines such as diazepam (Valium), alprazolam (Xanax), flunitrazepam (Rohypnol), clonazepam (Klonopin), flurazepam (Dalmane), lorazepam (Ativan), and chlordiazepoxide (Librium and Librax). These drugs, especially the benzodiazepines, are often used in combination with drugs such as heroin, cocaine, and the "club drugs."

The 2003 MTF showed a significant decline in the use of tranquilizers among tenth and twelfth graders. Most of the tranquilizer use involved Valium and Xanax. Sedative (including barbiturates) use among twelfth graders and college students had been rising steadily for about a decade before leveling and possibly beginning to decline in the past two years. Use continued to increase for young adults. The MTF reported that lifetime use of Rohypnol has been declining since 1999 (Johnston et al., 2004a, 2004b).

The NSDUH reported lifetime use of various benzodiazepines: Valium (6.2%), Xanax (4.0%), Klonopin (1.2%), and Rohypnol (0.2%). Young adults aged 18–25 reported the highest lifetime rates of use of these drugs.

The number of new initiates of nonmedical use of tranquilizers has increased from 431,000 in 1992 to 1.2 million in 2002. During this same time period, average age has dropped from 27.5 to 23.5 (SAMHSA, 2004d, 2004e).

DAWN ED mentions of barbiturates increased from 6793 in 1995 to 9783 in 2002, which is a 44% increase. Mentions of benzodiazepines increased from 71,548 in 1995 to 105,752 in 2002, which is a 38% increase. Alprazolam was the benzodiazepine most often mentioned (27,659 in 2002); notably, there had been a 62% increase in mentions of this drug since 1995. Clonazepam was the benzodiazepine that was used by 17,042 patients, and the number of mentions increased by 33% between 1995 and 2002. Diazepam was mentioned 11,193 times, and there has been no significant change in the number of mentions over the years (SAMHSA, 2003a). Approximately 78% of the visits involved two or more drugs. Alcohol was involved in more than twice as many benzodiazepine-related visits as marijuana, the second most frequently mentioned drug (Office of Applied Studies, 2004b).

In 1995 and 2002, patients aged 26–44 had the highest rates of ED visits involving benzodiazepines, but the greatest increase was for patients aged 18 and 19. In 1995, the rate was higher for female patients than for male patients (37 vs. 23 visits per 100,000); however, by 2002 there was no statistical difference between female and male patients. Half of the visits involving benzodiazepines were the result of suicide attempts, but visits attributed to drug dependence and drug-taking for psychic effects have been increasing (Office of Applied Studies, 2004c).

TEDS admission data show that the percent of admissions for tranquilizers has remained at 0.3–0.4% since 1992, and admissions for sedatives/hypnotics have remained at 0.2% (Exhibit 1.2). Admissions for tranquilizers tended to be female (50%), White (82%), and with an average age of 36. Admissions for sedatives also tended to be female (51%), White (81%), and age 35 (SAMHSA, 2004a). For both groups, secondary drugs of abuse included alcohol and marijuana (SAMHSA, 2004b).

According to 2002 DAWN ME data, benzodiazepines (e.g., diazepam, alprazolam, or an unnamed benzodiazepine) were listed in the top 10 drugs mentioned in drug abuse deaths in a majority of participating metropolitan areas (26 out of 31). Diazepam ranked among the top 10 drugs mentioned in deaths in 20 areas, including Detroit (112 mentions), Philadelphia (85), San Diego (53), St. Louis (45), Phoenix (43), and Dallas (42). Alprazolam ranked among the top 10 drugs in seven areas, including Las Vegas (34 mentions), Chicago (26), and Long Island (26; SAMHSA, 2004c). Alprazolam (Xanax) is the benzodiazepine most commonly identified by NFLIS laboratories (National Forensic Laboratory Information System, 2004).

At the June and December 2003 CEWG meetings, Xanax was reported as a major drug of abuse. In Miami, abuse of benzodiazepines was seen in all age groups, and it was a key "mixer" with other drugs. Xanax and Valium are problems in Philadelphia, with use of benzodiazepines also reported "up" in Los Angeles. Rohypnol use was reported "down" in Miami, "quiet" in St. Louis, and a continuing problem along the Texas border.

LSD

LSD (lysergic acid diethylamide) is one of the major drugs in the hallucinogen class. It was discovered in 1938 and is one of the most potent mood-changing chemicals. It is manufactured from lysergic acid, which is found in ergot, a fungus that grows on rye and other grains. It is odorless, colorless, and is sold in tablet, capsule, and liquid forms as well as on pieces of blotter paper that have absorbed the drug.

Lifetime LSD use among eighth, tenth, and twelfth graders has been trending downward since the mid-1990s, while use by college students peaked in 1998 and use by young adults peaked in 2000. The declines for tenth and twelfth graders between 2002 and 2003 were statistically significant (Exhibit 1.1; Johnston et al., 2004a, 2004b).

The NSDUH in 2003 reported that 10.3% of the US population aged 12 and older (24.4 million) had ever used LSD. Approximately 1.6% of those aged 12–17 had ever used LSD, as compared to 14.0% of those aged 18–25 and 10.8% of those aged 26 and older. In the past, LSD incidence rose to 844,000 new users in 1996 and then dropped to 272,000 new users in 2002. Average age of new LSD users has dropped from 19.6 in 1984 to 17.1 in 2002 (SAMHSA, 2004d, 2004e).

The number of mentions of LSD in the DAWN ED system decreased from 5182 in 1994 to 891 in 2002. In 2002, 87% were male, 75% White, 9% Black, and 9% Hispanic. Some 19% were aged 12–17, 57% were 18–25, 11% were 25–34, and 13% were 35 and older. The motives for using LSD included psychic effects (47%) and dependence (40%), and the known reasons for seeking help in the emergency departments included unexpected reaction (52%), overdose (22%), and seeking detoxification (18%). Other drugs mentioned in this DAWN ED episode included alcohol (45%), marijuana (43%), cocaine (20%), heroin (15%), and ecstasy (14%; SAMHSA, 2003a).

The TEDS system defined other hallucinogens as "hallucinogens, LSD, DMT, STP, mescaline, psilocybin, peyote, etc." Admissions for a primary problem with a hallucinogen have constituted 0.1–0.2% of all admissions since 1992 (Exhibit 1.2). In 2002, 73% of admissions were male, 75% were White, and the average age was 24 years. Forty-four percent were criminal justice referrals (SAMHSA, 2004a). Hallucinogen abusers also reported problems with other drugs: marijuana, 35%; alcohol, 18%; and cocaine, 14% (SAMHSA, 2004b). NFLIS laboratories reported that the proportion of seizures identified as LSD peaked in 1998 at 0.6% and then dropped to less than 0.1% in 2003.

At the June and December 2003 CEWG meetings, LSD indicators were reported as declining sharply in most CEWG areas. The drug has been mentioned less frequently and less in ethnographic reports in Atlanta, while in Texas the number of calls to Poison Control Centers concerning abuse or misuse of LSD dropped from 113 in 1999 to 20 in 2003.

PCP

Phencyclidine (PCP) is a dissociative chemical that distorts perceptions of sight and sound and produces feelings of detachment. It is often referred to as "angel dust," "fry," "amp," or "wack." It can be sprinkled directly on a joint and smoked, or a joint can be dipped into embalming fluid or formaldehyde into which the PCP has been dissolved.

According to the MTF, lifetime PCP use among US twelfth graders has declined since 1996, but use has increased slightly for young adults (Exhibit 1.1; Johnston et al., 2004a, 2004b). The NSDUH in 2003 reported that 3.0% of the US population aged 12 and older (740,000) had ever used PCP. Some 0.8% of those aged 12–17 had ever used PCP, as compared to 3.0% of those aged 18–25 and 3.3% of those aged 26 and older. The number of new initiates increased from 83,000 in 1990 to 191,000 in 2001 and then dropped to 131,000 in 2002. Average age dropped as well, from 22.2 in 1990 to 16.7 in 2002 (SAMHSA, 2004d, 2004e).

DAWN ED mentions of PCP per 100,000 have risen from 2.6 per 100,000 to 3.0 per 100,000, which is a 16% increase. Among the patients who presented to emergency departments in 2002, 64% were male, 30% White, 43% Black, and 12% Hispanic. Some 38% were between the ages of 18 and 25, 33% were 35 or older, and 21% were between 26 and 34 years. Thirty-eight percent took PCP for psychic reasons and 28% took it because of dependence (SAMHSA, 2003a).

Whereas other PCP indicators are rising, PCP admissions to treatment have remained stable at 0.2% since 1992 (Exhibit 1.2). In 2002, 49% of admissions were Black, 25% Hispanic, and 20% White; 67% were male. Average age was 29 years. Fifty percent were criminal justice referrals (SAMHSA, 2004a). Eighty-seven percent reported smoking PCP (usually on a cigarette or marijuana joint) and other problem substances included alcohol (24%), marijuana (31%), and crack cocaine (12%; SAMHSA, 2004b).

The mean number of male arrestees testing positive for PCP in 2003 was 1.8%. In Philadelphia, 12.3% tested positive, as did 11.0% in Washington, DC. In 12 of the 39 sites, there were no positives for PCP. Among female arrestees, the mean was 1.4%, with 12.7% of all female arrestees in Washington, DC, 6.3% of female arrestees in Cleveland, and 5.6% of female arrestees in Chicago testing positive. In 16 of 25 sites, no females tested positive for PCP (National Institute on Justice, 2004). PCP exhibits examined by NFLIS laboratories have remained at 0.3% of all exhibits since 2000 (National Forensic Laboratory Information System, 2004).

PCP indicators increased in four CEWG cities, and it was reported that the drug is available in most other areas. Emergency department rates, arrestees testing positive, treatment admissions, and forensic testing by law enforcement personnel were reported as consistently high in Washington, DC, and Philadelphia. Data reported during this panel discussion suggested a possible resurgence of PCP use and abuse in Hartford, CT, and Washington, DC, and a "cycling" of abuse in Los Angeles. PCP can be dissolved in embalming fluid, and individuals who smoke marijuana joints or cigarettes that have been dipped in embalming fluid may or may not be aware that the embalming fluid contains PCP (National Institute on Drug Abuse, 2004). In Newark, NJ, there was a significant increase in the rate of PCP emergency department mentions in 2002: seven mentions per 100,000. Of the 124 PCP mentions reported during this time period, nearly three-quarters (73%) were mentioned during multidrug episodes. Although PCP is not found in high quantities in Minneapolis/St. Paul, MN, it is identified in most indicator data, including emergency department mentions (which increased significantly from 2000 to 2002), police exhibits, and medical examiner data. In Philadelphia, PCP was detected in nearly 400 decedents from 1994 to 2003. It was the fifth most frequently detected drug during that multiple year period.

MDMA (ecstasy)

MDMA (3,4-methylenedioxymethamphetamine; also called Adam, E, ecstasy, X, eccie) is a synthetic, psychoactive drug with both stimulant and hallucinogenic properties similar to methamphetamine and mescaline. It has been a Schedule I drug since 1985. A similar compound, 3,4-methylenedioxyamphetamine (MDA), is also classified as a Schedule I drug.

The effects and pharmacological actions of 3,4-methylenedioxyethamphetamine (MDEA, called Eve) are reported to be similar, but not identical, to MDMA. Other drugs that appear in the ecstasy scene include *p*-methoxyamphetamine (paramethoxyamphetamine; PMA), a drug packaged as ecstasy and which is mistakenly assumed to be a by-product in the synthesis of MDMA. PMA shares the stimulant and hallucinogenic effects of MDMA as well as its risk of hyperthermia, and fatalities related to the use of PMA have been reported.

Many surveys and studies, such as the MTF, NSDUH, and DAWN, query about use of "MDMA" when the term "ecstasy" would be more appropriate, since users "hope" they are consuming MDMA but do not actually know what is in the pill unless a toxicological test has been run. In this chapter the term "ecstasy" will be used, except in discussing the NFLIS data, which reflect the results of chemical analyses.

Findings from the 2003 MTF indicate that lifetime, past year, and past month use of ecstasy peaked for eighth, tenth, and twelfth graders in 2000 and 2001 and has declined since (Exhibit 1.1). For all three grades, the declines between 2002 and 2003 in both annual prevalence and 30-day prevalence were statistically significant. The decline in prevalence of use appears related to perceptions of increased risk and decreased availability. In 2000, only 38% of twelfth graders said there was a great risk of harm associated with trying ecstasy once or twice; that proportion increased to 56% in 2003. The perceived availability of ecstasy as reported by the twelfth graders decreased from a high of 62% in 2001 to 58% in 2003, while the disapproval of people who tried ecstasy once or twice increased from 81% in 2001 to 85% in 2003 (Johnston et al., 2004a).

Recent MTFs also reported that for college students, lifetime and past year use peaked in 2001 and declined in 2002. For young adults aged 19–28, lifetime use peaked in 2003, past year use peaked in 2001, and past month use peaked in 2000. The decline in past year use from 2002 to 2003 among young adults was significant (Johnston et al., 2004b).

The NSDUH in 2003 reported that 4.6% of the US population aged 12 and over had ever used ecstasy, 0.9% had used it in the past year, and 0.2% had used it in the past month. Some 2.4% of those aged 12–17 had ever used ecstasy, compared to 14.8% of those aged 18–25 and 3.1% of those aged 26 and older. In the mid- to late-1990s, the number of new ecstasy users had consistently risen. Beginning in 1991, there were 165,000 new users. By 2001, the number of first-time ecstasy users had increased to 1.8 million. This trend reversed slightly in 2002, when there were 1.1 million new users. Average age of new initiates declined from 22.5 to 20.7 in this same time period (SAMHSA, 2004d, 2004e).

The number of mentions of ecstasy in emergency departments monitored by DAWN increased from 253 in 1994 to 5542 in 2001 and then dropped back to 4026 in 2002, a nonsignificant change. Fifty percent of the patients mentioning ecstasy in 2002 were male, and the race/ethnic distribution has changed. In 1999, 74% were White, as compared to 64% in 2002. In 2002, 12% were African American and 9% were Hispanic. Race/ethnicity was not reported for 15% of patients. Further, 18% were aged 12–17, 57% were 18–25, 17% were 26–34, and 8% were 35 and older. The motives for using ecstasy in 2002 were psychic effects (56%) or dependence (21%), and the reasons given for seeking emergency department services were unexpected reaction (39%) or overdose (30%). Other drugs mentioned in these episodes included alcohol (40%), marijuana (39%), and cocaine (20%; SAMHSA, 2003a).

The TEDS does not report numbers on admissions with a problem with ecstasy, but the Texas Commission on Alcohol and Drug Abuse collects these data on publicly funded Texas programs. Admissions for a primary, secondary, or tertiary problem with ecstasy have increased from 9 in 1989 to 502 in 2003. In comparison to users of other club drugs, those who entered treatment in 2003 for problems with ecstasy were more likely to be young (age 21), racially diverse (51% White, 28% Hispanic, 18% Black), and male (58%). Forty-one percent reported marijuana as their primary problem drug, as compared to 14% who reported ecstasy as their primary problem drug. Sixty-five percent were referred to treatment by the criminal justice system (Maxwell, 2004).

Ecstasy is not a major drug of abuse, based on law enforcement seizures. The NFLIS reported that in 2003, 0.6% of all items identified were MDMA, as compared to 36% that were cannabis, and 31% that were cocaine (Exhibit 1.4). Of the "club drug" items that were identified in 2003, 6039 were MDMA, 777 were MDA, and three were PMA (National Forensic Laboratory Information System, 2004).

MDA use was reported as early as the June 1980 meeting of the CEWG, and MDMA was first reported at the December 1985 meeting. At the June and December 2003 CEWG meetings, it was reported that in Atlanta ecstasy was no longer seen as a club drug, but was being used by low-income polydrug users and use had also spread to the African American community. Methamphetamine and ecstasy were being used in combination because the effects of ecstasy alone were "not enough," and ecstasy was being bought in larger quantities, with some users reported to be developing tolerance to the drug. "Trolling," which is using ecstasy and LSD together, was also reported. In Baltimore, ecstasy use was growing in the central city and the increase was said to be due to the hip-hop culture and rap songs about ecstasy. In Chicago, ecstasy use was reported as "down" and the price was stable; however, it was spreading to new groups of White suburban youth. In Detroit, ecstasy use was stable, particularly outside Detroit, where it is known as a "prom" drug. In Miami, ecstasy use was reported as "passé" but that, when it was used, it was used in combination with other drugs, including Viagra, primarily in the gay "party and play" club scene. This same "party and play" phenomenon was reported in San Francisco, where ecstasy use was reported "down."

In Minneapolis/St. Paul, ecstasy use was reported as level, and it was used in combination with ketamine and methamphetamine. Ecstasy and ketamine are often sold together in Philadelphia. In St. Louis, ecstasy was available in clubs and around colleges, and there were reports of gay males using Viagra and ecstasy ("party packs"). In New York City, ecstasy use was reported "up," especially among Hispanics and African Americans. Use was reported as stable in Boston. In San Diego, use of ecstasy was reported as declining, and it was also noted that Mexican methamphetamine was being pressed into pills that look like ecstasy. In Seattle, use was higher among young males having sex with males, and there were reports of depression among users. In Los Angeles, ecstasy use was reported as decreasing. In Texas, the proportion of White clients had decreased to 51%, while African American and Hispanic admissions were increasing, a further indication that ecstasy has spread beyond the White club culture.

GHB, GBL, and 1,4-BD

Gamma hydroxybutyrate (sodium hydroxybutyrate, sodium oxybutyrate, GHB), a naturally occurring fatty acid found in mammals, is a central nervous system depressant which has intoxicating effects and, at sufficiently high doses, anesthetic properties. In 1990, after reports of adverse events, the Food and Drug Administration ordered the removal of GHB from the market. GHB produces anterograde amnesia and may cause victims to lose consciousness and be unable to resist or recall sexual assault. Because of these problems, it is now a Schedule I drug.

GHB is known on the street by terms such as "fantasy," "liquid ecstasy," "liquid X," "Grievous Bodily Harm," "scoop," "cherry meth," "soap," "salty water," "organic quaalude," "G," "Growth Hormone Booster," "somatomax PM," "gamma OH," and "Georgia Home Boy." It is available as a powder or a liquid. Illegal GHB and its precursors, GBL and 1,4-BD, can be obtained over the Internet and sometimes are marketed as solvents or as dietary supplements in health food stores, gyms, raves, and nightclubs. Chemistry kits, reagents, and recipes are available on the Web to convert the precursors into GHB, and GHB itself can be ordered from Web sites in some other countries.

The MTF showed that past year use for eighth and twelfth graders peaked in 2000, while use by tenth graders peaked in 2002–2003 (Johnston et al., 2004a). Past year use by college students and by young adults was as low or lower than for secondary school students (Johnston et al., 2004b). The NSDUH did not survey for GHB.

DAWN ED mentions of GHB, GBL, or 1,4-BD increased from 56 in 1994 to a high of 4969 in 2000, and then declined to 3330 in 2002. Patients mentioning GHB in 2002 were male (66%), and 92% were White and 1% Black. Race/ethnicity was not reported for 7%. Of these patients, 54% were aged 18–25, 32% were 26–34, and 12% were 35 and older. GHB and alcohol have a synergistic effect that can produce serious side effects, including unconsciousness. Other drugs mentioned included alcohol (64%), cocaine (15%), and marijuana (14%). Of the known motives for using GHB, 80% reported psychic effects, and the reason for emergency department contact was overdose (61%) or unexpected reaction (36%; SAMHSA, 2004a).

GHB treatment admissions are not collected in the TEDS, but Texas treatment data reported 31 admissions in 2003 for a primary, secondary, or tertiary problem with GHB. Of these, the average age was 28, 77% were White, and 39% were male. For 45%, the primary drug of abuse was methamphetamine, and GHB was the primary drug for 16%. Methamphetamine is often used to stay awake while using GHB, and GHB can be used to "come down" from a speed binge. Some 45% were referred to treatment from the criminal justice system (Maxwell, 2004). The NFLIS reported that in 2003 there were 376 items identified as being GHB or GBL (National Forensic Laboratory Information System, 2004).

GHB was first reported at a CEWG meeting in December 1990. At the June and December 2003 CEWG meetings, reports of use of GHB varied across the nation. In Atlanta, it was prevalent in the gay male scene. In Chicago, levels of use of GHB were low, and it tended to be used by young heroin inhalers. In Miami, Minneapolis/St. Paul, Detroit, and San Francisco, use was reported as "down." In Los Angeles, typical users were older White males. Use in Texas was centered in the Dallas/Fort Worth metroplex area.

Ketamine

Ketamine, a derivative of phencyclidine hydrochloride, is an anesthetic that has been approved for human and animal use, both in trauma and emergency surgery as well as in veterinary medicine. Ketamine on the street is also known as "special K," "vitamin K," "K," "kit-kat," "keets," "super acid," "super K," and "jet."

Ketamine users try to achieve or "fall into" a "K-hole," which is described as physical immobilization and social detachment lasting up to an hour. It is characterized by a distorted sense of space, such as a small room appearing the size of a football field, and an indistinct awareness of time, such as a few minutes seeming like an hour. The K-hole ends rather abruptly but can be quickly reentered following another dose of ketamine.

Ketamine is a Schedule III controlled substance and is available in powder, tablet, and injectable forms. It is difficult to manufacture and most abusers acquire it through diversion of the prescription product or theft from veterinary supplies. Recreational users usually administer ketamine intranasally, although it is also injected.

The MTF reported past year use of ketamine peaked in 2000 for eighth grade students and in 2002 for tenth and twelfth graders (Johnson et al., 2004a). The decreases between 2002 and 2003 were not statistically significant. Use of ketamine by college students and young adults was as low or lower than for secondary students (Johnston et al., 2004b). The NSDUH did not ask about ketamine.

The number of mentions of ketamine in the DAWN ED system increased from 19 in 1994 to 679 in 2001, but dropped to 260 in 2002. Ketamine users in 2002 were male (77%); 67% were White, 8% Hispanic, and race/ethnicity was not reported for 26%. Twelve percent were aged 12–17, 56% were 18–25, 22% were 26–34, and 12% were 35 or older. The primary motive for using ketamine was psychic effects (68%), and the known reasons for seeking help in emergency departments included overdose (47%) and unexpected reaction (28%; SAMHSA, 2003a).

The TEDS does not collect data on ketamine admissions to treatment, but the Texas system reported 13 admissions with a primary, secondary, or tertiary problem with ketamine in 2003. Average age was 24, 77% were male, and 54% were White and 31% were Hispanic. Other drugs of abuse included alcohol, methamphetamine, marijuana, and powder cocaine (Maxwell, 2004). The NFLIS reported that while ketamine was a very small proportion of all drugs analyzed, the number of seizures increased from 18 items in 1998 to 696 in 2003 (National Forensic Laboratory Information System, 2004).

Abuse of ketamine was first reported at a CEWG meeting in December 1991. At the June and December 2003 CEWG meetings, ketamine use was reported as higher and demand was greater than availability in Detroit; use was down in Boston, Los Angeles, Newark, and San Francisco. In Texas, there were 8 calls in 1998 to Poison Control Centers about misuse or abuse of ketamine, and there were 17 calls in 2003.

Conclusion

Based on the extant data, there are some general statements that can be made regarding trends in drug use for 2004. Alcohol is the most widely used drug, with an economic cost of $166.5 billion to American society in 1995, as compared to an economic cost of $109.8 billion for drug abuse (Harwood et al., 1998). Binge and heavy drinking remains a problem, and alcohol is often misused in combination with other drugs. Another concern is that use by girls aged 12–17 now equals or surpasses that of boys. Inhalant use is commonly assumed to be a problem among adolescents, but indicator data show that inhalants are also abused by adults, although the problem tends to be unrecognized and inhalant abusers of all ages are underserved.

Crack cocaine use is high and relatively stable in many large US cities, but is spreading from African American to White and Hispanic populations. Indications of use of powder cocaine are lower but still problematic. Methamphetamine use can be characterized as a series of epidemics, with increasingly high levels in the West, growing problems (particularly in the rural areas) in the Midwest, and indications of increasing use on the East Coast. The drug is also of concern because of its use, along with risky sex, within the gay club scene. Marijuana is the most used illicit drug. Survey data, emergency department reports, and treatment admissions are now documenting an increase in marijuana users who are reporting adverse effects or meeting the criteria for dependence. Indicators also show an increase in marijuana users entering services as a result of referrals by the criminal justice system. Like cocaine, heroin use remains stable in many regions of the country. Because of the different types of heroin that are available throughout the USA, the route of administration differs regionally. On the West Coast, for example, heroin users are most likely to inject the drug, while on the East Coast, heroin users can also inhale ("snort") or smoke the drug.

In recent years, the use of prescription drugs, especially other opiates such as oxycodone and hydrocodone, has increased. This increase, which is partially due to the emergence of OxyContin, is growing among new users in their twenties and it is more of a problem in rural areas. Patterns of sedative/tranquilizer use vary. Benzodiazepine use has increased and these drugs are often abused in combination with other drugs, as shown by their presence in drug overdose deaths. Tranquilizer use has decreased among high school students, but has increased in individuals who access their local emergency department for a drug-related illness or injury. As a percentage of treatment admissions, tranquilizers and sedative/hypnotics are very low and stable.

In general, LSD use appears to be decreasing in the USA. Fewer secondary school students report annual or current LSD use; the number of new users in the general population has dropped; and the mentions of LSD among emergency department episodes has declined since 1994. PCP use is relatively low in most cities of the USA, with the exception of Washington, DC, and Philadelphia, but emergency department visits are increasing across the nation. The use of most club drugs, including MDMA (ecstasy), GHB (and its analogues), and ketamine, peaked between the late 1990s and 2001, and has been declining since. Initially, the use of these substances was concentrated in the rave and club scene, but their use has spread to the street scene and house parties.

References

Chadwick, O., & Anderson, H. (1989). Neuropsychological consequences of volatile substance abuse: A review. *Human Toxicology, 8*, 307–312.

Chadwick, O., Yule, W., & Anderson, R. (1990). The examination attainments of secondary school pupils who abuse solvents. *British Journal of Educational Psychology, 60*, 180–191.

Compton, W. M., Grant, B. F., Colliver, J. D., Glantz, M. D., & Stinson, F. S. (2004). Prevalence of marijuana use disorders in the United States; 1991–1992 and 2001–2002. *Journal of the American Medical Association, 291*, 2114–2121.

Drug Enforcement Administration (2003). *Illegal Drug Price and Purity Report: Drug Intelligence Report*, DEA-02058. Washington, DC: DEA.

Drug Enforcement Administration (2004a). *2003 Domestic monitoring program*, Special data run, May 2004. Washington, DC: DEA.

Drug Enforcement Administration (2004b). *National Forensic Laboratory Information System: Annual report 2003.* Arlington, VA: DEA, Office of Diversion Control.

Harwood, H. J., Fountain, D., & Livermore, G. (1998). *The economic costs of alcohol and drug abuse in the United States, 1992.* Rockville, MD: National Institute on Drug Abuse and National Institute on Alcoholism and Alcohol Abuse.

Johnston, L. D., O'Malley, P. M., Bachman, J. G., & Schulenberg, J. E. (2004a). *Monitoring the Future national results on adolescent drug use, 1975–2003. Volume I: Secondary school students* (NIH Publication No. 04–5507). Bethesda, MD: National Institute on Drug Abuse.

Johnston, L. D., O'Malley, P. M., Bachman, J. G., & Schulenberg, J. E. (2004b). *Monitoring the Future national survey results on drug use, 1975–2003. Volume II: College students and adults ages 19–40* (NIH Publication No. 04–5508). Bethesda, MD: National Institute on Drug Abuse.

Maxwell, J. C. (2001). Deaths related to the inhalation of volatile substances in Texas: 1988–1998. *American Journal of Drug and Alcohol Abuse, 27*, 689–698.

Maxwell, J. C. (2004). Substance abuse trends in Texas: June 2004. In *Epidemiologic trends in drug abuse, Proceedings of the Community Epidemiology Work Group.* Rockville, MD: National Institute on Drug Abuse.

National Forensic Laboratory Information System (2004). Special data run downloaded July 3, 2004 from http://www.deadiversion.usdoj.gov/nflis/index.html.

National Institute on Drug Abuse (2000). *Inhalant abuse. Research report series.* Rockville, MD: National Institute on Drug Abuse.

National Institute on Drug Abuse (2004). *Epidemiologic trends in drug abuse, Proceedings of the Community Epidemiology Work Group, June 2004.* Rockville, MD: National Institute on Drug Abuse.

National Institute on Justice (2004). *2003 Adult male and females, use of phencyclidine (PCP)*, Special data run May 12, 2004. Washington, DC: NIJ.

Office of Applied Studies (2004a). *The DAWN report: Amphetamine and methamphetamine emergency department visits: 1995–2002.* Rockville, MD: Substance Abuse and Mental Health Services Administration.

Office of Applied Studies (2004b). *The DAWN report: benzodiazepines in drug abuse-related emergency department visits: 1995–2002.* Rockville, MD: Substance Abuse and Mental Health Services Administration.

Office of Applied Studies (2004c). *The DAWN report: Demographic characteristics of benzodiazepine-involved ED visits*. Rockville, MD: Substance Abuse and Mental Health Services Administration.

Office of Applied Studies (2004d). *The DAWN report: Oxycodone, hydrocodone, and polydrug use, 2002*. Rockville, MD: Substance Abuse and Mental Health Services Administration.

Office of Applied Studies (2004e). *The DASIS report: Treatment admissions involving narcotic painkillers: 2002 Update*. Rockville, MD: Substance Abuse and Mental Health Services Administration.

Office of Applied Studies (2004f). *The DASIS report: Treatment admissions in urban and rural areas involving abuse of narcotic painkillers: 2002 Update*. Rockville, MD: Substance Abuse and Mental Health Services Administration.

Substance Abuse and Mental Health Services Administration (SAMHSA), Office of Applied Studies (2003). *Emergency department trends from the Drug Abuse Warning Network, final estimates 1995–2002*, DAWN Series D-24, DHHS Publication No. (SMA) 03-3780. Rockville, MD: SAMHSA.

Substance Abuse and Mental Health Services Administration (SAMHSA), Office of Applied Studies (2004a). *Treatment Episode Data Set (TEDS) highlights – 2002. National admissions to Substance Abuse Treatment Services*, DASIS Series S-22, DHHS Publication No. (SMA) 04-3946. Rockville, MD: SAMHSA.

Substance Abuse and Mental Health Services Administration (SAMHSA), Office of Applied Studies. (2004b). *Treatment Episode Data Set (TEDS)*, Special data run downloaded July 3, 2004 from http://wwwdasis.samhsa.gov/webt/quicklink/US92.htm.

Substance Abuse and Mental Health Services Administration (SAMHSA), Office of Applied Studies (2004c). *Mortality data from the Drug Abuse Warning Network, 2002*, DAWN Series D-25, DHHS Publication No. (SMA) 043875. Rockville, MD: SAMHSA.

Substance Abuse and Mental Health Services Administration (SAMHSA), Office of Applied Studies (2004d). *Results from the 2003 National Survey on Drug Use and Health: Detailed tables, prevalence estimates, standard errors, p-values, and sample size*. Downloaded from www.samhsa.gov.

Substance Abuse and Mental Health Services Administration (SAMHSA), Office of Applied Studies (2004e). *Overview of findings from the 2003 National Survey on Drug Use and Health*, NHSDA Series H-24, DHHS Publication No. SMA 04-3964. Rockville, MD: SAMHSA.

Zhang, Z. (2004). *Drug and alcohol use and related matters among arrestees: 2003*. Washington, DC: National Institute on Justice.

Part I

Popular Drugs of Misuse

2 Alcohol

Marlene Oscar-Berman and Ksenija Marinković

Introduction

Alcoholism is a multidimensional disorder involving excessive ethanol ingestion. The course of the disease is influenced by an interaction of environmental factors with specific biological components, and manifests in the form of behavior abnormalities. In this chapter, we begin with an overview of the acute and residual effects of alcoholism, including its prevalence and the risk factors for developing neuropsychological deficits. Risk factors include genetics and family history, age, gender, and physical as well as mental health conditions. Next, we review the cognitive and emotional effects of intoxication. Examples of these effects are given for attentional, semantic, and psychomotor functions. We also consider the regions of the brain that are most vulnerable to the effects of alcoholism, i.e., the frontal lobes, the cerebellum, and the limbic system. Brain imaging techniques hold great promise for localizing brain areas most affected by intoxication. We suggest that these techniques be used in combination with other methodologies for maximal benefits in the treatment of alcoholism and in charting the course of recovery of function. Ideally, the collective methodologies will include neuropsychological testing, electromagnetic recordings (e.g., event-related potentials and magnetoencephalography), and brain scans (especially structural and functional magnetic resonance imaging).

Definitions and overview of acute and residual effects of alcoholism

The American Psychiatric Association's *Diagnostic and Statistical Manual of Mental Disorders* (DSM-IV; APA, 1994) defines two alcohol use disorders, *alcohol abuse* and *alcohol dependence*. Abuse involves psychological, social, and work-related impairments or distress, causing problems with activities of daily living, in which alcohol consumption is implicated. Dependence stresses a disability (manifested by craving, tolerance, and physical dependence) in which drinking behaviors cannot be adequately restrained.

It is important to distinguish between the acute and the residual effects of alcoholism. The most obvious acute effect of ethanol consumption is intoxication. Residual neurobehavioral effects are those that remain after a person has been abstinent for at least a month. Researchers interested in studying the residual effects will restrict patient enrollment to alcoholics who have been abstinent for a minimum of four weeks; this is important for obtaining stable levels of performance.

Scope of the problem: Prevalence of brain-related deficits associated with alcoholism

Approximately half of the nearly 20 million people in the United States who are problem drinkers have not been diagnosed with cognitive impairments. The remaining problem drinkers have neuropsychological difficulties that range from mild to very severe. For example, up to 2 million alcoholics develop permanent and debilitating conditions that require lifetime custodial care (Rourke & Løberg, 1996). Examples of such conditions include alcohol-induced persisting amnesic disorder (also called alcoholic Korsakoff's syndrome) (Butters, 1981), and alcohol-induced persisting dementia (APA, 1994) which seriously affects many mental functions in addition to memory (e.g., language, reasoning, and problem-solving abilities).

Most alcoholics with neuropsychological impairments show at least some improvement in brain structure and functioning within a year of abstinence. However, some alcoholics require additional time, and others have permanent deficits (Bates, Bowden, & Barry, 2002; Gansler et al., 2000; Sullivan, 2000). To date, little is known about the rate and extent to which people recover specific structural and functional processes after they stop drinking. In contrast, a number of studies have identified various factors that increase the likelihood that alcohol misuse will result in brain deficits.

Alcoholism's effects on the brain and behavior are diverse, and they are moderated and/or mediated by many factors (Oscar-Berman, 2000; Parsons, 1996). Consequently, no single measuring instrument can establish definitive criteria for alcoholism or the putative neurobehavioral sequelae of the disease. Among the numerous factors influencing the expression and course of alcoholism are: demographic variables (e.g., age, level of education, gender), genetic background, temperament, family history of alcoholism, alcohol exposure in the prenatal and perinatal periods, the social and ethnic surroundings during childhood, alcohol use patterns (e.g., the age of onset of alcohol consumption, the type and amount of alcohol consumed, severity and duration of the dependency, duration of abstinence, nutritional status during periods of consumption), and the use or abuse of other psychoactive substances. Additionally, overall physical and mental health are important factors, because comorbid medical, neurological, and psychiatric conditions can interact to aggravate alcoholism's effects on the brain and behavior (Petrakis, Gonzalez, Rosenheck, & Krystal, 2002). Examples of common comorbid conditions include:

- medical conditions such as malnutrition and diseases of the liver and the cardiovascular system;
- neurological conditions such as head injury, inflammation of the brain (i.e., encephalopathy), and fetal alcohol syndrome (or fetal alcohol effects); and
- psychiatric conditions such as depression, anxiety, post-traumatic stress disorder, schizophrenia, and the use of medicines or other drugs.

These conditions also can contribute to further drinking.

Risk factors and comorbid conditions that influence alcohol-related brain damage

The manner in which alcoholism leads to brain and behavior abnormalities is not surprising, because of the many different factors having an influence on the outcome measures used by clinicians and researchers (Grant, 1987; Parsons, 1996). In this section, we consider the following critical influences: genetic background and family history of alcoholism; age; gender; and health status.

Genetics and family history

In 1989, based on the results of twin, family, and adoption studies showing that hereditary factors influence vulnerability to alcoholism, the National Institute on Alcohol Abuse and Alcoholism (NIAAA) funded Collaborative Studies on Genetics of Alcoholism (COGA). The goal of COGA is to identify specific genes that underlie this vulnerability. COGA investigators have successfully recruited over 3000 individuals from more than 300 extended families densely affected by alcoholism. The investigators have collected extensive clinical, neuropsychological, electrophysiological, biochemical, and genetic data. Evidence from these studies supports the idea that genes play an important role in alcoholism (e.g., see reviews by Dick & Bierut, 2006; Dick & Foroud, 2003; Schuckit, Smith, & Kalmijn, 2004).

At least 40% of the addictions to alcohol, tobacco, and other drugs have genetic influences (Bierut et al., 2002; Bowirrat & Oscar-Berman, 2005; McGue, 1999; Tsuang et al., 1998; Uhl & Grow, 2004). For example, offspring of monozygotic and dizygotic twins with a history of alcohol dependence were found to exhibit alcohol abuse or addiction more frequently than offspring of nonalcoholic fathers, and offspring of an alcohol-abusing monozygotic twin whose co-twin was alcohol dependent were more likely to be alcohol dependent than offspring of nonalcoholic twins (Jacob et al., 2003). However, in the absence of paternal alcoholism, offspring with high genetic risk (the unaffected father's co-twin is alcoholic) showed lower rates of alcoholism than children of alcoholics (Jacob et al., 2003).

The physiological basis of alcoholism is the subject of considerable research, along with the possible genetic underpinnings of its effects on ion channels (Davies et al., 2003). A complete picture of the basic mechanisms of alcohol ingestion has been difficult to achieve partly because, unlike other psychoactive drugs, ethanol does not selectively bind to specific receptor sites. Instead, it affects the state of the membranes and thus modifies a variety of ion channels or receptors. As noted by Dick and Foroud (2003), sequencing of the human genome will facilitate the development of a catalog of human genes. Based on the findings from this catalog, researchers can identify candidate genes to determine the degree to which they are associated with alcoholism. Once replicable associations are established, the next step will be to identify the causative genetic variants responsible for the role of that gene in alcohol dependence. It also will be important to understand how the relevant genes influence patterns of alcohol use and metabolism, as well as the manner in which the genes may contribute to comorbidity of alcoholism with other psychiatric disorders (Dick & Bierut, 2006).

Age

Neuropathological analyses provided some of the earliest insights into the relationship between alcoholism and aging. In *postmortem* specimens of brains of alcoholics, cerebral atrophy was found to resemble the brain shrinkage that occurs with normal chronological aging (Harper, 1998). The atrophy is most prominent in the frontal lobes, and it extends backwards to the parietal lobes. Other effects include ventricular enlargement and widening of the cerebral sulci of alcoholics in relation to increasing age (Fein et al., 2002; Pfefferbaum, Sullivan, Mathalon, & Lim, 1997; Sullivan, 2000).

Given the observed morphological similarities in the brains of alcoholic and aging individuals, more recent studies sought to characterize parallels in functional decline associated with alcoholism and aging (Gansler et al., 2000). Some investigators proposed that alcoholism is associated with premature aging. The Premature Aging hypothesis has been put forth in two versions (reviewed by Ellis & Oscar-Berman, 1989; Oscar-Berman & Schendan, 2000). The initial model, the "accelerated aging" (or "cumulative effects") model, purported that alcoholism is accompanied by the precocious onset of neuroanatomical and behavioral changes typically associated with advancing age. Essentially, alcoholics become "cognitively old" before their time; thus, alcoholics at all ages are impaired compared to age-matched nonalcoholic controls. The second version places the timing of the changes somewhat differently. In this view (the "increased vulnerability" interpretation), an aging brain is more vulnerable to the influences of toxic substances, including ethanol, than is the brain of a younger person. This version proposes that only older alcoholics (over age 50) are impaired compared to age-matched controls, not younger alcoholics.

Taken together, most of the evidence from neuropathological and neuroradiological investigations supports the increased vulnerability model of premature aging. That is, certain brain structures show greater reduction in size (or blood flow) in older alcoholics than in younger alcoholics: the cerebral cortex (Di Sclafani et al., 1995; Harris et al., 1999; Pfefferbaum et al., 1997), the corpus callosum (Pfefferbaum, Lim, Desmond, & Sullivan, 1996), the hippocampus (Laakso et al., 2000; Pfefferbaum et al., 1995), and the cerebellum (Harris et al., 1999; Sullivan, 2003). Although cortical changes have been reported throughout the brain, there is evidence that some cortical regions (especially the frontal lobes) are more consistently vulnerable to aging and alcoholism than other regions (e.g., Gansler et al., 2000; Gilman et al., 1996; Moselhy, Georgiou, & Kahn, 2001; Oscar-Berman & Hutner, 1993; Sullivan, 2000). Results of neurobehavioral investigations tend to support the view that aging increases one's vulnerability to alcohol-related decline (Gansler et al., 2000; Sullivan, 2000).

Gender

Until recently, research on gender differences in the biological effects of alcoholism had focused mainly on the reproductive system and hepatic injury rather than on the central nervous system. Evidence suggests that women alcoholics have increased menstrual disturbances, spontaneous abortions, and miscarriages, and women are more susceptible to alcoholic liver disease than men (NIAAA, 1997). Only in the last decade have gender differences been the focus of research on alcohol-related brain damage (Lancaster, 1995; NIAAA, 1997; Wuethrich, 2001), and the degree to which gender moderates the nature and extent of brain vulnerability remains controversial (Pfefferbaum, Rosenbloom, Serventi, & Sullivan, 2002; Sullivan, 2003). Parsons (1994) reported that although male and female alcoholics showed impaired performance on neuropsychological tests relative to same-sex controls, only the male alcoholics differed from their controls using event-related brain potentials (ERPs). Other investigators found that male and female alcoholics displayed similar electrophysiological abnormalities (Hill & Steinhauer, 1993).

Neuroimaging studies measuring gender differences in alcoholics' brain size and functioning have yielded contradictory evidence, with some studies showing women to be more susceptible than men to brain impairments, and other studies showing no such distinction. Using functional magnetic resonance imaging (fMRI), Tapert and colleagues (Tapert et al., 2001) found decreased activity in parietal and frontal cortex, particularly in the right hemisphere, in alcohol-dependent women during performance of a spatial working memory task. Using structural MRI, Kroft et al. (1991) found that the average ventricular volume in female alcoholics was within the typical range found in MRI studies of nonalcoholic females of similar ages. Using computerized tomography (CT) scans to measure brain atrophy, another group found evidence of a similar degree of brain shrinkage in men and women, despite shorter drinking histories in the women (Mann, Batra, Gunthner, & Schroth, 1992). Hommer et al. (1996) used structural MRI technology to measure the size of the corpus callosum in male and female alcoholics. The alcoholic women had smaller callosal areas than alcoholic men and nonalcoholic controls; alcoholic men did not differ from nonalcoholic male controls. Abnormalities in the structure of the corpus callosum can occur as a consequence of diffuse cortical damage and subsequent degeneration of cortical axons. Interestingly, the size of the corpus callosum is notably reduced with age in alcoholic men (Pfefferbaum et al., 1996). In another study, Pfefferbaum and his group measured white matter brain macrostructure in women alcoholics to determine whether observed abnormalities interact with age (Pfefferbaum et al., 2002). Although the alcoholic women did not differ from controls in any brain measures, in the alcoholics, greater length of sobriety was associated with more cortical white matter. Based on the results of a similar study employing Diffusion Tensor Imaging (a technique highly sensitive to microstructure damage) on separate subject groups, Pfefferbaum and Sullivan (2002) suggested that alcohol use by women causes white matter microstructural disruption that is not detectable with grosser measures of white matter mass, and may antedate its appearance.

Physical and mental health

The medical conditions most likely to influence neurobiological function include liver disease, cardiovascular disease, and malnutrition. Common neurological conditions in alcoholics are head injury, encephalopathy (inflammation of the brain), and fetal alcohol syndrome (or fetal alcohol effects). Frequently occurring psychiatric conditions include depression, anxiety, post-traumatic stress disorder, schizophrenia, and the use of other drugs (Petrakis et al., 2002). Additionally, and apart from individual characteristics and vulnerabilities of the alcoholic, there are specific "outcome measures" (results of evaluations and tests performed by researchers and clinicians). Certain tests that are used to measure alcohol's effects on brain and behavior are more sensitive than others, and different tests are aimed at assessing very distinct functions or structures. Finally, it is important to consider each person's motivation to perform well on the tests, and expectations about failure.

Cognitive and emotional effects of intoxication

Whether considering the acute or the residual consequences of ethanol ingestion, its effects reach across various cognitive, emotional, psychomotor, and social abilities (Rourke & Løberg, 1996). The type and extent of the abnormalities are dependent upon factors such as those noted above. Although alcohol intoxication affects functioning at multiple levels of the central nervous system, cognitive abilities in situations of increased complexity are most likely to be disrupted. Alcohol may interfere with cognitive assessment of the environment and the capacity to inhibit impulsive responses. These impairments may contribute to socially important effects of acute intoxication, as well as to the development of alcohol dependence itself. Indeed, in concert with studies on chronic alcoholics and populations at risk, studies using acute alcohol challenges are important as they may help to parse out the effects of alcohol neurotoxicity, genetic susceptibility, and environmental factors. An understanding of the dose- and task-related parameters of acute alcohol effects on the brain may offer insight into neural systems that are most susceptible to chronic alcohol abuse. Furthermore, studies of acute alcohol challenge are valuable, as they indicate the types of functions and the neural circuits that underlie impairments due to alcohol intoxication. The importance of such evidence derives from its direct applicability to driving situations, work-related hazards, and other societally relevant concerns.

Effects of alcohol depend on an individual's blood alcohol concentration (BAC), as low doses may have a stimulatory effect and higher levels may have depressant effects on behavior. In addition, effects can differ depending on the time lapsed since ingestion; the same BAC may result in different effects on the ascending versus descending limbs of the BAC curve (Pohorecky, 1977). Furthermore, there are significant interindividual differences in tolerance to acute intoxication. Even when people are subjected to the same environmental conditions, their responses to a given dose of alcohol vary significantly on metabolic, physiological, subjective, cognitive, motor, and other measures (Reed, 1985). The pharmacokinetics (time course of absorption, distribution, metabolism, and excretion of ethanol) vary significantly when alcohol is administered orally, but much less so under intravenous administration conditions (Grant, Millar, & Kenny, 2000). Furthermore, there are marked *intra*individual differences (Nagoshi & Wilson, 1989) in the consistency of responses of the same individual when measured at different points across time. In general, effects of alcohol intoxication follow a biphasic time course as the initial feelings of relaxation and exuberance give way to hangover, exhaustion, and depression, or vomiting and loss of consciousness in cases of higher doses. Impairments in mental functions such as attention or vigilance can be detected at BAC levels much lower than the legal intoxication levels, such as 0.02–0.03% (Koelega, 1995). Furthermore, consistent with the evidence obtained from chronic alcoholics, acute intoxication results in a disproportionate impairment of executive functions such as planning, working memory, or complex psychomotor control (Peterson, Rothfleisch, Zelazo, & Pihl, 1990). A more detailed picture of the neurophysiological basis of these effects emerges from neuroimaging studies.

Effects of alcohol on cognitive event-related potentials: Attentional Networks

Event-related potentials (ERPs) reflect moment-to-moment changes in the electrical activity of the brain as it relates to parameters of the stimuli occurring either in the environment or in internally generated thoughts. ERPs have been used extensively to investigate effects of acute intoxication as well as chronic abuse of alcohol (Porjesz & Begleiter, 1985, 1996). A commonly used "oddball" paradigm consists of frequently presented standard stimuli and rarely occurring task-relevant target (oddball) stimuli such as tones or light flashes. In addition, a task-irrelevant, novel stimulus is presented in some versions of the task (Marinković, Halgren, Klopp, & Maltzman, 2000; Rodriguez Holguin, Porjesz, Chorlian, Polich, & Begleiter, 1999). Infrequently occurring stimuli elicit a large positive potential termed P3 with a latency of about 300 ms in simple tasks. P3 amplitude is smaller under alcohol intoxication (Pfefferbaum, Horvath, Roth, Clifford, & Kopell, 1980; Porjesz & Begleiter, 1985), suggesting a disruption of the central processing of novel, task-irrelevant stimuli even at very low BAC levels (Grillon, Sinha, & O'Malley, 1995; Jääskeläinen, Schroger, & Näätänen, 1999; Marinković, Halgren, & Maltzman, 2001). This effect is inversely related to the alcohol dose (Rohrbaugh et al., 1987; Teo & Ferguson, 1986) and is modulated by task difficulty (Campbell, Marois, & Arcand, 1984). Furthermore, it has been shown that the P3 is not a unitary component but a composite of at least two deflections (termed P3a and P3b) differing in task correlates, latency, scalp topography, and generating structures (Halgren, 1990). The P3a is evoked in the frontocentral parts of the brain by novel, unexpected stimuli (Courchesne, Hillyard, & Galambos, 1975). It is highly correlated with sympathetic arousal, and is selectively affected by acute intoxication (Marinković et al., 2001) (see Figure 2.1).

Inasmuch as the P3a reflects orienting to novelty, these results indicate high susceptibility of the attentional domain relevant for processing of the significant stimuli to alcohol intoxication. Conversely, P3b is largest over the posterior scalp regions, it is elicited by task-relevant stimuli and may index cognitive closure of stimulus event processing (Knight,

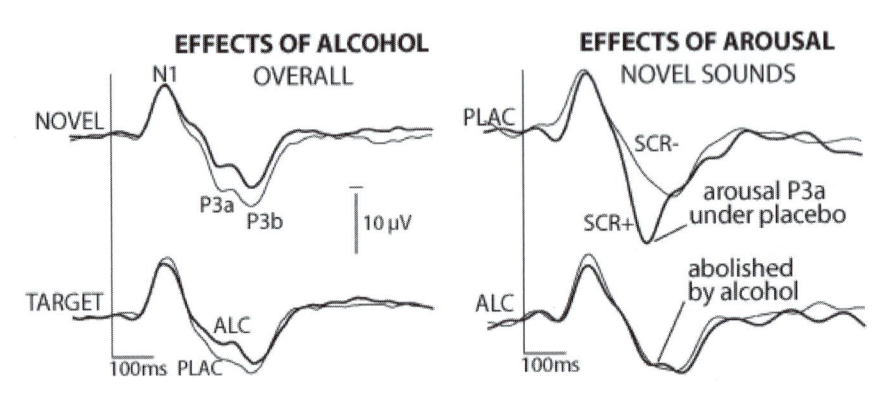

Figure 2.1 Group-average event-related potential (ERP) waveforms recorded at Fz. Alcohol (average BAC = 0.045%) decreases the late positive deflection to target and novel stimuli overall (left panel). The right panel shows group-average ERP waveforms to novel sounds in placebo and alcohol conditions depending on the presence (SCR+) or absence (SCR−) of skin conductance responses. Alcohol selectively abolished the arousal-related P3a. (Adapted from Marinković et al., 2001, with permission.)

Grabowecky, & Scabini, 1995). Consistent with this evidence, irreversible amplitude attenuation and sometimes latency increase of the P3 deflection (Porjesz & Begleiter, 1985, 1996) have been observed in chronic alcoholics. Furthermore, the role of genetics (Begleiter & Porjesz, 1999; Goodwin, 1977; Schuckit, 2000) in increasing the risk for alcoholism has promoted the search for biological markers that could help to identify such individuals and could potentially allow for early diagnosis, focused prevention, and treatment of alcoholism. Attenuated P3 amplitude has been documented in individuals at high risk for alcoholism, such as offspring of alcoholics, and has given rise to a vulnerability marker hypothesis whereby attenuated P3 may suggest predisposition to an array of disinhibitory disorders including alcohol dependence (Begleiter & Porjesz, 1999; Monteiro & Schuckit, 1988; Pfefferbaum, Ford, White, & Mathalon, 1991; Porjesz et al., 2005). Inasmuch as the commonly used "oddball" paradigm engages attentional brain circuits, this converging evidence also implicates their susceptibility to alcohol effects.

Semantic networks

Studies using semantic, more cognitively challenging tasks have explored alcohol effects on verbal, semantic, and memory brain networks. It has been established that the reaction speed and accuracy in word categorization and recognition tasks are impaired by acute alcohol intoxication (Haut, Beckwith, Petros, & Russell, 1989; Maylor, Rabbitt, & Kingstone, 1987). Some behavioral evidence suggests that alcohol impairs semantic processing (Maylor, Rabbitt, James, & Kerr, 1990). In light of this evidence, it is surprising to note that alcohol's effects on the brain during verbal cognitive processing have not been adequately studied, in spite of a proliferation of ERP studies of language processing. A negative ERP component with a latency of about 400–450 ms (N400 or N4) has been described (Kutas & Hillyard, 1980) which is sensitive to the semantic, but not orthographic, aspects of congruity with the preceding context. Novel words with an unexpected or incongruent meaning evoke a large N4 (such as "I like my tea with nails"). Conversely, semantic priming decreases N4 amplitude and latency (Nagy & Rugg, 1989; Smith & Halgren, 1987), suggesting its dependence on the ease of semantic contextual integration (Halgren, 1990; Holcomb, 1993). Recent studies indicate that alcohol intoxication affects verbal processing during early, prelexical, and late semantic stages, resulting in the increased difficulty of semantic access and integration (see Figure 2.2; Marinković, Halgren, & Maltzman, 2004). Neuroimaging studies indicate that the early, prelexical visual feature analysis is subserved by the ventrotemporal area, whereas the later stage of semantic and contextual integration relies on the distributed circuits that primarily encompass the left prefrontal and temporal regions (Buckner, Logan, Donaldson, & Wheeler, 2000; Marinković, 2004). Future studies will need to determine whether alcohol's effects on these stages of verbal processing are independent or merely cumulative, and to what degree they are modulated via attentional impairments.

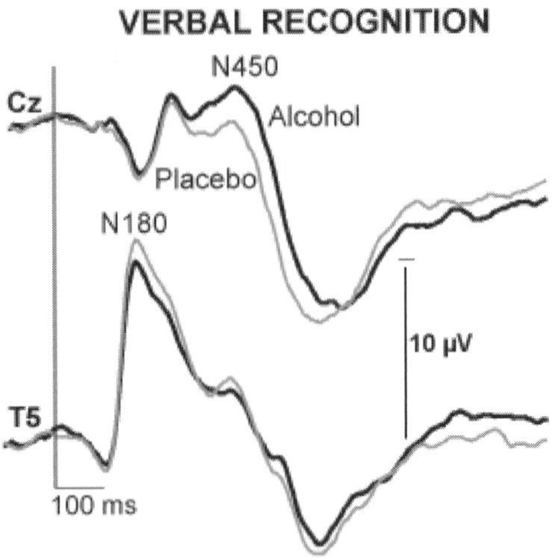

Figure 2.2 Alcohol affects the early (prelexical, peaking at 180 ms) and late (semantic, contextual, peaking at 450 ms) stages of verbal processing, as shown with group-average event-related potentials. (Adapted from Marinković et al., 2004, with permission.)

Psychomotor effects and impulsivity

Stimulus events evoke two seamlessly integrated brain-processing streams: one stream evaluates the stimulus ("input"), whereas the other prepares the response ("output"). Both of these aspects occur in parallel and form an integrated processing stream, but are rarely considered together. As outlined above, it has been shown that alcohol intoxication disrupts cognitive stimulus processing in the attentional and semantic domains. Research evidence suggests that alcohol impairs the psychomotor aspects of functioning as well.

It is a common belief that alcohol ingestion leads to impulsive or aggressive behavior. Indeed, laboratory research shows that alcohol intoxication increases the likelihood of aggressive behavior (Bushman & Cooper, 1990). However, careful examination of the doubtlessly complex interactions between alcohol intoxication and the multifaceted construct of aggression is still lacking. For instance, a behavior labeled as "aggressive" could include combinations of impulsivity, disinhibition, social or sexual inappropriateness, thought or decision-making impairments, or some other feature. Some evidence suggests that alcohol may have disinhibitory effects on behavior. Rather low alcohol doses (peak BAC of ~ 0.04%) decrease the latency of arousal to sexually explicit stimuli (Wilson & Niaura, 1984). Alcohol-induced disinhibition is also reflected in premature motor preparation based on incomplete stimulus evaluation (Marinković et al., 2000). The disinhibitory effects could result from the psychomotor stimulant properties of alcohol (Wise, 1988), or may reflect a disruption in the inhibitory control of behavior subserved by prefrontal regions (Peterson, Rothfleisch, Zelazo, & Pihl, 1990).

Indeed, alcohol decreases inhibitory control under the conditions of stop-signal imperative stimuli (Mulvihill, Skilling, & Vogel-Sprott, 1997) and a demanding continuous performance task (Dougherty et al., 1999), as moderately intoxicated subjects are impaired in withholding inappropriate responses.

Furthermore, these disinhibitory effects of alcohol are correlated with personality traits related to impulsivity and hyperactivity (Dougherty et al., 1999; Marinković et al., 2000), as well as with drinking problems (Nagoshi, Wilson, & Rodriguez, 1991). Disinhibition and antisocial traits are associated with increased risk for early-onset alcoholism (Mazas, Finn & Steinmetz, 2000) and sensation/novelty seeking is associated with increased drinking (Finn, Sharkansky, Brandt, & Turcotte, 2000). Indeed, a cluster of traits termed "antisocial personality disorder," inclusive of hyperactivity and impulsivity, correlates highly with chronic alcohol use (Regier et al., 1990). Research has indicated that the shared neurochemical markers may underlie the commonalities between alcohol abuse and traits subsumed in "antisocial personality disorder" (Virkkunen & Linnoila, 1993). This may be suggestive of a preexisting neurochemical milieu in certain individuals that is associated with the impulsive, hyperactive, or aggressive behaviors and which, in turn, is susceptible to alcohol. Thus, impulsive behavior may be a premorbid trait predisposing individuals to a spectrum of disorders including alcohol dependence (Pihl, Peterson, & Lau, 1993).

In addition to the "input" and "output" processing streams, there are also "self-monitoring" functions such as error monitoring and error correction. An ERP component termed error-related negativity (ERN) is evoked when an error is made on a task trial and is presumed to be generated by the anterior cingulate cortex (Coles, Scheffers, & Fournier, 1995). It has been recently shown that moderate intoxication reduces the ERN amplitude (Ridderinkhof et al., 2002). Because errors are detected via a complex system involving multiple stages of stimulus processing, response monitoring, and feedback loops, future research will have to establish which stages are most impaired by alcohol intoxication (Holroyd & Yeung, 2003).

Overall, the ERP literature suggests that significant alterations in brain function can be detected in both semantic and attentional domains at rather low alcohol doses and that the measures of brain function are more sensitive to alcohol-induced impairments than behavioral measures alone. Because they reflect neural events with a millisecond temporal resolution, the electromagnetic methods (ERPs and MEG – magnetoencephalography) can delineate alcohol-induced changes in distinct waveform components, and can consequently indicate alterations in *stages* of processing. However, the underlying neural substrate cannot be inferred unambiguously from ERP/MEG. In contrast, methods relying on hemodynamic changes in brain activity (such as functional magnetic resonance imaging – fMRI, or positron emission tomography – PET) are temporally limited as they reflect the neural activity only indirectly. Nevertheless, they can provide excellent spatial sampling and can thus indicate reliably *where* in the brain alcohol-induced changes are occurring.

Effects of inebriation revealed with hemodynamic methods (fMRI and PET)

As previously noted, MRI technology, which has been used to investigate structural brain abnormalities due to chronic alcohol use, revealed the presence of frontal lobe atrophy (Jernigan et al., 1991; Pfefferbaum et al., 1992; Sullivan, 2000). Few studies have utilized newer technologies, such as fMRI, to study the neurobiological effects of alcohol. Functional MRI, which measures hemodynamic changes resulting from increased metabolic demands of an activated brain region, has high spatial resolution and may offer insight into task- or alcohol-induced changes in the whole brain. However, it measures neural activity indirectly and the neurovascular coupling mechanisms are still poorly understood. Thus, alcohol-induced activation changes may be due to its vasoactive properties, rather than reflecting neural events. Consequently, additional studies are required to delineate the basic physiological interaction between alcohol intoxication and the resulting hemodynamic changes (Tracey, 2001).

The fMRI studies conducted thus far indicate a decrease in the activation levels (Levin et al., 1998; Seifritz et al., 2000), but the functional and regional specificity of these effects needs further investigation in view of alcohol's vasoactive properties. These results concur with PET, some studies showing that an alcohol-induced global decrease in glucose metabolism may be dose-related (de Wit, Metz, Wagner, & Cooper, 1990) and gender-specific (Wang et al., 2003). Another PET study (Volkow et al., 1988) reported decreased blood flow to cerebellum but increased blood flow to right temporal and prefrontal cortices at higher alcohol doses (1 g/kg). Other PET studies, however, reported a global increase in cerebral blood flow, but functionally- and regionally-specific blood flow reduction in the left prefrontal region during a verbal task (Wendt & Risberg, 2001). In a recent study using fMRI (Calhoun et al., 2004), two alcohol doses were administered to healthy subjects on separate occasions as they engaged in a visual perception task. In addition to a global activation decrease, there were dose-related changes in the prefrontal, insular, temporal, occipital, and parietal regions. Future fMRI studies of cognitive functions will reveal task-specific activation patterns and dose-related effects of alcohol intoxication with more precision.

PET also has been utilized successfully for the purpose of delineating the neural circuits of alcohol's reinforcing properties. For example, alcohol increases blood flow to the cerebral reward system, including the anterior cingulate and septum, medial temporal lobe, and lower brainstem (Ingvar et al., 1998). Moreover, a recent study showed that alcohol administration correlated with increased release of dopamine in the ventral striatum, which is similar to the effects observed during the administration of psychostimulants (Boileau et al., 2003). Future PET studies using alcohol challenge will reveal dose-specific changes in neurotransmitter function. They can be particularly valuable in revealing the neural basis of the rewarding properties of intoxication (alcohol-induced "high") and delineating possible mechanisms of alcohol dependence (Bowirrat & Oscar-Berman, 2005).

In general, hemodynamic brain scanning techniques are highly sensitive to localization of brain function. Moreover, these techniques will be instrumental in the development of pharmacological treatments that will target brain areas activated during inebriation. Furthermore, they will be helpful in charting the course of recovery of brain functioning with abstinence.

Vulnerable brain structures

Results of research employing techniques from pathology, neuroimaging, electrophysiology, and behavioral neuroscience have determined that the brain structures most vulnerable to the effects of alcoholism are the neocortex (especially the frontal lobes), the limbic system (especially the hippocampus and hypothalamus), and the cerebellum (Gansler et al., 2000; Sullivan, 2000) (see Figure 2.3). Each of these is considered in turn.

The frontal lobes

The frontal lobes are connected with all of the other lobes of the brain, and they receive and send fibers to numerous subcortical structures as well

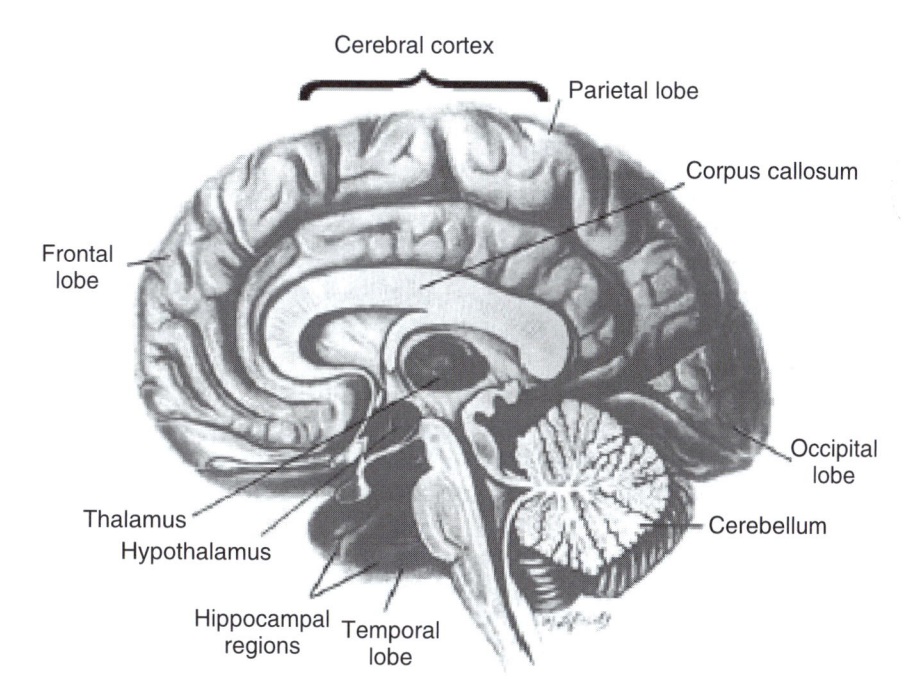

Figure 2.3 The human brain in cross-section.

(Fuster, 1997, 2006). While control of motor function takes place in the posterior region of the frontal lobes, the anterior region of the frontal lobes (prefrontal cortex) plays a kind of executive regulatory role within the brain (Goldberg, 2001; Lichter & Cummings, 2001). Executive functions (which depend upon many of our cognitive abilities, such as attention, perception, memory, and language) are defined differently by different theorists and researchers. Most agree, however, that executive functions are human qualities, including self-awareness, that allow us to be independent individuals with purpose and foresight about what we will do and how we behave. For example, executive abilities include judgment, problem-solving, decision-making, planning, and social conduct.

Damage to frontal brain systems consists of aberrations in personality, as well as cognitive changes such as those just mentioned. Frontal personality traits have been described in terms of "disinhibition" and lack of concern for the consequences of untoward behaviors. In comparison to dramatic personality changes, intellectual or cognitive changes are mild, but unmistakable. Frontal-system features have been only partially defined, but it is generally agreed that executive function deficits follow dorsolateral circuit damage, and that disinhibition and emotional changes follow orbitofrontal circuit lesions (Miller & Cummings, 1999).

Many studies have found the frontal lobes to be more susceptible to alcohol-related brain damage than other cerebral regions (Gansler et al., 2000; Moselhy et al., 2001; Ratti, Bo, Giardini, & Soragna, 2002; Sullivan, 2000). Studies of brain pathology at autopsy have revealed decreased neuron density in the frontal cortex of alcoholics (Harding, Wong, Svoboda, Kril, & Halliday, 1997). Harper (1998) and his collaborators established that 15–23% of cortical neurons are selectively lost from the frontal association cortex following chronic alcohol consumption. MRI studies have shown frontal lobe volume losses in alcoholic subjects (Pfefferbaum et al., 1997), and prefrontal neurobehavioral dysfunctioning has been frequently observed in alcoholics with and without the dense amnesia of Korsakoff's syndrome (Gansler et al., 2000; Oscar-Berman & Evert, 1997). Frontal abnormalities in alcoholics have been identified with fMRI scans (Tapert et al., 2001), reduced regional blood flow measurements (Melgaard et al., 1990), and with measurements of lower glucose metabolism throughout the brain (including prefrontal cortex) during alcohol intoxication (Volkow et al., 1995). Frontal lobe blood flow (Nicolás et al., 1993) and metabolism (Volkow et al., 1992) may decrease in alcoholics before significant shrinkage or major cognitive problems become detectable (Nicolás et al., 1993; Wang et al., 1993).

Cognitive functions and motor coordination may improve at least partially within three to four weeks of abstinence (Oscar-Berman & Evert, 1997; Sullivan, 2000), accompanied by at least partial reversal of brain shrinkage (O'Neill, Cardenas, & Meyerhoff, 2001; Pfefferbaum et al., 1995; Shear, Jernigan, & Butters, 1994) and some recovery of metabolic functions in the frontal lobes (Johnson-Greene, Adams, & Gilman, 1997) and cerebellum

(Martin, Nimmerrichter, Riddle, Welch, & Willcott, 1995; Seitz, Widmann, & Seeger, 1999). Frontal lobe blood flow continues to increase with abstinence, returning to approximately normal levels within four years (Gansler et al., 2000). Relapse to drinking leads to resumption of shrinkage (Pfefferbaum et al., 1995), continued declines in metabolism and cognitive function (Johnson-Greene et al., 1997), and evidence of neuronal cell damage (Martin et al., 1995).

The cerebellum

The cerebellum is a portion of the brain that coordinates movement of voluntary muscles, balance, and eye movements, and it also is essential to the neural circuitry subserving cognition and emotion (Schmahmann, 1997, 2000). The cerebellum contains about half of the brain's neurons, but the nerve cells are so small that the cerebellum accounts for only 10% of the brain's total weight. The cerebellum consists mainly of two large, tightly folded lobes, joined at the middle by the vermis. Also located anteriorly are the small flocculonodular lobes (flocculi). The cerebellum connects with the other brain structures through the cerebellar peduncles, located to the anterior of the cerebellum. Five different nerve cell types make up the cerebellum: stellate, basket, Purkinje, Golgi, and granule cells. The Purkinje cells are the only ones to send axons out of the cerebellum.

Atrophy of the cerebellum is commonly associated with alcoholism. White matter volume of the cerebellar vermis is significantly reduced (Baker, Harding, Halliday, Kril, & Harper, 1999; Pentney, Mullan, Felong, & Dlugos, 2002; Sullivan, 2003), and cerebellar vermian atrophy occurs in 25–40% of all alcoholics. Vermal white matter volume was reduced in ataxic alcoholics by 42%. It occurs even more often in people with additional thiamine deficiency, with 35–50% of those individuals showing evidence of superior vermian degeneration (Victor, 1992). Gross vermian atrophy is commonly seen *post-mortem* in alcoholics (Phillips, Harper, & Kril, 1987), and it also has been observed with *in vivo* neuroimaging techniques (Sullivan, 2003).

Over the past two decades, careful study has expanded the purview of the cerebellum to include influence on functions classically associated with frontal lobe functioning (Schmahmann, 2000; Sullivan, 2003). As noted in the previous section on frontal lobes, this part of the brain has executive control functions such as cognitive flexibility, speed in allocation of attentional resources, shifting ability, inhibition of perservative errors, abstractive and planning skills, and suppression of irrelevant information. Together, these observations suggest a functional role for frontocerebellar circuitry (Schmahmann, 1997). Thus, there is ample evidence for alcohol's untoward effects on the structure and function of the cerebellum and frontal lobes, and disruption of this circuitry is a potential mechanism underlying the behavioral impairment characteristic of alcoholism (Harris et al., 1999; Sullivan et al., 2003).

Alcoholics with Korsakoff's syndrome have shown a significant decrease in Purkinje cell density in the cerebellar vermis and molecular layer volume (Baker et al., 1999). A 36% reduction in Purkinje cell numbers in the flocculi suggests disruption of vestibulocerebellar pathways. This is of particular interest given recent data showing the importance of cerebellum in the organization of higher order cerebral functions (Schmahmann, 2000).

The limbic system

The limbic system is responsible for monitoring internal homeostasis, mediating memory and learning, and contributing to emotions. The limbic system also drives important aspects of sexual behavior, motivation, and feeding behaviors. Primary areas of the limbic system include the hippocampus, amygdala, septal nuclei, hypothalamus, and anterior cingulate gyrus. For the purpose of this chapter, because numerous studies of alcoholics have reported abnormalities in the amygdala, hippocampus, and hypothalamus, the discussion is focused on those brain regions.

Amygdala

The amygdala is a small almond-shaped structure, deep inside the anteroinferior region of the temporal lobe. It is a heterogeneous brain area consisting of 13 nuclei and cortical regions and their subdivisions (Pitkänen, Pikkarainen, Nurminen, & Ylinen, 2000; Sah, Faber, Lopez De Armentia, & Power, 2003). It connects with prefrontal cortex, the hippocampus, the septal nuclei, and the medial dorsal nucleus of the thalamus. These connections make it possible for the amygdala to play its important role on the mediation and control of major affective states such as love, fear, rage, anxiety, and general negative affectivity (Aggleton, 2000; Amaral et al., 2003; Pitkänen et al., 2000). The amygdala, being important in identifying danger, is fundamental for self-preservation.

Neuroimaging studies in humans have shown that the amygdala responds to facial expressions of many emotions, especially those with negative affective qualities such as sadness, anger, and fear (Blair, Morris, Frith, Perrettand, & Dolan, 1999; Breiter & Rosen, 1999; Wang, McCarthy, Song, & LaBar, 2005; Winston, O'Doherty, & Dolan, 2003). In fact, facial expressions convey such strong emotional information that merely observing anger or fearful faces elicits visceral responses, including increased heart rate and sweating (Ohman & Soares, 1998). Neuroimaging studies (Davis & Whalen, 2001) have illustrated that these fearful responses to facial expressions are processed and largely mediated by the amygdala (having connections to both early sensory processing areas and autonomic reflex centers). Furthermore, amygdala responses to fearful faces have been observed even in the absence of conscious awareness of their presentation to subjects (Whalen et al., 1998).

A number of studies have linked the amygdala to the processing of motivational significance of stimuli and to the control of emotion (Breiter & Rosen, 1999; Everitt, Cardinal, Parkinson, & Robbins, 2003; LeDoux, 2003; Rolls, 2000). The amygdala is controlled in part by the brain's dopamine system (Delaveau, Salgado-Pineda, Wicker, Micallef-Roll, & Blin, 2005), the same system that responds to alcohol and produces feelings of pleasure when good things happen. In a recent study using fMRI in our laboratory, we observed clear evidence of differences between abstinent long-term alcoholics and nonalcoholic controls in amygdala activation to emotional materials. The subjects were scanned while viewing emotional words and emotional facial expressions. Subjects were given either shallow processing instructions ("Decide if the word [or the face] appears in color or black/white") or semantic deep processing instructions ("Decide if the word is abstract or concrete," or "if the person is intelligent or not"). After each of the four conditions, subjects were tested for recognition of the stimuli ("Have you seen this face/word before?"). Results indicated group differences in activation of mesial temporal brain regions, depending upon whether the materials were faces or words, and whether the processing level was deep or shallow. These differences were most apparent in the amygdala (and in the hippocampus to a lesser extent) with face stimuli. Thus, the alcoholic group showed significantly reduced activity during the deep processing of emotional faces. Faces with negative and positive emotional expressions evoked stronger bilateral amygdala activity in the controls than in the alcoholics, whose responses were blunted. These results suggest that the alcoholics responded to the emotionally valenced stimuli in an undifferentiated manner. A similar lack of emotional differentiation by alcoholics also was observed in the hippocampus, although to a lesser degree than in the amygdala.

Hippocampus

The hippocampus is a horseshoe-shaped sheet of neurons located on the floor of each lateral ventricle within the temporal lobes and adjacent to the amygdala (Pitkänen et al., 2000). As part of the limbic system, it is intimately involved in motivation and emotion, and it also plays a central role in the formation of memories. The hippocampus consists of the complex interfolded layers of the dentate gyrus and Ammon's horn, which are continuous with the subiculum, which in turn merges with the parahippocampal gyrus. Although the idea that the hippocampus may play a role in brain mechanisms underlying anxiety is not new (Bannerman et al., 2002; Gray & McNaughton, 2000), there is now mounting evidence that the ventral hippocampus plays an important role in a brain system associated with fear and/or anxiety (Bannerman et al., 2002; Kjelstrup et al., 2002; McHugh, Deacon, Rawlins, et al., 2004). The anatomy of the hippocampus is closely associated with subcortical structures which contribute to the hypothalamic-pituitary-adrenal axis (Kjelstrup et al., 2002). A recent study also demonstrated that encoding of emotional memories depends on the hippocampus in conjunction with the amygdala, as well as their interaction with each other (Richardson, Strange, & Dolan, 2004).

The hippocampus may be a target site for the teratogenic effects of ethanol (West & Pierce, 1986, but see Harding et al., 1997). Morphological changes in this brain region may play a critical role in the mental deficiency and behavioral abnormalities of individuals with fetal alcohol syndrome or alcohol-related neurodevelopmental disorder (Roebuck, Mattson, & Riley, 1998). There is evidence that certain hippocampal neuronal cell types are particularly sensitive to ethanol teratogenicity. For example, in nonhuman animals, chronic exposure of the developing hippocampus to ethanol can result in selective damage, such as a decrease in the number of CA1 pyramidal cells (Abdollah, Catlin, & Brien, 1993; Bonthius & West, 1990; Gibson, Butters, Reynolds, & Brien, 2000; Miller, 1995). One study of human alcoholics aged 45 years and under reported an early neuronal loss of the dentate gyrus and the ammonic fields CA1–CA4 (Bengochea & Gonzalo, 1990). Another study discovered glial cell loss (especially astrocytes and oligodendrocytes) in the hippocampus of alcoholics (Korbo, 1999).

The results of a recent study suggested that the effect of ethanol on the survival of newly formed neurons in the adult rat hippocampus could result in impairment of hippocampal-dependent cognitive functions, or, alternatively, the changes in cognition observed in alcoholism could lead to decreased neuronal survival (Herrera et al., 2003). Neurogenesis is primarily a developmental process that involves the proliferation, migration, and differentiation into neurons of primordial stem cells of the central nervous system. Neurogenesis declines until it ceases in the young adult mammalian brain, with two exceptions: The olfactory bulb and the hippocampus produce new neurons throughout adult life. The ethanol-induced reductions in hippocampal neurogenesis can be attributed to two general mechanisms: an effect on cell proliferation or on cell survival. These changes in hippocampal structure could be part of the anatomical basis for cognitive deficits observed in alcoholism.

Structural neuroimaging studies have demonstrated a reduction of hippocampal volume in alcoholics (Agartz, Momenam, Rawlings, Kerich, & Hommer, 1999; Kurth et al., 2004; Pfefferbaum & Sullivan, 2002). The loss of hippocampal volume has been attributed to changes in white matter (Harding et al., 1997), but the incorporation of newly formed neurons to the dentate gyrus could also be affected by alcohol. One MRI study measured hippocampus volume in late-onset alcoholics (Type I) and violent early-onset alcoholics (Type II), compared to nonalcoholic controls (Laakso et al., 2000). The right, but not left, hippocampus was significantly smaller in both alcoholic groups. While there was no correlation between the hippocampal volumes with age in the control subjects, there was tendency toward decreased volumes with aging and also with the duration of alcoholism in the Type I alcoholics. In a study of teens (aged 15–17 years) with alcohol use disorders, Nagel, Schweinsburg, Phan, and Tapert (2005) found reduced left – but not right – hippocampal volume compared to healthy age-equivalent controls. The groups were equivalent in right hippocampal, intracranial gray and white matter volumes, and memory performance. The authors suggested that premorbid volumetric differences might account for some of the observed group differences in hippocampal volume. Reduction of hippocampal volume in alcoholics is reversible after short periods of abstinence (White, Matthews, & Best, 2000). Similarly, hippocampal-dependent cognitive functions have also shown reversibility after comparable periods of abstinence.

Hypothalamus

The hypothalamus literally means "under the thalamus." It is a small structure nestled within the limbic system directly above the brainstem. The hypothalamus plays a role in many regulatory functions, such as eating and drinking, temperature control, hormone regulation, and emotional functions. The hypothalamus has connections with many other brain regions, and is involved in learning (Simonov, 1986).

Alcohol-related damage to the mammillary bodies of the hypothalamus is considered to lead to Korsakoff's syndrome (Oscar-Berman & Evert, 1997). Lesions of the mammillary bodies or to other regions of the brain (basal forebrain, hippocampus, fornix, medial and anterior nuclei of the thalamus) are associated with memory impairments (Butters, 1981; Mesulam, 2000). The specific memory impairments include severe anterograde amnesia for recent events, and some retrograde amnesia, i.e., loss of memory for events that happened long ago (prior to the appearance of obvious symptomatology). Damage to basal forebrain structures (important in the production of neurotransmitters, which are needed for normal memory functions) may also be involved.

Amnesia, especially anterograde amnesia, or memory loss for recent events, is an intriguing and serious disorder. When amnesia occurs as a consequence of long-term alcoholism, it is referred to as alcohol-induced persisting amnestic disorder (APA, 1994), or alcoholic Korsakoff's syndrome. Patients with Korsakoff's syndrome are permanently unable to remember new information for more than a few seconds. Because new events are forgotten a few seconds after they occur, virtually nothing new is learned, and patients with Korsakoff's syndrome live perpetually in the past. However, in contrast to patients with alcoholic dementia, who have generalized cognitive decline (including widespread memory loss), patients with Korsakoff's syndrome retain old memories formed prior to the onset of alcohol-related brain damage.

Although anterograde amnesia is the most obvious presenting symptom in Korsakoff patients, these individuals have other cognitive impairments as well. Like patients with bilateral prefrontal cortical lesions, Korsakoff patients are abnormally sensitive to distractions (proactive interference). This sensitivity may be due to alcoholism-related prefrontal dysfunction, which impairs the ability to counteract the effects of cognitive interruptions. In addition to their memory problems and their sensitivity to interference, Korsakoff patients also tend to repeat unnecessary behaviors (perseverative responding), have restricted attention, retarded perceptual processing abilities, ataxia, and decreased sensitivity to reward contingencies (Oscar-Berman & Evert, 1997). These additional abnormalities reflect widespread cerebral atrophy accompanying sustained alcohol abuse. Thus, consideration should be given to sensory and cognitive deficits that may be integral to the disease process caused by chronic alcoholism.

Implications for treatment and recovery

Clinicians must consider a variety of treatment methods to promote cessation of drinking, maintenance of sobriety, and recovery of impaired functioning. Because alcoholism is associated with diverse changes to the brain and behavior, treatment professionals might find it most helpful to use a combination of neuropsychological observations and structural and functional brain imaging results in developing predictors of abstinence versus relapse, with the purpose of tailoring treatment methods to each individual patient. For example, the development of effective medications for controlling alcoholism relies upon knowledge about the neuroanatomical origins of neurotransmitters involved in craving, intoxication, and addiction. Neuroimaging methods have already provided significant insight into the nature of brain damage caused by heavy alcohol use, and the integration of results from different methods of neuroimaging will spur further advances in the diagnosis and treatment of alcoholism-related damage. Clinicians also can use brain imaging techniques to monitor the course of treatment because these techniques can reveal structural, functional, and biochemical changes in patients across time as a result of abstinence, therapeutic interventions, withdrawal, or relapse. Neuroimaging research already has shown that abstinence of less than a month can result in an increase in cerebral metabolism, particularly in the frontal lobes, and that continued abstinence can lead to at least partial reversal in loss of brain tissue (Gansler et al., 2000; Sullivan, 2000). Thus, through the combined efforts of scientists and clinicians, important strides already have been made in the diagnosis, prevention, and treatment of alcoholism, and hopefully there will be continued advances in the future.

Conclusions

Alcoholics are a diverse group. They experience different subsets of symptoms, and the disease has different origins and modulating influences for different people. Therefore, to understand the effects of alcoholism, it is important to consider the influence of a wide range of variables on a particular behavior or set of behaviors. The underpinnings of alcohol-induced brain defects are multivariate; to date, the available literature does not support the assertion that any one variable can consistently and completely account for these impairments.

The most plausible conclusion is that neurobehavioral deficits in some alcoholics result from prolonged ingestion of alcohol, which impairs the way the brain normally works, by people who are vulnerable to some forms of brain damage. The identification of these vulnerabilities is a primary focus of current research. In the search for answers, it is necessary to use as many kinds of tools as possible, keeping in mind that specific deficits can be observed only with certain methods, with specific paradigms, and with particular types of people with distinct risk factors. Such confluence of information can provide evidence linking structural damage, functional alterations, and the specific behavioral and neuropsychological effects of alcoholism. These measures also can determine the degree to which abstinence and treatment result in the reversal of atrophy and dysfunction.

Acknowledgments

This writing of this chapter was supported by National Institute on Alcohol Abuse and Alcoholism grants R37–AA07112, K05–AA00219, and K01–AA13402, by the Medical Research Service of the US Department of Veterans Affairs, and by the Alcohol Beverage Medical Research Foundation.

References

Abdollah, S., Catlin, M. C., & Brien, J. F. (1993). Ethanol neuro-behavioural teratogenesis in the guinea pig: Behavioural dysfunction and hippocampal morphological change. *Canadian Journal of Physiology and Pharmacology*, 71, 776–782.

Agartz, I., Momenam, R., Rawlings, R. R., Kerich, M. J., & Hommer, D. W. (1999). Hippocampal volume in patient with alcohol dependence. *Archives of General Psychiatry*, 56, 356–363.

Aggleton, J. P. (2000). *The amygdala: a functional analysis* (2nd ed.). Oxford: Oxford University Press.

Amaral, D. G., Bauman, M. D., Capitanio, J. P., Lavenex, P., Mason, W. A., Mauldin-Jourdain, M. L., et al. (2003). The amygdala: is it an essential component of the neural network for social cognition? *Neuropsychologia*, 41, 517–522.

APA (1994). *Diagnostic and statistical manual of mental disorders (DSM-IV)*. Washington, DC: American Psychiatric Association.

Baker, K. G., Harding, A. J., Halliday, G. M., Kril, J. J., & Harper, C. G. (1999). Neuronal loss in functional zones of the cerebellum of chronic alcoholics with and without Wernicke's encephalopathy. *Neuroscience, 19*, 429–438.

Bannerman, D. M., Deacon, R. M. J., Offen, S., Friswell, J., Grubb, M., & Rawlins, J. N. P. (2002). A double dissociation of function within the hippocampus: Spatial memory and hyponeophagia. *Behavioral Neuroscience, 116*, 884–901.

Bates, M. E., Bowden, S. C., & Barry, D. (2002). Neurocognitive impairment associated with alcohol use disorders: Implications for treatment. *Experimental and Clinical Psychopharmacology, 10*, 193–212.

Begleiter, H., & Porjesz, B. (1999). What is inherited in the predisposition toward alcoholism? A proposed model. *Alcoholism: Clinical and Experimental Research, 23*, 1125–1135.

Bengochea, O., & Gonzalo, L. M. (1990). Effect of chronic alcoholism on the human hippocampus. *Histology and Histopathology, 5*, 349–357.

Bierut, L. J., Saccone, N. L., Rice, J. P., Goate, A., Foroud, T., Edenberg, H., et al. (2002). Defining alcohol-related phenotypes in humans. The collaborative study on the genetics of alcoholism. *Alcohol Research and Health, 26*, 208–213.

Blair, R. J. R., Morris, J. S., Frith, C. D., Perrettand, D. I., & Dolan, R. J. (1999). Dissociable neural responses to facial expressions of sadness and anger. *Brain, 122*, 883–893.

Boileau, I., Assaad, J. M., Pihl, R. O., Benkelfat, C., Leyton, M., Diksic, M., et al. (2003). Alcohol promotes dopamine release in the human nucleus accumbens. *Synapse, 49*, 226–231.

Bonthius, D. J., & West, J. R. (1990). Alcohol-induced neuronal loss in developing rats: Increased brain damage with binge exposure. *Alcoholism: Clinical and Experimental Research, 14*, 107–118.

Bowirrat, A., & Oscar-Berman, M. (2005). Relationship between dopaminergic neurotransmission, alcoholism, and reward deficiency syndrome. *American Journal of Medical Genetics Part B (Neuropsychiatric Genetics), 118*, 29–37.

Breiter, H. C., & Rosen, B. R. (1999). Functional magnetic resonance imaging of brain reward circuitry in the human. In J. F. McGinty (Ed.), *Advancing from the ventral striatum to the extended amygdala* (Vol. 877, pp. 523–547). New York: New York Academy of Sciences.

Buckner, R. L., Logan, J., Donaldson, D. I., & Wheeler, M. E. (2000). Cognitive neuroscience of episodic memory encoding. *Acta Psychologica (Amsterdam), 105*, 127–139.

Bushman, B. J., & Cooper, H. M. (1990). Effects of alcohol on human aggression: An integrative research review. *Psychological Bulletin, 107*, 341–354.

Butters, N. (1981). The Wernicke-Korsakoff syndrome: a review of psychological, neuropathological and etiological factors. *Current Topics in Alcoholism, 8*, 205–232.

Calhoun, V. D., Altschul, D., McGinty, V., Shih, R., Scott, D., Sears, E., et al. (2004). Alcohol intoxication effects on visual perception: An fMRI study. *Human Brain Mapping, 21*, 298–299.

Campbell, K., Marois, R., & Arcand, L. (1984). Ethanol and the event-related evoked potentials. Effects of rate of stimulus presentation and task difficulty. *Annals of the New York Academy of Sciences, 425*, 551–555.

Coles, M. G., Scheffers, M. K., & Fournier, L. (1995). Where did you go wrong? Errors, partial errors, and the nature of human information processing. *Acta Psychologica (Amsterdam), 90*, 129–144.

Courchesne, E., Hillyard, S. A., & Galambos, R. (1975). Stimulus novelty, task relevance and the visual evoked potential in man. *Electroencephalography and Clinical Neurophysiology, 39,* 131–143.

Davies, A. G., Pierce-Shimomura, J. T., Kim, H., VanHoven, M. K., Thiele, T. R., Bonci, A., et al. (2003). A central role of the BK potassium channel in behavioral responses to ethanol in C. elegans. *Cell, 115,* 655–666.

Davis, M., & Whalen, P. J. (2001). The amygdala: vigilance and emotion. *Molecular Psychiatry, 6,* 13–34.

de Wit, H., Metz, J., Wagner, N., & Cooper, M. (1990). Behavioral and subjective effects of ethanol: Relationship to cerebral metabolism using PET. *Alcoholism: Clinical and Experimental Research, 14,* 482–489.

Delaveau, P., Salgado-Pineda, P., Wicker, B., Micallef-Roll, J., & Blin, O. (2005). Effect of levodopa on healthy volunteers' facial emotion perception: an FMRI study. *Clinical Neuropharmacology, 28,* 255–261.

Di Sclafani, V., Ezekiel, F., Meyerhoff, D. J., MacKay, S., Dillon, W. P., Weiner, M. W., et al. (1995). Brain atrophy and cognitive function in older abstinent alcoholic men. *Alcoholism: Clinical and Experimental Research, 19,* 1121–1126.

Dick, D. M., & Bierut, L. J. (2006). The genetics of alcohol dependence. *Current Psychiatry Reports, 8,* 151–157.

Dick, D. M., & Foroud, T. (2003). Candidate genes for alcohol dependence: A review of genetic evidence from human studies. *Alcoholism: Clinical and Experimental Research, 27,* 868–879.

Dougherty, D. M., Moeller, F. G., Steinberg, J. L., Marsh, D. M., Hines, S. E., & Bjork, J. M. (1999). Alcohol increases commission error rates for a continuous performance test. *Alcoholism: Clinical and Experimental Research, 23,* 1342–1351.

Ellis, R. J., & Oscar-Berman, M. (1989). Alcoholism, aging, and functional cerebral asymmetries. *Psychological Bulletin, 106,* 128–147.

Everitt, B. J., Cardinal, R. N., Parkinson, J. A., & Robbins, T. W. (2003). Appetitive behavior: impact of amygdala-dependent mechanisms of emotional learning. *Annals of the New York Academy of Sciences, 985,* 233–250.

Fein, G., Di Sclafani, V., Cardenas, V. A., Goldmann, H., Tolou-Shams, M., & Meyerhoff, D. J. (2002). Cortical gray matter loss in treatment-naive alcohol dependent individuals. *Alcoholism: Clinical and Experimental Research, 26,* 558–564.

Finn, P. R., Sharkansky, E. J., Brandt, K. M., & Turcotte, N. (2000). The effects of familial risk, personality, and expectancies on alcohol use and abuse. *Journal of Abnormal Psychology, 109,* 122–133.

Fuster, J. M. (1997). *The prefrontal cortex* (3rd ed.). New York: Lippincott-Raven.

Fuster, J. M. (2006). The cognit: A network model of cortical representation. *International Journal of Psychophysiology, 60,* 125–132.

Gansler, D. A., Harris, G. J., Oscar-Berman, M., Streeter, C., Lewis, R. F., Ahmed, I., et al. (2000). Hypoperfusion of inferior frontal brain regions in abstinent alcoholics: A pilot SPECT study. *Journal of Studies on Alcohol, 61,* 32–37.

Gibson, M. A., Butters, N. S., Reynolds, J. N., & Brien, J. F. (2000). Effects of chronic prenatal ethanol exposure on locomotor activity, and hippocampal weight, neurons, and nitric oxide synthase activity of the young postnatal guinea pig. *Neurotoxicology and Teratology, 22,* 183–192.

Gilman, S., Adams, K. M., Johnson-Greene, D., Koeppe, R. A., Junck, L., Kluin,

K. J., et al. (1996). Effects of disulfiram on positron emission tomography and neuropsychological studies in severe chronic alcoholism. *Alcoholism: Clinical and Experimental Research, 20*, 1456–1461.

Goldberg, E. (2001). *The executive brain: Frontal lobes and the civilized mind.* New York: Oxford University Press.

Goodwin, D. W. (1977). Genetic and experiential antecedents of alcoholism: a prospective study. *Alcoholism: Clinical and Experimental Research, 1*, 259–265.

Grant, I. (1987). Alcohol and the brain: Neuropsychological correlates. *Journal of Consulting and Clinical Psychology, 55*, 310–324.

Grant, S. A., Millar, K., & Kenny, G. N. (2000). Blood alcohol concentration and psychomotor effects. *British Journal of Anaesthesiology, 85*, 401–406.

Gray, J. A., & McNaughton, N. (2000). *The neuropsychology of anxiety: An enquiry into the functions of the septo-hippocampal system* (2nd ed.). Oxford, UK: Oxford University Press.

Grillon, C., Sinha, R., & O'Malley, S. S. (1995). Effects of ethanol on the processing of low probability stimuli: an ERP study. *Psychopharmacology (Berlin), 119*, 455–465.

Halgren, E. (1990). Human evoked potential. In A. A. Boulton, G. B. Baker, & C. Vanderwolf (Eds.), *Neuropsychological techniques: Applications to neural systems* (Vol. 15, pp. 147–275). Clifton, NJ: Humana.

Harding, A. J., Wong, A., Svoboda, M., Kril, J. J., & Halliday, G. M. (1997). Chronic alcohol consumption does not cause hippocampal neuron loss in humans. *Hippocampus, 7*, 78–87.

Harper, C. (1998). The neuropathology of alcohol-specific brain damage, or does alcohol damage the brain? *Journal of Neuropathology and Experimental Neurology, 57*, 101–110.

Harris, G. J., Oscar-Berman, M., Gansler, D. A., Streeter, C., Lewis, R. F., Ahmed, I., et al. (1999). Hypoperfusion of cerebellum and aging effects on cerebral cortex blood flow in abstinent alcoholics: A SPECT study. *Alcoholism: Clinical and Experimental Research, 23*, 1219–1227.

Haut, J. S., Beckwith, B. E., Petros, T. V., & Russell, S. (1989). Gender differences in retrieval from long-term memory following acute intoxication with ethanol. *Physiology and Behavior, 45*, 1161–1165.

Herrera, D. G., Yague, A. G., Johnsen-Soriano, S., Bosch-Morell, F., Collado-Morente, L., Muriach, M., et al. (2003). Selective impairment of hippocampal neurogenesis by chronic alcoholism: Protective effects of an antioxidant. *Proceedings of the National Academy of Sciences, 100*, 7919–7924.

Hill, S. Y., & Steinhauer, S. R. (1993). Event-related potentials in women at risk for alcoholism. *Alcohol, 10*, 349–354.

Holcomb, P. J. (1993). Semantic priming and stimulus degradation: implications for the role of the N400 in language processing. *Psychophysiology, 30*, 47–61.

Holroyd, C. B., & Yeung, N. (2003). Alcohol and error processing. *Trends in Neuroscience, 26*, 402–404.

Hommer, D., Momenan, R., Rawlings, R., Ragan, P., Williams, W., Rio, D., et al. (1996). Decreased corpus callosum size among alcoholic women. *Archives of Neurology, 53*, 359–363.

Ingvar, M., Ghatan, P. H., Wirsen-Meurling, A., Risberg, J., Von Heijne, G., Stone-Elander, S., et al. (1998). Alcohol activates the cerebral reward system in man. *Journal of Studies on Alcohol, 59*, 258–269.

Jacob, T., Waterman, B., Heath, A., True, W., Bucholz, K. K., Haber, R., et al. (2003).

Genetic and environmental effects on offspring alcoholism: new insights using an offspring-of-twins design. *Archives of General Psychiatry, 60*, 1265–1272.

Jernigan, T. L., Butters, N., DiTraglia, G., Schafer, K., Smith, T., Irwin, M., et al. (1991). Reduced cerebral grey matter observed in alcoholics using magnetic resonance imaging. *Alcoholism: Clinical and Experimental Research, 15*, 418–427.

Johnson-Greene, D., Adams, K. M., & Gilman, S. (1997). Effects of abstinence and relapse upon neuropsychological function and cerebral glucose metabolism in severe chronic alcoholism. *Journal of Clinical and Experimental Neuropsychology, 19*, 378–385.

Jääskeläinen, I. P., Schroger, E., & Näätänen, R. (1999). Electrophysiological indices of acute effects of ethanol on involuntary attention shifting. *Psychopharmacology (Berlin), 141*, 16–21.

Kjelstrup, K. G., Tuvnes, F. A., Steffenach, H. A., Murison, R., Moser, E. I., & Moser, M. B. (2002). Reduced fear expression after lesions of the ventral hippocampus. *Proceedings of the National Academy of Sciences, 99*, 10825–10830.

Knight, R. T., Grabowecky, M. F., & Scabini, D. (1995). Role of human prefrontal cortex in attention control. In H. H. Jasper, S. Riggio, & P. S. Goldman-Rakic (Eds.), *Epilepsy and the functional anatomy of the frontal lobe* (pp. 21–36). New York: Raven Press.

Koelega, H. S. (1995). Alcohol and vigilance performance: a review. *Psychopharmacology (Berlin), 118*, 233–249.

Korbo, L. (1999). Glial cells in the hippocampus of alcoholics. *Alcoholism: Clinical and Experimental Research, 23*, 164–168.

Kroft, C. L., Gescuk, B., Woods, B. T., Mello, N. K., Weiss, R. D., & Mendelson, J. H. (1991). Brain ventricular size in female alcoholics: An MRI study. *Alcoholism: Clinical and Experimental Research, 8*, 31–34.

Kurth, C., Wegerer, V., Reulbach, U., Lewczuk, P., Kornhuber, J., Steinhoff, B. J., et al. (2004). Analysis of hippocampal atrophy in alcoholic patients by a Kohonen feature map. *Neuroreport, 15*, 367–371.

Kutas, M., & Hillyard, S. A. (1980). Reading senseless sentences: brain potentials reflect semantic incongruity. *Science, 207*, 203–205.

Laakso, M. P., Vaurio, O., Savolainen, L., Repo, E., Soininen, H., Aronen, H. J., et al. (2000). A volumetric MRI study of the hippocampus in type 1 and 2 alcoholism. *Behavioral Brain Research, 109*, 177–186.

Lancaster, F. E. (1995). Gender differences in animal studies. Implications for the study of human alcoholism. *Recent Developments in Alcoholism, 12*, 209–215.

LeDoux, J. E. (2003). The emotional brain, fear, and the amygdala. *Cell and Molecular Neurobiology, 23*, 727–738.

Levin, J. M., Ross, M. H., Mendelson, J. H., Kaufman, M. J., Lange, N., Maas, L. C., et al. (1998). Reduction in BOLD fMRI response to primary visual stimulation following alcohol ingestion. *Psychiatry Research, 82*, 135–146.

Lichter, D. G., & Cummings, J. L. (2001). *Frontal-subcortical circuits in psychiatric and neurological disorders*. New York: The Guilford Press.

Mann, K., Batra, A., Gunthner, A., & Schroth, G. (1992). Do women develop alcoholic brain damage more readily than men? *Alcoholism: Clinical and Experimental Research, 16*, 1052–1056.

Marinković, K. (2004). Spatiotemporal dynamics of word processing in the human cortex. *Neuroscientist, 10*, 142–152.

Marinković, K., Halgren, E., Klopp, J., & Maltzman, I. (2000). Alcohol effects on movement-related potentials: a measure of impulsivity? *Journal of Studies on Alcohol, 61*, 24–31.

Marinković, K., Halgren, E., & Maltzman, I. (2001). Arousal-related P3a to novel auditory stimuli is abolished by moderately low alcohol dose. *Alcohol and Alcoholism, 36*, 529–539.

Marinković, K., Halgren, E., & Maltzman, I. (2004). Effects of alcohol on verbal processing: An ERP study. *Alcoholism: Clinical and Experimental Research, 28*, 415–423.

Martin, P. R., Nimmerrichter, A., Riddle, W. R., Welch, L. W., & Willcott, M. R. (1995). Brain proton magnetic resonance spectroscopy studies in recently abstinent alcoholics. *Alcoholism: Clinical and Experimental Research, 19*, 1078–1082.

Maylor, E. A., Rabbitt, P. M., James, G. H., & Kerr, S. A. (1990). Comparing the effects of alcohol and intelligence on text recall and recognition. *British Journal of Psychology, 81*, 299–313.

Maylor, E. A., Rabbitt, P. M., & Kingstone, A. (1987). Effects of alcohol on word categorization and recognition memory. *British Journal of Psychology, 78*, 233–239.

Mazas, C. A., Finn, P. R., & Steinmetz, J. E. (2000). Decision-making biases, antisocial personality, and early-onset alcoholism. *Alcoholism: Clinical and Experimental Research, 24*, 1036–1040.

McGue, M. (1999). The behavioral genetics of alcoholism. *Current Direction in Psychological Science, 8*, 109–115.

McHugh, S. B., Deacon, R. M. J., Rawlins, J. N. P., et al. (2004). Amygdala and ventral hippocampus contribute differentially to mechanisms of fear and anxiety. *Behavioral Neuroscience, 118*, 63–78.

Melgaard, B., Henriksen, L., Ahlgren, P., Danielsen, U. T., Sorensen, H., & Paulson, O. B. (1990). Regional cerebral blood flow in chronic alcoholics measured by single photon emission computerized tomography. *Acta Neurologica Scandinavica, 82*, 87–93.

Mesulam, M.-M. (2000). Behavioral neuroanatomy. Large-scale networks, association cortex, frontal syndromes, the limbic system, and hemispheric specialization. In M.-M. Mesulam (Ed.), *Principles of behavioral and cognitive neurology* (pp. 1–120). New York: Oxford.

Miller, B. L., & Cummings, J. L. (1999). *The human frontal lobes: Functions and disorders*. New York: Guilford Press.

Miller, M. W. (1995). Generation of neurons in the rat dentate gyrus and hippocampus: Effects of prenatal and postnatal treatment with ethanol. *Alcoholism: Clinical and Experimental Research, 19*, 1500–1509.

Monteiro, M. G., & Schuckit, M. A. (1988). Populations at high alcoholism risk: recent findings. *Journal of Clinical Psychiatry, 49*, 3–7.

Moselhy, H. F., Georgiou, G., & Kahn, A. (2001). Frontal lobe changes in alcoholism: A review of the literature. *Alcohol and Alcoholism, 36*, 357–368.

Mulvihill, L. E., Skilling, T. A., & Vogel-Sprott, M. (1997). Alcohol and the ability to inhibit behavior in men and women. *Journal of Studies on Alcohol, 58*, 600–605.

Nagel, B. J., Schweinsburg, A. D., Phan, V., & Tapert, S. F. (2005). Hippocampal volume among adolescents with alcohol use disorders without psychiatric comorbidity. *Psychiatry Research: Neuroimaging, 139*, 181–190.

Nagoshi, C. T., & Wilson, J. R. (1989). Long-term repeatability of human alcohol metabolism, sensitivity and acute tolerance. *Journal of Studies on Alcohol, 50*, 162–169.

Nagoshi, C. T., Wilson, J. R., & Rodriguez, L. A. (1991). Impulsivity, sensation seeking, and behavioral and emotional responses to alcohol. *Alcoholism: Clinical and Experimental Research, 15*, 661–667.

Nagy, M. E., & Rugg, M. D. (1989). Modulation of event-related potentials by word repetition: the effects of inter-item lag. *Psychophysiology, 26*, 431–436.

NIAAA. (1997). *Ninth special report to the US Congress on alcohol and health*. Bethesda, MD: NIAAA.

Nicolás, J. M., Catafau, A. M., Estruch, R., Lomeña, F. J., Salamero, M., Herranz, R., et al. (1993). Regional cerebral blood flow-SPECT in chronic alcoholism: Relation to neuropsychological testing. *Journal of Nuclear Medicine, 34*, 1452–1459.

O'Neill, J., Cardenas, V. A., & Meyerhoff, D. J. (2001). Effects of abstinence on the brain: quantitative magnetic resonance imaging and magnetic resonance spectroscopic imaging in chronic alcohol abuse. *Alcoholism: Clinical and Experimental Research, 25*, 1673–1682.

Ohman, A., & Soares, J. J. (1998). Emotional conditioning to masked stimuli: expectancies for aversive outcomes following nonrecognized fear-relevant stimuli. *Journal of Experimental Psychology: General, 127*, 69–82.

Oscar-Berman, M. (2000). Neuropsychological vulnerabilities in chronic alcoholism. In A. Noronha, M. J. Eckardt & K. Warren (Eds.), *Review of NIAAA's neuroscience and behavioral research portfolio* (Vol. 34, pp. 437–471). Bethesda, MD: US Department of Health and Human Services.

Oscar-Berman, M., & Evert, D. L. (1997). Alcoholic Korsakoff's syndrome. In P. D. Nussbaum (Ed.), *Handbook of neuropsychology and aging* (pp. 201–215). New York: Plenum Press.

Oscar-Berman, M., & Hutner, N. (1993). Frontal lobe changes after chronic alcohol ingestion. In W. A. Hunt & S. J. Nixon (Eds.), *Alcohol-induced brain damage* (Vol. 22, pp. 121–156). Rockville, MD: NIAAA.

Oscar-Berman, M., & Schendan, H. E. (2000). Asymmetries of brain function in alcoholism: Relationship to aging. In L. Obler & L. T. Connor (Eds.), *Neurobehavior of language and cognition: Studies of normal aging and brain damage* (pp. 213–240). New York: Kluwer Academic.

Parsons, O. A. (1994). Neuropsychological measures and event-related potentials in alcoholics: Interrelationships, long-term reliabilities, and prediction of resumption of drinking. *Journal of Clinical Psychology, 50*, 37–46.

Parsons, O. A. (1996). Alcohol abuse and alcoholism. In R. L. Adams, O. A. Parsons, J. L. Culbertson & S. J. Nixon (Eds.), *Neuropsychology for clinical practice* (pp. 175–201). Washington, DC: American Psychological Press.

Pentney, R. J., Mullan, B. A., Felong, A. M., & Dlugos, C. A. (2002). The total numbers of cerebellar granule neurons in young and aged Fischer 344 and Wistar-Kyoto rats do not change as a result of lengthy ethanol treatment. *Cerebellum, 1*, 79–89.

Peterson, J. B., Rothfleisch, J., Zelazo, P. D., & Pihl, R. O. (1990). Acute alcohol intoxication and cognitive functioning. *Journal of Studies on Alcohol, 51*, 114–122.

Petrakis, I. L., Gonzalez, G., Rosenheck, R., & Krystal, J. H. (2002). Comorbidity of alcoholism and psychiatric disorders. *Alcohol Research and Health, 26*, 81–89.

Pfefferbaum, A., Ford, J. M., White, P. M., & Mathalon, D. (1991). Event-related potentials in alcoholic men: P3 amplitude reflects family history but not alcohol consumption. *Alcoholism: Clinical Experimental Research, 15*, 839–850.

Pfefferbaum, A., Horvath, T. B., Roth, W. T., Clifford, S. T., & Kopell, B. S. (1980). Acute and chronic effects of ethanol on event-related potentials. *Advances in Experimental and Medical Biology, 126*, 625–639.

Pfefferbaum, A., Lim, K. O., Desmond, J. E., & Sullivan, E. V. (1996). Thinning of the corpus callosum in older alcoholic men: A magnetic resonance imaging study. *Alcoholism: Clinical and Experimental Research, 20*, 752–757.

Pfefferbaum, A., Lim, K. O., Zipursky, R. B., Mathalon, D. H., Rosenbloom, M. J., Lane, B., et al. (1992). Brain gray and white matter volume loss accelerates with aging in chronic alcoholics: a quantitative MRI study. *Alcoholism: Clinical and Experimental Research, 16*, 1078–1089.

Pfefferbaum, A., Rosenbloom, M., Serventi, K. L., & Sullivan, E. V. (2002). Corpus callosum, pons, and cortical white matter in alcoholic women. *Alcoholism: Clinical and Experimental Research, 26*, 400–406.

Pfefferbaum, A., & Sullivan, E. V. (2002). Microstructural but not macrostructural disruption of white matter in women with chronic alcoholism. *NeuroImage, 15*, 708–718.

Pfefferbaum, A., Sullivan, E. V., Mathalon, D. H., & Lim, K. O. (1997). Frontal lobe volume loss observed with magnetic resonance imaging in older chronic alcoholics. *Alcoholism: Clinical and Experimental Research, 21*, 521–529.

Pfefferbaum, A., Sullivan, E. V., Mathalon, D. H., Shear, P. K., Rosenbloom, M. J., & Lim, K. O. (1995). Longitudinal changes in magnetic resonance imaging brain volumes in abstinent and relapsed alcoholics. *Alcoholism: Clinical and Experimental Research, 19*, 1177–1191.

Phillips, S. C., Harper, C. G., & Kril, J. (1987). A quantitative histological study of the cerebellar vermis in alcoholic patients. *Brain, 110*, 301–314.

Pihl, R. O., Peterson, J. B., & Lau, M. A. (1993). A biosocial model of the alcohol-aggression relationship. *Journal of Studies on Alcohol (Supplement), 11*, 128–139.

Pitkänen, A., Pikkarainen, M., Nurminen, N., & Ylinen, A. (2000). Reciprocal connections between the amygdala and the hippocampus formation, perirhinal cortex, and postrhinal cortex in rat. A review. In H. E. Scharfman, R. Schwarcz, & M. P. Witter (Eds.), *The parahippocampal region: Implications for neurological and psychiatric diseases* (Vol. 911, pp. 369–391). New York: New York Academy of Sciences.

Pohorecky, L. A. (1977). Biphasic action of ethanol. *Biobehavioral Reviews, 1*, 231–240.

Porjesz, B., & Begleiter, H. (1985). Human brain electrophysiology and alcoholism. In R. E. Tarter & D. H. Van Thiel (Eds.), *Alcohol and the brain* (pp. 139–182). New York: Plenum Press.

Porjesz, B., & Begleiter, H. (1996). Effects of alcohol on electrophysiological activity of the brain. In H. Begleiter & B. Kissin (Eds.), *The pharmacology of alcohol and alcohol dependence* (pp. 207–247). New York: Oxford University Press.

Porjesz, B., Rangaswamy, M., Kamarajan, C., Jones, K. A., Padmanabhapillai, A., & Begleiter, H. (2005). The utility of neurophysiological markers in the study of alcoholism. *Clinical Neurophysiology, 116*, 993–1018.

Ratti, M. T., Bo, P., Giardini, A., & Soragna, D. (2002). Chronic alcoholism and the frontal lobe: Which executive functions are impaired? *Acta Neurologica Scandinavica, 105*, 276–281.

Reed, T. E. (1985). The myth of "the average alcohol response". *Alcohol, 2*, 515–519.

Regier, D. A., Farmer, M. E., Rae, D. S., Locke, B. Z., Keith, S. J., Judd, L. L., et al.

(1990). Comorbidity of mental disorders with alcohol and other drug abuse. Results from the Epidemiologic Catchment Area (ECA) study. *Journal of the American Medical Association, 264,* 2511–2518.

Richardson, M. P., Strange, B. A., & Dolan, R. J. (2004). Encoding of emotional memories depends on amygdala and hippocampus and their interactions. *Nature Neuroscience, 7,* 278–285.

Ridderinkhof, K. R., de Vlugt, Y., Bramlage, A., Spaan, M., Elton, M., Snel, J., et al. (2002). Alcohol consumption impairs detection of performance errors in mediofrontal cortex. *Science, 298,* 2209–2211.

Rodriguez Holguin, S., Porjesz, B., Chorlian, D. B., Polich, J., & Begleiter, H. (1999). Visual P3a in male alcoholics and controls. *Alcoholism: Clinical and Experimental Research, 23,* 582–591.

Roebuck, T. M., Mattson, S. N., & Riley, E. P. (1998). A review of the neuroanatomical findings in children with fetal alcohol syndrome or prenatal exposure to alcohol. *Alcoholism: Clinical and Experimental Research, 22,* 339–344.

Rohrbaugh, J. W., Stapleton, J. M., Parasuraman, R., Zubovic, E. A., Frowein, H. W., Varner, J. L., et al. (1987). Dose-related effects of ethanol on visual sustained attention and event-related potentials. *Alcohol, 4,* 293–300.

Rolls, E. T. (2000). Precis of the brain and emotion. *Behavioral and Brain Sciences, 23,* 177–234.

Rourke, S. B., & Løberg, T. (1996). The neurobehavioral correlates of alcoholism. In I. Grant & S. J. Nixon (Eds.), *Neuropsychological assessment of neuropsychiatric disorders* (2nd ed., pp. 423–485). New York: Oxford University Press.

Sah, P., Faber, E. S., Lopez De Armentia, M., & Power, J. (2003). The amygdaloid complex: anatomy and physiology. *Physiological Review, 83,* 803–834.

Schmahmann, J. D. (1997). *The cerebellum and cognition* (Vol. 41). San Diego: Academic Press.

Schmahmann, J. D. (2000). The role of the cerebellum in affect and psychosis. *Journal of Neurolinguistics, 13,* 189–214.

Schuckit, M. A. (2000). Genetics of the risk for alcoholism. *American Journal on Addictions, 9,* 103–112.

Schuckit, M. A., Smith, T. L., & Kalmijn, J. (2004). The search for genes contributing to the low level of response to alcohol: Patterns of findings across studies. *Alcoholism: Clinical and Experimental Research, 28,* 1449–1458.

Seifritz, E., Bilecen, D., Hanggi, D., Haselhorst, R., Radu, E. W., Wetzel, S., et al. (2000). Effect of ethanol on BOLD response to acoustic stimulation: implications for neuropharmacological fMRI. *Psychiatry Research, 99,* 1–13.

Seitz, D., Widmann, U., & Seeger, U. (1999). Localized protein magnetic resonance spectroscopy of the cerebellum in detoxifying alcoholics. *Alcoholism: Clinical and Experimental Research, 23,* 158–163.

Shear, P. K., Jernigan, T. L., & Butters, N. (1994). Volumetric magnetic resonance imaging quantification of longitudinal brain changes in abstinent alcoholics. *Alcoholism: Clinical and Experimental Research, 18,* 172–176.

Simonov, P. V. (1986). *The emotional brain.* New York: Plenum Press.

Smith, M. E., & Halgren, E. (1987). Event-related potentials during lexical decision: effects of repetition, word frequency, pronounceability, and concreteness. *Electroencephalography and Clinical Neurophysiology (Supplement), 40,* 417–421.

Sullivan, E. V. (2000). Neuropsychological vulnerability to alcoholism: Evidence from neuroimaging studies. In A. Noronha, M. Eckardt, & K. Warren (Eds.), *Review of*

NIAAA's neuroscience and behavioral research (Vol. 34, pp. 473–508). Bethesda, MD: NIAAA.

Sullivan, E. V. (2003). Compromised pontocerebellar and cerebellothalamocortical systems: Speculations on their contributions to cognitive and motor impairment in nonamnesic alcoholism. *Alcoholism: Clinical and Experimental Research, 27*, 1409–1419.

Sullivan, E. V., Harding, A. J., Pentney, R., Dlugos, C., Martin, P. R., Parks, M. H., et al. (2003). Disruption of frontocerebellar circuitry and function in alcoholism. *Alcoholism: Clinical and Experimental Research, 27*, 301–309.

Tapert, S. F., Brown, G. G., Kindermann, S. S., Cheung, E. H., Frank, L. R., & Brown, S. A. (2001). fMRI measurement of brain dysfunction in alcohol-dependent young women. *Alcoholism: Clinical and Experimental Research, 21*, 236–245.

Teo, R. K., & Ferguson, D. A. (1986). The acute effects of ethanol on auditory event-related potentials. *Psychopharmacology, 90*, 179–184.

Tracey, I. (2001). Prospects for human pharmacological functional magnetic resonance imaging (phMRI). *Journal of Clinical Pharmacology, 4*, 21S–28S.

Tsuang, M. T., Lyons, M. J., Meyer, J. M., Doyle, T., Eisen, S. A., Goldberg, J., et al. (1998). Co-occurrence of abuse of different drugs in men: the role of drug-specific and shared vulnerabilities. *Archives of General Psychiatry, 55*, 967–972.

Uhl, G. R., & Grow, R. W. (2004). The burden of complex genetics in brain disorders. *Archives of General Psychiatry, 61*, 223–229.

Victor, M. (1992). The effects of alcohol on the nervous system. In C. S. Lieber (Ed.), *Medical and nutritional complications of alcoholism: Mechanisms and management* (pp. 413–457). New York: Plenum Press.

Virkkunen, M., & Linnoila, M. (1993). Brain serotonin, type II alcoholism and impulsive violence. *Journal of studies on Alcohol (Supplement), 11*, 163–169.

Volkow, N. D., Hitzemann, R., Wang, G. J., Fowler, J. S., Burr, G., Pascani, K., et al. (1992). Decreased brain metabolism in neurologically intact healthy alcoholics. *American Journal of Psychiatry, 149*, 1016–1022.

Volkow, N. D., Hitzemann, R., Wang, G. J., Fowler, J. S., Burr, G., Pascani, K., et al. (1995). Monitoring the brain's response to alcohol with positron emission tomography. *Alcohol Health and Research World, 19*, 296–299.

Volkow, N. D., Mullani, N., Gould, L., Adler, S. S., Guynn, R. W., Overall, J. E., et al. (1988). Effects of acute alcohol intoxication on cerebral blood flow measured with PET. *Psychiatry Research, 24*, 201–209.

Wang, G. J., Volkow, N. D., Fowler, J. S., Franceschi, D., Wong, C. T., Pappas, N. R., et al. (2003). Alcohol intoxication induces greater reductions in brain metabolism in male than in female subjects. *Alcoholism: Clinical and Experimental Research, 27*, 909–917.

Wang, G. J., Volkow, N. D., Roque, C. T., Cestaro, V. L., Hitzemann, R. J., Cantos, E. L., et al. (1993). Functional importance of ventricular enlargement and cortical atrophy in healthy subjects and alcoholics as assessed with PET, MR imaging, and neuropsychologic testing. *Radiology, 186*, 59–65.

Wang, L., McCarthy, G., Song, A. W., & LaBar, K. S. (2005). Amygdala activation to sad pictures during high-field (4 tesla) functional magnetic resonance imaging. *Emotion, 5*, 12–22.

Wendt, P. E., & Risberg, J. (2001). Ethanol reduces rCFB activation of left dorsolateral prefrontal cortex during a verbal fluency task. *Brain and Language, 77*, 197–215.

West, J. R., & Pierce, D. R. (1986). Perinatal alcohol exposure and neuronal damage. In J. R. West (Ed.), *Alcohol and brain development* (pp. 120–157). New York: Oxford University Press.

Whalen, P. J., Rauch, S. L., Etcoff, N. L., McInerney, S. C., Lee, M. B., & Jenike, M. A. (1998). Masked presentations of emotional facial expressions modulate amygdala activity without explicit knowledge. *Journal of Neuroscience, 18*, 411–418.

White, A. M., Matthews, D. B., & Best, P. J. (2000). Ethanol, memory, and hippocampal function: A review of recent findings. *Hippocampus, 10*, 88–93.

Wilson, G. T., & Niaura, R. (1984). Alcohol and the disinhibition of sexual responsiveness. *Journal of Studies on Alcohol, 45*, 219–224.

Winston, J. S., O'Doherty, J., & Dolan, R. J. (2003). Common and distinct neural responses during direct and incidental processing of multiple facial emotions. *Neuroimage, 20*, 84–97.

Wise, R. A. (1988). Psychomotor stimulant properties of addictive drugs. *Annals of the New York Academy of Sciences, 537*, 228–234.

Wuethrich, B. (2001). Does alcohol damage female brains more? *Science, 291*, 2077–2079.

3 Benzodiazepines

Simon F. Crowe and Melinda J. Barker

Introduction

Following their introduction in the 1960s, the benzodiazepines quickly became the most widely used of all psychotropic drugs, with over a billion dollars worth sold each year (Lader & Petursson, 1983; Lucki & Rickels, 1986). They are commonly used in the treatment of anxiety, insomnia and panic disorder, and to a lesser extent to treat other conditions, including psychotic states, depression, social phobia, obsessive–compulsive disorder, drug withdrawal, and the side effects induced by antidepressants and neuroleptics (Coleman, 1985; Pollack, 1993). They are also used as anesthetics, muscle relaxants, and antiepileptics (Coleman, 1985).

According to the Drug Utilization Subcommittee of the Commonwealth Department of Health and Ageing, 6.95 million prescriptions for benzodiazepines were dispensed through pharmacies in Australia in 2001 alone (excluding inpatient subscribing: Barker, Jackson, Greenwood, & Crowe, 2003) and, although figures do vary, prevalence rates per capita are reported to be similar in the USA, UK, and Australia (National Health and Medical Research Council, 1991). Epidemiological data from one multinational survey indicate that the overall prevalence of the use of antianxiety agents varies from 7.4% in the Netherlands, 12.9% in the USA, to 17.6% in Belgium (Balter, Mannheimer, Mellinger, & Ulenhuth, 1984). One Australian survey in 1990 found that 22% of 20–39-year-olds had previously used benzodiazepines (Brown, 1995).

More recently, researchers in the Netherlands reported benzodiazepine use in 0.6% in their study of 80,000 general practice patients (Zandstra et al., 2002). Epidemiological data from a number of countries indicate that between 1.6% and 5% of the adult population use benzodiazepines on a long-term basis of one year or more (Balter et al., 1984; Chen, 1990; Mellinger, Balter, & Uhlenhuth, 1984).

Clearly benzodiazepine use is prevalent, yet the long-term consequence of this use has not been comprehensively studied. In this review we will examine a number of aspects of the action of the benzodiazepines, including their pathophysiological mechanisms, consideration of animal models and postmortem findings, the effects of intoxication and withdrawal of these agents both cognitively and psychologically, their residual effects both cognitively and psychologically, and the association between the neuropsychological findings and the imaging data, and we will conclude with a discussion of the effects of the benzodiazepines on driving.

Pathophysiology

A drug's half-life ($t_{1/2}$) refers to the amount of time it takes for the amount of the drug in the body to fall by 50%. The elimination of the drug is usually an exponential process with a constant amount of drug eliminated per unit time (Birkett, 1998). The benzodiazepines can be categorized by their duration of action: ultra-short acting ($t_{1/2}$ <2 hours), short acting ($t_{1/2}$ <6 hours), intermediate acting ($t_{1/2}$ = 6–24 hours) and long acting ($t_{1/2}$ >24 hours: Walls, 2004). The onset of the drug's activity and their duration of action are related to their absorption and uptake in the central nervous system (CNS) and to their metabolism by the liver. Sensitivity to the CNS depressant effects of the benzodiazepines differs widely with age, gender, physical or emotional state, and their use in concert with other drugs, including tobacco and alcohol (American Hospital Formulary Service, 1998).

Each of the benzodiazepines has a similar mode of action and there is little evidence to suggest that one benzodiazepine is superior to another in adequate dosage; however, pharmacokinetic differences between the drugs can be an important consideration in the drug chosen (American Hospital Formulary Service, 1998; Coleman, 1985). There does tend to be a preponderance of application of the different forms of the benzodiazepines, with those prescribed for their anxiolytic action including diazepam, alprazolam, chlordiazepoxide, lorazepam and oxazepam, those for their largely sedative action including nitrazepam, flunitrazepam, flurazepam, loprazolam, temazepam, lormetazepam, and the benzodiazepine-like agents zaleplon, zolpidem, and zopiclone, and those with an anticonvulsant effect including clonazepam.

This classification is however by no means exclusive, with a number of these agents comfortably fitting into each class of activity. For example diazepam, lorazepam, and midazolam each are commonly prescribed for their anxiolytic, hypnotic, and sedative properties (Keltner & Folks, 1997). These differences are mediated by the dose–response relationships between the drug and the individual, with antianxiety effects noted in lower doses, sedative, anticonvulsant, and muscular relaxation effects at moderate doses, and sleep induction and anterograde memory impairment noted at the highest doses.

The differing clinical effects of these drugs is either directly or indirectly mediated by their site of action (Roy-Byrne & Nutt, 1991), and it is proposed that benzodiazepine receptors in the cerebellum mediate their ataxic effects, receptors in the brainstem or cortex mediate their sedative effects, receptors in the forebrain and hippocampus mediate their amnestic effects, and receptors in the hippocampus and other limbic brain regions mediate their anxiolytic effects (Roy-Byrne & Nutt, 1991). Other benzodiazepine binding sites have also been identified in the adrenals, the pituitary, and the pineal gland, which has been suggested to indicate a role for these agents in neuroendocrinological regulation in response to environmental stress (Collomp et al., 1994).

Animal models

Despite their widespread adoption immediately following their introduction in the 1960s, the mechanism of action of the benzodiazepines remained unknown until 1977 (see Haefely, 1978, for a review), when it was discovered that they interacted with a specific binding site in the CNS, the gamma-aminobutyric acid (GABA) receptor complex. The complex was isolated, sequenced, and cloned in 1987 (Schofield et al., 1987), and it was subsequently visualized using electron microscopy in 1994 (Nayeem et al., 1994).

Benzodiazepines and the $GABA_A$ receptor complex

The central binding site for benzodiazepines is located on the supramolecular complex, which acts as the receptor for GABA, the dominant inhibitory neurotransmitter of the CNS. GABA is one of the most widespread neurotransmitters in the brain, released at perhaps 30% of all synapses (Sieghart, 1989), and helps to shape, integrate, and refine the information conveyed by excitatory neurotransmission. GABA tends to act as a "brake" on the brain, with too much transmission causing the individual to become drowsy and sedated, and too little making the individual become anxious and overexcited. The ubiquitous distribution of GABA receptors suggests the possibility of some level of GABAergic involvement in almost every CNS function (Davies, 1996). The overall level of activity in the CNS is mediated by the balance between excitatory inputs (as mediated mostly by the neurotransmitter glutamate) and inhibitory inputs (as mediated by GABA). If the balance between the two swings toward higher levels of GABA then sedation, amnesia, and ataxia ensue. A swing toward a preponderance of glutamate results in arousal, anxiety, restlessness, insomnia, and heightened reactivity (Nutt & Malizia, 2001).

Benzodiazepines occupy a specific binding site on the macromolecular protein complex that forms the GABA receptor (Tallman & Gallagher, 1985). The complex is a structure that spans the cell membrane and is composed of five protein subunits arranged in a rosette around a central pore which acts as a conduit for the transport of chloride and other anions into and out of the cell. There are several distinct receptor subtypes that bind GABA, including the $GABA_A$, $GABA_B$, and $GABA_C$ receptors. The $GABA_A$ receptor is directly linked to a gated chloride ion channel. GABA inhibits the firing of neurons by opening chloride-gated channels on the neuronal membrane. The opening of the channels hyperpolarizes the membrane potential, and consequently a greater depolarization is needed to trigger an action potential once the receptor has been activated (Kandel, 1995). Compounds that block the GABA$_A$ receptor, such as the antagonist bicuculline and the convulsant drug picrotoxin, directly decrease chloride ion flux and thus GABAergic transmission (Braestrup & Squires, 1978).

The GABA$_B$ and GABA$_C$ receptor subclasses are pharmacologically distinct from the GABA$_A$ receptor type and are bicuculline-insensitive (Paredes & Agmo, 1992). The GABA$_B$ receptor has been associated with more than one ionic channel. For example, stimulation of GABA$_B$ receptors in hippocampal pyramidal cells has been shown to increase K^+ current, and in dorsal root ganglion neurons the GABA$_B$ receptor appears to influence neurotransmitter release by inhibiting the calcium component of the action potential (Bormann, 1988). As only the GABA$_A$ receptor contains a binding site for the benzodiazepines, the other two subtypes are not relevant in the present context and will not be discussed further.

Binding of the benzodiazepines to the benzodiazepine–GABA receptor complex facilitates the inhibitory transmission of GABA by augmenting the ability of GABA to depress neuronal excitation (Nelson & Chouinard, 1996). The classical benzodiazepines enhance the effectiveness of the available levels of GABA by altering the conformation of the receptor complex, thereby lowering the concentration of GABA necessary for opening the channel. This increases the frequency of opening of the chloride channel, but does not alter the channel conductance or the duration of opening (Cooper, Bloom, & Roth, 1996).

The benzodiazepine receptor is a unique modulatory site since the type of ligand that binds to the site can either enhance or reduce GABA$_A$ receptor function (Davies, 1996). This action is quite different from other similar types of drugs which act on the GABA receptor, such as the barbiturates, chloral hydrate, chlormethiazole, and ethanol (each of which can both enhance levels of GABA and open the chloride channel). These drugs are thus fatal in overdose (whereas the benzodiazepines rarely are), probably as a result of their direct effect on the chloride channel. The benzodiazepines do not inhibit vital brain centres more than would be observed as a result of the naturally occurring GABA effect, thus reducing morbidity (Nutt & Malizia, 2001).

It has been suggested that an endogenous benzodiazepine may also be involved in neuronal processing, possibly as a result of the brain itself producing an anxiety-reducing compound. Benzodiazepines have been found in the preserved brains of individuals who have passed away long before the development of these drugs (Sangameswaran, Fales, Freidrich, & De Blas, 1986), plants, particularly fungi, have been noted to produce a range of benzodiazepines (Nutt & Malizia, 2001), and endogenous benzodiazepine agonists (endodiazepines) have been found in a rare congenital condition, idiopathic recurrent stupor (Tinuper et al., 1994).

Support for the notion that differences in benzodiazepine receptor affinity underlie the differences in their effect profiles comes from studies of the agent flumazenil (Ro 15-1788), a specific benzodiazepine receptor antagonist. This agent binds to the benzodiazepine site and has the opposite effect of the benzodiazepines, i.e. producing stimulation, anxiogenesis, and inducing convulsions. In human studies flumazenil is reported to block the sedative and psychomotor effects of benzodiazepines, but not their amnesic effects (Curran & Birch, 1991; Hommer, Weingartner, & Breier, 1993; Kirkby, Montgomery, Badcock, & Daniels, 1995). Treatment with flumazenil does not reverse the midazolam- or diazepam-induced amnesic effects on measures of explicit and implicit memory (Curran & Birch, 1991; Hommer et al., 1993). Birch and Miller (1995) for example found that flumazenil reversed the psychomotor effects of midazolam, but did not effectively reverse its amnesic action.

Research has also revealed that there are two subtypes of the central benzodiazepine receptor, BZ_1 and BZ_2 (Squires et al., 1988), which are differentially concentrated within the CNS. Both have similar regional distribution in the cerebellum, cerebral cortex, and substantia nigra, but BZ_2 is more prevalent in the nucleus acumbens, hippocampus, caudate, and putamen (Squires et al., 1988). Traditional benzodiazepines do not exhibit selectivity for these receptor subtypes, but benzodiazepine-like agents such as zolpidem have greater affinity for BZ_1 receptors. While these selective benzodiazepine sites show a different pattern of distribution, they still act via the GABA receptor complex and their distributions do overlap.

While considerable study of the actions of the benzodiazepines in animal models of anxiety has been undertaken, the principal focus of this research has largely surrounded the study of memory functioning (Farkas & Crowe, 2000). Compounds which activate the GABAergic system have been found to either enhance or impair memory on a wide variety of learning tasks in animals. In rats, post-training administration of the $GABA_A$-receptor antagonists bicuculline or picrotoxin enhances retention, while application of the agonist muscimol has been found to impair retention, particularly on aversively motivated tasks (Aranko, Mattila & Seppala, 1983; Balter et al., 1984; Brown, 1995; National Health and Medical Research Council, 1991). Decreasing the level of GABAergic transmission by the administration of bicuculline or flumazenil ameliorates the memory-impairing effects of midazolam (Adler, Angrist & Peselow, 1985; Patterson, 1990), and flumazenil also blocks the effects of diazepam on learning and memory tasks in mice and chicks (Curran, 1992; Farkas & Crowe, 2000). Interestingly, flumazenil blocks the effects of benzodiazepines on memory functioning in animal studies (Adler et al., 1985; Curran, 1992; Patterson, 1990), but does not do so in human studies (Ashton & Golding, 1989; Ciraulo & Sarid-Segal, 1991; Coleman, 1985; Nestoros, Nair, & Pulman, 1983).

One of the crucial issues concerning benzodiazepine-induced memory impairment in animal studies is the degree to which this effect occurs as a consequence of sedation, or whether there is a specific effect of these drugs on the processing of memory *per se*. Unfortunately the animal literature is yet to yield a definitive answer to this question.

Postmortem

Unfortunately little postmortem data regarding the effects of the benzodiazepines is available. This is largely because death from benzodiazepine overdose is actually quite rare in the absence of alcohol and other CNS depressants, with most patients recovering from benzodiazepine overdose quite rapidly (American Hospital Formulary Service, 1998). Pandey and colleagues (Pandey et al., 1997) have noted that postmortem analysis of Brodmann's area 10 in suicide victims indicated that the benzodiazepine receptors were upregulated in the anterior regions of the brains of suicide victims who had died by violent means. This study supports in part the work undertaken with suicide attempters (e.g. Jollant et al., 2005; Oquendo et al., 2003; van Heeringen, 2001), which proposes a connection between lethality, hypometabolism of the basal forebrain, impaired serotonergic activity, and impulsivity as measured by neuropsychological indicators in successful suicide attempters. Some suggestions have also been made that benzodiazepine receptors, as measured postmortem, may be involved in some of the symptoms of chronic schizophrenia (Kiuchi, Kobayashi, Takeuchi, Shimizu, Ogata, & Toru, 1989; Pandey et al., 1997).

Intoxication and withdrawal

It is now well accepted that, even with normal therapeutic doses, benzodiazepines are capable of causing both physiological and pharmacological dependence as evidenced by a withdrawal syndrome following discontinuation of the drug (Ashton, 1986, 1995; Chen, 1990; Lader, 1982). In some cases this can occur as quickly as days or weeks after the commencement of treatment (American Psychiatric Association, 1990; Miller, 1995). Furthermore, the longer the period of drug-taking, the higher the incidence of dependence. Abrupt withdrawal can lead to more severe symptoms, and these may develop and be more severe following long-term use of the shorter-acting benzodiazepines (Chen, 1990). Patients who become dependent upon benzodiazepines commonly display substance-seeking behavior (Ashton, 1995) and may increase their own dose and/or go to numerous doctors to obtain more of the drug, a practice sometimes referred to as "doctor shopping" (National Health and Medical Research Council, 1991). The National Health and Medical Research Council suggests that patients who are presenting for a chronic or ongoing condition are more likely to develop dependence.

Tolerance to the various actions of benzodiazepines does not develop at the same rate (Aranko et al., 1983; Seppala, Palva, Mattila, Korttila, & Shrotriya, 1980). Tolerance to the hypnotic effects of benzodiazepines can develop rapidly within a few weeks of regular treatment, with users no longer experiencing daytime drowsiness after only a few days. Tolerance to the anticonvulsant effects can also occur in a short period of time (less than 6 months), making the benzodiazepines less suitable for the long-term treatment of epilepsy (Ashton, 1995; Chen, 1990). Tolerance to the anxiolytic effects tends to develop more slowly (Ashton 1986, 1995), with some authors suggesting that tolerance to the amnestic effects may not develop at all in long-term users (Curran, 1992; Lucki, Rickels, & Geller, 1986).

If benzodiazepines have been taken regularly for any length of time, and particularly if high doses have been used, they should be discontinued gradually using a tapering approach (Greist, Jefferson, & Marks, 1998). Withdrawal side effects such as insomnia, irritability, anxiety, confusion, seizures, restlessness, lethargy, nausea, depression, agitation, tension, dysphoria, sweating, diarrhea, blurred vision, memory impairment, impaired concentration, ataxia, hallucinations, weight loss, acute psychosis, panic attacks, agoraphobia, flushing, gastrointestinal disturbances, paresthesia and muscle pain have all been reported to occur (American Hospital Formulary Service, 1998; Ashton, 1984; Greist, Jefferson, & Marks, 1998; Schweizer, 1995).

After stopping a short-half-life benzodiazepine, withdrawal symptoms typically begin to appear within 6–12 hours, peak within 2–4 days, and subside in 1–3 weeks (Schweizer, 1995). Withdrawal symptoms from a long-half-life benzodiazepine start within 24–48 hours, peak in 4–7 days and then subside in 2–4 weeks (Schweizer, 1995). Because of the high potential for withdrawal symptoms, patients are advised to consult their doctor before discontinuing benzodiazepine therapy (American Hospital Formulary Service, 1998).

It is suggested that withdrawal symptoms are difficult to distinguish from manifestations of the return of the illness or the so-called "rebound" phenomenon (American Hospital Formulary Service, 1998; American Psychiatric Association, 1990; Gudex, 1991; Roy-Byrne, 1991). Some authors describe a "discontinuance syndrome" in which there are three categories of symptoms – rebound, recurrence, and withdrawal (American Psychiatric Association, 1990; Roy-Byrne, 1991).

Rebound symptoms are a return of the original symptoms which are transient and more intense than those observed before treatment. Recurrence occurs if the cause of the original symptoms was not corrected and therefore the same pattern and intensity of symptoms recurs once the treatment is ceased. This type of discontinuation syndrome is likely when benzodiazepines have only been used for a brief period of time. Withdrawal refers to the development of new signs and symptoms that were not part of the disorder for which the benzodiazepines were originally prescribed (American Psychiatric Association, 1990). These symptoms are thought to be a corrective physiological reaction to the absence of the drug (Roy-Byrne, 1991). Gudex (1991) indicates that the larger and better organized studies focusing on withdrawal symptoms feature an incidence rate of between 40 and 80%. However if the definition is refined to include only new symptoms, then the incidence is closer to 50% (Gudex, 1991). The distinction between rebound and recurrence is a difficult one to make, as clinically they often co-occur, with the common pattern of discontinuance manifesting initially as an immediate worsening of symptoms shortly after the patient stops their benzodiazepine (rebound). The original symptoms then lessen, and after a few days return to the same or lower intensity and then persist (recurrence) (American Psychiatric Association, 1990). Symptoms likely to represent "true" withdrawal (i.e. new symptoms) include depersonalization, derealization, nausea, loss of appetite, depression, increased sensory perception, and abnormal perception or sensation of movement (Roy-Byrne, 1991).

Change in neurotransmitter activity at the receptor site is the most likely cause of withdrawal symptoms. Chronic benzodiazepine treatment has been reported to lead to a GABA downregulation (Ashton, 1989; Hutchinson, Smith, & Darlington, 1996). Abrupt discontinuation may lead to an acute reduction in GABA which leads to a more excited (less inhibited) CNS, resulting in an increase in irritability, myoclonus, seizures, and other symptoms (American Psychiatric Association, 1990).

Discontinuation symptoms can be minimized or even eliminated by using a method of gradual discontinuation (American Hospital Formulary Service, 1998; American Psychiatric Association, 1990; Bailey, Ward, & Musa, 1994; Greist et al., 1998). Some authors support a tapering schedule that reduces by a fixed percentage rather than a fixed amount (Roy-Byrne, 1991). Another method of discontinuation management includes pharmacologic treatment and, although there are limited data from controlled trials, substances that have been suggested to ease discontinuation effects include the beta-blockers, clonidine, and carbamazepine (Roy-Byrne, 1991).

Acute cognitive effects of the benzodiazepines

In examining the literature on short-term cognitive effects of benzodiazepines, it is difficult to compare the results from different studies as different benzodiazepines have been studied at various doses and via various routes of administration, with numerous areas of cognition assessed using a variety of assessment tools. Anterograde amnesia is a commonly noted effect of benzodiazepine treatment (American Psychiatric Association, 1990; Ashton, 1995; Kirkby et al., 1995). The onset and duration of the amnesia vary depending upon the benzodiazepine used, its dose and route of administration (Kirkby et al., 1995), and the type of memory assessment employed (Curran, 1991).

Other cognitive domains commonly affected include verbal fluency (Kirkby et al., 1995), psychomotor speed (Allen, Curran, & Lader, 1991; Curran, Schiwy, & Lader, 1987; Fleishaker, Garzone, Chambers, & Sirocco, 1995; Ghoneim, Mewaldt, & Hinrichs, 1984; Gorissen, Eling, van Luijtelaar, &

Coenen, 1995; Seppala et al., 1980), reaction time (Allen et al., 1991; Ghoneim, Hinrichs, & Mewaldt, 1984), effortful processing (Joyce & File, 1995), coordination and attention (Curran et al., 1987; Hommer et al., 1993; Seppala et al., 1980; Smirne, Ferini Strambi, Pirola, & Tancredi, 1989), working memory (Hommer et al., 1993), recall (Hommer et al., 1993; Joyce & File, 1995), short-term memory (Streufert et al., 1996), immediate memory (Hege, Ellinwood, Wilson, & Helligers, 1997; Smirne et al., 1989), episodic memory (Curran, Gorenstein, & Lader, 1993; Hommer et al., 1993; Mintzer et al., 2001), explicit memory (Stewart, Rioux, Connolly, & Dunphy, 1996), and implicit memory (Fleishaker et al., 1995). The severity of these effects tends to be dose dependent (Hommer, 1991).

Retrieval of information already in memory has been shown to be unaffected by the drug and memory for information that is part of semantic or procedural memory, or information that was acquired just prior to drug administration, is unaffected (Curran, 1991; Curran et al., 1987; Weingartner, Eckardt, Molchan, & Sunderland, 1992). In other words, retrograde amnesia has not been demonstrated to be a short-term effect of benzodiazepine use.

As noted with the animal literature, the cause of the memory effects has been argued by some to be linked to the sedative properties of the drug, while others have argued that the effects of these drugs on memory are due to their direct effects on the neurobiological systems that are involved in memory consolidation (Weingartner et al., 1992). What is clear, however, is that patients being prescribed a benzodiazepine should be warned about the possible effects on memory (American Hospital Formulary Service, 1998) as well as the possibility of impaired ability to perform activities requiring mental alertness or physical coordination, such as driving a car, when under the influence of the drug (American Psychiatric Association, 1990; Chen, 1990).

Acute psychological and other effects of the benzodiazepines

Apart from their well-documented effectiveness in the treatment of anxiety, insomnia, and panic disorder, the efficacy of benzodiazepines has been demonstrated with regard to the treatment of numerous other conditions, including psychotic states (Pollack, 1993), schizophrenia (Nestoros et al., 1983), obsessive–compulsive disorder (OCD: Insel & Murphy, 1981), catatonia (Salam, Pillai, & Beresford, 1987), social phobia (Munjack, Baltazar, & Bohn, 1990; Reiter, Pollack, & Rosenbaum, 1990), complex partial seizures (Pollack, 1993), withdrawal syndromes (Patterson, 1990), akathisia (Adler et al., 1985), tardive dyskinesia (Pollack, 1993), myoclonus (Garvey & Tollefson, 1987), and early tricyclic syndrome (Pollack, 1993). Benzodiazepines have also been used in the management of acute alcohol withdrawal (American Hospital Formulary Service, 1998; National Health and Medical Research Council, 1991), as well as during surgery, both preoperatively and as anesthetics or sedatives in producing anterograde amnesia during minor surgeries (National Health and Medical Research Council, 1991; Pollack, 1993), including gastroscopy and dental procedures. This latter action of the benzodiazepines has seen them also employed as "date rape" drugs as they have the benefit for the perpetrator of causing amnesia, disinhibition, and sedation of the victim, rendering subsequent testimony, if it is advanced, subject to significant scrutiny by the courts. In combination with other medications, benzodiazepines have also been used to treat nausea and vomiting associated with cancer chemotherapy and to relieve agitation in the management of neonatal opiate withdrawal (Pollack, 1993).

The literature reveals that there are several distinct populations that use benzodiazepines (American Psychiatric Association, 1990; Coffey, 1993; Schweizer, 1995). These include older patients with a high prevalence of medical, depressive, and psychotic states, patients with chronic anxiety and dysphoric symptoms, patients suffering panic disorder, patients with psychiatric illnesses, individuals who abuse illicit drugs and use benzodiazepines in combination with these other drugs, individuals with epilepsy, and children with anxiety conditions.

The number of known side effects of benzodiazepines is extensive. Most of the side effects already discussed are common to most types of benzodiazepines, with a proportion of side effects reported to occur only with a specific type of benzodiazepine therapy. The main adverse CNS effects are often an extension of the pharmacological activity of the drug. These include drowsiness, ataxia, fatigue, confusion, weakness, drowsiness, and vertigo (Bourin, du Tertre, & Payeur, 1993; Vgontzas, Kales, & Bixler, 1995). The major determinants of the frequency and severity of side effects include the drug's elimination half-life, receptor binding affinity, effects on the hypothalamic-pituitary-adrenal axis, as well as the interaction of these various factors (Vgontzas et al., 1995).

Other side effects reported to occur with benzodiazepine therapy include bizarre or abnormal behavior, agitation, visual and auditory hallucinations, paranoid ideation, panic, delirium, depression, sleepwalking, aggression, headache, vivid dreams, dysarthria, hiccups, nausea, gastrointestinal complaints, constipation, increased appetite, anorexia, weight gain or loss, dryness of the mouth, increased salivation, swollen tongue, bitter or metallic taste, increased or decreased libido, menstrual irregularities, failure to ovulate, genitourinary complaints, visual disturbances, joint pain, muscle cramps, palpitations, tachycardia, shortness of breath, and flushing (American Hospital Formulary Service, 1998; American Psychiatric Association, 1990; Griest et al., 1998). Although the list of side effects is long, it is relatively unlikely that the serious side effects will occur. Moreover, the mild side effects typically subside within the first few days of treatment (American Hospital Formulary Service, 1998).

Paradoxical CNS stimulation has been reported and tends to occur early in benzodiazepine therapy. The symptoms include talkativeness, restlessness, anxiety, mania, euphoria, sleep disturbance, nightmares, excitement, hyperactivity, and acute rage reactions. These paradoxical effects occur more frequently in psychiatric patients and hyperactive children and it is recommended that benzodiazepine therapy be ceased if these signs emerge (American Hospital Formulary Service, 1998). These authors also report an increase in suicidal ideation in previously depressed patients.

When taken during pregnancy, benzodiazepines are considered to be teratogenic. The results of retrospective studies suggest an increased risk of congenital malformations in babies whose mothers took a benzodiazepine during the first trimester of the pregnancy (American Hospital Formulary Service, 1998; Coleman, 1985). Babies of mothers who took diazepam during the pregnancy have been reported to experience withdrawal symptoms such as tremors, hypertonicity, irritability, and hyperactivity (Auerbach, Hans, Marcus, & Maeir, 1992), as well as an increased rate of oral cleft, dysmorphism, and CNS dysfunction (American Psychiatric Association, 1990). Because some of the mothers studied may have also been taking other illicit drugs, including alcohol and cocaine, it has been argued that there is in fact no increased risk of congenital malformation in babies who have only been exposed to benzodiazepine during development (Cohen & Rosenbaum, 1987). Other possible effects of benzodiazepines include prolonged CNS depression in neonates (American Hospital Formulary Service, 1998), changes in female breast tissue due to the effect on endocrine activity, including release of the hormone prolactin (Gudex, 1991), and changes in metabolism during submaximal exercise that does not influence performance (Collomp et al., 1994).

Residual effects

Although the benzodiazepines were initially thought to be quite safe, reports began to emerge as early as 1963 regarding the potential for addiction, abuse, and withdrawal difficulties related to the use of Librium, one of the first marketed benzodiazepines. The World Health Organization (WHO) reported in 1964 that Librium was addictive. In 1982/83, the WHO requested that the United Nations Commission on Narcotic Drugs (UNCND) limit the availability of benzodiazepines by classifying them as a "scheduled" drug. This effort was thwarted by heavy lobbying from the pharmaceutical companies (UNCND, 1984).

More recently, attitudes toward these drugs have changed in parallel with a growing concern, and the subsequent development of a body of literature, regarding dependence, withdrawal, and their long-term harmful effects. The National Health and Medical Research Council of Australia, for example, now recommends that the use of benzodiazepines is best avoided, but if necessary they should be prescribed for the shortest period of time at the lowest possible dose (National Health and Medical Research Council, 1991). In 1990 the American Psychiatric Association convened a task force to review the available information on benzodiazepines and concluded, ". . . concern is justified regarding their appropriate therapeutic use, toxicity, abuse, and risk of inducing a drug dependent state" (American Psychiatric Association, 1990, p. 55)

Estimates from surveys of different countries have indicated that between 1.6% and 5% of the adult population use benzodiazepines on a long-term basis of one year or more (Balter et al., 1984; Chen, 1990; Mellinger et al., 1984). Long-term users comprised approximately 37% of all users in an Australian survey (Lyndon & Russell, 1988). This figure is similar to the level of 31% reported in the UK (Ashton & Golding, 1989).

Many surveys of long-term benzodiazepine users in general practice settings have been conducted. The surveys characterize these patients as typically older (Simpson et al., 1990) and who take these drugs in normal doses (Hawley, Tattersall, Dellaportas, & Hallstrom, 1994), or as mainly older and female with high levels of emotional stress (Chen, 1990; Lader, 1984; Mellinger et al., 1984; Rodrigo, King, & Williams, 1988; Salinsky & Dore, 1987). Among the population of chronic benzodiazepines users, females consistently outnumber males with ratios varying from 1.6:1 to 4:1 (Ashton, 1995; Mellinger et al., 1984; Rodrigo et al., 1988; Salinsky & Dore, 1987; Simpson et al., 1990). Somewhat different characteristics were found in one comparison of long-term users in two settings in the UK which described those attending discontinuation trials as predominantly young married women taking moderate doses of anxiolytics, and those referred to hospital clinics with a high rate of psychiatric comorbidity (Hawley et al., 1994).

From the many population studies conducted, two opposing views regarding long-term use have emerged in the literature. Some reviewers conclude that benzodiazepine overuse has been exaggerated (Ciraulo & Sarid-Segal, 1991; Ulenhuth, 1988) and that most actual use of benzodiazepine is appropriate (Hollister, Conley, Britt, & Shuer, 1981; Romach et al., 1991; Woods, Katz, & Winger, 1992) or at least not widely abused (American Psychiatric Association, 1990). Others argue that this is simply not the case (Griffiths, 1995). According to Romach et al (1991), both views are supported by results from the respective studies of the differing user populations. It thus seems likely that studies of polydrug users, as compared to surveys of those who take these drugs in a supervised manner for anxiety or insomnia, would yield quite different results.

Residual cognitive effects of the benzodiazepines

As can clearly be noted from qualitative reviews of the literature on the acute and chronic cognitive effects of the benzodiazepines (see Barker et al., 2003; Stewart, 2005), the results are often inconsistent, contradictory, and difficult to interpret. This literature has been considered difficult to integrate due to the variety of study designs and methodologies used, the variety of tests employed, and the nature of the subject samples used, including their level of chronicity, their current treatment status, and the appropriate selection of comparison controls. Statistical meta-analysis has proven to be a powerful tool for amalgamating the results of conflicting studies in controversial areas such as this. By using meta-analytic techniques, a comprehensive analysis of all of the existing positive and negative findings can be performed, resulting in a succinct synthesis of findings across the literature (Durlak, 1995).

Our group has undertaken a number of meta-analyses of this literature: see Barker, Greenwood, Jackson and Crowe (2004a, 2004b) for a complete account of these findings, including the methods, selection criteria, and the papers analyzed.

The cognitive effects of long-term benzodiazepine use

In our first meta-analysis on this literature (Barker et al., 2004a), a total of 13 research studies that employed neuropsychological tests to evaluate cognitive performance after long-term use of benzodiazepine medication met the strict inclusion criteria. The neuropsychological tests employed in the studies were each categorized as measuring one of 12 cognitive domains. The effect sizes were calculated following the method established by Rosenthal (1991) using Cohen's d as the effect size index. The effect size represents the difference between the patient and the control group divided by the pooled standard deviation. Therefore, a negative effect size indicates that the patients are performing worse than the controls on assessment. Nine of the studies specified when the testing was carried out relative to the time since last dose. In five of the studies, testing took place at least one day since the last dose. In the remaining four, the testing took place either just prior to the normal daily dose or not within four hours of the normal daily dose. In those studies that examined the effect of the normal daily dose, the predose data were used in the meta-analysis.

The results of the study (see Figure 3.1) demonstrated that long-term benzodiazepine users performed consistently worse than controls across all cognitive categories examined, including sensory processing, psychomotor speed, nonverbal memory, visuospatial awareness, speed of processing, problem-solving, attention/concentration, verbal memory, general intelligence, motor control/performance, working memory, and verbal reasoning. Of the 95 effect sizes obtained from the 13 studies analyzed, the mean weighted effect size was −0.74 with a standard deviation of 0.25 (median = −0.68, range −1.30 to −0.42). It is clear from Figure 3.1 that the 95% confidence intervals do not span zero, indicating that all of the effects were significant and different from zero. According to Cohen (1988) effect sizes of $d = 0.20$, 0.50, and 0.80 are considered small, medium, and large in magnitude, respectively. Based on this taxonomy, these data demonstrate that moderate to large effect sizes were found across all categories of cognition surveyed following long-term benzodiazepine use.

Most investigations of the effects of long-term use of benzodiazepines undertaken to date tend to focus on only one or two specific areas of cognition. However, integrating all of the available evidence together using the

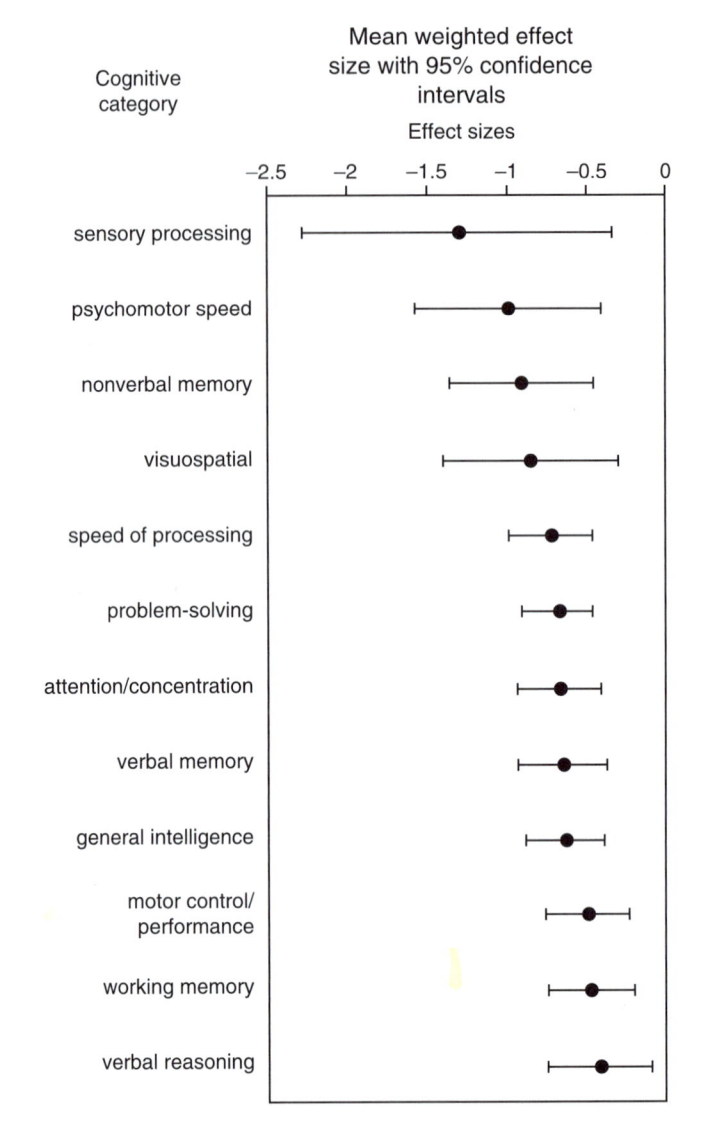

Figure 3.1 Weighted mean effect sizes and 95% confidence intervals for the performance of patients who were taking benzodiazepines on various tests of cognitive functioning. A negative effect size indicates that patients performed worse than controls. (From Barker et al., 2004a.)

meta-analytic technique indicates that it is the case that long-term benzodiazepine users are affected in a generalized, rather than a specific, manner with some areas being more affected than others.

Following on from the results of this meta-analysis we addressed two additional questions (Barker et al., 2004b): Does the cognitive function of long-term benzodiazepine users improve following withdrawal? and Are previous long-term benzodiazepine users still impaired at follow-up compared to controls or normative data?

Does the cognitive function of long-term benzodiazepine users improve following withdrawal?

For inclusion in the additional meta-analyses, studies needed to have conducted long-term follow-up assessments after the benzodiazepines had been discontinued. This occurred in 10 of the 13 independent studies analyzed previously. Effect sizes addressing the first question regarding improvement represent the difference between the patient group at initial assessment and their performance at follow-up assessment. Therefore, a positive effect size indicates improvement of function. The effect sizes addressing the second question regarding persistence of deficit after discontinuation represent the difference between the patients at follow-up assessment and controls at follow-up assessment or normative data. Therefore, a negative effect size represented poorer performance of long-term benzodiazepine users compared to controls or normative data.

From the 10 studies covering 12 categories (a maximum of 120 possible effect sizes), 44 effect sizes were obtained. The mean weighted effect size was 0.41 (median = 0.37) with a standard deviation of 0.22. When compared to their initial assessment, previous long-term benzodiazepine users appeared to improve across all of the cognitive domains examined at the follow-up assessment. All of the effect sizes were positive and ranged in magnitude from 0.06 to 0.70. It is clear from Figure 3.2 that the 95% confidence intervals do not span zero for five of the 11 effect sizes and therefore that these effects are significant and different from zero (it was not possible to calculate effect sizes for all 12 categories as only one test within the problem-solving category was used), indicating that the categories of visuospatial, attention/concentration, general intelligence, psychomotor speed, and nonverbal memory improved significantly for the benzodiazepine users when they discontinued.

Are previous long-term benzodiazepine users still impaired at follow-up compared to controls or normative data?

In this meta-analysis examining nine studies covering 12 categories (a maximum of 108 possible effect sizes: Barker et al., 2004b), 37 effect sizes were obtained. The mean weighted effect size was −0.48 (median = 0.48) with a standard deviation of 0.45. When compared to controls or norms, previous long-term benzodiazepine users performed more poorly across all cognitive categories, except sensory processing, when examined at follow-up assessment. Effect sizes ranged in magnitude from −1.50 to 0.26. It is clear from Figure 3.3 that the 95% confidence intervals do not span zero for eight of the 11 effect sizes (i.e. verbal memory, psychomotor speed, speed of processing, motor control/performance, visuospatial awareness, general intelligence,

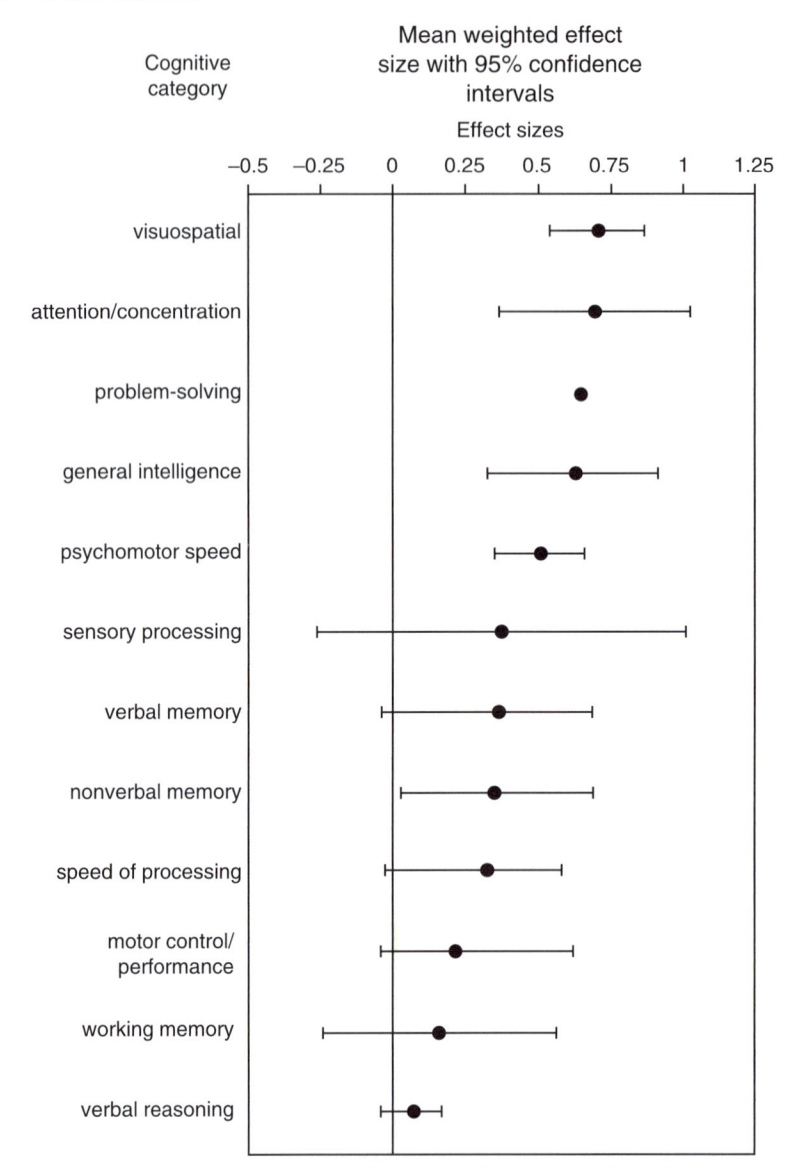

Figure 3.2 Weighted mean effect sizes and 95% confidence intervals for the performance of patients who had withdrawn from long-term benzodiazepine use. A positive effect size indicates that the previous benzodiazepine users improved on tests of various cognitive function at follow-up assessment. (From Barker et al., 2004b.)

attention/concentration, and nonverbal memory) and therefore that most of these effects are significant and different from zero (it was not possible to calculate effect sizes for all 12 categories as only one test within the problem-solving category was used).

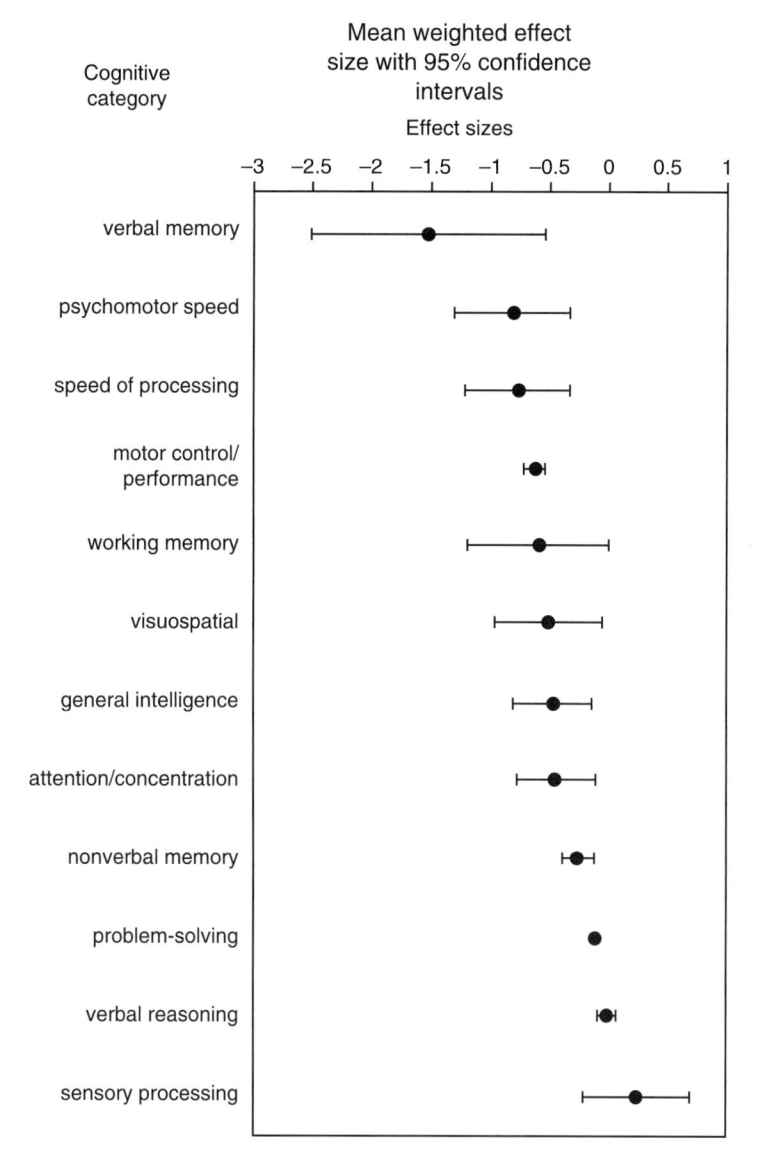

Figure 3.3 Weighted mean effect sizes and 95% confidence intervals for the performance of patients who had withdrawn from long-term benzodiazepine use on tests of various cognitive functions. A negative effect size indicates that the previous benzodiazepine users performed worse than controls or normative data. (From Barker et al., 2004b.)

The results of this meta-analysis indicate that, compared to controls or norms, previous long-term benzodiazepine users performed more poorly across all cognitive categories, except sensory processing, when examined at follow-up assessment. Effect sizes ranged in magnitude from −1.50 to 0.26.

The effect sizes found in this meta-analysis were substantial across most domains and many of the 95% confidence intervals did not span zero.

The results of the three meta-analyses reported here support extreme caution in the use of long-term benzodiazepine therapy. Although these findings suggest that previous long-term benzodiazepine use may lead to impairments in cognition, some degree of improvement in cognitive function after withdrawal is observed, suggesting that previous benzodiazepine users are likely to experience the benefit of improved cognitive functioning after withdrawal. However, the data do not support a full recovery, at least in the first six months following cessation and suggest that there may be some permanent deficits or deficits that take periods longer than six months to completely recover.

Methodological issues in studying long-term effects of withdrawal of the benzodiazepines

A number of methodological issues arise in consideration of the attempt to determine what the long-term effects of benzodiazepine use are. These include the fact that repeated-dose studies are too few in number to allow the drawing of any consistent conclusion due to their differences in the benzodiazepine used, the dose, and the cognitive measures employed (Golombok, Moodley, & Lader, 1988; Tata, Rollings, Collins, Pickering, & Jacobson, 1994). The between-subject design of many longitudinal studies introduces increased error variance and requires that a greater drug effect must be present for the observed differences to be significant (Golombok et al., 1988). Also, most withdrawal studies tend to be retrospective and cross-sectional and involve individualized medication regimes (Tata et al., 1994). Long-term studies should take into consideration factors such as time since last dose in order to separate the acute and chronic effects observed in long-term users, the schedule of drug use, the type of benzodiazepine used, and its half-life (Lucki & Rickels, 1986). Heterogeneity of samples with regard to psychiatric diagnoses, use of alcohol and other drugs, range of dosage, and an overinclusive definition of what is termed chronic use have all been cited as problematic issues in these studies (Gorenstein, Bernik, & Pompeia, 1994).

In a paper discussing further research into the effects of chronic benzodiazepine use, Tansella (1980) makes a number of suggestions with regard to issues of research methodology. Firstly, the most suitable subjects to study are suggested to be chronically anxious subjects who feature high trait anxiety rather than patients with high state anxiety or patients with low trait anxiety. Since there is no evidence of superiority of one benzodiazepine over another, the choice of which benzodiazepine to study should be based on prevalence of use and economics of the drug. Due to individual differences, it is likely to be more convenient to use a flexible dosage scheme rather than a fixed one. The use of placebo or a comparison medication is not practical in this area of research, and patients should be required to act as their own controls and be assessed before, during, and after withdrawal from benzodiazepine therapy. The author argues that a trial length of 6–8 weeks should be sufficiently long, thus limiting the number of patients dropping out, and the follow-up period should be at least two weeks.

While many of the above suggestions are worthwhile, a trial length of 6–8 weeks is not sufficient to be considered "long-term," and the follow-up period is too short to allow for any possible recovery. Because it is not ethical to place patients on benzodiazepines for an extended period of time, the most useful data are therefore likely to arise from between-patient studies of long-term users of more than two years, before and after withdrawal, and then followed up at least two years later to assess the persistence of any deficits. Unfortunately, valuable baseline data obtained before commencing benzodiazepines would not be available. Long-term users should be compared to both normal and anxious controls matched for age, sex, and education to account for the possible effects of anxiety on test performance as well as practice effects on the instruments used. Patients should be assessed at various intervals with a variety of well-standardized cognitive assessment tools that cover all the cognitive areas previously implicated in the literature. Conducting large-scale studies examining many areas of cognition is an unlikely scenario and therefore a series of smaller, methodologically sound studies, which comprehensively investigate a small number of cognitive domains, is a more feasible possibility. Provided that these data were presented in a manner amenable to meta-analyses, a thorough systematic and statistical evaluation of this area could then follow.

In the context of these methodological issues and the results of the meta-analyses noted above, we conducted an empirical evaluation of the functioning of previous long-term benzodiazepine users (Barker, Greenwood, Jackson, & Crowe, 2005). Five of the cognitive areas identified in the follow-up meta-analysis as having moderate to large effect sizes were chosen for further assessment. These were attention/concentration, motor control/performance, nonverbal memory, verbal memory, and visuospatial skills. The study was designed to overcome some of the methodological criticisms made of previous research. Twenty previous long-term benzodiazepine users of more than one year's duration, who had remained abstinent for over six months, were each matched closely to two controls (with and without anxiety) for age, sex, and education. General exclusion criteria were: heavy alcohol or drug use; head injury; stroke; or current antidepressant medication use.

The results of this study indicate that previous long-term benzodiazepine users, assessed after at least six months of abstinence, continued to display cognitive deficits in a number of areas, as compared to matched controls. Significant, moderate to large effect sizes were observed in the areas of verbal memory, motor control/performance and nonverbal memory when comparing the previous benzodiazepine users and the normal controls. Significant differences were also found on these measures between previous benzodiazepine users and the anxious control group.

The observation that the anxious control group and the normal control group performed similarly on most measures and significantly better than the previous benzodiazepine users implicates long-term benzodiazepine use as the most plausible explanation for the difference. On only one measure, the Milner Maze (nonverbal memory), did the anxious control group and normal control group differ. In addition, there was no difference between the previous benzodiazepine users and the anxious control group, indicating that elevated anxiety levels may have impacted negatively on performance for this measure.

The results of this study provide additional support for the hypothesis that long-term benzodiazepine use impacts negatively on cognitive functioning in a number of areas. Given that the length of abstinence from benzodiazepines in this study was between 1 and 29 years, the persisting cognitive effects observed indicate that the impairments may also be permanent. These findings have important implications for those considering taking benzodiazepine medication, as well as those considering prescribing these drugs. Informed decisions regarding this therapy should be made only after considering the potential long-term impact in conjunction with the proposed treatment benefits.

The absence of previous meta-analyses or very large-scale studies in this area has precluded consideration of the notion that long-term benzodiazepine use may produce a generalized negative effect on cognitive function. The focus on the impact of these drugs has historically been specific to particular categories of cognitive functioning, thus the possibility that there may be a generalized effect from long-term benzodiazepine has not been adequately evaluated. One possible explanation for this finding may be that the sedative effect of benzodiazepines, over a long period of time, has a lasting negative impact on basic arousal functions such as alertness, information processing speed, attention, and concentration. The impact of reduced performance in these areas may then manifest as poorer performance on a number of cognitive measures, resulting in the appearance of a generalized deficit (Golombok, 1989; Golombok et al., 1988; Sakol & Power, 1988).

Alternatively, it may be that higher-order functions, which tend to be more sensitive or susceptible to brain impairment, are specifically affected after long-term benzodiazepine use. As a result, measures that involve the integration, organization, or simultaneous processing of information would again be affected, leading to the generalized picture observed (Golombok et al., 1988).

Taken together, the results of this series of studies provide strong support for the hypothesis that long-term benzodiazepine use does lead to cognitive deficits. While the results of the meta-analyses do indicate that long-term benzodiazepine users show recovery of function in many areas after withdrawal, there remains a significant impairment in most areas of cognition in comparison to controls or normative data after discontinuation. The findings highlight the problems associated with long-term benzodiazepine therapy and suggest that previous benzodiazepine users are likely to experience improved cognitive functioning after withdrawal. However, the reviewed data did not support full restitution of function, at least in the first six months following cessation, and suggest that there may be some permanent deficits or deficits that take longer than six months to completely recover following withdrawal, if they recover at all.

Residual emotional effects of the benzodiazepines

The implications of these data for the informed and responsible prescription of benzodiazepines are numerous. Most importantly, patients and clinicians should be aware that both physiological and pharmacological dependence can develop rapidly with these drugs (American Psychiatric Association, 1990; Miller, 1995). Abrupt withdrawal can lead to more severe symptoms (Chen, 1990), and as a result patients may opt to continue benzodiazepine therapy to avoid withdrawal or rebound symptoms and risk possible long-term, irreversible cognitive impairments. The cognitive impairments implicated in benzodiazepines use may have serious consequences for the patient's ability to function optimally in daily life (Curran et al., 1994), and may extend into impairment of the skills necessary for safe driving or efficient functioning in the workplace (Lucki & Rickels, 1986; Unützer et al., 2001).

Although it may not be possible to determine a length of time for benzodiazepine therapy that is safe, it appears that a low dose over a short time has less effect, whereas a high dose for prolonged periods is more likely to be harmful (Golombok et al., 1988). Others have suggested that even at low therapeutic doses, long-term users of benzodiazepines display cognitive deficits that persist for weeks (Petursson, Gudjonsson, & Lader, 1983) or months after discontinuation (Gorenstein, Bernik, Pompeia, & Marcourakis, 1995). Closely monitored use of benzodiazepines may be a very effective treatment of acute anxiety states in the short term, however the risk of cognitive compromise as a result of long-term benzodiazepine therapy is not insubstantial.

Association between the neuropsychological and clinical profile and neuroimaging data

The data arising from computerized tomography (CT) studies undertaken with individuals who feature chronic benzodiazepine use yield contrasting results. Significantly higher mean ventricle-to-brain ratios were noted in 17 high- and low-dose benzodiazepine-dependent patients compared to matched controls. Furthermore, a dose-dependent effect of benzodiazepines on ventricular dilatation was observed (Schmauss & Krieg, 1987). Bergman, Borg, Engelbrektson, and Vikander (1989) found an increased prevalence of ventricular dilatation, most pronounced in the third ventricle, which they concluded indicated atrophy of the central parts of the brain. However the authors of this study urge caution in the interpretation of this result, as an earlier investigation undertaken by their group with a larger sample of participants did not show such a difference between the patient and control groups (Allgulander, Borg, & Vikander, 1984).

Mean ventricle : brain ratio was found to be increased in a group of 20 long-term benzodiazepine users when compared to matched controls, but was less severe than that seen in a group of alcoholic patients (Lader, Ron, & Petursson, 1984). No evidence of a relationship between CT scan appearances and the duration of benzodiazepine use was noted. In a subsequent study, some marginal abnormalities in CT scan appearance were reported in chronic benzodiazepine users when compared to control subjects, however no overall differences were found in relation to ventricle : brain ratios (Moodley, Golombok, Shine, & Lader, 1993).

Poser, Poser, Roscher, and Argyrakis (1983) report evidence of cerebral atrophy only in patients with a history of either alcohol or combined alcohol and benzodiazepine abuse but no significant difference was evident between controls and a group of benzodiazepine patients without a history of alcohol use. These authors conclude that isolated abuse of benzodiazepine is not associated with cerebral atrophy. Subsequent investigations of CT brain scans in long-term benzodiazepine users have similarly concluded that there is no association between long-term benzodiazepine use and brain abnormalities (Busto, Bremner, Knight, terBrugge, & Sellers, 2000; Perera, Powell, & Jenner, 1987). Although the greater resolution provided by magnetic resonance imaging (MRI) would allow better identification of areas affected by benzodiazepine use if these changes did actually exist, no such study was able to be located in a comprehensive search of the current literature.

Positron emission tomography (PET) studies have demonstrated a global decrease in brain activity following benzodiazepine administration (Bagary et al., 2000; Forster, Juge, & Morel, 1982), with some studies suggesting regional differences in blood flow, particularly in the right hemisphere, most notably of the frontal lobe (Matthew, Wilson, & Daniel, 1985). Veselis and colleagues (1997) found decreased cerebral blood flow in the insula, the cingulate gyrus, multiple areas of the prefrontal cortex, the thalamus, and the parietal and temporal association areas. The authors concluded that these dose-related changes on blood flow occur in regions associated with arousal, attention, and memory. A number of other studies have demonstrated similar reductions in cerebral blood flow to regions of the brain, including the left dorsolateral prefrontal cortex, bilateral orbitofrontal cortex, left middle temporal gyrus and right hippocampus (Reinsel et al., 2000), the basal forebrain and amygdaloid complexes (Kajimura et al., 2004), the anterior cingulate cortex, cerebellum, and precuneus (Mintzer et al., 2001), and the prefrontal, superior temporal, and parieto-occipital regions (Bagary et al., 2000).

In a study measuring regional cerebral blood flow during non-REM sleep, Kajimura and colleagues (2004) noted that blood flow to the basal forebrain and amygdaloid complex was decreased during non-REM sleep in the participants given benzodiazepines. The authors considered that this hypnotic effect may be due to deactivation of the control of wakefulness mediated by the forebrain and that the anxiolytic effect could be caused by a deactivation of the emotional centre.

Studies conducted in individuals featuring a variety of anxiety-related conditions indicate some interesting aspects of the mechanism of these agents. In the study conducted by Malizia and colleagues (Malizia, Cunningham, Bell, Liddle, Jones, & Nutt, 1998), radioactively labeled flumazenil (i.e. the receptor antagonist) was used to map $GABA_A$–benzodiazepine receptor binding. They noted that there was a significant overall reduction in flumazenil binding in patients with panic disorder relative to controls. Previous study using this technique has indicated that patients with panic disorder given an intravenous dose of 2 mg of flumazenil (a dose which has been demonstrated to occupy more than half of the receptors in the brain) provoked panic in most of the patients but not in the control participants (Nutt, Glue, Lawson, & Wilson, 1990).

Similar results were noted using a radioactively labeled compound related to flumazenil, iomazenil, using single positron emission tomography (SPECT: see Malizia, 1999), which indicated a similar decrease in binding in the patients diagnosed with panic disorder as compared to controls. Tiihonen and colleagues (1997) noted a localized reduction in benzodiazepine binding in the temporal lobe of patients with the diagnosis of generalized anxiety disorder.

These findings led Nutt and Malizia (2001) to speculate, "These findings are consistent with the idea that some anxiety disorders may be due to defective neuroinhibitory processes. The greatest decreases observed in benzodiazepine binding occurred in areas thought to be involved in the experience of anxiety in man, such as the orbitofrontal and temporal cortex and insula" (Nutt & Malizia, 2001, p. 392). This result was also supported by their PET study finding using an anxiety induction, in which they noted that the anxiolytic effects of the benzodiazepines were closely related to their ability to modulate brain metabolism in the insula and ventromedial prefrontal cortex, along with other locations (Malizia, 2000).

Benzodiazepines and driving

Given the deleterious and global effects of benzodiazepines on cognition, it seems reasonable to be concerned regarding the capability of users to complete various activities of daily living, most notably the capacity to drive an automobile or to operate heavy machinery. Consistent evidence has emerged from the literature that patients taking benzodiazepines have an increased risk of being involved in road traffic accidents (Barbone et al., 1998; Verster, Veldhuijzen, & Volkerts, 2004).

The important aspects of the agents which impact upon their influence on driving surround four important factors: the benzodiazepine used; the dose, temporal aspects of drug administration, and demographic factors with regard to the person operating the vehicle.

The effects of the benzodiazepines on unimpaired healthy control participants indicate that these agents do indeed impact upon the behavioral skills involved in driving. The greatest effects are noted with those tasks that require higher-level cognitive functioning, such as executive functioning, with simple perceptual-type tasks being the least affected of all (de Visser et al., 2003). The most significant cognitive and emotional effects of these agents, in order of severity, are: sedation and impairment of fine motor performance, memory impairment, and disinhibition.

A particularly concerning aspect of the laboratory simulation experiments with the benzodiazepines is that the effects in the laboratory are not easily extrapolated to real-world driving situations. More ecologically valid studies which use real-world driving assessment, however, have also demonstrated that the hypnotic benzodiazepines produce next-day sedative effects and can impair driving for up to 17 hours after bedtime administration (Verster et al., 2004). Other benzodiazepine agents produced significant driving impairment in the morning sessions only.

The impairment of motor performance noted with these agents has been numerously reported in the literature (Allen et al., 1991; Curran et al., 1987; Fleishaker et al., 1995; Ghoneim, Mewaldt, & Hinrichs, 1984; Gorissen et al., 1995; Seppala et al., 1980). This includes significant effects upon driving, engaging in dangerous physical activities, and in the use of hazardous machinery (American Psychiatric Association 1990; Chen 1990; Woods et al., 1992). These effects are most pronounced in the initial phases of treatment.

As noted above (Curran 1992; Lucki et al., 1986), the effects of the benzodiazepines with regard to memory impairment (a desirable aspect of their action in surgical procedures) indicate that these are dose related and there does not seem to be much by way of development of tolerance. These memory effect are most commonly encountered with the rapid-onset compounds.

The disinhibitory effect of these agents is particularly concerning in those individuals with risk factors for externalizing behaviors, including individuals with histories of aggression, impulsivity, and the borderline and antisocial personality disorders (Walls, 2004), and it is easy to speculate that as a result of the combined drug–individual interaction these individuals may be more prone to express these behaviors in the context of the stresses associated with driving, possibly culminating in acts of "road rage." MacDonald, Wells, Giesbrecht, and Cherpitel (1999), for example, have noted that individuals who had suffered violent as opposed to accidental injuries were significantly more likely to test positive for benzodiazepines although not nearly so many as tested positive for alcohol.

Another interesting aspect of the benzodiazepines is that they may on occasions elicit paradoxical effects. These might include agitation, restlessness, increased aggression, and behaviors out of character for the individual. These paradoxical effects tend to be more common with flunitrazepam, clonazepam, alprazolam, and midazolam and tend to occur more commonly when the agents are applied in higher than usual doses (but still within therapeutic ranges), in abusers of benzodiazepines, and particularly if they are used in concert with other CNS depressants such as alcohol (Walls, 2004).

Risk studies undertaken with these agents show that benzodiazepine users had a fivefold increase in risk of hospital admission in comparison to non-using controls (Skegg, Richards, & Doll, 1979). Barbone and colleagues (1998) used a record-linkage database to examine the association of prescription between psychotropic drugs and road traffic accidents. The drugs examined were tricyclic antidepressants, selective serotonin reuptake inhibitors, benzodiazepines, and other tranquilizers. The users of anxiolytic benzodiazepines were at significantly increased risk of involvement in a road traffic accident. The users of hypnotic benzodiazepines were not found to show an increased risk, which the authors hypothesized was due to the night-time-only dose. There was insufficient evidence of an association with other psychotropic drugs.

Specific effects of the benzodiazepines on driving

The benzodiazepine used

The risk for drivers over 65 is much higher when they take long-acting and larger quantities of benzodiazepine (Thomas, 1998). Verster, Volkerts, and Verbaten (2002) note that alprozolam is a particularly problematic agent in this regard. Their comprehensive review of samples submitted to the Washington State Toxicological Laboratory between January 1998 and December 2003 indicated that lorazepam was also capable of causing significant impairment of driving skill as well as of psychomotor abilities, and did so in a manner independent of the concentration detected (Clarkson, Gordon, & Logan, 2004; van Laar, Volkerts, & Verbaten, 2001).

Clearly, the appropriate use of a benzodiazepine requires a balance between obtaining the optimal sedative effect when it is needed at bedtime and reducing the residual sedating effects the morning after. Staner and colleagues' (2005) results on the next-day driving ability of insomniac patients after repeated benzodiazepine administration indicate that the residual effects of the hypnotics increased with their half-lives. Some authors further suggest that increased risk of crash involvement may be limited to long-half-life benzodiazepines (Hemmelgarn, Suissa, Huang, Boivin, & Pinard, 1997), while agents such as zaleplon were reported to have little or no residual effect when administered in the middle of the night to as late as 1 hour before waking, and did not impair driving skill as assessed by actual driving 4 hours after administration (Patat, Paty, & Hindmarch, 2001).

Dose

In their study of the association between concentration of benzodiazepines and apprehension of drivers by law enforcement officers, Bramness, Skurtveit and Mørland (2002) note that the blood level of benzodiazepine was the only characteristic related to impairment, indicating that there is a direct drug concentration effect of the benzodiazepines and possibly indicating that determination of a legal limit for benzodiazepines in relationship to driving may be possible.

Temporal aspects of drug administration

Two aspects of the timing of the use of the benzodiazepines are of relevance: time since the dose was taken and the time since therapy with the agents was begun. On road driving, research has shown that impairments of driving decrease during the day following the dose, such that morning driving was found to be more affected than afternoon driving (Verster et al., 2004). The relative risk of accident involving elderly drivers increases by 45% in the first week following commencement of the benzodiazepines, particularly if they were prescribed the long-acting agents (Hemmelgarn et al., 1997). Relative risk of hospitalization following road traffic accident increased 6.5-fold with initiation of therapy in 78,000 patients (Neutel, 1995).

Demographic factors with regard to the person operating the vehicle

Risk studies in Australia (Drummer, 2004; Drummer et al., 2004) indicate that there is a significant enhancement in odds ratio by 27% over drug-free drivers for individuals using benzodiazepines, however this effect is more marked with other drugs. It has been suggested that the elderly comprise a significant proportion of long-term users (Ayd, 1994). Furthermore, the altered elimination of metabolites, resulting from normal age-related decreases in liver function, can lead to the elderly being more sensitive to the effects of benzodiazepines (Ayd, 1994; Chen, 1990; Kruse, 1990; Madhusoodanan & Bogunovic, 2004; Sheikh, 1992).

Elderly users may also be more likely to experience side effects such as amnesia, impaired attention, ataxia, psychomotor slowing, and delayed recall, with reports of confusion, dysarthria, disorientation, increased likelihood of falls, agitation, and wandering behaviour resembling dementia (Ayd, 1994; Chen, 1990; Kruse, 1990; Salzman, Fisher, Nobel, & Glassman, 1992; Sheikh, 1992; Sumner, 1998; Wengel, Burke, Ranno, & Roccaforte, 1993) commonly noted. One study of drivers over 65 found benzodiazepines to be positively related with at-fault crash involvement, with an odds-ratio of 5.2 (95% CI 0.9–30.0; McGwinn, Sims, Pulley, & Roseman, 2000).

Summary and conclusion

The implications for the informed and responsible prescription of benzodiazepines are numerous. Most importantly, patients and clinicians should be aware that both physiological and pharmacological dependence can develop rapidly to these drugs. Abrupt withdrawal can lead to more severe symptoms, and as a result patients may opt to continue benzodiazepine therapy to avoid these withdrawal or rebound symptoms and risk long-term, potentially irreversible cognitive impairments. While many unanswered questions remain, and further research is required, the results of the studies reviewed call for caution to be exercised in the administration of benzodiazepine medication. The well-established acute effects of memory loss and sedation have important implications for an individual's daily functioning, particularly during activities involving driving or operating machinery, or in the elderly population who may suffer an increased likelihood of falls due to daytime sedation.

Although it may not be possible to determine a length of time for benzodiazepine therapy that is safe, it appears that a low dose over a short time has less effect, whereas a high dose for prolonged periods is more likely to be harmful. However, even at low therapeutic doses, long-term users of benzodiazepines display pervasive cognitive deficits that persist for months after discontinuation. Closely monitored use of benzodiazepines may be a very effective treatment of acute anxiety states in the short term, but the risks of long-term benzodiazepine therapy to cognitive functioning are now beyond dispute.

References

Adler, L., Angrist, B., & Peselow, E. (1985). Efficacy of propranolol in neuroleptic induced akathisia. *Journal of Clinical Psychopharmacology*, 5, 164–166.

Allen, D., Curran, H. V., & Lader, M. (1991). The effects of repeated doses of clomipramine and alprazolam on physiological, psychomotor and cognitive functions in normal subjects. *European Journal of Clinical Pharmacology*, 40, 355–362.

Allgulander, C., Borg, S., & Vikander, B. (1984). A 4–6 year follow up of 50 patients with primary dependence on sedative and hypnotic drugs. *American Journal of Psychiatry*, 141, 1580–1582.

American Hospital Formulary Service (1998). *AHFS Drug Information 98*. Bethesda, MD: AHFS.

American Psychiatric Association (1990). *Benzodiazepine dependence, toxicity, and abuse*. Washington, DC: APA.

Aranko, K., Mattila, M. J., & Seppala, T. (1983). Development of tolerance and cross-tolerance to the psychomotor actions of lorazepam and diazepam in man. *British Journal of Pharmacology*, 15, 545–552.

Ashton, H. (1984). Benzodiazepine withdrawal: an unfinished story. *British Medical Journal*, 288, 1135–1140.

Ashton, H. (1986). Adverse effects of prolonged benzodiazepine use. *Adverse Drug Reaction Bulletin*, 118, 440–443.

Ashton, H. (1989). Risks of dependence on benzodiazepine drugs: a major problem of long term treatment. *British Medical Journal*, 298, 103–104.

Ashton, H. (1995). Toxicity and adverse consequences of benzodiazepine use. *Psychiatric Annals*, 25, 158–165.

Ashton, H., & Golding, J. G. (1989). Tranquillizers: prevalence, predictors and possible consequences. Data from a large United Kingdom survey. *British Journal of Addiction, 84*, 541–546.

Auerbach, J. G., Hans, S. L., Marcus, J., & Maeir, S. (1992). Maternal psychotropic medication and neonatal behavior. *Neurotoxicology and Teratology, 14*, 399–406.

Ayd, F. J. (1994). Prescribing anxiolytics and hypnotics for the elderly. *Psychiatric Annals, 24*, 91–97.

Bagary, M., Fluck, E., File, S. E., Joyce, E., Lockwood, G., & Grasby, P. (2000). Is benzodiazepine-induced amnesia due to deactivation of the left prefrontal cortex? *Psychopharmacology, 150*, 292–299.

Bailey, L., Ward, M., & Musa, M. N. (1994). Clinical pharmacokinetics of benzodiazepines. *Journal of Clinical Pharmacology, 34*, 804–811.

Balter, M. B., Mannheimer, D. I., Mellinger, G. D., & Ulenhuth, E. H. (1984). A cross-national comparison of anti-anxiety/sedative drug use. *Current Medical Research Opinion, 8*, 5–20.

Barbone, F., McMahon, A. D., Davey, P. G., Morris, A. D., Reid, I. C., McDevitt, D. G., & MacDonald, T. M. (1998). Association of road-traffic accidents with benzodiazepine use. *Lancet, 352*, 1331–1336.

Barker, M. J., Greenwood, K. M., Jackson, M., & Crowe, S. F. (2004a). The cognitive effects of long-term Benzodiazepine use: A meta-analysis. *CNS Drugs, 18*, 37–48.

Barker, M. J., Greenwood, K. M., Jackson, M., & Crowe, S. F. (2004b). Persistence of cognitive effects after withdrawal from long-term benzodiazepine use: A meta-analysis. *Archives of Clinical Neuropsychology, 19*, 437–454.

Barker, M. J., Greenwood, K. M., Jackson, M., & Crowe, S. F. (2005). An evaluation of persisting cognitive effects after withdrawal from long-term benzodiazepine use. *Journal of the International Neuropsychological Society, 11*, 281–289.

Barker, M. J., Jackson, M., Greenwood, K. M., & Crowe, S. F. (2003). Cognitive effects of benzodiazepine use: A review. *Australian Psychologist, 38*, 202–213.

Bergman, H., Borg, S., Engelbrektson, K., & Vikander, B. (1989). Dependence on sedative-hypnotics: neuropsychological impairment, field dependence and clinical course in a 5-year follow-up study. *British Journal of Addiction, 84*, 547–553.

Birch, B. R. P., & Miller, R. A. (1995). An assessment of resedation following flumazenil-induced antagonism of intravenous midazolam: Comparison of psychomotor and amnesic recovery with a non-sedated reference group. *Journal of Psychopharmacology, 9*, 103–111.

Birkett, D. J. (1998). *Pharmacokinetics made easy*. Sydney, Australia: McGraw-Hill.

Bormann, J. (1988). Electrophysiology of GABA-A and GABA-B receptor subtypes. *Trends in Neurosciences, 11*, 112–116.

Bourin, M., du Tertre, A. C., & Payeur, R. (1993). Evaluation of safety and side effects in the process of anti-anxiety drug development. *European Psychiatry, 8*, 285–291.

Braestrup, C., & Squires, R. F. (1978). Pharmacological characterization of benzodiazepine receptors in the brain. *European Journal of Pharmacology, 48*, 263–270.

Bramness, J. G., Skurtveit, S., & Mørland, J. (2002). Clinical impairment of benzodiazepines – relation between benzodiazepine concentrations and impairment in apprehended drivers. *Drug and Alcohol Dependence, 68*, 131–141.

Brown, H. (1995). *Young people and the use of prescription pills (benzodiazepines)*. Victoria: Art Offset.

Busto, U., Bremner, K. E., Knight, K., terBrugge, K., & Sellers, E. M. (2000). Long-term benzodiazepine therapy does not result in brain abnormalities. *Journal of Clinical Psychopharmacology, 20*, 2–6.

Chen, Y. (1990). Long-term benzodiazepine treatment: Is it ever justified? *Human Psychopharmacology: Clinical and Experimental, 5*, 301–312.

Ciraulo. D. A., & Sarid-Segal, O. (1991). Benzodiazepines: Abuse liability. In P. Roy-Byrne & D. S. Cowley (Eds.), *Benzodiazepines in clinical practice: Risks and benefits* (pp. 157–174). Washington, DC: American Psychiatric Press.

Clarkson, J. E., Gordon, A. M., & Logan, B. K. (2004). Lorazepam and driving impairment. *Journal of Analytical Toxicology, 28*, 475–480.

Coffey, B. J. (1993). Review and update: Benzodiazepines in childhood and adolescence. *Psychiatric Annals, 23*, 332–339.

Cohen, J. (1988). *Statistical power analyses for the behavioral sciences* (2nd ed.). Hillsdale, NJ: Lawrence Erlbaum Associates.

Cohen, L. S., & Rosenbaum, J. F. (1987). Clonazepam: New uses and potential problems. *Journal of Clinical Psychiatry, 48S*, 50–55.

Coleman, V. (1985). *Life without tranquillizers*. London: Judy Piatkus Publishers.

Collomp, K.., Fortier, M., Cooper, S., Long, A., Ahmaidi, S., Prefaut, C., et al. (1994). Performance and metabolic effects of benzodiazepine during submaximal exercise. *Journal of Applied Physiology, 77*, 828–833.

Cooper, J. R., Bloom, F. E., & Roth, R. H. (1996). Amino acid transmitters. In *The biochemical basis of neuropharmacology* (7th ed., pp. 126–193). New York: Oxford University Press.

Curran, H. V. (1991). Benzodiazepines, memory and mood: a review. *Psychopharmacology, 105*, 1–8.

Curran, H. V. (1992). Memory functions, alertness and mood of long-term benzodiazepine users: A preliminary investigation of the effects of a normal daily dose. *Journal of Psychopharmacology, 6*, 69–75.

Curran, H. V., & Birch, B. R. P. (1991). Differentiating the sedative psychomotor and amnesic effects of benzodiazepines: A study with midazolam and the benzodiazepine antagonist, flumazenil. *Psychopharmacology, 103*, 519–523.

Curran, H. V., Bond, A., O'Sullivan, G., Bruce, M., Marks, I., Lelliot, P., et al. (1994). Memory functions, alprazolam and exposure therapy: a controlled longitudinal study of agoraphobia with panic disorder. *Psychological Medicine, 24*, 969–976.

Curran, H. V., Gorenstein, C., & Lader, M. (1993). Comparative amnesic and sedative effects of lorazepam and oxazepam in healthy volunteers. *Journal of Psychopharmacology, 7*, 249–256.

Curran, H. V., Schiwy, W., & Lader, M. (1987). Differential amnesic properties of benzodiazepines: A dose–response comparison of two drugs with similar elimination half-lives. *Psychopharmacology, 92*, 358–364.

Davies, M. F. (1996). The pharmacology of the gamma-aminobutyric acid system. In A. Baskys & G. Remington (Eds.), *Brain mechanisms and psychotropic drugs* (pp. 101–116). Boca Raton, FL: CRC Press.

De Visser, S. J., van der Post, J. P., de Waal, P. P., Cornet, F., Cohen, A. F., & van Gerven, J. M. A. (2003). Biomarkers for the effects of benzodiazepines in healthy volunteers. *British Journal of Clinical Pharmacology, 55*, 39–50.

Drummer, O. H. (2004). Postmortem toxicology of drugs of abuse. *Forensic Science International, 142*, 101–113.

Drummer, O. H., Gerostamoulos, J., Batziris, H., Chu, M., Caplehorn, J., Robertson, M. D., & Swann, P. (2004). The involvement of drugs in drivers of motor vehicles killed in Australian road traffic crashes. *Accident Analysis and Prevention, 36*, 239–248.

Durlak, J. A. (1995). *School-based prevention programs for children and adolescents.* Thousand Oaks, CA: Sage Publications.

Farkas, L., & Crowe, S. F. (2000). The role of the benzodiazepine–GABA system in the memory processes of the day-old chick. *Pharmacology, Biochemistry and Behavior, 65*, 223–231.

Fleishaker, J. C., Garzone, P. D., Chambers, J. H., & Sirocco, K. (1995). Comparison of the spectrum of cognitive effects of alprazolam and adinazolam after single doses in healthy subjects. *Psychopharmacology, 120*, 169–176.

Forster, A., Juge, O., & Morel, D. (1982). Effects of midazolam on cerebral blood flow in human volunteers. *Anesthesiology, 56*, 453–455.

Garvey, M. J., & Tollefson, G. D. (1987). Occurrence of myoclonus in patients treated with cyclic antidepressants. *Archives of General Psychiatry, 44*, 269–272.

Ghoneim, M. M., Hinrichs, J. V., & Mewaldt, S. P. (1984). Dose–response analysis of the behavioral effects of diazepam: I. Learning and memory. *Psychopharmacology, 82*, 291–295.

Ghoneim, M. M., Mewaldt, S. P., & Hinrichs, J. V. (1984). Dose–response analysis of the behavioral effects of diazepam: II. Psychomotor performance, cognition and mood. *Psychopharmacology, 82*, 296–300.

Golombok, S. (1989). Causes, effects and treatment of long-term benzodiazepine use: A review of psychological perspectives. *Human Psychopharmacology: Clinical and Experimental, 4*, 15–20.

Golombok, S., Moodley, P., & Lader, M. (1988). Cognitive impairment in long-term benzodiazepine users. *Psychological Medicine, 18*, 365–374.

Gorenstein, C., Bernik, M. A., & Pompeia, S. (1994). Differential acute psychomotor and cognitive effects of diazepam on long-term benzodiazepine users. *International Clinical Psychopharmacology, 9*, 145–153.

Gorenstein, C., Bernik, M. A., Pompeia, S., & Marcourakis, T. (1995). Impairment of performance associated with long-term use of benzodiazepines. *Journal of Psychopharmacology, 9*, 313–318.

Gorissen, M., Eling, P., van Luijtelaar, G., & Coenen, A. (1995). Effects of diazepam on encoding processes. *Journal of Psychopharmacology, 9*, 113–121.

Greist, J. H., Jefferson, J. W., & Marks, I. M. (1998). *Medications. Anxiety and its treatment: Help is available.* Washington, DC: American Psychiatric Press.

Griffiths, R. R. (1995). Commentary on review by Woods and Winger. Benzodiazepines: long-term use among patients is a concern and abuse among polydrug abusers is not trivial. *Psychopharmacology, 118*, 116–117.

Gudex, C. (1991). Adverse effects of benzodiazepines. *Social Science and Medicine, 33*, 587–596.

Haefely, W. E. (1978). Central action of benzodiazepines: general introduction. *British Journal of Psychiatry, 133*, 231–238.

Hawley, C. J., Tattersall, M., Dellaportas, C., & Hallstrom, C. (1994). Comparison of long-term benzodiazepine users in three settings. *British Journal of Psychiatry, 165*, 792–796.

Hege, S. G., Ellinwood, E. H. J., Wilson, W. H., & Helligers, C. A. M. (1997). Psychomotor effects of the anxiolytic abecarnil: A comparison with lorazepam. *Psychopharmacology, 131*, 101–107.

Hemmelgarn, B., Suissa, S., Huang, A., Boivin, J., & Pinard, G. (1997). Benzodiazepine use and the risk of motor vehicle crash in the elderly. *Journal of the American Medical Association, 278*, 27–31.

Hollister, L. E., Conley, F. K., Britt, R. H., & Shuer, L. S. (1981). Long-term use of benzodiazepines. *Journal of the American Medical Association, 246,* 1568–1570.
Hommer, D. W. (1991). Benzodiazepines: Cognitive and psychomotor effects. In P. Roy-Byrne & D. S. Cowley (Eds.), *Benzodiazepines in clinical practice: Risks and benefits.* Washington DC: American Psychiatric Press.
Hommer, D., Weingartner, H. J., & Breier, A. (1993). Dissociation of benzodiazepine-induced amnesia from sedation by flumazenil pre-treatment. *Psychopharmacology, 112,* 455–460.
Hutchinson, M. A., Smith, P. F., & Darlington, C. L. (1996). The behavioural and neuronal effects of the chronic administration of benzodiazepine anxiolytic and hypnotic drugs. *Progress in Neurobiology, 49,* 73.
Insel, T. R., & Murphy, D. L. (1981). The psychopharmacologic treatment of obsessive-compulsive disorder. *Journal of Clinical Psychopharmacology, 1,* 304–311.
Jollant, F., Bellvier, F., Leboyer, M., Astruc, B., Torres, S., Verdier, R., et al. (2005). Impaired decision making in suicide attempters. *American Journal of Psychiatry, 162,* 304–310.
Joyce, E. M., & File, S. E. (1995). Temazepam impairs effortful but not automatic processing of stimulus elements. *Human Psychopharmacology Clinical and Experimental, 10,* 449–453.
Kajimura, N., Nishikawa, M., Uchiyama, M., Kato, M., Watanabe, T., Nakajima, T., et al. (2004). Deactivation by benzodiazepine of the basal forebrain and amygdala in normal humans during sleep: a placebo-controlled [^{15}O]H$_2$O PET study. *American Journal of Psychiatry, 161,* 748–751.
Kandel, E. R. (1995). Synaptic integration. In E. R. Kandel, J. H. Schwartz, & T. M. Jessell (Eds.), *Essentials of neural science and behaviour.* Norwalk, CT: Appleton & Lange.
Keltner, N. L., & Folks, D. G. (1997). *Psychotropic drugs* (2nd ed.). St. Louis, MO: Mosby.
Kirkby, K. C., Montgomery, I. M., Badcock, R., & Daniels, B. A. (1995). A comparison of age-related deficits in memory and frontal lobe function following oral lorazepam administration. *Journal of Psychopharmacology, 9,* 319–325.
Kiuchi, Y., Kobayashi, T., Takeuchi, J., Shimizu, H., Ogata, H., & Toru, M. (1989). Benzodiazepine receptors increase in post-mortem brain of chronic schizophrenics. *European Archives of Psychiatry and Neurological Sciences, 239,* 71–78.
Kruse, W. H. (1990). Problems and pitfalls in the use of benzodiazepines in the elderly. *Drug Safety, 5,* 328–344.
Lader, M. H. (1982). Psychological effects of buspirone. *Journal of Clinical Psychiatry, 43,* 62–67.
Lader, M. H (1984). Short-term versus long-term benzodiazepine therapy. *Current Medical Research Opinion, 8,* 120–126.
Lader, M., & Petursson, H. (1983). Long term effects of benzodiazepines. *Neuropharmacology, 22,* 527–533.
Lader, M. H., Ron, M., & Petursson, H. (1984). Computerized axial tomography in long term benzodiazepine users. *Psychological Medicine, 14,* 203–206.
Lucki, I., & Rickels, K. (1986). The behavioral effects of benzodiazepines following long-term use. *Psychopharmacology Bulletin, 22,* 424–433.
Lucki, I., Rickels, K., & Geller, A. M. (1986). Chronic use of benzodiazepines and psychomotor and cognitive test performance. *Psychopharmacology, 88,* 426–433.

Lyndon, R. W., & Russell, J. D. (1988). Benzodiazepine in a rural general practice population. *Australian and New Zealand Journal of Psychiatry, 22*, 292–298.

MacDonald, S., Wells, S., Giesbrecht, N., & Cherpitel, C. J. (1999). Demographic and substance use factors related to violent and accidental injuries: results from an emergency room study. *Drug and Alcohol Dependence, 55*, 53–61.

Madhusoodanan, S., & Bogunovic, O. J. (2004). Safety of benzodiazepines in the elderly. *Expert Opinion on Drug Safety, 3*, 485–493.

Malizia, A. L. (1999). What do brain imaging studies tell us about anxiety disorders? *Journal of Psychopharmacology, 13*, 372–378.

Malizia, A. L. (2000). Positron emitting ligands in the study of the clinical psychopharmacology of anxiety and anxiety disorders. MD thesis, Faculty of Medicine, University of Bristol, UK.

Malizia, A. L., Cunningham, V. J., Bell, C. M., Liddle, P. F., Jones, T., & Nutt, D. J. (1998). Decreased brain $GABA_A$–benzodiazepine receptor binding in panic disorder: Preliminary results from a quantitative PET study. *Archives of General Psychiatry, 55*, 715–720.

Matthew, R. J., Wilson, W. H., & Daniel, D. G. (1985). The effect of non-sedating doses of diazepam on regional blood flow. *Biological Psychiatry, 20*, 1109–1116.

McGwinn, G., Sims, R. V., Pulley, L., & Roseman, J. M. (2000). Relations among chronic medical conditions, medications and automobile crashes in the elderly: a population-based case–control study. *American Journal of Epidemiology, 152*, 424–431.

Mellinger, G. D., Balter, B. B., & Uhlenhuth, E. H. (1984). Prevalence and correlates of the long-term regular use of anxiolytics. *Journal of the American Medical Association, 251*, 375–379.

Miller, N. S. (1995). Liability and efficacy from long-term use of benzodiazepines: Documentation and interpretation. *Psychiatric Annals, 25*, 166–173.

Mintzer, M. Z., Griffiths, R. R., Contoreggi, C., Kames, A. S., London, E. D., & Ernst, M. (2001). Effects of triazolam on brain activity during episodic memory encoding: A PET study. *Neuropsychopharmacology, 25*, 744–756.

Moodley, P., Golombok, S., Shine, P., & Lader M. (1993). Computerized axial brain tomograms in long-term benzodiazepine users. *Psychiatry Research, 48*, 135–144.

Munjack, D. J., Baltazar, P. L., & Bohn, P. B. (1990). Clonazepam in the treatment of social phobia. *Journal of Clinical Psychiatry, 51*, 34–40.

National Health and Medical Research Council (1991). *Guidelines for the prevention and management of benzodiazepine dependence.* Canberra: Australian Government Publishing Service.

Nayeem, N., Green, T. P., Martin, J. L., et al. (1994). Quaternary structure of the native $GABA_A$ receptor determined by electron microscopic image analysis. *Journal of Neurochemistry, 62*, 815–818.

Nelson, J., & Chouinard, G. (1996). Benzodiazepines: Mechanisms of action and clinical indications. In A. Baskys & G. Remington (Eds.), *Brain mechanisms and psychotropic drugs.* Boca Raton, FL: CRC Press.

Nestoros, J. N., Nair, N. P. V., & Pulman, J. R. (1983). High doses of diazepam improve neuroleptic-resistant chronic schizophrenic patients. *Psychopharmacology, 81*, 42–47.

Neutel, C. I. (1995). Risk of traffic accident injury after a prescription for a benzodiazepine. *Annals of Epidemiology, 5*, 239–244.

Nutt, D. J., Glue, P., Lawson, C. W., & Wilson, S. (1990). Flumazenil provocation of panic attacks: evidence for altered benzodiazepine receptor sensitivity in panic disorders. *Archives of General Psychiatry, 47*, 917–925.

Nutt, D. J., & Malizia, A. L. (2001). New insights into the role of the GABA(A)–benzodiazepine disorder. *British Journal of Psychiatry, 179*, 390–396.

Oquendo, M. A., Placidi, G. P., Malone, K. M., Campbell, C., Keilp, J., Brodsky, B., et al. (2003). Positron emission tomography of regional brain metabolic responses to a serotonergic challenge and lethality of suicide attempts in major depression. *Archives of General Psychiatry, 60*, 14–22.

Pandey, G., Conley, R., Pandey, S., Goel, S., Roberts, R. C., Tamminga, C. A., et al. (1997). Benzodiazepine receptors in the post-mortem brain of suicide victims and schizophrenic subjects. *Psychiatry Research, 71*, 137–149.

Paredes, R. G., & Agmo, A. (1992). GABA and behavior: the role of receptor sub-types. *Neuroscience and Biobehavioral Review, 16*, 145–170.

Patat, A., Paty, I., & Hindmarch, I. (2001). Pharmacodynamic profile of zapelon, a new non-benzodiazepine hypnotic agent. *Human Psychopharmacology: Clinical and Experimental, 16*, 369–392.

Patterson, J. F. (1990). Withdrawal from alprazolam dependency using clonazepam: clinical observations. *Journal of Clinical Psychiatry, 51*, 47–49.

Perera, K. M., Powell, T., & Jenner, F. A. (1987). Computerized axial tomographic studies following long-term use of benzodiazepines. *Psychological Medicine, 17*, 775–777.

Petursson, H., Gudjonsson, G. H., & Lader, M. H. (1983). Psychometric performance during withdrawal from long-term benzodiazepine treatment. *Psychopharmacology, 81*, 345–349.

Pollack, M. H. (1993). Innovative uses of benzodiazepines in psychiatry. *Canadian Journal of Psychiatry, 38*, 122–126.

Poser, W., Poser, S., Roscher, D., & Argyrakis, A. (1983). Do benzodiazepines cause cerebral atrophy? *Lancet, 1*, 715.

Reinsel, R. A., Veselis, R. A., Dnistrian, A. M., Feshchenko, V. A., Beattie, B. J., & Duff, M. R. (2000). Midazolam decreases cerebral blood flow in the left prefrontal cortex in a dose-dependant fashion. *International Journal of Neuropharmacology, 3*, 117–127.

Reiter, S. R., Pollack, M. H., & Rosenbaum, J. F. (1990). Clonazepam for the treatment of social phobia. *Journal of Clinical Psychiatry, 51*, 470–472.

Rodrigo, E. K., King, M. B., & Williams, P. (1988). Health of long term benzodiazepine users. *British Medical Journal, 296*, 603–606.

Romach, M., Busto, U., Sobell, L. C., Sobell, M. B., Somer, G., & Sellers, E. M. (1991). Long-term alprazolam use: Abuse, dependence or treatment? *Psychopharmacology Bulletin, 27*, 391–395.

Rosenthal, R. (1991). *Meta-analytic procedures of social research* (revised ed.). London, UK: Sage Publications.

Roy-Byrne, P. P. (1991). Benzodiazepines: Dependence and withdrawal. In P. Roy-Byrne & D. S. Cowley (Eds.), *Benzodiazepines in clinical practice: Risks and benefits* (pp. 133–153). Washington, DC: American Psychiatric Press.

Roy-Byrne, P. P., & Nutt, D. J. (1991). Benzodiazepines: Biological mechanisms. In P. Roy-Byrne & D. S. Cowley (Eds.), *Benzodiazepines in clinical practice: Risks and benefits* (pp. 5–18). Washington, DC: American Psychiatric Press.

Sakol, M. S., & Power, K. G. (1988). The effects of long-term benzodiazepine treatment and graded withdrawal on psychometric performance. *Psychopharmacology, 95,* 135–138.

Salam, S. A., Pillai, A. K., & Beresford, T. P. (1987). Lorazepam for psychogenic catatonia. *American Journal of Psychiatry, 144,* 1082–1083.

Salinsky, J. V., & Dore, C. J. (1987). Characteristics of long term benzodiazepine users in general practice. *Journal of the Royal College of General Practitioners, 37,* 202–204.

Salzman, C., Fisher, J., Nobel, K., & Glassman, R. (1992). Cognitive improvement following benzodiazepine discontinuation in elderly nursing home residents. *International Journal of Geriatric Psychiatry, 7,* 89–93.

Sangameswaran, L., Fales, H. M., Friedrich, P., & De Blas, A. L. (1986). Purification of a benzodiazepine from bovine brain and detection of benzodiazepine-like immunoreactivity in the human brain. *Proceedings of the National Academy of Sciences of the USA, 83,* 9236–9241.

Schmauss, C., & Krieg, J. C. (1987). Enlargement of cerebrospinal fluid spaces on long-term benzodiazepine abusers. *Psychological Medicine, 17,* 869–873.

Schofield, P. R., Darlison, M. G., Fujita, N., Burt, D. R., Stephenson, F. A., Rodriguez, H., et al. (1987). Sequence and functional expression of the $GABA_A$ receptor shows a ligand-gated receptor superfamily. *Nature, 328,* 221–227.

Schweizer, E. (1995). Generalized anxiety disorder: Longitudinal course and pharmacologic treatment. *Psychiatric Clinics of North America, 18,* 843–857.

Seppala, T., Palva, E., Mattila, M. J., Korttila, K., & Shrotriya, R. C. (1980). Tofisopam, a novel 3,4-benzodiazepine: multiple dose effects on psychomotor skills and memory. Comparison with diazepam and interactions with ethanol. *Psychopharmacology, 69,* 209–218.

Sheikh, J. I. (1992). Problems associated with long-term benzodiazepine use in the elderly. In C. A. Shamoian (Ed.), *Psychopharmacological treatment complications in the elderly* (pp. 71–87). Washington, DC: American Psychiatric Press.

Sieghart, W. (1989). Multiplicity of $GABA_A$–benzodiazepine receptors. *Trends in Pharmacological Science, 10,* 407–411.

Simpson, R. J., Power, K. G., Wallace, L. A., Butcher, M. H., Swanson, V., & Simpson, E. C. (1990). Controlled comparison of the characteristics of long-term benzodiazepine users in general practice. *British Journal of General Practice, 40,* 22–26.

Skegg, D. C. G., Richards, S. M., & Doll, R. (1979). Minor tranquillisers and road accidents. *British Medical Journal, 1,* 917–919.

Smirne, S., Ferini Strambi, L., Pirola, R., & Tancredi, O. (1989). Effects of flunitrazepam on cognitive functions. *Psychopharmacology, 98,* 251–256.

Squires, R. F., Benson, D. I., Braestrup, C., Coupet, J., Klepner, C. A., Myers, V., & Beer, B. (1988). Some properties of brain specific benzodiazepine receptors: New evidence for multiple receptors. *Pharmacology, Biochemistry and Behavior, 10,* 825–830.

Staner, L., Ertle, S., Boeijinga, P., Rinaudo, G., Arnal, M. A., Muzet, A., & Luthringer, R. (2005). Next-day residual effects of hypnotics in DSM-IV primary insomnia: a driving simulator study with simultaneous electroencephalogram monitoring. *Psychopharmacology, 181,* 790–798.

Stewart, S. A. (2005). The effects of benzodiazepines on cognition. *Journal of Clinical Psychiatry, 66,* 9–13.

Stewart, S. H., Rioux, G. F., Connolly, J. F., & Dunphy, S. C. (1996). Effects of oxazepam and lorazepam on implicit and explicit memory: Evidence for possible influences of time course. *Psychopharmacology, 128,* 139–149.

Streufert, S., Satish, U., Pogash, R., Gingrich, D., Landis, R., Lonardi, L., et al. (1996). Effects of Alprazolam on complex human functioning. *Journal of Applied Social Psychology, 26,* 1912–1930.

Sumner, D. D. (1998). Benzodiazepine-induced persisting amnestic disorder: are older adults at risk? [published erratum appears in *Archives of Psychiatric Nursing, 12,* 237]. *Archives of Psychiatric Nursing, 12,* 119–125.

Tallman, J., & Gallagher, D. W. (1985). The GABAergic system: A locus of benzodiazepine action. *Annual Review of Neuroscience, 8,* 21.

Tansella, C. Z. (1980). The long-term treatment with benzodiazepines: suggestions for further research. *International Pharmacopsychiatry, 15,* 99–104.

Tata, P. R., Rollings, J., Collins, M., Pickering, A., & Jacobson, R. R. (1994). Lack of cognitive recovery following withdrawal from long-term benzodiazepine use. *Psychological Medicine, 24,* 203–213.

Thomas, R. E. (1998). Benzodiazepine use and motor vehicle accidents. Systematic review of reported association. *Canadian Family Physician, 44,* 799–808.

Tiihonen, J., Kuikka, J., Rasanen, P., Lepola, U., Koponen, H., Liuska, A., et al. (1997). Cerebral benzodiazepine receptor binding and distribution in generalized anxiety disorder: a fractal analysis. *Molecular Psychiatry, 6,* 463–471.

Tinuper, P., Montagna, P., Plazzi, G., Avoni, P., Cerullo, A., Cortelli, P., et al. (1994). Idiopathic recurring stupor. *Neurology, 44,* 621–625.

Ulenhuth, E. H. (1988). Risks and benefits of long-term benzodiazepine use. *Journal of Clinical Psychopharmacology, 8,* 161–167.

UNCND (United Nations Commission on Narcotic Drugs) (1984). Benzodiazepines and pentazocine scheduled under convention on psychotropic substances. *Lancet, 1,* 637.

Unützer, J., Rubenstein, L., Katon, W. J., Tang, L., Duan, N., Lagomasino, I., & Wells, K. (2001). Two-year effects of quality improvement programs on medication management for depression. *Archives of General Psychiatry, 58,* 935–942.

Van Heeringen, C. (2001). Suicide, serotonin and the brain. *Crisis, 22,* 66–70.

Van Laar, M., Volkerts, E., & Verbaten, M. (2001). Subchronic effects of the GABA-agonist lorazepam and the 5-HR2A antagonist ritanserin on driving performance, slow wave sleep and daytime sleepiness in healthy volunteers. *Psychopharmacology (Berlin), 154,* 189–197.

Verster, J. C., Veldhuijzen, D. S., & Volkerts, E. R. (2004). Residual effects of sleep medication on driving ability. *Sleep Medicine Reviews, 8,* 309–325.

Verster, J. C., Volkerts, E. R., & Verbaten, M. N. (2002). Effects of alprazolam on driving ability, memory functioning and psychomotor performance: a randomized, placebo-controlled study. *Neuropsychopharmacology, 27,* 260–269.

Veselis, R. A., Reinsel, R. A., Beattie, B. J., Mawlawi, O. R., Feshchenko, V. A., Di Resta, G. R., Larson, S. M., & Blasberg, R. G. (1997). Midazolam changes cerebral blood flow in discrete brain regions: an H2150 positron emission tomography study. *Anesthesiology, 87,* 1106–1117.

Vgontzas, A. N., Kales, A., & Bixler, E. O. (1995). Benzodiazepine side effects: role of pharmacokinetics and pharmacodynamics. *Pharmacology, 51,* 205–223.

Walls, C. (2004). Benzodiazepines: Effects on human performance and behavior. Paper presented at the International Council on Alcohol, Drugs and Traffic Safety Meeting, Florida, 2004.

Weingartner, H., Eckardt, M., Molchan, S. E., & Sunderland, T. (1992). Measurement and interpretation of changes in memory in response to drug treatments. Special Feature: Neuropsychological factors in mental disorders and their treatments. *Psychopharmacology Bulletin, 28*, 331–340.

Wengel, S. P., Burke, W. J., Ranno, A. E., & Roccaforte, W. H. (1993). Use of benzodiazepines in the elderly. *Psychiatric Annals, 23*, 325–331.

Woods, J. H., Katz, J. L., & Winger, G. (1992). Benzodiazepines: Use, abuse, and consequences. *Pharmacology Review, 44*, 147–151.

Zandstra, S. M., Furer, J. W., van de Lisdonk, E. H., Van't Hof, M., Bor, J. H. J., van Weel, C., et al. (2002). Different study criteria affect the prevalence of benzodiazepine use. *Social Psychiatry and Psychiatric Epidemiology, 37*, 139–144.

4 Cocaine

Karen I. Bolla and Jean L. Cadet

Introduction

Cocaine is a potent stimulant that is addictive and widely used. There is evidence that cocaine was first used over 4000 years ago by South American natives to relieve fatigue. Current use in the United States is estimated at 2 million current cocaine users, 567,000 of whom are "crack users" (USDHHS, 2002). Because of its wide use and highly addictive properties cocaine has been used as a prototype to further our understanding of addiction. A large number of studies have evaluated treatment issues related to cocaine dependence with varying degrees of success. One of the shortcomings of the extant treatment approaches has been the lack of integration of neurobiological functioning, including neuropsychological profiles, within these therapeutic frameworks. In order to remedy these problems, researchers have sought to characterize the neurobiological impairments associated with cocaine dependence. The purpose of this chapter is to summarize the current knowledge regarding the neurobiological and neuropsychological abnormalities associated with heavy cocaine use and offer suggestions as to how these findings might be relevant to treatment outcomes.

This chapter will present an overview on the neurobiology of heavy cocaine use. The term "heavy cocaine use" will be used in place of the Cocaine Use Disorders terms "cocaine abuse" or "cocaine dependence" in the Diagnostic and Statistical Manual of Mental Disorders (DSM-IV). Topics covered in this chapter on the neurologic sequelae of cocaine use include: the pre-clinical neurobiology/psychopharmacology of cocaine, the clinical neurobiology of cocaine use in humans, the acute (with administration) and residual (after abstinence) effects of cocaine use on cerebrovascular function, neurocognitive function, metabolic function (cerebral blood flow and glucose metabolism), and brain structure, and the psychology of cocaine dependence abuse.

Neurobiology of cocaine

Although cocaine can nonselectively block transport of the monoamines dopamine, serotonin, and norepinephrine (Reith & Selmeci, 1992; Amara &

Kuhar, 1993), the effect of cocaine on dopamine uptake sites is thought to be responsible for the behavioral and reinforcing effects of the drug as well as the potential for abuse by human addicts (Bergman, Madras, Johnson, & Spealman, 1989; Madras, Fahey, Bergman, Canfield, & Spealman, 1989; Ritz, Lamb, Goldberg, & Kuhar, 1987; Volkow et al., 1997). Binding of cocaine to these recognition sites causes inhibition of dopamine transport, resulting in the accumulation of dopamine in the synaptic cleft (Hurd, Kehr, & Ungerstedt, 1988; Pettit & Justice, Jr., 1989, 1991). The accumulated dopamine then binds to dopamine receptors (D1-like and D2-like binding sites) that are located in cells postsynaptic to dopamine terminals (Civelli, Bunzow, Grandy, Zhou, & Vantol, 1991; Sokoloff et al., 2001). (Figure 4.1).

Administration of dopamine uptake inhibitors, direct dopamine agonists, and dopamine antagonists in various combinations with or without co-administration of cocaine causes cocaine-induced changes in dopamine tone that are associated with changes in behavior (Mello & Negus, 1996). For example, Ritz et al. (1987) demonstrated a significant correlation between dopamine transporter occupancy and the reinforcing effects of a number of dopamine transporter inhibitors from distinct structural classes. Moreover, Volkow and colleagues (1997) showed that the subjective "high" experienced by human cocaine users is mediated by dopamine transporter occupancy.

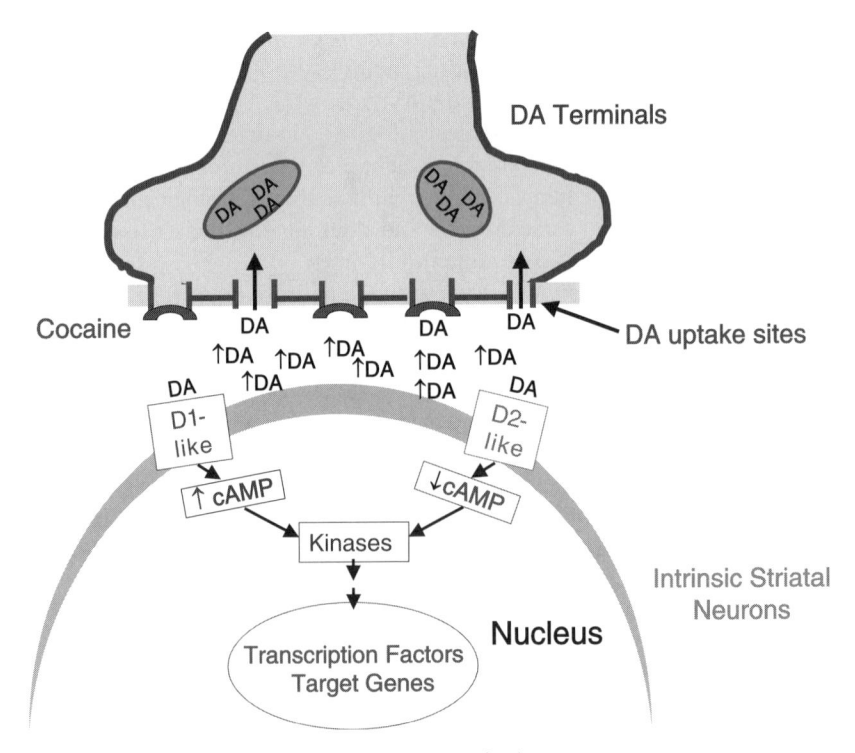

Figure 4.1 Illustration of dopamine (DA) terminals.

A number of paradigms have been used to study the effects of cocaine, including reinstatement, self-administration, and drug discrimination models (Lu, Shepard, Scott, & Shaham, 2003; Mantsch, Yuferov, Mathieu-Kia, Ho, & Kreek, 2004; Porrino, Daunais, Smith, & Nader, 2004). For example, the cocaine reinstatement model is thought to closely mimic relapse to cocaine abuse (Lu et al., 2003). In a reinstatement procedure, self-administration is extinguished, followed by presentation of drug and/or environmental stimuli. In humans, triggers of relapse have been reported to engender reinstatement of drug-seeking behavior. These include cues and stressful events (Goeders, 2002).

Acute administration of cocaine in rodents and primates has profound metabolic effects on the ventral striatum (Porrino, 1993; Porrino, Lyons, Smith, Daunais, & Nader, 2004; Lyons, Friedman, Nader, & Porrino, 1996). This outcome is consistent with postmortem assays of normal human brains, which revealed that cocaine binds to dopamine uptake sites in the basal ganglia and to serotonin uptake sites in the frontal cortex and hippocampus (Biegon et al., 1992). Acute administration of cocaine *increases* metabolic activity in rats, primarily in subcortical brain regions (London et al., 1986; Porrino, 1993), while in nonhuman primates glucose utilization is *decreased* in the limbic system, including the nucleus accumbens, limbic cortex, orbitofrontal cortex and other prefrontal cortices, and part of the hippocampus formation (Lyons et al., 1996).

This interspecies difference in the effects of cocaine on brain metabolism may be attributed to more complex neuroanatomical architecture in the primate as compared to the rodent. These results suggest that the central action of cocaine in the primate involves corticostriatal activity, originating in limbic cortex and projecting to the ventral striatum. It is through these projections that the reinforcing effects of cocaine may be mediated, in part, by limbic cortical structures (Lyons et al., 1996). The discrepancy in findings between rodent and primate studies illustrates the limitations of animal models of the neurobiological consequences of chronic cocaine use and justifies the need to investigate the chronic effects of cocaine in humans.

Clinical neurobiology of cocaine use in humans

Heavy use of cocaine is associated with alterations of neurotransmitter systems in humans. These alterations can manifest as abnormalities in regional cerebral blood flow and cerebral glucose metabolism in the prefrontal cortex and in other limbic areas, which, in turn, provide the substrates for neurobehavioral effects [i.e., psychiatric (depression, compulsive behavior), cognitive deficits] associated with heavy cocaine use. It is also very likely that cocaine-induced neurological abnormalities, such as atrophy and/or cell death as a result of ischemic events, can also manifest as neuropsychological impairment (Bolla, Cadet, & London, 1998; Cadet & Bolla, 1996). The

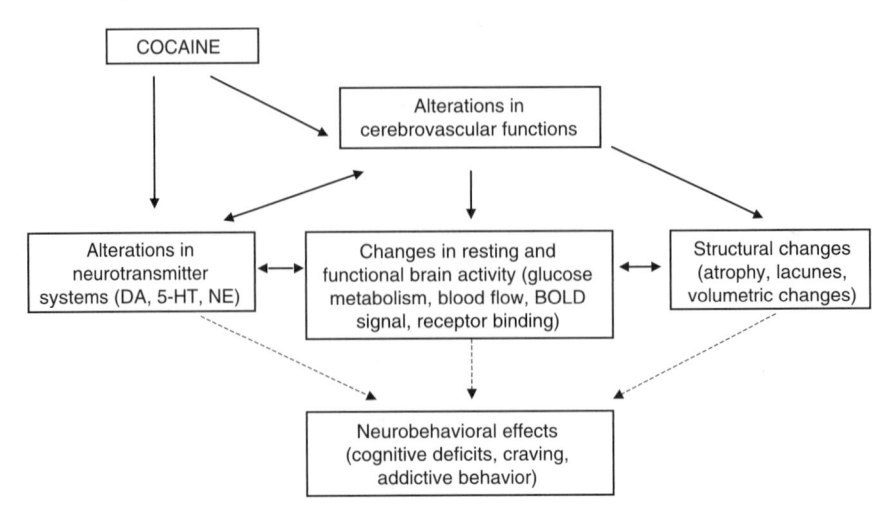

Figure 4.2 A neurobiological model of the effects of cocaine on neurotransmitters, functional brain activity, brain structure, and neurobehavior (*solid lines:* neurobiological effects; *broken lines:* contribution to neurobehavioral effects; DA = dopamine; 5-HT = serotonin; NE = norepinephrine).

neurobiological model presented in Figure 4.2 summarizes the effects of cocaine on the brain.

Overview of functional neuroimaging

Unlike x-ray or magnetic resonance imaging (MRI), functional neuroimaging methods provide an index of brain function, not just anatomy. Several neuroimaging techniques are currently available to investigate brain functioning in humans, including single proton emission computed tomography (SPECT), positron emission tomography (PET) and functional magnetic resonance imaging (fMRI). SPECT involves the detection of gamma rays emitted singly from radioactive atoms, called radionuclides, such as technetium-99m and thallium-201. When PET is utilized, a number of different metabolic processes can be imaged depending on the radiotracer administered. For example, glucose metabolism can be imaged using [^{18}F]fluorodeoxyglucose (FDG), while global and regional cerebral blood flow can be imaged using an $H_2^{15}O$ radiotracer. Global and regional cerebral blood flow (CBF and rCBF) are regulated by the requirements of cerebral metabolism (Roy & Sherrington, 1980). In animals, normal human subjects, and patients with brain disease (Nilsson, Rehncrona, & Siesjo, 1978), rates of rCBF are related to regional cerebral metabolic rates for glucose (Des Rosiers et al., 1974), and, in some cases (i.e., during hard exercise), rCBF is coupled to the regional cerebral metabolic rate for oxygen in the cerebral cortex (Raichle et al., 1976). Regional CBF can be either increased or decreased in neuropathological states, such as dementia (Ingvar & Lassen, 1979) and stroke (Schieve &

Wilson, 1953). In addition, specific brain receptors such as dopamine D2 receptors and synaptic dopamine concentration can be studied using compounds such as [^{11}C] raclopride. Each of the aforementioned techniques mentioned involve the administration of a radioactive compound and, as a result, only a limited number of PET studies can be performed over a 12-month period. Moreover, this limitation hinders researchers' capacity to conduct longitudinal studies.

Functional MRI overcomes this limitation because the technique does not rely on the administration of a radioactive compound. Functional MRI is based on the premise that the supply of oxygenated blood increases with neural activity and that the hemoglobin supply is depleted as a result of intense activity. Therefore, the fMRI brain image reflects the relative distribution of oxygenated blood throughout the brain during the recording interval or the BOLD signal (blood oxygen level dependent contrast).

The development of neuroimaging techniques has made it possible to visualize brain activity in humans during both a resting state and a cognitive activation state. The use of these potent imaging techniques has advanced our understanding of the immediate and residual effects of cocaine on the brain. For example, cocaine-induced hypoperfusion has been reported in several compartments of the frontal lobe as detected using SPECT (Levin et al., 1994; Pearlson et al., 1993) and PET (Bolla et al., 2004). PET studies have described reduced frontal metabolism that persists even after 3–4 months of abstinence from cocaine (London et al., 1990; Volkow et al., 1988, 1992). London et al. (1990) have also reported reduced cerebral metabolism after injections of cocaine that causes euphoric responses in cocaine-addicted patients. The brain regions most often reported to be affected in cocaine abusers are the orbitofrontal cortex (OFC), the anterior cingulate cortex (ACC), the dorsolateral prefrontal cortex (DLPFC), amygdala, putamen, and cerebellum.

Possible mechanisms of cocaine addiction in humans

Prefrontal brain regions, including the OFC, ACC, DLPFC, and amygdala, are activated during intoxication, craving, and binging, and deactivated during withdrawal (Goldstein & Volkow, 2002). These same brain regions are also involved in critical behaviors such as decision-making, control and inhibition of inappropriate responses, conflict monitoring, and evaluation of the saliency of a stimuli or reward. Based on this brain–behavior relationship, Goldstein and Volkow (2002) have proposed that drug addiction is a syndrome of impaired response inhibition and salience attribution (I-RISA syndrome of drug addiction). This model conceptualizes addiction as a dysregulation of cognitive and emotional processes that results in the overvaluing of drug reinforcers, the undervaluing of alternative reinforcers, and difficulty with the inhibitory cognitive control that culminates as an inability to abstain from drug taking.

Based on this logic, the heavy use of cocaine, because of repeated ischemic events due to its vasoconstrictive properties, might have caused a state comparable to what is observed with lacunar infarcts in the white matter of the brain. This might, in turn, cause neurological states akin to deconnection syndromes between regions within cerebral hemispheres. Nevertheless, given the complexity of the abnormalities observed in the brains of heavy cocaine users, it is likely that intercerebral hemispheric disconnections are important contributors to the impaired inhibition syndrome.

The powerful reinforcing effects of cocaine are at least partly related to the pleasurable feelings it produces. The lateral OFC is sensitive to punishment and overrides behavior based on the previous rewarding values of stimuli and responses, whereas the medial OFC is involved in reward and guessing situations when the outcomes are undetermined (O'Doherty, Kringelbach, Rolls, Hornak, & Andrews, 2001). Furthermore, the OFC was found to be involved in positive reinforcement (Rolls & Baylis, 1994), and neurons in this region increased their firing rate during rewarding electrical stimulation to other brain regions (Mora, Avrith, & Rolls, 1980; Rolls, Burton, & Mora, 1980). In contrast to positive stimuli, aversive olfactory stimulation increased rCBF in the left OFC in humans (Zald & Kim, 1996). These findings suggest that OFC may play a role in processing both positive and negative emotional stimuli. Cocaine abuse is also associated with repetitive compulsive acts that perpetuate drug-seeking behaviors. It is notable that patients who suffer from obsessive–compulsive disorder (OCD) also have metabolic abnormalities in OFC as well as in the ACC (Baxter et al., 1987; Benkelfat et al., 1990). Thus, it is plausible that cocaine-induced abnormalities in OFC and ACC might contribute to the compulsive behaviors observed in addicted individuals.

The ACC appears to be a key anatomical region in the developmental process of addiction. It is also important in the proper and efficient functioning of frontolimbic attentional networks. The cingulate cortex, like the OFC, is involved in positive reinforcement in animal studies (Dworkin & Smith, 1992). The ACC may also participate in the modulation of the execution of appropriate responses and the suppression of inappropriate responses or incorrect actions (conflict monitoring) (Bush et al., 1999; Paus et al., 1993). In a study by Bolla et al. (2004), 23-day abstinent cocaine abusers were required to suppress inappropriate responses on a modified Stroop task. No correlation was found between the Stroop interference score and activation in the ACC in heavy cocaine users, an association that was significant in the non-drug-using control group. These findings suggest ACC dysfunction in chronic cocaine abusers.

The ACC may also be involved in memory consolidation. A "memory" of the positive drug experience may contribute to attention bias and perpetuate cocaine use, which may in turn lead to a feeling of craving when the drug is discontinued after repeated administration (Johanson & Fischman, 1989). The exact neurobiological substrates for consolidation of this "memory" are unknown, but probably involve the ACC as well as other brain regions.

The DLPFC plays a role in maintaining attentional demands of the task as well as planning and working memory. Heavy cocaine users showed less activation relative to nondrug users in the right DLPFC during performance of a decision-making task (Bolla et al., 2003b) and during performance on the Stroop task (Bolla et al., 2004). In summary, cumulative evidence suggests that prefrontal brain regions, specifically the OFC, ACC, and DLPFC, are likely involved in the development and maintenance of cocaine addiction.

Acute and residual effects of cocaine use on cerebrovascular function, neurocogntive function, metabolic function, and brain structure

Acute cerebrovascular effects of cocaine administration

Cocaine use is associated with increased risk for stroke. For example, dose-related cerebral vasoconstriction was detected using magnetic resonance angiography with intravenous administration of cocaine in healthy cocaine users (Kaufman et al., 1998). Vasoconstriction was seen with low-dose cocaine (0.4 and 0.2 mg/kg) when no other risk factors (i.e., polysubstance use, hypertension, cerebrovascular disease) were present. When outcome was stratified by self-reports of lifetime frequency of use (3–10 times, 11–40 times, > 40 times), an even stronger dose-related effect was found. This finding suggests that greater lifetime use of cocaine is associated with a greater vasoconstriction. The findings from Kaufman and colleagues (1998) are consistent with the findings from epidemiological studies showing that cocaine use is a risk factor for stroke (Broderick et al., 2003).

Acute neurocognitive effects of cocaine administration

Few studies have documented the manner in which cocaine affects neuropsychological functioning immediately following administration. Intravenous administration of cocaine (0.325 mg/kg and 0.65 mg/kg) was associated with improved performance on an attentional task (Rapid Visual Information Processing Task) in a sample of eight participants who had a DSM-IV diagnosis of cocaine dependence (Johnson, Oldman, Goodall, Chen, & Cowen, 1996; Johnson et al., 1998). Similar results were observed with intranasal cocaine administration on a measure of attention and speed of information processing (Digit Symbol Substitution) in a sample of eight recreational cocaine users under controlled laboratory conditions (Higgins et al., 1990). Thus, cocaine may enhance performance in a manner similar to that reported for amphetamine (Johnson et al., 1996). This similarity is logical because both cocaine and amphetamine act as stimulants to the central nervous system.

Acute metabolic effects of cocaine administration

In the last decade, substance abuse researchers have utilized various neuroimaging techniques to document the neurobiological alterations that occur as a result of heavy cocaine use. For instance, acute administration of cocaine reduced absolute and regional CBF (Holman et al., 1993; Pearlson et al., 1993; Volkow et al., 1988; Weber et al., 1993; Wallace et al., 1994, 1996). In one study, blood flow after cocaine administration was reduced by about 30% of baseline, probably as a result of the vasoconstrictive properties of cocaine (Wallace et al., 1994). Cerebral glucose utilization, as measured by PET and [^{18}F]fluorodeoxyglucose, was also reduced when cocaine was administered to volunteers with histories of intravenous cocaine abuse (London et al., 1990). Significant decreases were found in most brain regions assayed. Moreover, fMRI revealed that activation was observed in a number of limbic and paralimbic regions (Breiter et al., 1997); for example, administration of cocaine produced increases in signal in the ventral tegmentum, pons, basal forebrain, caudate, the cingulate cortex, and the lateral prefrontal cortex, among other brain regions. The increase in signal in these brain regions was correlated with rush ratings. Areas that showed increased signal and a correlation with rush ratings were nucleus accumbens/subcallosal cortex, the right parahippocampal gyrus, and some regions of the lateral prefrontal cortex (Breiter et al., 1997). This study was able to demonstrate that cocaine administration results in a dynamically changing brain network that is associated with euphoria and craving.

Residual cerebrovascular effects of heavy cocaine use

With the advent of the use of free-base cocaine (crack) in 1983, the number of reports of cocaine-related ischemic and hemorrhagic strokes increased dramatically (Daras, Tuchman, & Marks, 1991; Klonoff, Andrews, & Obana, 1989; Kosten, 1998; Levine & Welch, 1988; Levine et al., 1990, 1991; Sloan & Mattioni, 1992). While hemorrhagic strokes are more likely to occur in cocaine abusers who have preexisting risk factors for stroke (i.e. arteriovenous malformations, vascular disease, cardiac sources of emboli), the presence of an underlying structural lesion is not a necessary factor for the occurrence of other types of strokes. In some cases, sudden increases in arterial pressure occurring in already constricted vessels might be enough to cause hemorrhagic strokes. Other neurological abnormalities that might be secondary or concurrent with cocaine-induced vascular accidents include new-onset seizures (Sanchez-Ramos, 1993).

To determine possible causes for the increased incidence of strokes in abstinent crack users, Herning, King, Better, and Cadet (1999) used transcranial Doppler sonography to assess neurovascular functioning. Blood flow velocities were reduced in the middle and anterior cerebral arteries. Furthermore, the pulsatility index, a measure of vasoconstriction, was increased in cocaine users relative to controls at 72 hours of abstinence. These effects persisted even after 28 days of abstinence from drug use. These findings identify cocaine-induced vasoconstriction that persists for at least a month after cessation of cocaine administration.

The distribution of these changes in vascular resistance in the anterior cerebral artery provides a partial explanation for the observation that the prefrontal lobe appears to be especially vulnerable to cocaine-induced vascular accidents. Other factors, such as the vasoconstrictive actions of cocaine and the cocaine metabolites, benzoylecgonine (Powers & Madden, 1990) and norcocaine (Isner & Chokshi, 1989), also contribute to the increased incidence of ischemic strokes in cocaine users. Cocaine-induced vasoconstriction could result in cellular damage via production of oxygen-based radicals generated during the period of reperfusion in a manner similar to hypoxia-induced neuronal apoptosis.

Residual cognitive effects of chronic cocaine use

The findings from studies characterizing the neuropsychological sequelae of heavy cocaine use are equivocal. Some studies report deficits on measures of psychomotor speed, basic motor functioning, abstract reasoning, visual and verbal learning and memory, attention, and executive functioning (Azrin, Millsaps, Schneider, & Mittenberg, 1995; Block, Erwin, & Ghoneim, 2002; Bolla, Rothman, & Cadet, 1999; Manschreck et al., 1990; Meek, Clark, & Solana, 1989; Melamed & Bleiberg, 1986; Mittenberg & Motta, 1993; Negrete & Murphy, 1967; O'Malley, Adamse, Heaton, & Gawin, 1992; Rosselli, Ardila, Lubomski, Murray, & King, 2001; Selby, Azrin, Ireland, & Morgan, 1995; Smelson, Roy, Santana, & Engelhart, 1999), whereas others report minimal effects (Coffey, Dansky, Carrigan, & Brady, 2000; Tumeh et al., 1991; Volkow et al., 1992; Weber et al., 1990). Interestingly, there have also been reports of better performance in cocaine users relative to a control group on measures of motor speed (finger tapping) and visual learning and memory (Bolla et al., 1999; Hoff et al., 1991; O'Malley et al., 1992).

The discrepancies in the findings across studies most likely occurred as a result of the following factors: differences in the amount and/or duration of cocaine use, route of administration of cocaine (i.e., smoking versus snorting), the length of abstinence when tested, sensitivity of the neuropsychological tests administered, lack of a control group, a poorly matched control group, small sample size, and/or poor control for factors such as severity of depression, age, estimated premorbid level of intelligence, sex distribution, and personality characteristics (e.g., Antisocial Personality Disorder). In studies using similar methods that controlled for these factors, decrements in neurocognitive performance have been reported consistently. For example, in 4-week-abstinent cocaine abusers, after controlling for age, education, and intellectual ability, amount of cocaine used (grams per week) was associated with dose-related decrements on tests measuring executive/

attention functioning, impulsivity, visuoperception, psychomotor speed, manual dexterity, and verbal learning and memory (Bolla, Funderburk, & Cadet, 2000b; Bolla et al., 1999). Of note, deficits were only observed in the heaviest cocaine users (> 4 grams per week).

In a novel attempt to control for intellectual premorbid functioning, performance on the Iowa Test of Achievement in the fourth grade was used to equate a group of nondrug-using controls with a 3-month-abstinent drug-using group (Block et al., 2002). Drug users who used other drugs in addition to cocaine showed poorer Iowa Test scores in the fourth grade compared to the controls, demonstrating that premorbid intellectual ability may be associated with onset of cocaine use. After controlling for premorbid intellectual functioning, deficits on measures of memory and abstraction persisted even after 3 months of abstinence. Few improvements were observed over this 3-month period.

Other well-controlled prospective studies have reported persistent cognitive decrements in abstinent cocaine users. Even after up to 6 months of abstinence, cognitive deficits have been reported in executive functioning, spatial processing, memory, concentration, and motor function (Ardila, Rosselli, & Strumwasser, 1991; Di, Tolou-Shams, Price, & Fein, 2002; O'Malley & Gawin, 1990; O'Malley et al., 1992). Some studies have even shown a dose-related effect between cognitive performance and amount and duration of cocaine use (Bolla et al., 1999; Di et al., 2002). Thus, neurocognitive deficits associated with cocaine use appear to be dose-related and persistent even after 6 months of abstinence.

In studies conducted to examine the relationship between changes in cognitive function with increasing length of abstinence, mixed results were reported. van Gorp and colleagues (van Gorp et al., 1999) conducted a 45-day longitudinal study in abstinent cocaine-dependent individuals and matched controls. Both the cocaine and control groups improved their performance to the same degree on a test of verbal learning and memory, however the controls improved more than the drug-using group on a test of nonverbal declarative memory test. On a motor control task the cocaine group improved more because the control group showed a ceiling effect. Another study of outpatient 28-day abstinent cocaine abusers also showed linear improvements over time in affect, craving, and cognitive abilities (Coffey et al., 2000).

Interpreted collectively, studies on the neurocognitive effects of chronic cocaine abuse suggest that the long-term neurological sequelae of chronic cocaine abuse may be subtle and specific, rather than general. Problems with executive functioning (attention/planning/mental flexibility) are the most frequently reported cognitive difficulties. This cognitive domain relates primarily to the functional integrity of the frontal lobe (Lezak, 1995; Ohnishi et al., 1995; Stuss & Benson, 1986). In fact, performance on a classical test of frontal lobe function, the Stroop, correlates with changes in cerebral metabolism and blood flow in the ACC in heavy cocaine users (Bolla et al., 2004; Strickland et al., 1993; Volkow et al., 1993).

In the last 5 years, a subset of researchers has focused on the connection between decision-making impairments and vulnerability to substance abuse/dependence (Bechara & Damasio, 2002; Monterosso, Ehrman, Napier, O'Brien, & Childress, 2001). For example, impairments in decision-making have been reported in cocaine users (Bartzokis et al., 2000; Bolla et al., 2003a; Grant, Contoreggi, & London, 2000; Monterosso et al., 2001). The precise link between decision-making defects and cocaine use has not been defined; however, it is reasonable to speculate that there is an association.

Structural changes associated with chronic cocaine use

Abnormalities in brain structure and tissue composition have been reported in chronic cocaine abusers (Amass, Nardin, Mendelson, Teoh, & Woods, 1992; Bartzokis et al., 2000; Franklin et al., 2002; Langendorf et al., 1996; Liu, Matochik, Cadet, & London, 1998; Matochik, London, Eldreth, Cadet, & Bolla, 2003; Pascual-Leone, Dhuna, & Anderson, 1991). When computerized tomography measurements of habitual cocaine abusers were compared to those of first-time users and controls, habitual users had a greater degree of cerebral atrophy that correlated with duration of cocaine abuse on one measure (maximal frontal horn width) (Pascual-Leone et al., 1991). Polysubstance users who reported that cocaine was their drug of choice had smaller total volume of the bilateral prefrontal lobe (Liu et al., 1998). Similarly, a relatively new technique called voxel-based morphometry (VBM) showed lower grey matter tissue density in the insula, temporal cortex, and frontal regions, including the ACC (infragenual and perigenual regions) and medial and lateral OFC relative to a nondrug-using comparison group (Franklin et al., 2002; Matochik et al., 2003). Interestingly, Matochik and colleagues (2003) found structural abnormalities in the same regions that showed alterations in rCBF (PET: $H_2^{15}O$) in the same 25-day-abstinent cocaine users (Bolla et al., 2003b, 2004). Duration of cocaine use was also correlated with lower white matter density in the left and right subgyral frontal white matter.

These observations support the work of Bartzokis et al. (2002), who suggested that brain maturation may be arrested in chronic cocaine users such that the positive correlation that is normally found between white matter volume and age in the temporal and frontal lobes in normal individuals (Bartzokis et al., 2001) was absent in cocaine users (Bartzokis et al., 2002). When diffusion tensor imaging was used to specifically examine the integrity of white matter in frontal brain regions in cocaine dependence, cocaine users showed compromised white matter integrity in the inferior frontal brain regions (Lim, Choi, Pomara, Wolkin, & Rotrosen, 2002). These findings are consistent with the idea that cocaine dependence involves alterations in OFC connectivity and supports the idea that cocaine abuse is associated with the development of a cerebral deconnection syndrome (Geschwind & Kaplan, 1998).

As previously suggested, cocaine-associated structural abnormalities might be due to cocaine-induced vasoconstriction and secondary ischemia and cortical atrophy. In cases where there might be shrinkage without cell death, these neurological effects of cocaine may be partially reversible with abstinence (Kosten et al., 1998; Langendorf et al., 1996). Nevertheless, these vascular and structural abnormalities might form some of the substrates for the cognitive deficits observed in cocaine-addicted patients, as described below.

The psychology of cocaine dependence/abuse

Emotional functioning and personality disorders

Cocaine dependence is associated with a variety of changes in affect and personality, some of which are short-lived and others are relatively permanent. For example, the depressed mood reportedly associated with cocaine withdrawal may account for a portion of the cognitive difficulties found in chronic cocaine abusers (Gawin & Kleber, 1986; Hoff et al., 1991). Those heavy cocaine users that remained depressed following withdrawal showed decreased blood flow in the left frontal lobe as measured using SPECT (Gunnarsdottir et al., 2000), a pattern similar to that found in Major Depressive Disorder (Drevets et al., 1997).

There are numerous reports of comorbid personality disorders in heavy cocaine users. For example, Antisocial Personality Disorder (ASPD) has frequently been reported in cocaine abusers (Rosselli et al., 2001). In some studies, the presence of ASPD was associated with poorer cognitive function (Stein, Hollander, & Cohen, 1993) whereas another study found no association between personality profile and cognition in a subgroup of the cocaine abusers studied (Rosselli et al., 2001). Since the prefrontal cortex may be intimately involved in heavy cocaine use, it may be especially important to study ASPD in cocaine abusers because a relationship between ASPD and frontal lobe dysfunction has been demonstrated using neuropsychological testing (Stein et al., 1993) and event-related potentials (Bauer, O'Connor, & Hesselbrock, 1994).

Physiological and psychological withdrawal

Cocaine withdrawal is associated with alterations in physiological and psychological functioning. It is likely that disturbances in monoaminergic systems and/or in specific brain regions that regulate drive and affect also underlie, at least to some degree, the neuropsychiatric abnormalities, such as cognitive impairment, emotional disturbances, and craving, reported by a subset of heavy cocaine users during withdrawal (Dackis & Gold, 1985; Volkow et al., 1988, 1993). For example, individuals in acute withdrawal from cocaine report cravings that are strongly associated with hypermetabolism in the OFC and other prefrontal cortices (Volkow et al., 1991). Although it is not possible to directly measure the levels of brain monoamines in abstinent cocaine abusers, there seems to be a relationship between decreased D2 receptor availability and decreased glucose metabolism in several frontal brain regions, particularly the OFC and cingulate gyri (ACC) (Volkow et al., 1993). In addition, decreased D2 receptor availability has been reported to be related to years of cocaine abuse. Decreased D2 receptor availability could reflect downregulation of postsynaptic D2 receptors in response to repeated elevations in synaptic dopamine when cocaine is administered (Volkow et al., 1993). With abstinence from cocaine, metabolic abnormalities were found in the OFC and ACC, brain regions that receive dopaminergic afferents (Volkow et al., 1993).

Because neurotransmitter-mediated dysregulation of the prefrontal cortex and limbic system is associated with alterations in CBF and glucose metabolism in the OFC and ACC, the overall reinforcing and addictive properties of cocaine may be related to functional alterations in these brain structures. For example, the repeated use of cocaine may result in cocaine-induced dopaminergic overstimulation of systems that subsume reward and other affective and cognitive pathways, whereas acute cessation of drug administration might lead to activation of the OFC and other prefrontal brain regions with subsequent or co-incident increases in the drive to repeatedly self-administer cocaine; however, with more prolonged abstinences from cocaine use, these regions might become hypometabolic. Subsequent administration of cocaine could then reactivate these frontal brain regions, resulting in the vicious cycle of compulsive cocaine self-administration. The presence of disconnected interhemispheric and intrahemispheric pathways would also make it difficult to control these compulsive self-destructive acts.

Craving

It is critical to determine the physical and psychological mechanisms of craving to understand treatment relapse in the drug abusers. Heavy cocaine users are hypersensitive to environmental cues that relate to their cocaine use. Initial findings suggest that neuropsychological abnormalities are associated with increased levels of craving. For example, a relationship was found between attentional bias, obsessive thoughts about cocaine, and craving, such that slower reaction times were observed on cocaine-related cues in contrast to neutral cues for cocaine users who had more obsessive thoughts about cocaine and who reported higher craving (Franken, Kroon, & Hendriks, 2000). When cocaine users were kept in an inpatient setting for 4 weeks, cocaine cues also produced alterations in mood, increased craving, and increases in physiological arousal (Childress, Ehrman, McLellan, & O'Brien, 1988; Robbins, Joyce, & Sahakian, 1992). Also, if cocaine cues are presented during a negative mood state, the cocaine-dependent outpatients report higher levels of craving and withdrawal before and after exposure to the cue (Robbins, Ehrman, Childress, Cornish, & O'Brien, 2000).

Residual alterations in metabolic function associated with heavy cocaine use and functional neuroimaging (PET)

Over the last decade, functional neuroimaging has been utilized to characterize the brain alterations that occur as a result of heavy cocaine use. For example, in abstinent chronic cocaine abusers, resting FDG-PET scans showed that cerebral glucose metabolism was higher in the medial orbitofrontal cortex and basal ganglia during the first week of abstinence from cocaine as compared with metabolism in normal subjects, but then fell below normal levels for at least the next 3–6 months (Kosten et al., 1998; Volkow et al., 1991, 1992, 1993). In cocaine abusers who were abstinent for 1–6 weeks, glucose utilization also correlated mildly with an estimate of weekly dose of cocaine and years of cocaine use (Volkow et al., 1992). Nevertheless, the relationship between magnitude of cocaine use and decreases in frontal lobe metabolism suggests that the use of cocaine contributes to alterations in brain metabolism.

Compared to studies measuring metabolic glucose activity, studies of rCBF showed similar, although not identical, defects in prefrontal cortex in abstinent cocaine abusers (Mena et al., 1990; Tumeh et al., 1991; Volkow et al., 1988). During the first 10 days of abstinence, rCBF was decreased in the prefrontal cortex (Volkow et al., 1988) and remained depressed when scanned at 3 weeks of abstinence (Kosten et al., 1998). These rCBF deficits could reflect vasospasm in cerebral arteries exposed chronically to the sympathomimetic actions of cocaine (Volkow et al., 1988). Greater deficits are observed in rCBF than in glucose utilization when both are examined in the same cocaine-abusing individual (Volkow et al., 1988). The discrepancy may reflect the direct actions of cocaine on cerebral vessels. In one of the few studies that attempted to correlate a behavior measure (Bechara, Damasio, Damasio, & Anderson, 1994) with brain activation, 21–55-day-abstinent cocaine users ($n = 13$) showed a correlation between *resting* ACC and left DLPFC blood flow using SPECT and performance on the Iowa Gambling Task (Adinoff et al., 2003). However, no correlation was found between task performance and baseline or resting rCBF in the OFC. The absence of a correlation is probably related to the use of *resting* state instead of an *activation* state and small sample size. Left DLPFC was lower in the cocaine users relative to a comparison group. The results of a number of studies appear to be consistent: heavy cocaine users have metabolic abnormalities in prefrontal brain regions. Frontal lobe deficits in rCBF may be related to selective sensitivity to cocaine in the anterior and middle cerebral arteries.

In contrast to resting state studies, there are a few published papers that utilized activation protocols involving cocaine cues in studies of cocaine users. For example, an FDG-PET activation study showed that exposure to cocaine-related cues was associated with increased levels of self-reported craving and activation of a number of brain regions, including the temporal lobe, DLPFC, and medial OFC (Bonson et al., 2002; Grant et al., 1996).

Furthermore, self-reports of craving were positively correlated with metabolic increases in the DLPFC, medial temporal lobe (amygdala), and the cerebellum. Childress et al. (1999) used assays of rCBF with an $H_2^{15}O$-labeled water radiotracer to investigate the response to exposure to cocaine-related and neutral videotapes in heavy cocaine users. Self-reported increased craving accompanied increases in limbic (amygdala and ACC) rCBF and decreases in basal ganglia rCBF. Using fMRI, Maas and colleagues (1998) showed that exposure to cocaine-related cues was associated with significant activation in the ACC and left DLPFC (but not the amygdala) in the cocaine users. Additionally, self-reported levels of craving were correlated with activation in these regions. In conclusion, both cortical and limbic subcortical regions activate when exposed to cocaine cues. These regions include portions of the temporal lobe, the DLPFC, and the OFC. Brain regions that are correlated with self-reports of craving include the amygdala (Childress et al., 1999; Grant et al., 1996; Maas et al., 1998), DLPFC (Grant et al., 1996; Maas et al., 1998), cerebellum (Grant et al., 1996), and the ACC (Childress et al., 1999; Weinstein et al., 1998).

To date, there are few studies that utilized a cognitive task activation paradigm to investigate the association between neuropsychological impairments and neuroanatomical abnormalities in chronic cocaine users. In one study, a $H_2^{15}O$ rCBF PET imaging cognitive activation paradigm was used in heavy cocaine users who were abstinent for 25 days. Image acquisition occurred during the administration of a decision-making task (Bechara et al., 1994) that was used specifically to activate the OFC (Bolla et al., 2003a). Cocaine abusers showed greater activation in the right OFC and less activation in the right DLPFC and left medial prefrontal cortex compared to a control group. Better task performance was associated with greater activation in the right OFC in both groups. Grams per week of cocaine used were negatively correlated with activation in the left OFC. The results of this study are shown in Figure 4.3. These results are in contrast with those of Adinoff et al. (2003), who failed to find a correlation between Iowa Gambling Task performance and resting rCBF in the OFC. In contrast with resting state studies, activation studies are, by nature, dynamic and therefore capture changes that would not be captured by a resting state protocol.

Greater activation in the cocaine group relative to the controls was thought to reflect differences in the anticipation of reward, while less activation in the DLPFC and MPFC was interpreted to reflect differences in planning and working memory. The same group of cocaine users was also scanned while they performed a modified version of the Stroop test that was selected to engage the ACC and DLPFC (Bolla et al., 2004). Heavy cocaine users showed less activation in the left ACC and the right LPFC and greater activation in the right ACC than nondrug users. Collectively, these results show that heavy cocaine users have persistent disruption of prefrontal cortical functions even after almost 4 weeks of abstinence. These alterations occurred in brain regions that control executive functions, including

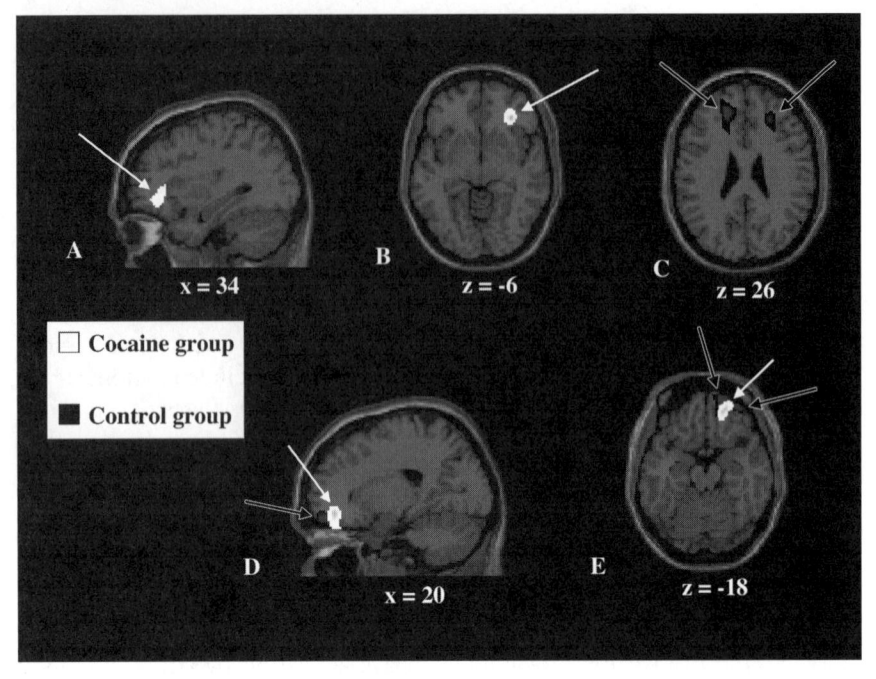

Figure 4.3 Sagittal and axial views of the brain. Cocaine abusers showed more activation than controls in the right orbitofrontal cortex (A, B) and less activation than controls in the right dorsolateral prefrontal cortex and left medial prefrontal cortex (C) during performance on the Iowa Gambling Task (active task minus control task). (D, E) Significant correlation between better performance on the Iowa Gambling Task and greater activation in the right medial orbitofrontal cortex in the cocaine abusers and control group. (Reprinted from Bolla et al. (2003a) with permission from Elsevier.)

decision-making, and could interfere with attempts to stop drug use and undermine treatment.

Functional magnetic resonance imaging (fMRI)

Functional MRI is a relatively new technique. As a result, there are few published studies using samples of heavy cocaine users. In the few studies that have been conducted in cocaine users, the results are similar to those found with PET and SPECT. To test whether cocaine craving was related to a dedicated neural circuit, cue-induced cocaine craving was explored in cocaine users (Garavan et al., 2000). Of 13 brain regions identified as possible integral sites for craving, only three (ACC, right inferior parietal lobe, and caudate/ lateral dorsal nucleus) showed greater activation while viewing a cocaine film than while viewing a film with explicit sexual content. These findings suggest that cocaine users activate similar anatomical substrates for evocative stimuli, irrespective of the content (i.e., cocaine cues and sexual content). Larger responses to the sexually explicit scenes were observed in the nondrug users. The authors concluded that cocaine acts on normal reward/emotional circuitry and that cocaine craving is related to users' memory of the reinforcing effects of cocaine (Garavan et al., 2000).

Disassociation between neuroimaging activation maps and neurocognitive performance

It is surprising that heavy cocaine users may show persistent changes in brain metabolism and structure with no detectable neurocognitive effects. For example, few neurocognitive effects were found in heavy cocaine users even though they showed significantly decreased rCBF in specific regions of the prefrontal lobe (Bolla et al., 2004; Tumeh et al., 1991; Volkow et al., 1988; Weber et al., 1990). This paradoxical finding is reported often when neuroimaging is used in combination with measures of neurobehavioral performance. There are a number of explanations for this phenomenon, including:

(1) Alternate neural substrates are used to perform the task adequately.
(2) Under conditions of decreased CBF, there are compensatory increases in the rate of oxygen extraction which may overcome performance difficulties (Wide et al., 1983).
(3) The neurobehavioral performance measures may have been flawed in some way when the behavioral task was adapted to conform to the limitations of the scanner environment.
(4) Traditionally, the number of subjects included in an imaging study is small (3–15) compared to studies that examine neurocognitive performance as the primary outcome. Thus, while the statistical power is ample for detecting metabolic changes, it may not be sufficient for detecting behavioral differences.

Combination of alcohol and cocaine

Not surprisingly, many heavy cocaine users also use other substances, including alcohol. At present, it is unclear whether the interaction of alcohol and cocaine is associated with greater levels of neuropsychological impairment than cocaine alone. Most studies have found that the interaction of the two substances is associated with greater neuropsychological impairment (Bolla et al., 2000b; Carroll, Rounsaville, & Bryant, 1993; Pennings, Leccese, & Wolff, 2002; Selby & Azrin, 1998), though other studies have not (Easton & Bauer, 1997; Higgins, Budney, Bickel, Foerg, & Badger, 1994; Robinson, Heaton, & O'Malley, 1999). These additive, dose-related effects were apparent at 1–3 days of abstinence and persisted even after 4 weeks of abstinence (Bolla, Funderburk, & Cadet, 2000a). The cognitive domains that were most affected were short- and long-term memory and visual motor functions

(Selby & Azrin, 1998). Additional evidence supporting the conclusion that the combination of alcohol and cocaine has more negative effects than either substance alone comes from a neuroimaging study showing that additional reductions in rCBF are observed when both alcohol and cocaine were used (Kosten et al., 1998).

The mechanism for the negative effects associated with the combination of alcohol and cocaine is believed to involve the formation of cocaethylene that acts as a potent neurotoxin. As mentioned previously, some studies have reported fewer effects with the combined use of cocaine and alcohol (Easton & Bauer, 1997; Higgins et al., 1994; Robinson et al., 1999). One explanation for these findings most likely involves confounding differences in drug administration and dose. For example, those using large amounts of cocaine may use less alcohol, and vice versa. Since most drug abusers use combinations of drugs, this area deserves further research.

Treatment

To date, two studies have investigated the association between neuropsychological functioning and treatment outcome. Aharonovich, Nunes, and Hasin (2003) found that those who completed cognitive–behavioral treatment (completers) had better cognitive performance at baseline in all cognitive domains, assessed by a computerized reaction time battery, than noncompleters. The cognitive domains that seemed to be the most predictive of treatment outcome included attention, reasoning, and spatial processing. In addition, treatment completers were more accurate and performed faster than treatment non-completers. In contrast, other investigators have found no neuropsychological differences between relapsers and nonrelapsers (Di et al., 2002).

Another line of investigation with important treatment implications involves individual differences in cerebral perfusion. There is preliminary evidence from a report of two cases that cerebral perfusion during early abstinence from cocaine may correlate with the ability to learn information which would prove beneficial for cognitive–behavioral therapy (Gottschalk, Beauvais, Hart, & Kosten, 2001). This conclusion is based on the finding that these cases demonstrated an association between response to cognitive–behavioral therapy (CBT) and improvement in cerebral perfusion. One could then speculate that early screening of brain function (i.e., cerebral perfusion) in treatment-seeking cocaine abusers could discriminate treatment responders. These results need to be replicated and extended.

Conclusions

The accumulated evidence supports the notion that chronic heavy cocaine use is associated with alterations in neurocognitive function, brain metabolism, and brain structure, most notably in the prefrontal cortex. Nevertheless, it remains to be determined whether heavy cocaine use is a result of a dysfunctional brain or cocaine acts as a neurotoxicant to cause brain dysfunction. Evidence that heavy cocaine use contributes, at least partly, to the development of neurobehavioral difficulties comes from studies showing a negative relationship between test scores and amount and duration of cocaine use, and between test scores and length of abstinence (Ardila et al., 1991; Bolla et al., 1999; Di et al., 2002; Mittenberg & Motta, 1993). It is also very likely that drug abusers might demonstrate some premorbid differences from nonsubstance abusers (Block et al., 2002). Factors that may predispose an individual to heavy cocaine use include lower intellectual abilities, attention problems (ADHD), impulsivity, ASPD, major depression, and schizophrenia.

Although one needs to consider the possibility that the existence of neurological impairment in these patients might antedate their cocaine use, the determination of cause and effect appears to be irrelevant from a clinical perspective if one is attempting to develop treatment strategies that might overcome the behavioral manifestations of existing neuropathological abnormalities. Finally, it is important to continue to explore the basic and clinical neurobiology of cocaine use because greater understanding of the neurological underpinnings of cocaine use should translate into better prevention and treatment of cocaine dependence/abuse. In turn, this knowledge can then be generalized to those who abuse substances other than cocaine.

Future directions

While previous work shows abnormalities in cerebral blood flow and metabolism in abstinent cocaine abusers, few have attempted to directly examine the behavioral correlates of these alterations in functional brain activity. In addition, there are only a few published studies that have used a cognitive activation task during PET scan or fMRI acquisition to increase the sensitivity and specificity of detecting subtle brain changes in heavy cocaine users. Studies of this type are critical to identify the neurobiological bases of behavioral deficits seen in cocaine abusers.

Cognitive deficits in cocaine abusers, specifically in the area of executive functioning (i.e., attention), may perpetuate addictive behavior by making self-monitoring and changing inappropriate behaviors difficult. Hence, a heavy cocaine user with these deficits would likely fail attempts to discontinue self-destructive, drug-seeking behavior. It is also paramount to identify specific executive processing deficits associated with heavy cocaine use. For example, if cocaine abusers have deficits in executive function, are these related to difficulties with sustained attention, divided attention, planning, or the use of feedback to change incorrect current behavior to subsequent correct behavior? Multiple neurocognitive tests measuring slightly different aspects of executive functioning should be developed and utilized in order to answer this question. Knowledge of specific deficits of cognitive processing in chronic cocaine users would prove helpful in designing appropriate drug treatment programs. In addition, knowledge of strengths and weaknesses in other cognitive domains, such as motor speed, could ultimately guide vocational rehabilitation programs to integrate unemployed individuals, who have suffered from uncontrolled heavy cocaine use, into the work force.

Assessment of neurocognitive strengths and weaknesses in chronic cocaine users has significant clinical utility. While neurocognitive assessment prior to the initiation of treatment is far from routine, the importance of obtaining a baseline level of cognitive and intellectual functioning is beginning to be realized. For example, deficits in attention could be a major factor when the cocaine user is expected to sustain attention during a 50- or 60-minute therapy session. Poor memory could make consolidation of the treatment material difficult. Executive function impairment would make it difficult to apply coping strategies to resist the impulse to use cocaine.

The association between neuropsychological functioning and treatment outcome is an area of investigation that holds paramount importance for the development of better treatments for cocaine abusers. Although most treatment centers do not screen for neuropsychological deficits prior to starting treatment, these assessments should be mandatory because intact cognitive abilities such as memory, decision-making, verbal skills, and abstract problem-solving are necessary for maximum benefit from treatment. As a result of the recent paradigm shift that posits addictive processes as a "brain disorder," new therapeutic efforts hold greater promises for those who abuse cocaine as well as those who abuse other illicit substances.

References

Adinoff, B., Devous, M. D., Sr., Cooper, D. B., Best, S. E., Chandler, P., Harris, T. et al. (2003). Resting regional cerebral blood flow and gambling task performance in cocaine-dependent subjects and healthy comparison subjects. *American Journal of Psychiatry*, *160*, 1892–1894.

Aharonovich, E., Nunes, E., & Hasin, D. (2003). Cognitive impairment, retention and abstinence among cocaine abusers in cognitive–behavioral treatment. *Drug and Alcohol Dependence*, *71*, 207–211.

Amara, S. G., & Kuhar, M. J. (1993). Neurotransmitter transporters: recent progress. *Annual Review of Neuroscience*, *16*, 73–93.

Amass, L., Nardin, R., Mendelson, J. H., Teoh, S. K., & Woods, B. T. (1992). Quantitative magnetic resonance imaging in heroin- and cocaine-dependent men: a preliminary study. *Psychiatry Research*, *45*, 15–23.

Ardila, A., Rosselli, M., & Strumwasser, S. (1991). Neuropsychological deficits in chronic cocaine abusers. *International Journal of Neuroscience*, *57*, 73–79.

Azrin, R. L., Millsaps, C., Schneider, B., & Mittenberg, W. (1995). Abstinent cocaine abusers' neuropsychological functioning on the SMW-R and WAIS-R. *Clinical Neuropsychology*, *9*, 289.

Bartzokis, G., Beckson, M., Lu, P. H., Edwards, N., Bridge, P., & Mintz, J. (2002).

Brain maturation may be arrested in chronic cocaine addicts. *Biological Psychiatry, 51*, 605–611.

Bartzokis, G., Beckson, M., Lu, P. H., Nuechterlein, K. H., Edwards, N., & Mintz, J. (2001). Age-related changes in frontal and temporal lobe volumes in men: a magnetic resonance imaging study. *Archives of General Psychiatry, 58*, 461–465.

Bartzokis, G., Lu, P. H., Beckson, M., Rapoport, R., Grant, S., Wiseman, E. J., et al. (2000). Abstinence from cocaine reduces high-risk responses on a gambling task. *Neuropsychopharmacology, 22*, 102–103.

Bauer, L. O., O'Connor, S., & Hesselbrock, V. M. (1994). Frontal P300 decrements in antisocial personality disorder. *Alcoholism: Clinical and Experimental Research, 18*, 1300–1305.

Baxter, L. R. J., Phelps, M. E., Mazziotta, J. C., Guze, B. H., Schwartz, J. M., & Selin, C. E. (1987). Local cerebral glucose metabolic rates in obsessive–compulsive disorder: A comparison with rates in unipolar depression and in normal controls. *Archives of General Psychiatry, 44*, 211–218.

Bechara, A., Damasio, A. R., Damasio, H., & Anderson, S. W. (1994). Insensitivity to future consequences following damage to human prefrontal cortex. *Cognition, 50*, 7–15.

Bechara, A., & Damasio, H. (2002). Decision-making and addiction (part I): impaired activation of somatic states in substance dependent individuals when pondering decisions with negative future consequences. *Neuropsychologia, 40*, 1675–1689.

Benkelfat, C., Nordahl, T. E., Semple, W. E., King, A. C., Murphy, D. L., & Cohen, R. M. (1990). Local cerebral glucose metabolic rates in Obsessive–Compulsive Disorder: Patients treated with Clomipramine. *Archives of General Psychiatry, 47*, 840–848.

Bergman, J., Madras, B. K., Johnson, S. E., & Spealman, R. D. (1989). Effects of cocaine and related drugs in nonhuman primates. III. Self-administration by squirrel monkeys. *Journal of Pharmacology and Experimental Therapeutics, 251*, 150–155.

Biegon, A., Dillon, K. A., Volkow, N. D., Hitzemann, R. J., Fowler, J. S., & Wolf, A. P. (1992). Quantitative autoradiography of cocaine binding sites in human brain postmortem. *Synapse, 10*, 126–130.

Block, R. I., Erwin, W. J., & Ghoneim, M. M. (2002). Chronic drug use and cognitive impairments. *Pharmacology, Biochemistry and Behavior, 73*, 491–504.

Bolla, K., Eldreth, D., London, E. D., Kiehl, K. A., Mouratidis, M., Contoreggi, C., et al. (2003a). Orbitofrontal cortex dysfunction in abstinent cocaine abusers performing a decision-making task. *NeuroImage, 19*, 1085–1094.

Bolla, K. I., Cadet, J.-L., & London, E. D. (1998). The neuropsychiatry of chronic cocaine use. *Journal of Neuropsychology and Clinical Neurosciences, 10*, 280–289.

Bolla, K. I., Eldreth, D. A., London, E. D., Kiehl, K. A., Mouratidis, M., Contoreggi, C., et al. (2003b). Orbitofrontal cortex dysfunction in abstinent cocaine abusers performing a decision-making task. *NeuroImage, 19*, 1085–1094.

Bolla, K. I., Ernst, M., Kiehl, K. A., Mouratidis, M., Eldreth, D. A., Contereggi, C., et al. (2004). Prefrontal cortical dysfunction in abstinent cocaine abusers. *Journal of Neuropsychiatry and Clinical Neuroscience, 16*, 456–464.

Bolla, K. I., Funderburk, F. R., & Cadet, J.-L. (2000a). Differential effects of cocaine and cocaine alcohol on neurocognitive performance. *Neurology, 54*, 2285–2292.

Bolla, K. I., Funderburk, F. R., & Cadet, J.-L. (2000b). Differential effects of cocaine and cocaine + alcohol on neurocognitive performance. *Neurology, 54*, 2285–2292.

Bolla, K. I., Rothman, R. B., & Cadet, J.-L. (1999). Dose-related neurobehavioral effects of chronic cocaine use. *Journal of Neuropsychiatry and Clinical Neurosciences, 11*, 361–369.

Bonson, K. R., Grant, S., Contoreggi, C., Links, J., Metalfe, J., Weyl, L. H., et al. (2002). Neural systems and cue-induced cocaine craving. *Neuropsychopharmacology, 26*, 376–386.

Breiter, H. C., Gollub, R. L., Weisskoff, R. M., Kennedy, D. N., Makris, N., Berke, J. D., et al. (1997). Acute effects of cocaine on human brain activity and emotion. *Neuron, 19*, 591–611.

Broderick, J. P., Viscoli, C. M., Brott, T., Kernan, W. N., Brass, L. M., Feldmann, E., et al. (2003). Major risk factors for aneurysmal subarachnoid hemorrhage in the young are modifiable. *Stroke, 34*, 1375–1381.

Bush, G., Frazier, J. A., Rauch, S. L., Seidman, L. J., Whalen, P. J., Jenike, M. A., et al. (1999). Anterior cingulate cortex dysfunction in attention-deficit/hyperactivity disorder revealed by fMRI and the counting stroop. *Biological Psychiatry, 45*, 1542–1552.

Cadet, J.-L., & Bolla, K. I. (1996). Chronic cocaine use as a neuropsychiatric syndrome: A model for debate. *Synapse, 22*, 28–34.

Carroll, K. M., Rounsaville, B. J., & Bryant, K. J. (1993). Alcoholism in treatment-seeking cocaine abusers: clinical and prognostic significance. *Journal of Studies in Alcohol, 54*, 199–208.

Childress, A., Ehrman, R., McLellan, A. T., & O'Brien, C. (1988). Conditioned craving and arousal in cocaine addiction: a preliminary report. *NIDA Research Monographs, 81*, 74–80.

Childress, A. R., Mozley, P. D., McElgin, W., Fitzgerald, J., Reivich, M., & O'Brien, C. P. (1999). Limbic activation during cue-induced cocaine craving. *American Journal of Psychiatry, 156*, 11–18.

Civelli, O., Bunzow, J. R., Grandy, D. K., Zhou, Q. Y., & Vantol, H. H. M. (1991). Molecular biology of the dopamine receptors. *European Journal of Pharmacology – Molecular Pharmacology Section, 207*, 277–286.

Coffey, S. F., Dansky, B. S., Carrigan, M. H., & Brady, K. T. (2000). Acute and protracted cocaine abstinence in an outpatient population: a prospective study of mood, sleep and withdrawal symptoms. *Drug and Alcohol Dependence, 59*, 277–286.

Dackis, C. A. & Gold, M. S. (1985). New concepts in cocaine addiction: The dopamine depletion hypothesis. *Neuroscience and Behavior Review, 9*, 469.

Daras, M., Tuchman, A. J., & Marks, S. (1991). Central Nervous System infarction related to cocaine abuse. *Stroke, 22*, 1320–1325.

Des Rosiers, M. H., Kennedy, C., Patlak, C. S., Pettigrew, K. D., & Sokolov, L. (1974). Relationship between local cerebral blood flow and glucose utilization in the rat. *Neurology, 24*, 389.

Di, S. V., Tolou-Shams, M., Price, L. J., & Fein, G. (2002). Neuropsychological performance of individuals dependent on crack-cocaine, or crack-cocaine and alcohol, at 6 weeks and 6 months of abstinence. *Drug and Alcohol Dependence, 66*, 161–171.

Drevets, W. C., Price, J. L., Simpson, J. R., Jr., Todd, R. D., Reich, T., Vannier, M., et al. (1997). Subgenual prefrontal cortex abnormalities in mood disorders. *Nature, 386*, 824–827.

Dworkin, S. I., & Smith, J. E. (1992). Cortical regulation of self-administration. In P. W. Kalivanas & H. A. Samson (Eds.), *Neurobiology of drug and alcohol addiction* (p. 274). New York: New York Academy of Sciences.

Easton, C., & Bauer, L. O. (1997). Neuropsychological differences between alcohol-dependent and cocaine-dependent patients with or without problematic drinking. *Psychiatry Research, 71*, 97–103.

Franken, I. H. A., Kroon, L. Y., & Hendriks, V. M. (2000). Influence of individual differences in craving and obsessive cocaine thoughts on attentional processes in cocaine abuse patients. *Addictive Behaviors, 25*, 99–102.

Franklin, T. R., Acton, P. D., Maldjian, J. A., Gray, J. D., Croft, J. R., Dackis, C. A., et al. (2002). Decreased gray matter concentration in the insular, orbitofrontal, cingulate, and temporal cortices of cocaine patients. *Biological Psychiatry, 51*, 134–142.

Garavan, H., Pankiewicz, J., Bloom, A., Cho, J. K., Sperry, L., Ross, T. J., et al. (2000). Cue-induced cocaine craving: neuroanatomical specificity for drug users and drug stimuli. *American Journal of Psychiatry, 157*, 1789–1798.

Gawin, F. H., & Kleber, H. D. (1986). Abstinence symptomatology and psychiatric diagnosis in cocaine abusers. Clinical observations. *Archives of General Psychiatry, 43*, 107–113.

Geschwind, N., & Kaplan, E. (1998). A human cerebral deconnection syndrome: a preliminary report. 1962. *Neurology, 50*, 1201.

Goeders, N. E. (2002). Stress and cocaine addiction. *Journal of Pharmacology and Experimental Therapeutics, 301*, 785–789.

Goldstein, R. Z., & Volkow, N. D. (2002). Drug addiction and its underlying neurobiological basis: neuroimaging evidence for the involvement of the frontal cortex. *American Journal of Psychiatry, 159*, 1642–1652.

Gottschalk, C., Beauvais, J., Hart, R., & Kosten, T. (2001). Cognitive function and cerebral perfusion during cocaine abstinence. *American Journal of Psychiatry, 158*, 540–545.

Grant, S., Contoreggi, C., & London, E. D. (2000). Drug abusers show impaired performance in a laboratory test of decision-making. *Neuropsychologia, 38*, 1180–1187.

Grant, S., London, E. D., Newlin, D. B., Villemagne, V. L., Liu, X., Contoreggi, C., et al. (1996). Activation of memory circuits during cue-elicited cocaine craving. *Proceedings of the National Academy of Sciences, 93*, 12040–12045.

Gunnarsdottir, E. D., Pingitore, R. A., Spring, B. J., Konopka, L. M., Crayton, J. W., Milo, T., et al. (2000). Individual differences among cocaine users. *Addictive Behaviors, 25*, 641–652.

Herning, R. I., King, D. E., Better, W. E., & Cadet, J.-L. (1999). Neurovascular deficits in cocaine abusers. *Neuropsychopharmacology, 21*, 110–118.

Higgins, S. T., Bickel, W. K., Hughes, J. R., Lynn, M., Capeless, M. A., & Fenwick, J. W. (1990). Effects of intranasal cocaine on human learning, performance and physiology. *Psychopharmacology (Berlin), 102*, 451–458.

Higgins, S. T., Budney, A. J., Bickel, W. K., Foerg, F. E., & Badger, G. J. (1994). Alcohol dependence and simultaneous cocaine and alcohol use in cocaine-dependent patients. *Journal of Addictive Diseases, 13*, 177–189.

Hoff, A. L., Riordan, H., Alpert, R., & Volkow, N. (1991). Cognitive function in chronic cocaine abusers. *Journal of Clinical and Experimental Neuropsychology, 13*, 60.

Holman, B. L., Mendelson, J., Garada, B., Teoh, S. K., Hallgring, E., Johnson, K. A., et al. (1993). Regional cerebral blood flow improves with treatment in chronic cocaine polydrug users. *Journal of Nuclear Medicine, 34*, 723–727.

Hurd, Y. L., Kehr, J., & Ungerstedt, U. (1988). In vivo microdialysis as a technique to monitor drug transport: correlation of extracellular cocaine levels and dopamine overflow in the rat brain. *Journal of Neurochemistry, 51,* 1314–1316.

Ingvar, D. H., & Lassen, N. A. (1979). Activity distribution in the cerebral cortex in organic dementia as revealed by measurements of regional cerebral blood flow. In F. Hochmeister & C. Muller (Eds.), *Brain function in old age* (pp. 268–277). New York: Springer Verlag.

Isner, J. M., & Chokshi, S. K. (1989). Cocaine and vasospasm. *New England Journal of Medicine, 321,* 1604–1606.

Johanson, C. E., & Fischman, M. W. (1989). The pharmacology of cocaine related to its abuse. *Pharmacological Reviews, 41,* 3–52.

Johnson, B., Overton, D., Wells, L., Kenny, P., Abramson, D., Dhother, S., et al. (1998). Effects of acute intravenous cocaine on cardiovascular function, human learning, and performance in cocaine addicts. *Psychiatry Research, 77,* 35–42.

Johnson, B. A., Oldman, D., Goodall, E. M., Chen, Y. R., & Cowen, P. J. (1996). Effects of GR 68755 on D-amphetamine-induced changes in mood, cognitive performance, appetite, food preferences, and caloric and macronutrient intake in humans. *Behavioral Pharmacology, 6,* 216–227.

Kaufman, M. J., Levin, J. M., Ross, M. H., Lange, N., Rose, S. L., Kukes, T. J., et al. (1998). Cocaine-induced cerebral vasoconstriction detected in humans with magnetic resonance angiography. *Journal of the American Medical Association, 279,* 376–380.

Klonoff, D. C., Andrews, B. T., & Obana, W. G. (1989). Stroke associated with cocaine use. *Archives of Neurology, 46,* 989–993.

Kosten, T. R. (1998). Pharmacotherapy of cerebral ischemia in cocaine dependence. *Drug and Alcohol Dependence, 49,* 133–144.

Kosten, T. R., Cheeves, C., Palumbo, J., Seibyl, J. P., Price, L. H., & Woods, S. W. (1998). Regional cerebral blood flow during acute and chronic abstinence from combined cocaine-alcohol abuse. *Drug and Alcohol Dependence, 50,* 187–195.

Langendorf, F. G., Anderson, D. C., Tupper, D. E., Rottenberg, D. A., & Weisman, I. D. (1996). *Brain atrophy and chronic cocaine abuse: Background and work in progress,* Research Monograph 163. Rockville, MD: US Department of Health and Human Services.

Levin, J. M., Holman, B. L., Mendelson, J. H., Teoh, S. K., Garada, B., Johnson, K. A., et al. (1994). Gender differences in cerebral perfusion in cocaine abuse: Technetium-99m-HMPAO SPECT study of drug-abusing women. *Journal of Nuclear Medicine, 35,* 1902–1909.

Levine, S. R., Brust, J. C. M., Futrell, N., Ho, K. L., Blake, D., Millikan, C. H., et al. (1990). Cerebrovascular complications of the use of the "crack" form of alkaloidal cocaine. *New England Journal of Medicine, 323,* 699–704.

Levine, S. R., Brust, J. C. M., Futrell, N., Brass, L. M., Blake, D., Fayad, P., et al. (1991). A comparative study of the cerebrovascular complications of cocaine: Alkaloidal versus hydrochloride – a review. *Neurology, 41,* 1173–1177.

Levine, S. R., & Welch, K. M. (1988). Cocaine and stroke. *Stroke, 19,* 779–783.

Lezak, M. D. (1995). *Neuropsychological Assessment* (3rd ed.). New York: Oxford University Press.

Lim, K. O., Choi, S. J., Pomara, N., Wolkin, A., & Rotrosen, J. P. (2002). Reduced frontal white matter integrity in cocaine dependence: a controlled diffusion tensor imaging study. *Biological Psychiatry, 51,* 890–895.

Liu, X., Matochik, J. A., Cadet, J.-L., & London, E. D. (1998). Smaller volume of prefrontal lobe in polysubstance abusers: a magnetic resonance imaging study. *Neuropsychopharmacology, 18*, 243–252.

London, E. D., Cascella, N. G., Wong, D. F., Phillips, R. L., Dannals, R. F., Links, J. M., et al. (1990). Cocaine induced reduction of glucose utilization in human brain. *Archives of General Psychiatry, 47*, 567–574.

London, E. D., Wilderson, G., Goldberg, S. R., & Risner, M. E. (1986). Effects of L-cocaine on local cerebral glucose utilization in the rat. *Neuroscience Letters, 68*, 73–78.

Lu, L., Shepard, J. D., Scott, H. F., & Shaham, Y. (2003). Effect of environmental stressors on opiate and psychostimulant reinforcement, reinstatement and discrimination in rats: a review. *Neuroscience and Biobehavior Review, 27*, 457–491.

Lyons, D., Friedman, D. P., Nader, M. A., & Porrino, L. J. (1996). Cocaine alters cerebral metabolism within the ventral striatum and limbic cortex of monkeys. *Journal of Neuroscience, 16*, 1230–1238.

Maas, L. C., Lukas, S. E., Kaufman, M. J., Weiss, R. D., Daniels, S. L., Rogers, V. W., et al. (1998). Functional magnetic resonance imaging of human brain activation during cue-induced cocaine craving. *American Journal of Psychiatry, 155*, 124–126.

Madras, B. K., Fahey, M. A., Bergman, J., Canfield, D. R., & Spealman, R. D. (1989). Effects of cocaine and related drugs in nonhuman primates. I. [^{3}H]cocaine binding sites in caudate-putamen. *Journal of Pharmacology and Experimental Therapeutics, 251*, 131–141.

Manschreck, T. C., Schneyer, M. L., Weisstein, C. C., Laughery, J., Rosenthal, J., Celada, T., et al. (1990). Freebase cocaine and memory. *Comprehensive Psychiatry, 31*, 369–375.

Mantsch, J. R., Yuferov, V., Mathieu-Kia, A. M., Ho, A., & Kreek, M. J. (2004). Effects of extended access to high versus low cocaine doses on self-administration, cocaine-induced reinstatement and brain mRNA levels in rats. *Psychopharmacology (Berlin), 175*, 26–36.

Matochik, J., London, E. D., Eldreth, D., Cadet, J.-L., & Bolla, K. (2003). Frontal cortical tissue composition in abstinent cocaine abusers: A magnetic resonance imaging study. *NeuroImage, 19*, 1095–1102.

Meek, P. S., Clark, H. W., & Solana, V. L. (1989). Neurocognitive impairment: The unrecognized component of dual diagnosis in substance abuse treatment. *Journal of Psychoactive Drugs, 21*, 153–160.

Melamed, J. I., & Bleiberg, J. (1986). Neuropsychological deficits in free-base cocaine abusers after cessation of use. Paper presented at the Annual Meeting of the American Psychiatric Association, Washington, DC.

Mello, N. K., & Negus, S. S. (1996). Preclinical evaluation of pharmacotherapies for treatment of cocaine and opioid abuse using drug self-administration procedures. *Neuropsychopharmacology, 14*, 375–424.

Mena, I., Miller, B., Garrett, K., Leedom, L., Khalkhali, I., & Djenderedjian, A. (1990). Neurospect in cocaine abuse. *European Journal of Nuclear Medicine, 16*, 5137.

Mittenberg, W., & Motta, S. (1993). Effects of chronic cocaine abuse on memory and learning. *Archives of Clinical Neuropsychology, 8*, 477–483.

Monterosso, J., Ehrman, R., Napier, K. L., O'Brien, C. P., & Childress, A. R. (2001). Three decision-making tasks in cocaine-dependent patients: do they measure the same construct? *Addiction, 96*, 1825–1837.

Mora, F., Avrith, D. B., & Rolls, E. T. (1980). An electrophysiological and behavioral study of self-stimulation in the orbitofrontal cortex of the rhesus monkey. *Brain Research Bulletin, 5*, 111–115.

Negrete, J. C., & Murphy, H. B. M. (1967). Psychological deficit in chewers of coca leaf. *Bulletin of Narcotics, 19*, 11–18.

Nilsson, B., Rehncrona, S., & Siesjo, B. K. (1978). Coupling of cerebral metabolism and blood flow in epileptic seizures, hypoxia, and hypoglycaemia. *Ciba Foundation Symposium, 56*, 199–218.

O'Doherty, J., Kringelbach, M. L., Rolls, E. T., Hornak, J., & Andrews, C. (2001). Abstract reward and punishment representations in the human orbitofrontal cortex. *Nature Neuroscience, 4*, 95–102.

O'Malley, S., Adamse, M., Heaton, R. K., & Gawin, F. H. (1992). Neuropsychological impairment in chronic cocaine abusers. *American Journal of Drug and Alcohol Abuse, 18*, 131–144.

O'Malley, S. S., & Gawin, F. H. (1990). Abstinence symptomatology and neuropsychological impairment in chronic cocaine abusers. *NIDA Research Monograph, 101*, 271–276.

Ohnishi, T., Hoshi, H., Nagamachi, S., Jinnouchi, S., Flores, L. G., II, Futami, S., et al. (1995). High resolution SPECT to assess hippocampal perfusion in neuropsychiatric diseases. *Journal of Nuclear Medicine, 36*, 1163–1169.

Pascual-Leone, A., Dhuna, A., & Anderson, D. C. (1991). Cerebral atrophy in habitual cocaine abusers: A planimetric CT study. *Neurology, 41*, 34–38.

Paus, T., Petrides, M., Evans, A., & Meyer, E. (1993). Role of human anterior cingulate cortex in the control of oculomotor, manual, and speech responses: A positron emission tomography study. *Journal of Neurophysiology, 70*, 453–469.

Pearlson, G. D., Jeffery, P. J., Harris, G. J., Ross, C. A., Fischman, M. W., & Camargo, E. E. (1993). Correlation of acute cocaine-induced changes in local cerebral blood flow with subjective effects. *American Journal of Psychiatry, 150*, 495–497.

Pennings, E. J., Leccese, A. P., & Wolff, F. A. (2002). Effects of concurrent use of alcohol and cocaine. *Addiction, 97*, 773–783.

Pettit, H. O., & Justice, J. B., Jr. (1989). Dopamine in the nucleus accumbens during cocaine self-administration as studied by in vivo microdialysis. *Pharmacology, Biochemistry and Behavior, 34*, 899–904.

Pettit, H. O., & Justice, J. B., Jr. (1991). Effect of dose on cocaine self-administration behavior and dopamine levels in the nucleus accumbens. *Brain Research, 539*, 94–102.

Porrino, L. J. (1993). Functional effects of cocaine depend upon route of administration. *Psychopharmacology, 112*, 343–351.

Porrino, L. J., Daunais, J. B., Smith, H. R., & Nader, M. A. (2004). The expanding effects of cocaine: studies in a nonhuman primate model of cocaine self-administration. *Neuroscience and Biobehavior Review, 27*, 813–820.

Porrino, L. J., Lyons, D., Smith, H. R., Daunais, J. B., & Nader, M. A. (2004). Cocaine self-administration produces a progressive involvement of limbic, association, and sensorimotor striatal domains. *Journal of Neuroscience, 24*, 3554–3562.

Powers, R. H., & Madden, J. A. (1990). Vasoconstrictive effects of cocaine metabolites, and structural analogs on cat cerebral arteries. *FASEB Journal, 4*, A1095 (abstract).

Raichle, M. E., Grubb, R., Gado, M. H., Eichling, J. O., & Ter-Pogossian, M. M. (1976). Correlation between regional cerebral blood flow and oxidative mechanisms. *Archives of Neurology, 33*, 523–526.

Reith, M. E., & Selmeci, G. (1992). Radiolabeling of dopamine uptake sites in mouse striatum: comparison of binding sites for cocaine, mazindol, and GBR 12935. *Naunyn Schmiedebergs Archives of Pharmacology, 345*, 309–318.

Ritz, M. C., Lamb, R. J., Goldberg, S. R., & Kuhar, M. J. (1987). Cocaine receptors on dopamine transporters are related to self-administration of cocaine. *Science, 237*, 1219–1223.

Robbins, S. J., Ehrman, R. N., Childress, A. R., Cornish, J. W., & O'Brien, C. P. (2000). Mood state and recent cocaine use are not associated with levels of cocaine cue reactivity. *Drug and Alcohol Dependence, 59*, 33–42.

Robbins, T. W., Joyce, E. M., & Sahakian, B. J. (1992). Neuropsychology and neuro-imaging of affective disorders. In Paykel ES (Ed.), *Handbook of affective disorders* (pp. 289–310). London: Churchill Livingston.

Robinson, J. E., Heaton, R. K., & O'Malley, S. S. (1999). Neuropsychological functioning in cocaine abusers with and without alcohol dependence. *Journal of the International Neuropsychology Society, 5*, 10–19.

Rolls, E. T., & Baylis, L. L. (1994). Gustatory, olfactory, and visual convergence within the primate orbitofrontal cortex. *Journal of Neuroscience, 14*, 5437–5452.

Rolls, E. T., Burton, M. J., & Mora, F. (1980). Neurophysiological analysis of brain-stimulation reward in the monkey. *Brain Research, 194*, 339–357.

Rosselli, M., Ardila, A., Lubomski, M., Murray, S., & King, K. (2001). Personality profile and neuropsychological test performance in chronic cocaine-abusers. *International Journal of Neuroscience, 110*, 55–72.

Roy, C. W., & Sherrington, C. S. (1980). On the regulation of the blood supply of the brain. *Journal of Physiology (London), 11*, 85–108.

Sanchez-Ramos, J. R. (1993). Psychostimulants. *Neurology Clinics, 11*, 535–553.

Schieve, J. F., & Wilson, W. P. (1953). The influence of age, anesthesia and cerebral arteriosclerosis on cerebral vascular activity to Co-2. *American Journal of Medicine, 15*, 171–174.

Selby, M. J., & Azrin, R. L. (1998). Neuropsychological functioning in drug abusers. *Drug and Alcohol Dependence, 50*, 39–45.

Selby, M. J., Azrin, R. L., Ireland, S. J., & Morgan, M. J. (1995). Differential recovery of neuropsychological functioning in alcohol, cocaine, and polysubstance abusers (abstract). *Archives of Clinical Neuropsychology, 10*, 390.

Sloan, M. A., & Mattioni, T. A. (1992). Concurrent myocardial and cerebral infarctions after intranasal cocaine use. *Stroke, 23*, 427–430.

Smelson, D. A., Roy, A., Santana, S., & Engelhart, C. (1999). Neuropsychological deficits in withdrawn cocaine-dependent males. *American Journal of Drug and Alcohol Abuse, 25*, 377–381.

Sokoloff, P., Le Foll, B., Perachon, S., Bordet, R., Ridray, S., & Schwartz, J. C. (2001). The dopamine D3 receptor and drug addiction. *Neurotoxicity Research, 3*, 433–441.

Stein, D. J., Hollander, E., & Cohen, L. (1993). Neuropsychiatric impairment in impulsive personality disorders. *Psychiatry Research, 48*, 257–266.

Strickland, T. L., Mena, I., Villanueva-Meyer, J., Miller, B. L., Cummings, J., Mehringer, C. M., et al. (1993). Cerebral perfusion and neuropsychological consequences of chronic cocaine use. *Journal of Neuropsychiatry and Clinical Neurosciences, 5*, 419–427.

Stuss, D. T., & Benson, D. F. (1986). *The frontal lobes*. New York: Raven Press.

Tumeh, S. S., Nagel, S. J., English, R. J., Moore, M., & Holman, L. (1991). Use of SPECT perfusion brain scintigraphy to investigate effects of cocaine on the brain.

In G. G. Nahas & G. Latour (Eds.), *Physiopathology of illicit drugs: Cannabis, cocaine opiates* (pp. 143–151). Oxford: Pergamon Press.
USDHHS (2002). *Overview of Findings from the 2002 National Survey on Drug Use and Health*, NHSDA Series H-21, DHHS Publication No. SMA03-3774. Rockville, MD: U.S. Department of Health and Human Services, Substance Abuse and Mental Health Services Administration Office of Applied Studies.
Van Gorp, W. G., Wilkins, J. N., Hinkin, C. H., Moore, L. H., Hull, J., Horner, M. D., et al. (1999). Declarative and procedural memory functioning in abstinent cocaine abusers. *Archives of General Psychiatry, 56*, 85–89.
Volkow, N. D., Fowler, J. S., Wang, G. J., Hitzemann, R., Logan, J., Schlyer, D., et al. (1993). Decreased dopamine D2 receptor availability is associated with reduced frontal metabolism in cocaine abusers. *Synapse, 14*, 169–177.
Volkow, N. D., Fowler, J. S., Wolf, A. P., Hitzemann, R., Dewey, S., Bendriem, B., et al. (1991). Changes in brain glucose metabolism in cocaine dependence and withdrawal. *American Journal of Psychiatry, 148*, 621–626.
Volkow, N. D., Hitzemann, R., Wang, G. J., Fowler, J. S., Wolf, A. P., Dewey, S. L., et al. (1992). Long-term frontal metabolic changes in cocaine abusers. *Synapse, 11*, 184–190.
Volkow, N. D., Mullani, H., Gould, K. L., Adler, S., & Krajewski, K. (1988). Cerebral blood flow in chronic cocaine abusers: A study with positron emission tomography. *British Journal of Psychiatry, 152*, 641–648.
Volkow, N. D., Wang, G. J., Fischman, M. W., Foltin, R. W., Fowler, J. S., Abumrad, N. N., et al. (1997). Relationship between subjective effects of cocaine and dopamine transporter occupancy. *Nature, 386*, 827–830.
Wallace, E. A., McMahon, T., Zubal, G., Wisniewski, G., van Dyck, C. H., Pfau, S. E., et al. (1994). Regional cerebral blood flow effects of acute cocaine infusion. In L. S. Harris (Ed.), *Problems of drug dependence*, National Institute on Drug Abuse Research Monograph 141, NIH Publication 94-3749. Washington, DC: US Government Printing Office.
Wallace, E. A., Wisniewski, G., Zubal, G., vanDyck, C. H., Pfau, S. E., Smith, E. O., et al. (1996). Acute cocaine effects on absolute cerebral blood flow. *Psychopharmacology (Berlin), 128*, 17–20.
Weber, D. A., Franceschi, D., Ivanovic, M., Atkins, H. L., Cabahug, C., Wong, C. T., et al. (1993). SPECT and planar brain imaging in crack abuse: iodine-123-iodoamphetamine uptake and localization. *Journal Nuclear Medicine, 34*, 899–907.
Weber, D. A., Klieger, P., Volkow, N. D., et al. (1990). SPECT regional cerebral blood flow (rCBF) studies in crack users and control participants. *Journal of Nuclear Medicine, 31*, 876–877.
Weinstein, A., Feldtkeller, B., Malizia, A., Wilson, S., Bailey, J., & Nutt, D. (1998). Integrating the cognitive and physiological aspects of craving. *Journal of Psychopharmacology, 12*, 31–38.
Wide, R. J., Bernardi, S., Frackowiak, R., et al. (1983). Serial observation on the pathophysiology of acute stroke; The transition from ischemia to infarction as reflected in regional oxygen extraction. *Brain, 106*, 197–222.
Zald, D. H., & Kim, S. W. (1996). Anatomy and function of the orbital frontal cortex, I: anatomy, neurocircuitry; and obsessive–compulsive disorder. *Journal of Neuropsychiatry and Clinical Neurosciences, 8*, 125–138.

5 Marijuana

Raul Gonzalez, Eileen M. Martin, and Igor Grant

A brief introduction to cannabis and its use

Notes on cannabis and its history

The cannabis plant (*Cannabis sativa*) is an annual flowering herb, often referred to as hemp or marijuana. The leaves, stems, and flowering tops have over 60 unique compounds (botanical cannabinoids) that interact with the human body in complex ways, though Δ-9-tetrahydrocannabinol (THC) is the most potent psychoactive constituent in cannabis. Cannabis use dates back to ancient times, when it was thought to have been used by several Eurasian and Middle Eastern civilizations as a medical treatment and as an agent for the induction of altered states of consciousness. The first mention of cannabis as a psychoactive and medicinal substance appears during the 1st and 2nd millennium BC, in the first-known herbal medicine texts in China.

In recent years, perhaps no other illicit recreational drug has received as much social, political, medical, and scientific attention. Whereas some denounce the plant as a neurotoxin that is associated with an array of consequences, including psychosis, cognitive dysfunction, addiction, and all manner of social depravity, others tout cannabis as a benign healing herb. This debate is longstanding (for extensive reviews see Booth, 2003; Guy, Whittle, & Robson, 2005; Iversen, 2000).

Cannabis has repeatedly been classified and reclassified as a recommended medicine and as an outlawed intoxicant. For instance, in the United States, reports documenting the medicinal properties of cannabis were published during the 19th century. Decades later, the 1937 Marihuana Tax Act criminalized the use of cannabis in the United States, yet it remained in the United States Pharmacopoeia until 1941, exemplifying the lack of consensus on its utility and harm.

Methods of consumption, THC content, and pharmacodynamics

Cannabis can be prepared and ingested in various ways. The leaves and flowers of the plant are often dried before consumption. Higher potency can be attained by compressing resin from the flowering heads of the plant to make hashish or by extracting THC with alcohol to make tinctures and oils. Cannabis preparations are often smoked using cigarette paper to envelop the substance before consumption or it can be smoked directly from a pipe. Apparatus is available that allows individuals to "vaporize" cannabis using a heating element that lets scorching air pass through the dried plant at a temperature that creates a THC vapor without combusting the plant itself. Cannabis can also be eaten. Users have attempted various uncommon methods of delivering THC to the bloodstream, which have included injecting cannabis preparations, placing tinctures on the eyes, or inserting cannabis into the rectum. Additionally, pharmaceutical companies have developed new systems of administration for delivery of cannabinoids or their synthetic analogues to the central nervous system (e.g., transdermal patches, eye drops, sublingual preparations).

Blood plasma levels of THC and its psychoactive effects depend on the potency and method of consumption. Factors influencing potency include the plant strain and method of growing, as well as how cannabis is prepared and consumed. The THC content of dried cannabis leaves and flowering tops typically ranges from 0.5 to 4%; however, the THC content of "sinsemilla" (seedless flowering tops of the female cannabis plant) can reach 20%. The THC levels in hashish and cannabis oil range from 10% to 50%.

Some scientists have suggested that the current potency of cannabis substantially exceeds the potency of cannabis during the 1960s and 1970s, though the findings on this issue are inconsistent and their significance is questioned. For example, a study of cannabis samples seized by the government in New Zealand between 1976 and 1996 reported no changes in average THC content across the 20 years (Poulsen & Sutherland, 2000). In contrast, in the United States, the THC content of cannabis samples seized between 1980 and 1997 rose steadily from less than 1.5% THC during 1980 to 4.47% in 1997 (ElSohly et al., 2000). Furthermore, commercial grade cannabis and sinsemilla confiscated in the United States during 2002 averaged 5.11% and 11.43% THC concentration, respectively (National Drug Intelligence Center, 2005).

Increasing levels of THC in cannabis and greater availability of more potent strains have been cited as a partial contributor to emergent cannabis-related health problems, such as increased psychiatric diagnoses of dependence and abuse (e.g., Compton, Grant, Colliver, Glantz, & Stinson, 2004). John P. Waters, the director of the United States White House Office of National Drug Control Policy, coined the phrase "This is not your father's marijuana," in an effort to convey the dangers associated with using the newly grown forms of cannabis. Others have criticized such claims, however. These critics note that potent strains have been available for many years, recent overall increases in potency have been small, and that smokers adjust the amount of cannabis consumed and frequently titrate their THC exposure to achieve the wanted effects (Earleywine, 2004; Hall & Swift, 2000; Mikuriya & Aldrich, 1988).

The pharmacokinetic and pharmacodynamic properties of THC and other cannabinoids have been well studied and vary according to route of administration (for a recent review, see Grotenhermen, 2003). When cannabis is smoked, THC is detectable in plasma within seconds. Peak concentration is attained in 3–10 minutes. Bioavailability is typically between 10 and 25%, and these values can vary depending on the users' amount of smoking experience. In contrast, consumption of cannabis in pill form results in erratic absorption of THC, with peak concentrations detectable in plasma between 1 to 6 hours and widely varying bioavailability.

It is noteworthy that THC is lipophilic, therefore repeated use of cannabis results in storage of THC in fatty tissue with subsequent slow release into the bloodstream. However, the amount and rate of THC released into the bloodstream from fat stores after cessation of use are not thought to be of enough magnitude or released rapidly enough to produce psychoactive effects. Estimates of THC half-life in plasma after cannabis consumption vary a great deal, ranging from several hours to several weeks depending on the method of use, potency of the preparation, and chronicity of use. Each of these factors is important to consider when attempting to assess last cannabis use through urine toxicology testing.

Prevalence of cannabis use

Despite its illegal status in many countries, prevalence of cannabis use worldwide from 2001 to 2003 is nearly 3.7% (146 million) for individuals 15–64 years old, compared with 0.3% for cocaine and 0.4% for opiates (United Nations Office on Drugs and Crimes, 2004). The highest annual prevalence of cannabis use was reported in Australia/Oceania (16.4%). North America, Africa, and Western Europe reported prevalences of 10.3%, 7.7%, and 6.7%, respectively. The lowest annual prevalences of cannabis use were reported in Eastern Europe (3.6%), South America (2.4%), and Asia (1.9%).

During 2003, in the United States alone, roughly 97 million (33%) Americans over the age of 12 reported ever using cannabis. Twenty-five million (12%) reported use during the last year and about 15 million (5%) during the last month (Substance Abuse and Mental Health Services Administration, 2003). Most Americans first try cannabis before age 18. During 2004, 51.1% of 12th graders reported use (Johnston, O'Malley, Bachman, & Schulenberg, 2005; Substance Abuse and Mental Health Services Administration, 2003). Cannabis use in America is most prevalent among adolescents and young adults between the ages of 15 and 29. Compared to the 30–49 year age group, almost twice as many Americans aged 15–29 reported cannabis use during the past year (approximately 15 million vs. 8 million) and the past month (approximately 9 million vs. 5 million) (Substance Abuse and Mental Health Services Administration, 2003). Fewer than 1.5 million Americans over 50 years old reported using marijuana during the past year.

In Europe, use of cannabis is also most prevalent among young adults

(European Monitoring Centre for Drugs and Drug Addiction, 2004). The proportion of individuals who have tried cannabis on at least one occasion differs substantially across countries. Estimates during 1999–2003 range from about 5% to 10% in Belgium, Estonia, and Portugal, with up to 24–31% prevalence in Denmark, Spain, France, and the United Kingdom. Cannabis use "in the last 12 months" among individuals between the ages of 15 to 34 were lowest in Sweden (1%), with higher rates reported for Estonia (4%), Hungary (5.4%), Poland (6.3%), Portugal (6.3%), Finland (7.1%), Slovakia (7.7%), Latvia (8.1%), Norway (8.1%), Ireland (8.7%), Greece (8.8%), Italy (9.2%), Netherlands (11.8%), Germany (13%), Denmark (13.1%), France (17%), Spain (17.3%), United Kingdom (20%), and Switzerland (22.1%). It is interesting to note that residents of European countries generally reported less lifetime cannabis use than the United States, despite many of them having less strict laws regarding possession of cannabis for personal use.

Laws governing cannabis use

Many countries (and states in the USA) have considered whether it would be prudent to modify the current statutes governing cannabis use. A number of factors underlie this consideration, including the high prevalence of use, the cost of enforcing prohibition, and the growing body of scientific evidence suggesting that controlled cannabis use provides therapeutic benefits with a tolerable margin of safety. In the USA, the government considers cannabis to have a strong potential for abuse and no accepted medical value, hence it is classified as a Schedule I drug by Title II of the Comprehensive Drug Abuse Prevention and Control Act of 1970. Cannabis receives the same classification status as heroin and LSD, whereas cocaine and methamphetamine receive less stringent regulations (Schedule II). Twelve states in the USA have passed laws to lessen criminal penalties for the possession or use of cannabis under various circumstances, but the federal government does not recognize these laws and retains the right to prosecute. Similarly, the European Union and United Nations classify cannabis as a controlled narcotic drug, but specific laws regarding use and possession differ across member nations. The general trend in many European countries has been to focus on "harm reduction" rather than criminalization. Alternative methods to prosecution include campaigns to discourage individuals from using cannabis, educating them about its potential dangers, and providing treatment for those with problems. Individuals distributing large amount of cannabis are more likely to be prosecuted, whereas those with small amounts for personal use may be reprimanded or left alone. Canada has been moving toward a position on cannabis that more resembles that of many European countries rather than the approach employed in the United States. Although the current public sentiment suggests a movement toward more lenient cannabis possession laws, the legal status of cannabis use remains an issue of intense dispute.

A brief introduction to cannabis neuropharmacology

Cannabinoid receptors and endogenous agonists in the brain

Increased interest in cannabis is evident in the scientific, sociopolitical, and legal realms. Published investigations on the central nervous system (CNS) and behavioral effects of cannabis increased by 100% from the 1980s to the 1990s. Further, the number of studies between 2000 and mid-2005 (at the time this chapter was written) already exceeds the total number published during the 1990s. Cannabis research increased significantly following the discovery and cloning of cannabinoid receptors CB_1 in mammalian brain (Devane, Dysarz, Johnson, Melvin, & Howlett, 1988; Howlett, Johnson, Melvin, & Milne, 1988; Matsuda, Lolait, Brownstein, Young, & Bonner, 1990) and CB_2 outside of the CNS (Munro, Thomas, & Abu-Shaar, 1993).

The cannabinoid (CB) receptors are in the family of G-protein-coupled receptors. Such proteins are involved in second messenger signaling, and modulate chemical reactions inside cells. The CB_1 receptors are diversely distributed in human brain tissue, where it is thought to be the most plentiful G-protein-coupled receptor (Biegon & Kerman, 2001; Herkenham et al., 1990; Herkenham, Lynn, de Costa, & Richfield, 1991). Highest concentrations of CB_1 are reported in basal ganglia, cerebellum, hippocampus, and amygdala, with lower concentrations in thalamus and brainstem (Abood & Martin, 1996; Breivogel & Childers, 1998; Glass, Dragunow, & Faull, 1997; Pertwee, 1997). The CB_1 receptors are also found peripherally in humans, but in much lower concentrations. The CB_2 receptors, on the other hand, are present mainly in immune tissues and cells (Galiegue et al., 1995; Munro et al., 1993). To date, CB_1 is thought to be the only cannabinoid receptor found in brain. More recent evidence, however, suggests the possibility of a third cannabinoid receptor (CB_3) in the brain (Breivogel, Griffin, Di Marzo, & Martin, 2001; Di Marzo et al., 2000; Fride et al., 2003).

The discovery of cannabinoid receptors in mammals prompted the search for naturally occurring ligands in the brain. Several endogenous metabolites of arachidonic acid (an essential fatty acid found in cell membranes and the brain) that are active at cannabinoid receptors have been identified (reviewed in De Petrocellis, Cascio, & Di Marzo, 2004; Freund, Katona, & Piomelli, 2003; Martin, Mechoulam, & Razdan, 1999; Piomelli, 2003). Anandamide (*N*-arachidonoyl-ethanolamine: Devane et al., 1992) and 2-AG (2-arachidonoyl-glycerol: Mechoulam et al., 1995; Sugiura et al., 1995) were the first endogenous cannabinoid receptor agonists with similar binding activity to THC to be identified and have been the most frequently studied. Several additional endogenous compounds reputedly bind with cannabinoid receptors; these include noladin ether (2-arachidonoyl-glyceryl ether: Hanus et al., 2001), virhodamine (*O*-arachidonoyl-ethanolamine: Porter et al., 2002), and NADA (*N*-arachidonoyl-dopamine: Bisogno et al., 2000; Huang et al., 2002).

Functioning of the cannabinoid signaling system in the CNS

The endocannabinoid system exerts its effects on the brain by regulating neurotransmission. Cannabinoid receptors in brain inhibit adenylyl cyclase and affect second messenger signaling through cAMP – they can decrease Ca^{2+} influx and increase K^+ conductance (reviewed in Pertwee, 1997; McAllister & Glass, 2002). Modulation of signaling by activity at CB_1 receptors has been implicated in many neurotransmitter systems, but is well understood to produce both inhibitory and excitatory signals by affecting GABAergic and glutamatergic systems (reviewed in Freund et al., 2003; Piomelli, 2003).

Several mechanisms for cannabinoid receptor function have been proposed. The CB_1 receptors in hippocampus are thought to be important in a critical process of GABAergic retrograde (postsynaptic to presynaptic) rapid signaling, termed depolarization-induced suppression of inhibition (DSI: reviewed in Davies, Pertwee, & Riedel, 2002; Maejima, Ohno-Shosaku, & Kano, 2001). A similar process, depolarization-induced suppression of excitation (DSE), may be mediated by cannabinoid receptors on glutamatergic neurons (reviewed in Maejima et al., 2001). Cannabis is thought to exert effects on cognition and behavior via signal modulation in structures that have the greatest level of CB_1 receptor density – the cognitive and behavioral functions associated with such brain structures would theoretically be most affected (reviewed in Freund et al., 2003; Iversen, 2000; Piomelli, 2003).

Interestingly, not all the mechanisms by which cannabis affects brain function are thought to be potentially harmful. Indeed, under specific circumstances cannabinoids are neuroprotective (Grundy, 2002; Guzman, Sanchez, & Galve-Roperh, 2001; Marsicano, Moosmann, Hermann, Lutz, & Behl, 2002; Mechoulam, 2002; Mechoulam, Panikashvili, & Shohami, 2002). For example, cannabinoids can inhibit the release of the excitatory neurotransmitter glutamate and production of reactive oxygen species (ROS), both of which are damaging to neurons in excess. Moreover, several cannabinoids, including THC, dampen experimentally induced excitotoxic injury in rodent brain tissue (reviewed in van der Stelt et al., 2002). Cannabinoids reduce damaging ROS through their powerful antioxidant properties, which have been demonstrated with cannabidiol, THC, and synthetic cannabinoids (reviewed in Hampson et al., 2000). Some cannabinoids have attenuated brain injury in several animal models of ischemia and show promise for management of traumatic brain injury in humans (reviewed in Biegon, 2004). The CB_1 receptors on sympathetic terminals inhibit norepinephrine release and may be involved in control of blood pressure (Pacher, Batkai, & Kunos, 2005).

Cannabis-associated mental health symptomatology

Mental health symptoms associated with acute intoxication

The acute effects of cannabis ingestion on mood, perception, and overall mental state have been well described. The majority of individuals report pleasant subjective characteristics of the cannabis "high," including euphoria, relaxation, heightened sensory experiences, and a proclivity for laughter. Common additional effects are light-headedness, rapid pulse, sedation, and psychomotor slowing. However, acute intoxication of cannabis has also been associated with more severe undesirable effects, including hypotension, paranoid thinking, anxiety, panic attacks, unpleasant feelings of depersonalization, and undesirable hallucinations. A recent comprehensive review of naturalistic and laboratory studies of cannabis intoxication concluded that subjective effects and behavioral features of cannabis intoxication vary considerably both within and across individuals (Green, Kavanagh, & Young, 2003) and are influenced by set (a person's expectations and psychic state) and setting. The review found that the majority of individuals in most studies reported pleasant effects, though multiple individual and environmental factors likely affect whether a person judges their subjective experience to be pleasant or not. After smoking a single cannabis cigarette initial psychophysiological effects are experienced within minutes, peak in the first hour, and dissipate several hours later.

The cannabis "withdrawal syndrome"

At present, it is unclear as to the presence and severity of mood and/or cognitive disturbance(s) emerging after cessation from cannabis use. "Cannabis withdrawal" is recognized formally in the most recent versions of the International Classification of Diseases (ICD-10), but not in the Diagnostic and Statistical Manual of the American Psychiatric Association (DSM-IV-TR). The putative effects of ceasing cannabis use have been studied extensively in both humans and animals, however the result of these studies is inconsistent with respect to the identification of a pattern of symptoms that occurs consistently following the cessation of cannabis abstinence. The disparities in the findings across studies often occur as a result of variability in the methods used by investigators to induce and measure "withdrawal." Furthermore, the relatively lengthy half-life of THC and its slow systemic elimination may attenuate withdrawal, thereby complicating findings.

There is substantial consensus that an acute withdrawal syndrome can be induced in animals receiving cannabis by administration of a potent CB_1 antagonist (SR 141716A); in contrast, the findings of studies in which animals undergo natural discontinuation from cannabis have yielded inconsistent results. Recent reviews of animal studies that utilized experimentally-induced withdrawal reported that findings depend on multiple factors, including the specific species examined, cannabinoid agonists used, and dosing schedules (Maldonado, 2002; Tanda & Goldberg, 2003).

Both reviews present evidence for cannabis tolerance and withdrawal. Maldonado (2002) tempers this conclusion by noting a lack of proof for strong reinforcing effects of cannabis, whereas Tanda and Goldberg (2003) report that new studies with squirrel monkeys demonstrate THC's reinforcing properties through self-administration. Nevertheless, the high doses and treatment schedules of animal studies may not generalize to humans (Maldonado, 2002).

There is extensive debate regarding the presence, onset, course, and character of symptoms that potentially emerge with cessation of cannabis use by humans. A review by Smith (2002) presents evidence from several outpatient and residential laboratory studies that show undesirable emotional and physical symptoms among cannabis users, but finds the data suspect based on its methodological failings. Limitations observed included disparate methods of cannabis administration, lack of suitable control groups, absence of an *a priori* definition for cannabis withdrawal, inconsistent reports of the symptoms characteristic of withdrawal, poor quantification of symptom severity, and cannabis using groups not thought to be representative of the general population of cannabis users. Smith concluded that further examination is warranted to determine if the unpleasant effects many users seemingly experience when abstaining from cannabis constitute a withdrawal syndrome.

In light of new evidence, Budney and colleagues (2004) have reexamined the conclusions of Smith (2002). Both reviews agree that early studies of cannabis withdrawal produced inconsistent findings of indeterminate significance; however, if the findings from several well-controlled inpatient laboratory and outpatient studies are considered separately, it was consistently observed that chronic daily cannabis smokers reliably display unfavorable symptoms upon abstinence that emerge by 48 hours after cessation of use, peak between 2 and 6 days, remit within 1–2 weeks, and are corroborated by family and friends.

Based on the results of these studies, Budney and others (2004) proposed criteria for a cannabis withdrawal syndrome. According to Budney et al., individuals meet the diagnostic criteria for cannabis withdrawal when they experience the following symptoms: "significant distress or dysfunction" from at least four symptoms classified as common (i.e., anger and aggression, decreased appetite or weight loss, irritability, nervousness/anxiety, restlessness, sleep difficulties) or uncommon (i.e., chills, depressed mood, stomach pain, shakiness, and sweating). The authors report that the criteria were formulated on the basis of investigations in which the samples were comprised of chronic daily cannabis smokers. They emphasize the need for more research to determine the quantity, frequency, and duration of cannabis use that is necessary to elicit a withdrawal syndrome.

Cannabis addiction: Potential for abuse and dependence

The issue of a cannabis withdrawal syndrome has often been used to guide sociopolitical arguments regarding the dangers and legal status of the drug; in particular, the presence of withdrawal symptoms is utilized as evidence of cannabis "addiction." It is noteworthy that current scientific and diagnostic practices no longer view tolerance and withdrawal as necessary for establishing a substance "addiction." The common feature of addiction as proposed by Dr Alan I. Leshner, former director of the National Institute on Drug Abuse, is an "uncontrollable, compulsive drug seeking and use, even in the face of negative health and social consequences." Such behaviors are the hallmark features used to diagnose "abuse" and "dependence" in commonly used classification systems. "Cannabis abuse" and "cannabis dependence" are treated as mental health diagnoses in the ICD-10 and DSM-IV-TR. Both classification systems require individuals to meet minimal criteria marking continued substance use despite causing specific adverse effects in a person's functioning.

The National Survey on Drug Use and Health (NSDUH, formerly NHSDA) during 2003 found that 2.5 million Americans aged 12 and over met the DSM-IV criteria for cannabis dependence and another 2.5 million met the criteria for cannabis abuse. When taken together, these numbers indicate that of all Americans that reported using cannabis in their lifetime, 5% met the criteria for cannabis abuse or dependence during 2003 compared to 4% for cocaine, 5% for heroin, and 12% for alcohol. Others have found that the risk of developing cannabis dependence among those who have tried the drug (conditional dependence) is 9%, but 32% for tobacco, 23% for heroin, 17% for cocaine, and 15% for alcohol. Thus, current evidence suggests that a sizable minority of all cannabis users is at significant risk for cannabis dependence or abuse, but the vast majority of cannabis users never meet such criteria. Future studies need to be conducted in order to identify risk factors for the onset of cannabis dependence and whether such vulnerabilities are specific to cannabis or any number of substances.

Associations between cannabis use and other mental health conditions

During 2003, the NSDUH reported that 17.2% of American adults using cannabis in the past year had a serious mental illness, compared to 7.8% of those who did not report using illegal drugs (Substance Abuse and Mental Health Services Administration, 2003). Estimates such as these provide valuable information, but they do not prove direct mental health consequences from cannabis use. Several fairly recent review articles have qualitatively summarized findings from the published scientific literature examining associations between cannabis and mental health conditions (Degenhardt, Hall, & Lynskey, 2003; Johns, 2001; Leweke, Gerth, & Klosterkotter, 2004; Macleod et al., 2004). Although cannabis use and psychopathology are often correlated, there appears to be no conclusive evidence to suggest that cannabis use can cause mental health problems in the absence of other confounding problems. Below we discuss conclusions from these reviews and methodological challenges that have made it difficult to make causal inferences regarding cannabis use and psychopathology.

Many investigators have examined links between cannabis use and psychotic symptoms or schizophrenia. Evidence exists to suggest that some individuals with no prior history of mental illness can develop transient psychotic episodes after very high doses of cannabis ingestion (Johns, 2001; Leweke et al., 2004). However such investigations have been deemed to suffer for numerous methodological weaknesses, including a lack of urine toxicology testing to rule out the presence of other drugs (Johns, 2001; Leweke et al., 2004). Further, Leweke et al. (2004) find no conclusive evidence for a distinct mental health entity called "cannabis psychosis" that produces symptoms specific to cannabis use. Johns (2001) concluded that studies of how cannabis modulates symptoms of individuals with schizophrenia have produced mixed and often contradictory results and no strong evidence implicates cannabis as a cause of schizophrenia. Leweke et al. (2004), however, note that cannabis might affect the symptomatology and course of schizophrenia, but further studies are needed to obtain more definitive findings.

The possibility that cannabis might cause or affect symptoms of depression has been extensively examined and recently reviewed (Degenhardt et al., 2003). As previously noted, cannabis use is correlated with psychopathology – the same observation has been made concerning depression. In their review of cross-sectional and longitudinal investigations of depression and cannabis use, Degenhardt and colleagues (2003) report that cannabis use was often found to be associated with a greater risk of depression later in life, particularly when use begins in adolescence. Longitudinal evidence did not support a "self-medication" hypothesis, where depression predicted later cannabis use. However, the authors conclude that when findings from all investigations are taken together, the evidence for cannabis to cause depression remains mixed due to many confounding variables. If a causal relationship exists, the authors thought it likely to be seen when individuals use cannabis heavily at an early age, but note that it probably, "makes, at most, a modest contribution to the population prevalence of depression."

The results of many investigations examining connections between cannabis use and psychopathology have been difficult to interpret due to several common limitations (Degenhardt et al., 2003; Macleod et al., 2004). Use of alcohol and other illegal psychoactive substances is often reported among cannabis users, but many investigations have failed to employ urine toxicology testing. Further complicating interpretation, many studies use participant samples seeking treatment for their cannabis use, because it has become problematic in their lives. Such samples are not thought to be representative of the vast majority of cannabis users. Establishing strong evidence of causation has also been hindered by reliance on cross-sectional designs. Many studies linking cannabis use with mental health problems have often poorly examined or controlled for factors that may differ between cannabis users and controls, which may account for differences in mental health symptoms. Such factors include economic disadvantage, low education, other substance use, parental level of education, family history of psychopathology, and mental health symptoms present prior to onset of cannabis use.

Not all investigations on this topic are hindered by these limitations. Macleod and colleagues (2004) reviewed only longitudinal studies with individuals 25 years old and younger in the general population. Causation can be more readily inferred from such investigations and confounds are more adequately controlled, thus they are more likely to clarify and address adequately the role of cannabis use in causing mental health problems. Unfortunately, only 16 of the 48 studies they recovered met their criteria for a "high quality" investigation (e.g., low chance of selection bias, adjustments for confounds, assessment of drug exposure using validated instruments). Equivocal findings were observed among studies implicating cannabis use with psychological problems and antisocial behavior. However, cannabis use was associated with lower educational attainment and more prevalent use of other drugs. The authors concluded that an association likely exists between cannabis use and poorer psychosocial outcomes, but found no clear evidence to suggest that it is causal or of a large magnitude.

The impact of cannabis use on neurocognitive functioning

Considerations in neurocognitive studies of cannabis use

The effects of cannabis use on neurocognitive functioning have been studied with various methods, such as examining brain activity, either at rest or when undergoing a cognitive challenge, using electroencephalography (EEG), positron emission tomography (PET), single photon emission computed tomography (SPECT), or functional magnetic resonance imaging (fMRI). Investigators have also relied on the results obtained by individuals on neuropsychological measures of various mental abilities, which include tests of processing speed, motor functions, attention, reaction time, visuospatial abilities, and executive and verbal functions. Below, we discuss findings of neuroimaging and neuropsychological studies of cannabis users, but first we present important methodological considerations that must be considered when interpreting the results of these investigations.

Regardless of the specific methods employed, to discuss the findings and relevance of neurocognitive studies, one must consider the length of abstinence from cannabis among participants in the study at the time the study is conducted. In their review, Pope et al. (1995) present a classification scheme that divides the effects of cannabis on neurocognition into two types: acute effects and residual effects. *Acute effects* on neurocognitive functions refer to the time when an individual is intoxicated with cannabis and several hours thereafter; that is, when a person is "high" and experiencing the psychoactive, intoxicating effects of the drug. *Residual effects* of cannabis use refer to changes in neurocognitive functioning that persists after cessation of cannabis use and after acute intoxication has subsided. Pope and others (1995) make a distinction between two types of residual effects. The first is referred to as a *"drug residue effect,"* which is used to describe cognitive changes that are apparent after acute effects have abated but cannabis products (i.e., THC and other cannabinoids) are still detectable in the individual. During this time, a cannabis withdrawal may be experienced, as we discussed in the previous section of this chapter. The second type of residual effect consists of changes in neurocognitive functioning as a result of cannabis use that persist despite no traces of cannabis in a person's system (i.e., after the drug has been completely eliminated). Pope et al. refer to this as a *"CNS alteration."* Others have referred to these stages as *acute, subacute*, and *chronic* effects of cannabis use, respectively (e.g., Solowij, 1999).

Because the term subacute can refer to severity of symptoms, their duration, or both in medical practice, we prefer the designation *intermediate duration disorder*. First proposed by Grant and Judd (1976), intermediate duration refers to neurobehavioral changes that slowly improve over many months. Such slow resolution of symptoms most likely reflects gradual processes of metabolic recalibration (e.g., changes in concentrations, conformation, or activity of proteins involved in receptor function, ligand turnover, or cellular metabolism) that occur after pressure from an exogenous psychoactive substance is released. If neurobehavioral deficits improve, but ultimately some abnormality persists indefinitely, then the term *persistent disorder* is appropriate (Reed & Grant, 1990).

To establish residual neurocognitive effects of cannabis, it is critical to rule out multiple potential confounds. These include, but are not limited to, acute effects, effects from other substances, preexisting differences between heavy or light cannabis users (i.e., premorbid differences), or other risk factors that differ between the population of heavy versus light or noncannabis users (e.g., academic achievement, occupational achievement, impoverished home environment). Later, we will discuss the methodological limitations of the existing literature in more detail.

Acute effects

As previously discussed, individuals experience a variety of subjective acute effects from cannabis use, which are due to seemingly transient changes in brain functioning from the actions of THC and possibly other cannabinoids on cannabinoid receptors in the brain. EEG, PET, SPECT, and fMRI have been used to study these acute changes, and the findings have been reviewed by others (Loeber & Yurgelun-Todd, 1999). Most studies conducted to date have examined regional cerebral blood flow (rCBF) or metabolism using radiolabeled molecules (usually oxygen or glucose). Nearly all of the studies reported increased rCBF among experienced cannabis users when challenged with intravenous THC or smoked marijuana compared to their drug-free baseline, when administered a placebo, or when compared to participants with no cannabis use. This effect is consistent with known vasodilatory effects of cannabinoids and contrasts with reduced regional flow associated with many other drugs of abuse, including cocaine, methamphetamine, and alcohol. Increased rCBF is most often seen in frontal, limbic, and cerebellar regions. Similarly, relative to controls, more rCBF primarily in "paralimbic" brain regions (i.e., orbital and mesial frontal lobes, insula, temporal poles, anterior cingulate, and cerebellum) have been observed when participants performed a task of attention after smoking cannabis, despite no significant differences on task performance compared to controls (O'Leary et al., 2002). Several studies have found correlations between rCBF and subjective feelings of intoxication, but the specific feeling reported and the specific region to which it is correlated have been inconsistent (Mathew, Wilson, Turkington, & Coleman, 1998; Mathew et al., 1999). Increased rCBF has been observed 30 minutes after a low-dose intravenous infusion of THC and found to persist beyond 120 minutes (Mathew et al., 2002). Results of EEG studies with humans intoxicated with cannabis are less consistent and sometimes yield contradictory findings, but most suggest changes in brain wave activity that are consistent with drowsiness (reviewed in Solowij, 1999).

Iverson (2000) provides a brief overview of studies that have specifically examined cognitive functioning during acute intoxication with cannabis. The subjective effects that individuals report when intoxicated include a distorted sense of time, perceptual changes, depersonalization, and psychomotor slowing, all of which could conceivably affect performance on neuropsychological measures administered during intoxication. However, Iverson indicated that individuals' subjective reports during intoxication do not generally correlate with their objective neuropsychological performance. For example, despite subjective reports of changes in cognition, intoxicated persons tend to perform fairly well on simple tests of attention. The ability to remember overlearned facts or autobiographical information (i.e., well-established memories) does not appear to be affected. Performance deficits are often noted on measures of declarative memory (e.g., hearing and then immediately repeating a list of words) and short-term recollection of recently presented information (e.g., a digit span test). The most consistent impairments, however, are reported to occur on measures that require sustained attention or on those that require active maintenance and mental manipulation of information (i.e., working memory). Intoxicated individuals will perform even more poorly on these measures of complex attention when presented with additional distracting stimuli.

In summary, studies of acute cannabis intoxication show that participants experience subjective changes in their cognition. Brain imaging studies generally demonstrate increased blood flow and metabolic rate in multiple brain regions (see Loeber & Yurgelun-Todd, 1999). On measures of neuropsychological performance, intoxicated cannabis users often show deficits in learning and remembering newly presented information, sustained attention, and on tasks of working memory. However, a consistent correspondence between functional neuroimaging results and neuropsychological functioning has not been established among acutely intoxicated cannabis users. Further, most of these investigations have examined individuals several hours to days after their last cannabis use, rather than during acute intoxication.

As it happens, few studies have examined neurocognitive functioning in acutely intoxicated cannabis users. These studies essentially addressed the following question: Do individuals that are acutely intoxicated with cannabis show differences in brain function? Most researchers agree that cannabis intoxication results in neurobiological changes that affect cognition, mood, and behavior. From a public-health standpoint, these investigations have also not been deemed as pertinent as those examining residual effects, which have been researched intensely and their methodologies and findings scrutinized and debated.

Residual (nonacute) effects

Neuroimaging and brain function

Loeber and Yurgelun-Todd (1999) also reviewed nine imaging studies (i.e., Mathew, Tant, & Burger, 1986; Mathew, Wilson, Coleman, Turkington, & Degrado, 1997; Mathew & Wilson, 1993; Mathew, Wilson, Humphreys, Lowe, & Wiethe, 1992; Mathew, Wilson, & Tant, 1989; Tunving, Thulin, Risberg, & Warkentin, 1986; Volkow et al., 1991, 1996; Solowij, Michie, & Fox, 1991) of brain function among abstinent cannabis users and concluded that findings were inconsistent (see also Crippa et al., 2005). Interpretation of the findings was constrained by disparate imaging methodologies, differences in cannabis use histories among participants, rigor with which abstinence has been ensured, the degree to which investigators controlled for other drug or alcohol use, demographic differences among participants, and varying length of abstinence among participants that have ranged from 12 hours to 3 months. These caveats notwithstanding, three of the four investigations that examined resting rCBF among abstinent users of cannabis relative to controls reported lower resting rCBF among the cannabis users, which contrasts with the increases in blood flow typically observed among acutely intoxicated individuals. These conclusions have been substantiated by a more recent study (Block et al., 2000), which reports that frequent cannabis users exhibit a relatively circumscribed decrease in cerebellar CBF relative to controls after approximately 27 hours of supervised abstinence. However, most studies report that rCBF differences are no longer present after approximately 2 weeks of abstinence, which supports the notion of a time-limited change in brain functioning (i.e., CBF and metabolism). Such findings suggest a residual (or drug residue) effect from cannabis use, but no permanent "CNS alterations." At present, however, the association between these functional changes and neurocognition is unclear.

More recent studies have investigated changes in cerebral metabolism in response to a cognitive challenge. Consistent with the findings reported on acute cannabis intoxication, these studies often find group differences in brain functioning despite no differences on task performance compared to controls. Block et al. (2002) examined brain metabolism and verbal memory, using O^{15}-labeled water, among frequent cannabis users abstinent for 16–28 hours. Relative to demographically matched controls, cannabis users required more presentations to learn a word-list during the first testing session (approximately 16 hours after last cannabis use) and demonstrated poorer recollection of word-list items during the second testing session (approximately 28 hours after the previous testing session). On the other hand, they remembered the same number of items as controls when tested with a new word-list during the second testing session. However, when recalling word-list items during the second testing session, cannabis users demonstrated decreased metabolism in prefrontal cortical regions, increased metabolism in cerebellum, and a different lateralization pattern of hippocampal metabolism relative to controls. An additional study compared oxygen metabolism among 11 frequent cannabis users abstinent at testing and matched controls while performing a modified version of the Stroop Color Word Task that requires inhibiting an automatic, dominant but inappropriate response (Eldreth, Matochik, Cadet, & Bolla, 2004). Although no between-group differences were observed on task performance, cannabis users showed decreased metabolism in left prefrontal regions and increased metabolism in hippocampus, bilaterally, after 25 days of verified abstinence – suggesting that cannabis users needed to recruit a more extensive neural network to achieve comparable performances to controls.

Findings from fMRI studies similarly report discordance between changes in function and neurocognitive performance. Kanayama, Rogowska, Pope, Gruber, and Yurgelun-Todd (2004) reported that a group of 12 frequent heavy cannabis users with recent abstinence from cannabis (between 6 and 36 hours) generally showed more widespread activation involving prefrontal, striatal, and temporal brain regions during a working memory task than a group of ten matched controls. Groups showed a similar level of task performance. In another investigation by this group, decreased activation in supplementary motor cortex and anterior cingulate was observed among nine recently abstinent (4–36 hours) heavy cannabis users during a finger tapping task relative to 16 controls despite no differences between groups on task performance (Pillay et al., 2004). Further, brain activation did not correlate with levels of THC metabolites in urine. Gruber and Yurgelun-Todd (2005) measured brain activation using fMRI with nine heavy cannabis users who tested positive for cannabinoids in urine and with nine controls who completed a modified version of the Stroop Color Word paradigm. Groups showed normal levels of performance and did not differ significantly on any task parameters, though cannabis users tended to make more errors during the most demanding task condition. However, pattern of activation in prefrontal regions differed between groups. Participants in this study were very heavy users that approximately consumed, on average, 39 cannabis joints a week and tested positive for cannabinoids in urine. Although specific information on time of last cannabis use prior to undergoing testing and neuroimaging was not provided, it is likely that these individuals had used cannabis very recently.

Neuropsychological studies

Studies of neuropsychological functioning that employ more comprehensive test batteries, compared with the single task typically used in functional neuroimaging, have provided more detailed evidence regarding characteristics and severity of cognitive deficits among cannabis users. This topic has been the subject of numerous reviews (e.g., Grant & Mohns, 1975; Iversen, 2000; Pope et al., 1995; Solowij, 1998, 1999). Interpretations of the totality of findings of available investigations have sometimes been disparate, possibly due to the manner in which reviewers interpret the impact of methodological limitations on a study's findings. Pope and colleagues have provided one of the more comprehensive and detailed qualitative reviews on this topic (Pope et al., 1995). They found limited evidence of possible drug residue effects among cannabis users abstinent for 12–24 hours after last use. Evidence of CNS alterations (i.e., longer-term toxic effects) was inconclusive. Studies reporting statistically significant findings tended to show decreased performance on tests of attention, memory, and visuomotor abilities among cannabis users. The authors noted that methodology was typically flawed among many existing studies, thus limiting the potential significance of their reported findings to a great extent.

Clearly, neuropsychological investigations of residual cannabis effects have been challenging to conduct due to the methodological rigor needed to yield readily interpretable and conclusive findings. Gonzalez, Carey, and Grant (2002) provided an updated qualitative review of the literature focusing on methodological issues of existing studies and presented "minimal criteria" that studies of residual cannabis use must meet in order to yield interpretable effects. These included: (1) a study sample of subjects whose predominant or exclusive drug of abuse was cannabis; (2) an appropriate control group with limited or no cannabis use history; (3) use of valid and standardized neuropsychological tests; (4) abstinence from all substances of abuse at testing; (5) reported length of abstinence from cannabis; (6) adequate controls for effects of other substance use among cannabis users; and (7) obtained and controlled for neurological and mental health history. Without these standards in between-group studies, any potential significant effects of cannabis that are found could be due to common confounds.

A review of the 40 published studies examining residual neuropsychological functioning among cannabis users that were retrieved after a very comprehensive review of the published literature found that only 13 studies met all minimal methodological standards (Gonzalez et al., 2002). More than half failed to meet two or more criteria. Although the methodological shortcomings in most studies served to increase the chances of finding deficits among cannabis users, it was surprising to find that among the 40 studies only 55% found at least some impairment in a given cognitive ability among cannabis users. Most reported deficits in tests of attention (45%) and motor functions (35%). Less than one-third of studies reported finding evidence for impairments in perceptual/motor, abstraction/executive, simple reaction time, learning, and verbal domains.

In order to improve interpretability of published findings and arrive at quantitative estimates of a possible residual effect of cannabis use, a meta-analysis was conducted by Grant, Gonzalez, Carey, Natarajan, and Wolfson (2003) using the same pool of investigations uncovered by Gonzalez and colleagues (2002). In addition to meeting the criteria presented by Gonzalez et al. (2002), studies included in Grant et al. (2003) also needed to provide the necessary statistical information to conduct a meta-analysis. Only 11 studies met all criteria (i.e., Block & Ghoneim, 1993; Carlin & Trupin, 1977; Croft, Mackay, Mills, & Gruzelier, 2001; Ehrenreich et al., 1999; Gouzoulis-Mayfrank et al., 2000; Hamil, 1996; Pope & Yurgelun-Todd, 1996; Pope, Gruber, Hudson, Huestis, & Yurgelun-Todd, 2001; Rodgers, 2000; Solowij, 1995; Solowij et al., 2002) and an additional four studies (i.e., Deif, El, & Fawzy, 1993; Grant, Rochford, Fleming, & Stunkard, 1973; Rochford, Grant, & LaVigne, 1977; Wig & Varma, 1977) violated only one criterion despite very forgiving standards for deciding if each criterion was met. Analyses were first conducted only for the 11 studies meeting all criteria and then for the 15 studies, which included the four investigations violating only one criterion. For both analyses an effect size of a "residual cannabis effect" was calculated separately for each of eight neuropsychological domains and for all neuropsychological tests combined. Both sets of analyses showed evidence of slightly poorer overall performance by cannabis users relative to controls that was statistically significant, but of small magnitude (effect sizes $d =$ $-.15$ and $-.16$, respectively). Analyses of specific neuropsychological domains showed statistically significant effect sizes were only found for two domains: "learning" and "forgetting/retrieval." Again, the magnitude of the "cannabis effect" was small regardless of whether the 11 or 15 studies were examined.

Participant characteristics of cannabis users and the specific methodologies of studies included in the meta-analysis help to guide understanding of the types of cannabis users and conditions under which the results of the meta-analysis are likely to generalize. Abstinence among cannabis users across studies ranged from about 24 hours to several months and most participants in the studies were daily cannabis smokers. Some investigations only included individuals seeking treatment for cannabis problems, whereas other recruited from the community. Thus, findings from the meta-analysis might reflect in part a "withdrawal syndrome / drug residue effect." More importantly, several factors may have served to increase the likelihood of finding poorer performance among cannabis users. Specifically, "minimal standards" criteria were used to filter studies that made no attempts to control for certain confounds; however, several investigations were given "the benefit of the doubt," thus introducing the potential for minor confounds. Because studies that report statistically significant findings are more likely to be submitted to journals and published, such studies are more readily available for meta-analysis than those with no significant differences found between cannabis users and nonusers. Finally, the issue of premorbid differences between cannabis users and controls remains a key hindrance in revealing a "cannabis effect." For example, individuals who go on to use cannabis may differ from nonusers on important variables that are pertinent to cognitive functioning. Cannabis users may be different in quality of educational experiences, family socioeconomic status, vulnerability to mental health conditions, or neurocognitive factors that may predispose the individual to drug use. These factors are even more troublesome when cannabis users included in a study are only those seeking treatment for dependence or other problems associated with their cannabis user, since such individuals represent only a small percentage of all cannabis users. Others have also discussed some of these limitations (e.g., Pope, 2002).

Since the publication of the meta-analysis, several manuscripts have emerged examining residual neurocognitive effects of cannabis using novel neurocognitive protocols and probes that have provided new information to the existing body of work on this topic (e.g., McDonald, Schleifer, Richards, & de Wit, 2003; Whitlow et al., 2004; Bolla, Brown, Eldreth, Tate, & Cadet, 2002; Kelleher, Stough, Sergejew, & Rolfe, 2004). These investigations have reported mixed findings, noting deficits among cannabis in disparate cognitive abilities. Some of the studies are limited by many of the confounds and limitations to interpretation that have been previously discussed; however, three notable investigations have appeared since the publication of the meta-analysis that avoid many of the aforementioned confounds through the use of sophisticated longitudinal and tightly controlled research designs. Fried, Watkinson, James, and Gray (2002) examined the neuropsychological effects of cannabis use with participants from the Ottawa Prenatal Prospective Study, which was initiated during 1978 and followed participants since birth to assess effects of maternal drug use. This longitudinal design allowed consideration of an individual's actual (rather than estimated) neuropsychological functioning before and after initiation of regular cannabis use. These investigators examined the IQ test performance of 113 individuals at ages 9–12 and again at 17–20 years. At follow-up, all subjects were classified into subgroups according to severity of current and previous cannabis use: (1) current regular heavy cannabis smokers (>5 joints/week); (2) current regular light smokers (<5 joints/week); (3) former regular smokers (no regular use for at least 3 months and no more than 2 joints in the last 2 months); and (4) a control group who never used cannabis regularly. Individuals were fairly well matched with adequate control of pertinent confounds and all cannabis users reported abstinence for at least 1 day prior to testing. Relative to their baseline, current heavy cannabis users demonstrated a statistically significant (but minimal) decrease in IQ scores of approximately 4 points. These investigators recently examined performance on tests of more specific cognitive abilities using a similar study design (Fried, Watkinson, & Gray, 2005). Again, statistically significant differences were found only between the "current regular heavy cannabis users" and nonusing controls. Deficits were evident on measures of immediate and delayed memory, information processing speed, and full-scale IQ. However, effect sizes were fairly small for each of these comparisons and Type I error was not controlled despite numerous statistical comparisons (none of which yielded p values > .01). Importantly, unlike the heaviest cannabis-using group, current light users and former heavy users were not found to differ significantly from controls. Finally, Lyons and others (2004) used a comprehensive battery of neuropsychological tests to examine 54 monozygotic male twin pairs discordant for history of cannabis use. Twin pairs were genetically identical, were raised in the same home, and did not differ on history of alcohol, other drug use, or indices of achievement (e.g., employment, educational attainment, school grades, and academic difficulties). Individuals with a history of cannabis, on average, first began regular use of cannabis at about 21 years of age (range = 19–43) for an average duration of about 6 years (range 1–22 years). No participants reported using cannabis at least 1 year prior to testing, with last regular use occurring about 27 years ago on average (range 19–43 years). Of over 50 different indices of neuropsychological performance examined, statistically significant differences of very small magnitude (effect size = .19) were only observed on the Block Design subtest of the WAIS-R, a measure of visuoconstructional abilities.

Overall, findings do not support that cannabis use causes permanent "CNS alterations." Among heavy cannabis users there is some evidence for minor cognitive deficits that may last several weeks after abstinence. Such deficits are likely consistent with a drug-residue effect or may be part of a withdrawal syndrome.

Overview on the medical use of cannabis

The location and presumed functions of cannabinoid receptors have made them likely targets for treatments of various symptoms and disorders, including pain (Farquhar-Smith et al., 2000; Hohmann & Herkenham, 1999), anxiety (Arevalo, de Miguel, & Hernandez-Tristan, 2001; Haller, Bakos, Szirmay, Ledent, & Freund, 2002; Martin, Ledent, Parmentier, Maldonado, & Valverde, 2002), gastric problems (Di Carlo & Izzo, 2003; Kunos & Pacher, 2004), emesis (Van Sickle et al., 2001), and feeding behaviors (Fride & Shohami, 2002; Fride et al., 2001). Other preclinical investigations suggest that cannabinoid agonists may also prove useful in the treatment of cancerous tumor growth and neuroinflammation, whereas cannabinoid antagonists may serve to alleviate addiction and improve cardiovascular health. Furthermore, as previously indicated in this chapter, cannabinoids have been demonstrated to dampen excitoxic damage to brain tissue and are potent antioxidants.

Preclinical investigations coupled with anecdotal evidence from patients and their physicians have prompted research into therapeutic applications through cannabinoids and manipulation of the endocannabinoid system in humans. The House of Lords Select Committee on Science and Technology of the British Parliament in 1998 and the Senate Special Committee on Illegal Drugs of the Parliament of Canada in 2002 have noted that cannabis likely has medical applications and urged that clinical trials be conducted on its effectiveness in the treatment of various conditions (Canadian Senate Report, 2002; House of Lords Committee on Science and Technology, 1998). During 2003, the Netherlands changed its laws to allow the prescription of cannabis through pharmacies. As previously noted, several states in the USA have enacted legislation to facilitate the use of cannabis as medicine. For example, Proposition 215 was passed in California during 1996 to allow patient access to cannabis under medical supervision. In 1999, the legislature of the State of California established the Center for Medicinal Cannabis Research at the University of California, which currently supports approximately 12 clinical studies examining the therapeutic effectiveness of smoked cannabis on patients suffering from several disorders. However, the prescription of cannabis outside of research settings remains illegal in the USA, with the US Supreme Court's ruling that Federal law, which declares cannabis to be a harmful substance with no medical use, preempts state laws.

Several investigators have reviewed and commented on the literature regarding therapeutic uses for cannabis, cannabinoids, and synthetic analogues. Clinical trials to date have yielded mixed results on the effectiveness of cannabinoids on symptoms of various disorders in humans. Some investigators have demonstrated that THC administration was associated with the relief of cancer-associated pain (Noyes, Brunk, Baram, & Canter, 1975) and a synthetic cannabinoid reduced pain with postoperative trauma (Jain, Ryan, McMahon, & Smith, 1981). However, others have noted no benefit of THC on pain (Clark, Janal, Zeidenberg, & Nahas, 1981; Raft, Gregg, Ghia, & Harris, 1977). New oral-mucosal sprays (Sativex and GW2000-02), which are derived from extracts of the whole cannabis plant, have produced mixed results in their ability to reduce neuropathic pain (Berman, Symonds, & Birch, 2004). In patients with multiple sclerosis, Sativex reduced bladder dysfunction (Brady et al., 2004) and self-reported spasticity (Wade, Makela, Robson, House, & Bateman, 2004), but did not reduce the most troubling symptoms self-reported by patients (Wade et al., 2004). Overall, results from studies examining benefits of cannabis compounds on symptoms of multiple sclerosis have been inconsistent. THC and several synthetic analogues, including FDA-approved dronabinol, may reduce the nausea and vomiting often associated with chemotherapy (Chang et al., 1981; Gralla et al., 1984; Orr, McKernan, & Bloome, 1980; Sallan, Cronin, Zelen, & Zinberg, 1980; Steele, Gralla, Braun, & Young, 1980; Tyson et al., 1985;

Vinciguerra, Moore, & Brennan, 1988). Dronabinol is also approved as an appetite stimulant by the FDA, being shown to increase appetite and produce weight gain in patients with cancer cachexia (Gorter, 1991) and AIDS wasting (Beal et al., 1995, 1997; Struwe et al., 1993).

Recent years have witnessed accelerated research on the development of synthetic cannabinergic compounds, including CB_1 and CB_2 agonists, antagonists, and endocannabinoid deactivation inhibitors (see Grant, Makriyannis, Mechoulam, & Piomelli, 2005). Dexanabinol (HU-211), a synthetic cannabinoid analogue, has proven promising in improving the outcome of severe traumatic brain injury in preclinical models and is undergoing Phase III clinical trials (Knoller et al., 2002). Rimonabant (SR141716A), a CB_1 antagonist, is being tested and shows promise in the treatment of obesity and hyperlipidemia (Van Gaal, Rissanen, Scheen, Ziegler, & Rossner, 2005). CB_1 antagonists may also be valuable in treating addictions, as endocannabinoid signaling has been implicated in the brain's reward pathway. The CB_2 selective antagonist AM 1241 has demonstrated analgesic effects in neuropathic pain models. Preclinical work is in progress to determine the hypertensive potential of inhibitors of endocannabinoid breakdown (e.g., agents that block the enzyme fatty-acid amide hydrolase [FAAH]).

Despite unclear findings from the previously noted published clinical trials of cannabis itself, the cannabinoid system continues to be a promising target for therapeutic interventions. Future testing and additional clinical trials may bring additional medicines based on modulating the cannabinoid system to market. Possible deleterious systemic effects of smoking cannabis on lungs and cerebrovascular functions (which are beyond the scope of this chapter) may preclude its use as an accepted medicine in its natural, smoked form. However, the efficient administration and titration of cannabinoids afforded through smoking cannabis continues to make it a preferred mode of medicinal consumption for many at this moment. Safe and efficient delivery of cannabinoids that result in more predictable bioavailability will be critical. The current literature suggests that administration of botanical cannabinoids in low and monitored doses will likely result in no significant mental health or neurocognitive difficulties among most adults, though a minority of individuals may be vulnerable. The safety and dangers of medical cannabis are likely to be no worse than many other medications currently not on Schedule I (e.g., opiates and benzodiazepines). However, additional investigations will have to be carried out with synthetic cannabinoids and antagonists to determine if their margin of safety is comparable to the botanical cannabinoids.

Summary and conclusions

> The only permanent feature of Cannabis research seems to be that it comes in and out of fashion every several decades.
>
> (Raphael Mechoulam, 2000)

Currently, research on cannabis, its recreational use, and search for clinical applications is in fashion. The widespread use of cannabis throughout most of the world, particularly among young adults in western countries, makes it critical to understand possible harm that may come from its use and its specific effects on the brain, its functioning, and resulting behavior. Despite the long history of human use of cannabis, our understanding of the effects this substance has on the brain and its functioning remains far from well understood. The scientific literature is replete with debates and disparate interpretation of findings across and within disciplines. Nevertheless, a substantial amount of new knowledge in recent years has done much to further our understanding. An endogenous cannabinoid signaling system in the mammalian brain has been discovered and continues to be characterized with increasing detail. Insight into this system has produced hypotheses on mechanisms by which botanical and synthetic cannabinoids can harm, protect, and alter brain function depending on the situation.

The current characteristics of cannabis usage and individual vulnerability to neurocognitive effects are not conclusive. However, methodological improvements in mental health and neurocognitive investigations of cannabis use have nevertheless enhanced our understanding of these issues. In this regard, several conclusions are suggested based on current scientific findings. Acute intoxication with cannabis clearly affects cognitive functions and may result in symptoms that resemble mental health conditions among a subset of users (e.g., transient psychotic symptoms); however, most users find the acute psychoactive effects of cannabis to be pleasurable. Evidence suggesting that cannabis can cause or exacerbate mental illness has been weak, usually of small magnitude, and difficult to interpret due to confounds. Nevertheless, available evidence suggests that some individuals become dependent on cannabis and a "withdrawal syndrome" that is characterized primarily by mood complaints can be elicited by cessation of use. However, available evidence suggests that these conditions occur primarily among the heaviest and most frequent active users of cannabis. Though such individuals represent only a minority of cannabis users, the high prevalence of cannabis use means that millions of people may be affected. Future studies need to examine how patterns of cannabis use (e.g., frequency, duration, amount, potency, recency of use) and subject characteristics affect vulnerability to cannabis-associated mental health complaints (including dependence and abuse). Furthermore, much is left to be learned on genetic factors that may predispose cannabis users toward cannabis dependence, mental health complications, and neuropsychological impairments.

The findings from neuropsychological investigations also suggest that problems are more reliably detected among heavy, frequent, long-term users of cannabis, with deficits most apparent in areas of learning and remembering new information. However, such deficits in cognitive functioning diminish over several days of abstinence and return to baseline about a month after cessation of use. Further, the clinical and functional significance of these effects have been questioned due to their small magnitude. Thus, current findings suggest that ongoing heavy users of cannabis experience neuropsychological functioning that is lower than expected compared with their non-using peers. More limited use of cannabis (as might be relevant to medical applications) is not likely to result in detectable neurocognitive impairment. As in studies examining the mental health sequelae of cannabis use, future neuropsychological studies of cannabis will need to focus on the specific factors that mediate or moderate how cannabis use affects neurocognition.

Converging evidence suggests that limited cannabis use for documented medicinal purposes is unlikely to result in significant mental health or neuropsychological harm and its margin of safety is likely to be consistent with other currently approved medicines. This perspective is not without controversy, but findings from the scientific literature have prompted advocacy of medical applications of cannabis. At present, results of clinical trials have been inconclusive. Nevertheless, the endocannabinoid signaling system remains a potentially significant target for a range of therapeutic interventions, including THC, non-THC botanical cannabinoids or synthetic compounds.

This chapter has focused on presenting brief overviews of pertinent scientific topics regarding the effects of cannabis on brain functioning, with an emphasis on mental health and neurocognitive sequelae. Scientific evidence is just one of many factors that influence public opinion on the harms and benefits of recreational or medical use of cannabis. A detailed review of all scientific and sociopolitical issues pertaining to cannabis use is well beyond the scope of this chapter and many interesting and important publications pertaining to cannabis use could not be included and discussed. Clearly, much is still left to be learned on how this ancient herb affects human brain and behavior, as well as the differing individual factors and varied conditions under which it can bestow beneficial or harmful effects. We can anticipate that public acceptance and opinions toward cannabis use will continue to evolve and fluctuate over time, while the scientific knowledge base continues to grow.

References

Abood, M. E., & Martin, B. R. (1996). Molecular neurobiology of the cannabinoid receptor. *International Review of Neurobiology, 39,* 197–221.

Arevalo, C., de Miguel, R., & Hernandez-Tristan, R. (2001). Cannabinoid effects on anxiety-related behaviours and hypothalamic neurotransmitters. *Pharmacology Biochemistry and Behavior, 70,* 123–131.

Beal, J. E., Olson, R., Laubenstein, L., Morales, J. O., Bellman, P., Yangco, B., et al. (1995). Dronabinol as a treatment for anorexia associated with weight-loss in patients with AIDs. *Journal of Pain and Symptom Management, 10,* 89–97.

Beal, J. E., Olson, R., Lefkowitz, L., Larenstein, L., Bellman, P., Yangco, B., et al. (1997). Long-term efficacy and safety of dronabinol for acquired immunodeficiency syndrome-associated anorexia. *Journal of Pain and Symptom Management, 14*, 7–14.

Berman, J. S., Symonds, C., & Birch, R. (2004). Efficacy of two cannabis based medicinal extracts for relief of central neuropathic pain from brachial plexus avulsion: Results of a randomised controlled trial. *Pain, 112*, 299–306.

Biegon, A. (2004). Cannabinoids as neuroprotective agents in traumatic brain injury. *Current Pharmaceutical Design, 10*, 2177–2183.

Biegon, A., & Kerman, I. A. (2001). Autoradiographic study of pre- and postnatal distribution of cannabinoid receptors in human brain. *Neuroimage, 14*, 1463–1468.

Bisogno, T., Melck, D., Bobrov, M. Y., Gretskaya, N. M., Bezuglov, V. V., De Petrocellis, L., et al. (2000). N-acyl-dopamines: Novel synthetic CB1 cannabinoid-receptor ligands and inhibitors of anandamide inactivation with cannabimimetic activity in vitro and in vivo. *Biochemical Journal, 351*, 817–824.

Block, R. I., & Ghoneim, M. M. (1993). Effects of chronic marijuana use on human cognition. *Psychopharmacology, 110*, 219–228.

Block, R. I., O'Leary, D. S., Hichwa, R. D., Augustinack, J. C., Ponto, L. L. B., Ghoneim, M. M., et al. (2000). Cerebellar hypoactivity in frequent marijuana users. *Neuroreport, 11*, 749–753.

Block, R. I., O'Leary, D. S., Hichwa, R. D., Augustinack, J. C., Ponto, L. L. B., Ghoneim, M. M., et al. (2002). Effects of frequent marijuana use on memory-related regional cerebral blood flow. *Pharmacology Biochemistry and Behavior, 72*, 237–250.

Bolla, K. I., Brown, K., Eldreth, D., Tate, K., & Cadet, J. L. (2002). Dose-related neurocognitive effects of marijuana use. *Neurology, 59*, 1337–1343.

Booth, M. (2003). *Cannabis: A history*. New York: St. Martin's Press.

Brady, C. M., DasGupta, R., Dalton, C., Wiseman, O. J., Berkley, K. J., & Fowler, C. J. (2004). An open-label pilot study of cannabis-based extracts for bladder dysfunction in advanced multiple sclerosis. *Multiple Sclerosis, 10*, 425–433.

Breivogel, C. S., Griffin, G., Di Marzo, V., & Martin, B. R. (2001). Evidence for a new G protein-coupled cannabinoid receptor in mouse brain. *Molecular Pharmacology, 60*, 155–163.

Breivogel, C. S., & Childers, S. R. (1998). The functional neuroanatomy of brain cannabinoid receptors. *Neurobiology of Disease, 5*, 417–431.

Budney, A. J., Hughes, J. R., Moore, B. A., & Vandrey, R. (2004). Review of the validity and significance of cannabis withdrawal syndrome. *American Journal of Psychiatry, 161*, 1967–1977.

Canadian Senate Report (2002). *Our position for a Canadian public policy – Report of the Senate Special Committee on Illegal Drugs*. Ottawa, Ontario: Canadian Parliament.

Carlin, A. S., & Trupin, E. W. (1977). The effect of long-term chronic marijuana use on neuropsychological functioning. *International Journal of the Addictions, 12*, 617–624.

Chang, A. E., Shiling, D. J., Stillman, R. C., Goldberg, N. H., Seipp, C. A., Barofsky, I., et al. (1981). A prospective evaluation of delta-9-tetrahydrocannabinol as an anti-emetic in patients receiving adriamycin and cytoxan chemotherapy. *Cancer, 47*, 1746–1751.

Clark, W. C., Janal, M. N., Zeidenberg, P., & Nahas, G. G. (1981). Effects of moderate and high-doses of marihuana on thermal pain – A sensory decision-theory analysis. *Journal of Clinical Pharmacology, 21*, S299–S310.

Compton, W. M., Grant, B. F., Colliver, J. D., Glantz, M. D., & Stinson, F. S. (2004). Prevalence of marijuana use disorders in the United States: 1991–1992 and 2001–2002. *Journal of the American Medical Association, 291,* 2114–2121.

Crippa, J. A., Lacerda, A. L., Amaro, E., Busatto, F. G., Zuardi, A. W., & Bressan, R. A. (2005). [Brain effects of cannabis – neuroimaging findings]. *Revista Brasileira de Psiquiatria, 27,* 70–78.

Croft, R. J., Mackay, A. J., Mills, A. T. D., & Gruzelier, J. G. H. (2001). The relative contributions of ecstasy and cannabis to cognitive impairment. *Psychopharmacology, 153,* 373–379.

Davies, S. N., Pertwee, R. G., & Riedel, G. (2002). Functions of cannabinoid receptors in the hippocampus. *Neuropharmacology, 42,* 993–1007.

De Petrocellis, L., Cascio, M. G., & Di Marzo, V. (2004). The endocannabinoid system: A general view and latest additions. *British Journal of Pharmacology, 141,* 765–774.

Degenhardt, L., Hall, W., & Lynskey, M. (2003). Exploring the association between cannabis use and depression. *Addiction, 98,* 1493–1504.

Deif, A., El, S. A., & Fawzy, R. K. (1993). Neurological, psychiatric and CT evaluation of chronic cannabis smokers. *Journal of the Medical Research Institute, 14,* 151–160.

Devane, W. A., Dysarz, F. A., III, Johnson, M. R., Melvin, L. S., & Howlett, A. C. (1988). Determination and characterization of a cannabinoid receptor in rat brain. *Molecular Pharmacology, 34,* 605–613.

Devane, W. A., Hanus, L., Breuer, A., Pertwee, R. G., Stevenson, L. A., Griffin, G., et al. (1992). Isolation and structure of a brain constituent that binds to the cannabinoid receptor. *Science, 258,* 1946–1949.

Di Carlo, G., & Izzo, A. A. (2003). Cannabinoids for gastrointestinal diseases: potential therapeutic applications. *Expert Opinion on Investigational Drugs, 12,* 39–49.

Di Marzo, V., Breivogel, C. S., Tao, Q., Bridgen, D. T., Razdan, R. K., Zimmer, A. M., et al. (2000). Levels, metabolism, and pharmacological activity of anandamide in CB1 cannabinoid receptor knockout mice: Evidence for non-CB1, non-CB2 receptor-mediated actions of anandamide in mouse brain. *Journal of Neurochemistry, 75,* 2434–2444.

Earleywine, M. (2004). Marijuana arrests and increase in marijuana use disorders. *Journal of the American Medical Association, 292,* 802.

Ehrenreich, H., Rinn, T., Kunert, H. J., Moeller, M. R., Poser, W., Schilling, L., et al. (1999). Specific attentional dysfunction in adults following early start of cannabis use. *Psychopharmacology, 142,* 295–301.

Eldreth, D. A., Matochik, J. A., Cadet, J. L., & Bolla, K. I. (2004). Abnormal brain activity in prefrontal brain regions in abstinent marijuana users. *Neuroimage, 23,* 914–920.

ElSohly, M. A., Ross, S. A., Mehmedic, Z., Arafat, R., Yi, B., & Banahan, B. F. (2000). Potency trends of Delta(9)-THC and other cannabinoids in confiscated marijuana from 1980–1997. *Journal of Forensic Sciences, 45,* 24–30.

European Monitoring Centre for Drugs and Drug Addiction (2004). *Annual Report 2004: The state of the drugs problem in the European Union and Norway.* Luxembourg: Office for Official Publications of the European Communities.

Farquhar-Smith, W. P., Egertova, M., Bradbury, E. J., McMahon, S. B., Rice, A. S. C., & Elphick, M. R. (2000). Cannabinoid CB1 receptor expression in rat spinal cord. *Molecular and Cellular Neuroscience, 15,* 510–521.

Freund, T. F., Katona, I., & Piomelli, D. (2003). Role of endogenous cannabinoids in synaptic signaling. *Physiological Reviews, 83*, 1017–1066.

Fride, E., Foox, A., Rosenberg, E., Faigenboim, M., Cohen, V., Barda, L., et al. (2003). Milk intake and survival in newborn cannabinoid CB1 receptor knockout mice: Evidence for a "CB3" receptor. *European Journal of Pharmacology, 461*, 27–34.

Fride, E., & Shohami, E. (2002). The endocannabinoid system: Function in survival of the embryo, the newborn and the neuron. *Neuroreport, 13*, 1833–1841.

Fride, E., Ginzburg, Y., Breuer, A., Bisogno, T., Di Marzo, V., & Mechoulam, R. (2001). Critical role of the endogenous cannabinoid system in mouse pup suckling and growth. *European Journal of Pharmacology, 419*, 207–214.

Fried, P., Watkinson, B., James, D., & Gray, F. (2002). Current and former marijuana use: Preliminary findings of a longitudinal study of effects on IQ in Young adults. *Canadian Medical Association Journal, 166*, 887–891.

Fried, P. A., Watkinson, B., & Gray, R. (2005). Neurocognitive consequences of marihuana – A comparison with pre-drug performance. *Neurotoxicology and Teratology, 27*, 231–239.

Galiegue, S., Mary, S., Marchand, J., Dussossoy, D., Carriere, D., Carayon, P., et al. (1995). Expression of central and peripheral cannabinoid receptors in human immune tissues and leukocyte subpopulations. *European Journal of Biochemistry, 232*, 54–61.

Glass, M., Dragunow, M., & Faull, R. L. M. (1997). Cannabinoid receptors in the human brain: A detailed anatomical and quantitative autoradiographic study in the fetal, neonatal and adult human brain. *Neuroscience, 77*, 299–318.

Gonzalez, R., Carey, C., & Grant, I. (2002). Nonacute (residual) neuropsychological effects of cannabis use: A qualitative analysis and systematic review. *Journal of Clinical Pharmacology, 42*, 48S–57S.

Gorter, R. (1991). Management of anorexia-cachexia associated with cancer and HIV infection. *Oncology, 5*, 13–17.

Gouzoulis-Mayfrank, E., Daumann, J., Tuchtenhagen, F., Pelz, S., Becker, S., Kunert, H. J., et al. (2000). Impaired cognitive performance in drug free users of recreational ecstasy (MDMA). *Journal of Neurology, Neurosurgery and Psychiatry, 68*, 719–725.

Gralla, R. J., Tyson, L. B., Bordin, L. A., Clark, R. A., Kelsen, D. P., Kris, M. G., et al. (1984). Antiemetic therapy – A review of recent studies and a report of a random assignment trial comparing metoclopramide with delta-9-tetrahydrocannabinol. *Cancer Treatment Reports, 68*, 163–172.

Grant, I., Gonzalez, R., Carey, C., Natarajan, L., & Wolfson, T. (2003). Non-acute (residual) neurocognitive effects of cannabis use: A meta-analytic study. *Journal of the International Neuropsychological Society, 9*, 679–689.

Grant, I., & Judd, L. L. (1976). Neuropsychological and EEG Disturbances in polydrug users. *American Journal of Psychiatry, 133*, 1039–1042.

Grant, I., Makriyannis, A., Mechoulam, R., & Piomelli, D. (2005). Future Directions in Cannabinoid Therapeutics: "From the bench to the clinic". *Neuropharmacology, 48*, 1067–1171.

Grant, I., & Mohns, L. (1975). Chronic cerebral effects of alcohol and drug abuse. *International Journal of the Addictions, 10*, 883–920.

Grant, I., Rochford, J., Fleming, T., & Stunkard, A. (1973). A neuropsychological assessment of the effects of moderate marihuana use. *Journal of Nervous and Mental Disease, 156*, 278–280.

Green, B., Kavanagh, D., & Young, R. (2003). Being stoned: A review of self-reported cannabis effects. *Drug and Alcohol Review, 22*, 453–460.

Grotenhermen, F. (2003). Pharmacokinetics and pharmacodynamics of cannabinoids. *Clinical Pharmacokinetics, 42*, 327–360.

Gruber, S. A., & Yurgelun-Todd, D. A. (2005). Neuroimaging of marijuana smokers during inhibitory processing: A pilot investigation. *Cognitive Brain Research, 23*, 107–118.

Grundy, R. I. (2002). The therapeutic potential of the cannabinoids in neuroprotection. *Expert Opinion on Investigational Drugs, 11*, 1365–1374.

Guy, G., Whittle, B. A., & Robson, P. J. (2005). *The medicinal use of cannabis and cannabinoids*. London: Pharmaceutical Press.

Guzman, M., Sanchez, C., & Galve-Roperh, I. (2001). Control of the cell survival/death decision by cannabinoids. *Journal of Molecular Medicine, 78*, 613–625.

Hall, W., & Swift, W. (2000). The THC content of cannabis in Australia: Evidence and implications. *Australian and New Zealand Journal of Public Health, 24*, 503–508.

Haller, J., Bakos, N., Szirmay, M., Ledent, C., & Freund, T. F. (2002). The effects of genetic and pharmacological blockade of the CB1 cannabinoid receptor on anxiety. *European Journal of Neuroscience, 16*, 1395–1398.

Hamil, W. L. (1996). Auditory learning and memory performance among veterans with a history of stimulant abuse. *Dissertation Abstracts International: Section B: The Sciences and Engineering, 56*, 5806.

Hampson, A. J., Grimaldi, M., Lolic, M., Wink, D., Rosenthal, R., & Axelrod, J. (2000). Neuroprotective antioxidants from marijuana. *Annals of the New York Academy of Sciences, 899*, 274–282.

Hanus, L., Abu-Lafi, S., Fride, E., Breuer, A., Vogel, Z., Shalev, D. E., et al. (2001). 2-Arachidonyl glyceryl ether, an endogenous agonist of the cannabinoid CB1 receptor. *Proceedings of the National Academy of Sciences of the United States of America, 98*, 3662–3665.

Herkenham, M., Lynn, A. B., de Costa, B. R., & Richfield, E. K. (1991). Neuronal localization of cannabinoid receptors in the basal ganglia of the rat. *Brain Research, 547*, 267–274.

Herkenham, M., Lynn, A. B., Little, M. D., Johnson, M. R., Melvin, L. S., de Costa, B. R., et al. (1990). Cannabinoid receptor localization in brain. *Proceedings of the National Academy of Sciences of the United States of America, 87*, 1932–1936.

Hohmann, A. G., & Herkenham, M. (1999). Localization of central cannabinoid CB1 receptor messenger RNA in neuronal subpopulations of rat dorsal root ganglia: A double-label in situ hybridization study. *Neuroscience, 90*, 923–931.

House of Lords Select Committee on Science and Technology (1998). *Cannabis: The scientific and medicinal evidence*. London: The Stationery Office.

Howlett, A. C., Johnson, M. R., Melvin, L. S., & Milne, G. M. (1988). Nonclassical cannabinoid analgetics inhibit adenylate-cyclase – Development of a cannabinoid receptor model. *Molecular Pharmacology, 33*, 297–302.

Huang, S. M., Bisogno, T., Trevisani, M., Al Hayani, A., De Petrocellis, L., Fezza, F., et al. (2002). An endogenous capsaicin-like substance with high potency at recombinant and native vanilloid VR1 receptors. *Proceedings of the National Academy of Sciences of the United States of America, 99*, 8400–8405.

Iversen, L. L. (2000). *The science of marijuana*. New York: Oxford University Press.

Jain, A. K., Ryan, J., McMahon, F. G., & Smith, G. (1981). Evaluation of intramuscular levonantradol and placebo in acute postoperative pain. *Journal of Clinical Pharmacology, 21*, 3205–3326.

Johns, A. (2001). Psychiatric effects of cannabis. *British Journal of Psychiatry, 178*, 116–122.

Johnston, L. D., O'Malley, P. M., Bachman, J. G., & Schulenberg, J. E. (2005). *Monitoring the future national results on adolescent drug use: Overview of key findings, 2004*. Bethesda, MD: National Institute on Drug Abuse.

Kanayama, G., Rogowska, J., Pope, H. G., Gruber, S. A., & Yurgelun-Todd, D. A. (2004). Spatial working memory in heavy cannabis users: A functional magnetic resonance imaging study. *Psychopharmacology, 176*, 239–247.

Kelleher, L. M., Stough, C., Sergejew, A. A., & Rolfe, T. (2004). The effects of cannabis on information-processing speed. *Addictive Behaviors, 29*, 1213–1219.

Knoller, N., Levi, L., Shoshan, I., Reichenthal, E., Razon, N., Rappaport, Z. H., et al. (2002). Dexanabinol (HU-211) in the treatment of severe closed head injury: A randomized, placebo-controlled, phase II clinical trial. *Critical Care Medicine, 30*, 548–554.

Kunos, G., & Pacher, P. (2004). Cannabinoids cool the intestine. *Nature Medicine, 10*, 678–679.

Leweke, F. M., Gerth, C. W., & Klosterkotter, J. (2004). Cannabis-associated psychosis – Current status of research. *CNS Drugs, 18*, 895–910.

Loeber, R. T., & Yurgelun-Todd, D. A. (1999). Human neuroimaging of acute and chronic marijuana use: Implications for frontocerebellar dysfunction. *Human Psychopharmacology: Clinical and Experimental, 14*, 291–304.

Lyons, M. J., Bar, J. L., Panizzon, M. S., Toomey, R., Eisen, S., Xian, H., et al. (2004). Neuropsychological consequences of regular marijuana use: a twin study. *Psychological Medicine, 34*, 1239–1250.

Macleod, J., Oakes, R., Copello, A., Crome, L., Egger, M., Hickman, M., et al. (2004). Psychological and social sequelae of cannabis and other illicit drug use by young people: A systematic review of longitudinal, general population studies. *Lancet, 363*, 1579–1588.

Maejima, T., Ohno-Shosaku, T., & Kano, M. (2001). Endogenous cannabinoid as a retrograde messenger from depolarized postsynaptic neurons to presynaptic terminals. *Neuroscience Research, 40*, 205–210.

Maldonado, R. (2002). Study of cannabinoid dependence in animals. *Pharmacology and Therapeutics, 95*, 153–164.

Marsicano, G., Moosmann, B., Hermann, H., Lutz, B., & Behl, C. (2002). Neuroprotective properties of cannabinoids against oxidative stress: Role of the cannabinoid receptor CB1. *Journal of Neurochemistry, 80*, 448–456.

Martin, B. R., Mechoulam, R., & Razdan, R. K. (1999). Discovery and characterization of endogenous cannabinoids. *Life Sciences, 65*, 573–595.

Martin, M., Ledent, C., Parmentier, M., Maldonado, R., & Valverde, O. (2002). Involvement of CB1 cannabinoid receptors in emotional behaviour. *Psychopharmacology, 159*, 379–387.

Mathew, R. J., Tant, S., & Burger, C. (1986). Regional cerebral blood flow in marijuana smokers. *British Journal of Addictions, 81*, 567–571.

Mathew, R. J., & Wilson, W. H. (1993). Acute changes in cerebral blood-flow after smoking marijuana. *Life Sciences, 52*, 757–767.

Mathew, R. J., Wilson, W. H., Chiu, N. Y., Turkington, T. G., Degrado, T. R.,

& Coleman, R. E. (1999). Regional cerebral blood flow and depersonalization after tetrahydrocannabinol administration. *Acta Psychiatrica Scandinavica, 100,* 67–75.

Mathew, R. J., Wilson, W. H., Coleman, R. E., Turkington, T. G., & Degrado, T. R. (1997). Marijuana intoxication and brain activation in marijuana smokers. *Life Sciences, 60,* 2075–2089.

Mathew, R. J., Wilson, W. H., Humphreys, D. F., Lowe, J. V., & Wiethe, K. E. (1992). Changes in middle cerebral-artery velocity after marijuana. *Biological Psychiatry, 32,* 164–169.

Mathew, R. J., Wilson, W. H., & Tant, S. R. (1989). Acute changes in cerebral blood-flow associated with marijuana smoking. *Acta Psychiatrica Scandinavica, 79,* 118–128.

Mathew, R. J., Wilson, W. H., Turkington, T. G., & Coleman, R. E. (1998). Cerebellar activity and disturbed time sense after THC. *Brain Research, 797,* 183–189.

Mathew, R. J., Wilson, W. H., Turkington, T. G., Hawk, T. C., Coleman, R. E., DeGrado, T. R., et al. (2002). Time course of tetrahydrocannabinol-induced changes in regional cerebral blood flow measured with positron emission tomography. *Psychiatry Research: Neuroimaging, 116,* 173–185.

Matsuda, L. A., Lolait, S. J., Brownstein, M. J., Young, A. C., & Bonner, T. I. (1990). Structure of a cannabinoid receptor and functional expression of the cloned cDNA. *Nature, 346,* 561–564.

McAllister, S. D., & Glass, M. (2002). CB1 and CB2 receptor-mediated signalling: A focus on endocannabinoids. *Prostaglandins, Leukotrienes and Essential Fatty Acids, 66,* 161–171.

McDonald, J., Schleifer, L., Richards, J. B., & de Wit, H. (2003). Effects of THC on behavioral measures of impulsivity in humans. *Neuropsychopharmacology, 28,* 1356–1365.

Mechoulam, R. (2000). Looking back at cannabis research. *Current Pharmaceutical Design, 6,* 1313–1322.

Mechoulam, R. (2002). Discovery of endocannabinoids and some random thoughts on their possible roles in neuroprotection and aggression. *Prostaglandins, Leukotrienes and Essential Fatty Acids, 66,* 93–99.

Mechoulam, R., Benshabat, S., Hanus, L., Ligumsky, M., Kaminski, N. E., Schatz, A. R., et al. (1995). Identification of an endogenous 2-monoglyceride, present in canine gut, that binds to cannabinoid receptors. *Biochemical Pharmacology, 50,* 83–90.

Mechoulam, R., Panikashvili, D., & Shohami, E. (2002). Cannabinoids and brain injury: therapeutic implications. *Trends in Molecular Medicine, 8,* 58–61.

Mikuriya, T. H., & Aldrich, M. R. (1988). Cannabis 1988 – Old drug, new dangers the potency question. *Journal of Psychoactive Drugs, 20,* 47–55.

Munro, S., Thomas, K. L., & Abu-Shaar, M. (1993). Molecular characterization of a peripheral receptor for cannabinoids. *Nature, 365,* 61–65.

National Drug Intelligence Center (2005). *National Drug Threat Assessment 2005.* Washington, DC: US Department of Justice.

Noyes, R., Jr., Brunk, S. F., Baram, D. A., & Canter, A. (1975). Analgesic effect of delta-9-tetrahydrocannabinol. *Journal of Clinical Pharmacology, 15,* 139–143.

O'Leary, D. S., Block, R. I., Koeppel, J. A., Flaum, M., Schultz, S. K., Andreasen, N. C., et al. (2002). Effects of smoking marijuana on brain perfusion and cognition. *Neuropsychopharmacology, 26,* 802–816.

Orr, L. E., McKernan, J. F., & Bloome, B. (1980). Antiemetic effect of tetrahydrocannabinol. Compared with placebo and prochlorperazine in chemotherapy-associated nausea and emesis. *Archives of Internal Medicine, 140*, 1431–1433.

Pacher, P., Batkai, S., & Kunos, G. (2005). Blood pressure regulation by endocannabinoids and their receptors. *Neuropharmacology, 48*, 1130–1138.

Pertwee, R. G. (1997). Pharmacology of cannabinoid CB1 and CB2 receptors. *Pharmacology and Therapeutics, 74*, 129–180.

Pillay, S. S., Rogowska, J., Kanayama, G., Jon, D. I., Gruber, S., Simpson, N., et al. (2004). Neurophysiology of motor function following cannabis discontinuation in chronic cannabis smokers: An fMRI study. *Drug and Alcohol Dependence, 76*, 261–271.

Piomelli, D. (2003). The molecular logic of endocannabinoid signaling. *Nature Reviews in Neuroscience, 4*, 873–884.

Pope, H. G. (2002). Cannabis, cognition, and residual confounding. *Journal of the American Medical Association, 287*, 1172–1174.

Pope, H. G., Jr., Gruber, A. J., & Yurgelun-Todd, D. (1995). The residual neuropsychological effects of cannabis: The current status of research. *Drug and Alcohol Dependence, 38*, 25–34.

Pope, H. G., Jr., & Yurgelun-Todd, D. (1996). The residual cognitive effects of heavy marijuana use in college students. *Journal of the American Medical Association, 275*, 521–527.

Pope, H. G., Gruber, A. J., Hudson, J. I., Huestis, M. A., & Yurgelun-Todd, D. (2001). Neuropsychological performance in long-term cannabis users. *Archives of General Psychiatry, 58*, 909–915.

Porter, A. C., Sauer, J. M., Knierman, M. D., Becker, G. W., Berna, M. J., Bao, J. Q., et al. (2002). Characterization of a novel endocannabinoid, virhodamine, with antagonist activity at the CB1 receptor. *Journal of Pharmacology and Experimental Therapeutics, 301*, 1020–1024.

Poulsen, H. A., & Sutherland, G. J. (2000). The potency of cannabis in New Zealand from 1976 to 1996. *Science and Justice, 40*, 171–176.

Raft, D., Gregg, J., Ghia, J., & Harris, L. (1977). Effects of intravenous tetrahydrocannabinol on experimental and surgical pain – Psychological correlates of analgesic response. *Clinical Pharmacology and Therapeutics, 21*, 26–33.

Reed, R., & Grant, I. (1990). The long term neurobehavioral consequences of substance abuse: Conceptual and methodological challenges for future research. In J. W. Spencer & J. J. Boren (Eds.), *Residual effects of abused drugs on behavior*, National Institute on Drug Abuse Research Monograph 101. Washington, DC: U.S. Government Printing Office.

Rochford, J., Grant, I., & LaVigne, G. (1977). Medical students and drugs: Further neuropsychological and use pattern considerations. *International Journal of the Addictions, 12*, 1057–1065.

Rodgers, J. (2000). Cognitive performance amongst recreational users of "ecstasy". *Psychopharmacology, 151*, 19–24.

Sallan, S. E., Cronin, C., Zelen, M., & Zinberg, N. E. (1980). Anti-emetics in patients receiving chemotherapy for cancer – Randomized comparison of delta-9-tetrahydrocannabinol and prochlorperazine. *New England Journal of Medicine, 302*, 135–138.

Smith, N. T. (2002). A review of the published literature into cannabis withdrawal symptoms in human users. *Addiction, 97*, 621–632.

Solowij, N. (1995). Do cognitive impairments recover following cessation of cannabis use? *Life Sciences, 56,* 2119–2126.

Solowij, N. (1998). *Cannabis and cognitive functioning.* Cambridge: Cambridge University Press.

Solowij, N. (1999). Long-term effects of cannabis on the central nervous system. In H. Kalant, W. Corrigall, W. Hall, & R. Smart (Eds.), *The health effects of cannabis.* Toronto: Addiction Research Foundation.

Solowij, N., Michie, P. T., & Fox, A. M. (1991). Effects of long-term cannabis use on selective attention – An event-related potential study. *Pharmacology, Biochemistry and Behavior, 40,* 683–688.

Solowij, N., Stephens, R. S., Roffman, R. A., Babor, T., Kadden, R., Miller, M., et al. (2002). Cognitive functioning of long-term heavy cannabis users seeking treatment. *Journal of the American Medical Association, 287,* 1123–1131.

Steele, N., Gralla, R. J., Braun, D. W., & Young, C. W. (1980). Double-blind comparison of the anti-emetic effects of nabilone and prochlorperazine on chemotherapy-induced emesis. *Cancer Treatment Reports, 64,* 219–224.

Struwe, M., Kaempfer, S. H., Geiger, C. J., Pavia, A. T., Plasse, T. F., Shepard, K. V., et al. (1993). Effect of dronabinol on nutritional-status in HIV-infection. *Annals of Pharmacotherapy, 27,* 827–831.

Substance Abuse and Mental Health Services Administration (2003). *National Survey on Drug Use and Health.* Rockville, MD: United States Department of Health and Human Services.

Sugiura, T., Kondo, S., Sukagawa, A., Nakane, S., Shinoda, A., Itoh, K., et al. (1995). 2-Arachidonoylgylcerol – A possible endogenous cannabinoid receptor-ligand in brain. *Biochemical and Biophysical Research Communications, 215,* 89–97.

Tanda, G., & Goldberg, S. R. (2003). Cannabinoids: Reward, dependence, and underlying neurochemical mechanisms – A review of recent preclinical data. *Psychopharmacology, 169,* 115–134.

Tunving, K., Thulin, S. O., Risberg, J., & Warkentin, S. (1986). Regional cerebral blood-flow in long-term heavy cannabis use. *Psychiatry Research, 17,* 15–21.

Tyson, L. B., Gralla, R. J., Clark, R. A., Kris, M. G., Bordin, L. A., & Bosl, G. J. (1985). Phase 1 trial of levonantradol in chemotherapy-induced emesis. *American Journal of Clinical Oncology, 8,* 528–532.

United Nations Office on Drugs and Crimes (2004). *World drug report.* New York: United Nations Publications.

Van der Stelt, M., Veldhuis, W. B., Maccarrone, M., Bar, P. R., Nicolay, K., Veldink, G. A., et al. (2002). Acute neuronal injury, excitotoxicity, and the endocannabinoid system. *Molecular Neurobiology, 26,* 317–346.

Van Gaal, L. F., Rissanen, A. M., Scheen, A. J., Ziegler, O., & Rossner, S. (2005). Effects of the cannabinoid-1 receptor blocker rimonabant on weight reduction and cardiovascular risk factors in overweight patients: 1-year experience from the RIO-Europe study. *Lancet, 365,* 1389–1397.

Van Sickle, M. D., Oland, L. D., Ho, W., Hillard, C. J., Mackie, K., Davison, J. S., et al. (2001). Cannabinoids inhibit emesis through CB1 receptors in the brainstem of the ferret. *Gastroenterology, 121,* 767–774.

Vinciguerra, V., Moore, T., & Brennan, E. (1988). Inhalation marijuana as an antiemetic for cancer-chemotherapy. *New York State Journal of Medicine, 88,* 525–527.

Volkow, N. D., Gillespie, H., Mullani, N., Tancredi, L., Grant, C., Ivanovic, M., et al.

(1991). Cerebellar metabolic-activation by delta-9-tetrahydro-cannabinol in human brain – A study with positron emission tomography and F-18 2-fluoro-2-deoxyglucose. *Psychiatry Research – Neuroimaging, 40*, 69–78.

Volkow, N. D., Gillespie, H., Mullani, N., Tancredi, L., Grant, C., Valentine, A., et al. (1996). Brain glucose metabolism in chronic marijuana users at baseline and during marijuana intoxication. *Psychiatry Research – Neuroimaging, 67*, 29–38.

Wade, D. T., Makela, P., Robson, P., House, H., & Bateman, C. (2004). Do cannabis-based medicinal extracts have general or specific effects on symptoms in multiple sclerosis? A double-blind, randomized, placebo-controlled study on 160 patients. *Multiple Sclerosis, 10*, 434–441.

Whitlow, C. T., Liguori, A., Livengood, L. B., Hart, S. L., Mussat-Whitlow, B. J., Lamborn, C. M., et al. (2004). Long-term heavy marijuana users make costly decisions on a gambling task. *Drug and Alcohol Dependence, 76*, 107–111.

Wig, N. N., & Varma, V. K. (1977). Patterns of long-term heavy cannabis use in North India and its effects on cognitive functions: A preliminary report. *Drug and Alcohol Dependence, 2*, 211–219.

6 MDMA

*Ari Kalechstein, William E. Fantegrossi,
Ronald L. Cowan, and James J. Mahoney*

Introduction

In 1914, two years after filing their initial application, the German pharmaceutical company (Merck) received a patent for the novel, ring-substituted amphetamine derivative 3,4-methylenedioxymethamphetamine (MDMA, see Figure 6.1D) (Shulgin, 1990). Despite persistent colloquial rumors that the compound was intentionally synthesized as an appetite suppressant, a psychotherapeutic, or a "psychological warfare agent," the Merck patent contains no mention of MDMA's pharmacological properties, nor does it state any intended pharmaceutical uses. Indeed, MDMA does not appear to have been studied at all until the 1950s. These toxicological studies, performed at the University of Michigan under a classified contract with the United States Army, were conducted during 1953 and 1954, declassified in 1969, and published in 1973 (Shulgin, 1986). In these experiments, MDMA was coded as EA-1475 (for Edgewood Arsenal, where this batch of compound was synthesized), and was one of seven compounds (each structurally related to the phenethylamine hallucinogen mescaline) studied and shown to have various behavioral and lethal effects in mice, rats, guinea pigs, dogs, and rhesus monkeys (Hardman, Haavik, & Seevers, 1973).

As early as 1976, MDMA appears to have diffused into the general drug culture due to the efforts of two groups of underground chemists, first in Boston, then later in Texas (Beck & Rosenbaum, 1994). During this time, MDMA could be legally purchased in various clubs and bars, and developed a reputation as a "new psychedelic" (Millman & Breeder, 1994). It was also during this time that the street name "ecstasy" was first applied to MDMA, eventually replacing the previous (and presumably less marketable) designations "Adam" and "empathy" (Parrott & Yeomans, 1995).

The purpose of this chapter is to provide a comprehensive review regarding MDMA. This includes sections on preclinical pharmacology, human neuroimaging studies, and studies examining the neuropsychological consequences of MDMA. Following the review, the discussion will survey the literature that examined the utility of MDMA as a treatment for social phobia.

Preclinical pharmacology

This section will delineate the effects of MDMA at the cellular level. The findings of these studies were based on animal models of MDMA use (typically rodents or primates). This section begins with a review of the basic chemistry of MDMA, which is noteworthy insofar as it is similar to, but distinct from, that of other classes of drugs (e.g., stimulants and hallucinogens). We then discuss the role of serotonin in response to MDMA, the behavioral effects of MDMA in animals, and the neurotoxic effects of MDMA in animals.

Chemistry

MDMA is structurally related to both the amphetamine-type stimulants and the mescaline-type hallucinogens. The basic chemical backbone for both groups of compounds is phenethylamine (Figure 6.1A). The general structure–activity rule determining pharmacological actions for the substituted phenethylamines is that substituents on the aromatic ring, particularly oxygen-containing groups, tend to establish hallucinogenic activity, whereas substitutions on the amine group, particularly in the presence of an unsubstituted aromatic ring, confer psychostimulant activity to the resulting compounds (Glennon, 1989). Amphetamine (Figure 6.1B), for example, is a central stimulant with little in the way of hallucinogenic effects unless very large doses are taken over some period of time. Compounds with this basic structure typically act by increasing relevant levels of central dopamine and function as behavioral stimulants. Mescaline (Figure 6.1C), on the other hand, has only weak central stimulant effects, and is a potent hallucinogen. Drugs possessing this basic structure typically act through serotonin (5-HT) receptors and are behavioral hallucinogens.

The importance of these chemical comparisons becomes clear when MDMA's structure (Figure 6.1D) is considered. This compound has chemical properties common to both the central stimulants and the hallucinogens; thus, in the absence of further information, it would be difficult to predict the behavioral effects of MDMA. The current scientific thinking on MDMA is that it represents a prototypical compound from a unique pharmacological class (Nichols, 1986). In this regard, MDMA and its analogues do not tend to exhibit behavioral effects congruent with those of amphetamine-like drugs. For example, neither the discriminative stimulus effects nor the observed abuse patterns of these compounds are consistent with those of the central stimulants. MDMA is usually taken intermittently, in the context of raves or dance parties, rather than in a compulsive binge pattern characteristic of the central stimulants. Furthermore, MDMA does not appear to be as reinforcing as cocaine or methamphetamine in rhesus monkeys (Fantegrossi, Ullrich, Rice, Woods, & Winger, 2002). On the other hand, MDMA and its analogues also lack some of the aspects of the traditional serotonergic

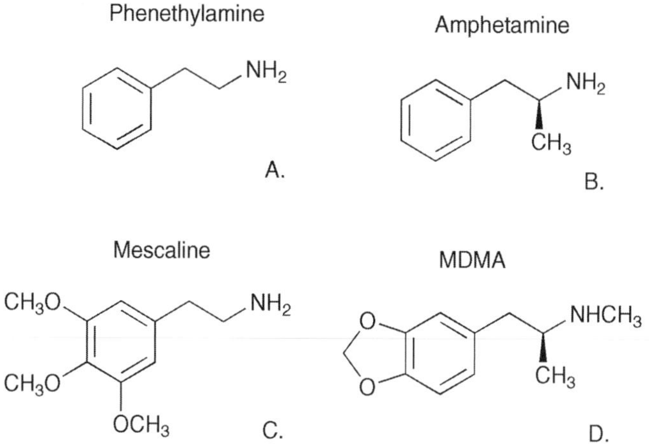

Figure 6.1 Chemical structures of phenethylamine (A), amphetamine (B), mescaline (C), and MDMA (D).

hallucinogens. MDMA does not produce frank hallucinations like those of mescaline, although it does produce "sensory distortions" at the doses taken by humans. MDMA also has clear and consistent reinforcing effects in non-human primates (Fantegrossi et al., 2002), which the phenylisopropylamine and indolealkylamine hallucinogens lack (Fantegrossi, Woods, & Winger, 2004).

Mechanism of action

Interest in the study of ring-substituted amphetamine analogues began as early as 1967 when Naranjo and co-workers published a report describing the lack of hallucinogenic effects of 3,4-methylenedioxyamphetamine (MDA) (Naranjo, Shulgin, & Sargent, 1967). Subsequent investigations into the pharmacological properties of MDA distinguished this compound from both the classical hallucinogens and the psychostimulants (Nichols, 1986). One of the most robust structure–activity laws for the hallucinogenic amphetamines states that N-methylation dramatically attenuates or abolishes psychedelic activity (Shulgin, 1978). But in the case of MDMA (the N-methyl derivative of MDA), pharmacological activity is retained at a potency only slightly less than that of MDA (Nichols, 1986). Additionally, for every other hallucinogenic amphetamine studied, it was determined that the $R(-)$ isomer is responsible for biological activity (Nichols & Glennon, 1984; Shulgin, 1973); however, with MDA and MDMA *both* enantiomers are active and possess distinct pharmacological effects (Fantegrossi et al., 2003, 2004a; Fischer, Zernig, Schatz, Humpel, & Saria, 2000; Nichols, 1986). These disparate findings lead Nichols to remark, "Either MDMA is not a hallucinogen or else it is a hallucinogen acting in a completely unexpected way that is different from the other substituted amphetamines ... One wonders whether it should be called a hallucinogen at all, based on its unusual pharmacology" (Nichols, 1986).

Nichols and colleagues were the first to study the biochemical effects of MDMA and related compounds in their endeavor to develop quantitative structure–activity relationships for the psychedelic drugs. In rat synaptosomes, the effects of the MDMA enantiomers on 5-HT release were quantified and compared to those of the stereoisomers of MDA. In these experiments, both isomers of MDA were shown to release 5-HT with equal potency, $S(+)$-MDMA was demonstrated to be approximately equipotent to the MDA isomers, and $R(-)$-MDMA was shown to be least potent in terms of 5-HT release (Nichols, Lloyd, Hoffman, Nichols, & Yim, 1982). Nichols later noted that the few other drugs known to share this mechanism have vastly different psychopharmacological effects in humans (Nichols, 1986). For example, the subjective effects reported following administration of the 5-HT releaser fenfluramine include dysphoria and sedation (Griffith, Nutt, & Jasinski, 1975), whereas MDMA is said to produce "an easily controlled altered state of consciousness, with emotional and sensual overtones" (Shulgin, 1986). Further studies by the Nichols group extended previous results by demonstrating blockade of 5-HT, dopamine and norepinephrine reuptake by the MDMA isomers, again in rat synaptosomes (Nichols, 1986). These experiments also revealed a modest stereoselectivity, with $S(+)$-MDMA producing slightly (2–4-fold) lower IC_{50} values for all three monoamines (Nichols, 1986). The stereoselective effects of the MDMA enantiomers are even more pronounced in behavioral assays, and will be discussed below in some detail.

The binding profile of MDMA was further established by the studies of Battaglia and associates. Their *ex vivo* radioligand binding experiments described a rank order of affinities for racemic MDMA at various central receptor systems, such that: affinity for 5-HT transporters > $α_2$-adrenoceptors = 5-HT_2 serotonin receptors = M-1 muscarinic receptors = H-1 histamine receptors > norepinephrine transporters = M-2 muscarinic receptors = $α_1$-adrenoceptors = β-adrenoceptors ≥ dopamine transporters = 5-HT_1 serotonin receptors >> D_2 dopamine receptors > D_1 dopamine receptors (Battaglia, Brooks, Kulsakdinun, & De Souza, 1988). Further experiments with the enantiomers revealed that $R(-)$-MDMA has higher affinity for postsynaptic 5-HT receptors than does $S(+)$-MDMA, while $S(+)$-MDMA has higher affinity for 5-HT transporters than does $R(-)$-MDMA (Battaglia & De Souza, 1989), perhaps explaining the previously observed stereoselective effects of the enantiomers on 5-HT release (Nichols et al., 1982). Since the initial publication of these studies, more receptor-selective tools have become available, and a reassessment of the affinities of MDMA and its enantiomers for various brain recognition sites using these improved methods should be encouraged.

The preferential effects of MDMA on central 5-HT systems were further elucidated by Rudnick and Wall. Their studies distinguished between

MDMA's effects at plasma membrane 5-HT transporters and vesicular transporters, and demonstrated that MDMA is a substrate for both systems (Rudnick & Wall, 1992). Their results also implied that MDMA causes 5-HT release via a 5-HT/MDMA exchange, perhaps analogous to amphetamine's effects on dopamine transporters (Rudnick & Wall, 1992). Further experiments demonstrated similar releasing effects on dopamine (Schmidt & Taylor, 1987), norepinephrine (Rothman et al., 2001), and acetylcholine (Acquas et al., 2001; Fischer et al., 2000), although all of these effects are lesser in magnitude than those observed with 5-HT release. Finally, recent evidence has shown that MDMA has agonist activity at the rat trace amine receptor TAR1, a property shared by the structurally related psychostimulant amphetamine (Bunzow et al., 2001). This convoluted cluster of effects led Parrot to describe the neuropharmacological effects of MDMA as "a minefield of potential drug interactions" (Parrott, 2001); however, the widely accepted classification of MDMA as (primarily) an indirect serotonin agonist seems to be well supported.

Role of endogenous 5-HT

It has become clear that preventing MDMA-induced 5-HT release, either by depleting endogenous 5-HT stores or by blocking plasma membrane 5-HT transporters, can attenuate many of the physiological, neurochemical, and behavioral effects of MDMA. For example, it has been shown that MDMA-induced 5-HT release and hyperthermia can be attenuated by depleting vesicular 5-HT stores via pretreatment with reserpine (Sabol & Seiden, 1998). Interestingly, the head twitch response elicited by $S(+)$-MDMA in the mouse is profoundly reduced by prior treatment with the 5-HT synthesis inhibitor *para*-chlorophenylalanine (*p*-CPA), although this pretreatment regimen does not alter twitch behavior elicited by $R(-)$-MDMA (Fantegrossi et al., 2004a). Furthermore, the hyperthermic effects of $S(+)$-MDMA are attenuated in the *p*-CPA-treated mouse, although the effects of the racemate on core temperature are preserved (Fantegrossi et al., 2004a). These studies exemplify the dramatic stereoselectivity of MDMA effects observed *in vivo*, and suggest that both 5-HT release and direct 5-HT agonism are implicated in this compound's behavioral effects, which are likely mediated by different mechanisms across multiple measures.

Role of 5-HT transporters

Serotonin selective reuptake inhibitors (SSRIs) have been shown to exert a long-lasting protective effect against MDMA-induced 5-HT neurodegeneration (Sanchez et al., 2001) and have proven efficacious in blocking MDMA-induced 5-HT depletion (Schmidt & Taylor, 1987) and locomotor stimulant effects (Callaway, Wing, & Geyer, 1990). The effects of SSRIs on MDMA-induced lethality are less clear: Fluoxetine attenuated lethality when administered prior to racemic MDMA, but was ineffective against the lethal effects of either isomer in the mouse (Fantegrossi et al., 2003). Furthermore, although fluoxetine attenuated both the hyperthermic and locomotor stimulant effects of racemic MDMA in the mouse, it *potentiated* locomotor stimulation induced by $S(+)$-MDMA, and did not block the induction of hyperthermia induced by this isomer (Fantegrossi et al., 2003). However, in humans, Liechti and colleagues have shown that SSRIs can attenuate MDMA-induced increases in prepulse inhibition of the startle reflex (Liechti, Geyer, Hell, & Vollenweider, 2001), block MDMA's effects on heart rate and blood pressure (Liechti & Vollenweider, 2000), and profoundly attenuate many of the drug's subjective effects (Liechti, Saur, Gamma, Hell, & Vollenweider, 2000).

Role of postsynaptic 5-HT receptors

Despite the above data highlighting the importance of 5-HT release, it is obvious that this can only be the first step in the initiation of MDMA's effects. The binding of released 5-HT to its diverse postsynaptic receptor population must therefore more proximally mediate the various behavioral and physiological effects of MDMA. Accordingly, converging evidence from diverse fields, including data from behavioral studies, electrophysiological studies, and radioligand binding studies, indicates that central 5-HT systems, specifically 5-HT$_2$ receptors, play a major role in the mediation of hallucinogen effects (Sadzot et al., 1989). Consistent with this finding, the behavioral effects of many hallucinogen-like drugs can be blocked by 5-HT$_2$ antagonists.

For example, administration of three non-selective 5-HT$_{1/2}$ antagonists attenuated the rate-decreasing effects of lysergic acid diethylamide (LSD) and 2,5-dimethoxy-4-methylamphetamine (DOM) on food-reinforced-responding in rats (Mokler, Commissaris, Warner, & Rech, 1983). Additionally, the discriminative stimulus effects of DOM, mescaline, LSD, and 5-methoxy N,N-dimethyltryptamine (5-OMe DMT) were blocked in rats by two 5-HT$_2$ antagonists (Glennon, Young, & Rosecrans, 1983). More germane to the present discussion, MDMA-induced locomotor stimulation was shown to be attenuated in rats by the selective 5-HT$_{2A}$ antagonist M100907 (Kehne et al., 1996), and human studies have indicated that many of the subjective effects of orally administered MDMA are attenuated by pretreatments with the nonselective 5-HT$_{2A/2C}$ antagonist ketanserin (Liechti et al., 2000). In a similar fashion, ketanserin and M100907 attenuate MDMA self-administration by the rhesus monkey at doses that do not alter responding for cocaine (Fantegrossi et al., 2002). Also consistent with this pattern of effects, MDMA-induced dopamine release has been shown to be potentiated by 5-HT$_2$ agonists (Gudelsky, Yamamoto, & Nash, 1994) and attenuated by 5-HT$_2$ antagonists (Schmidt, Sullivan, & Fadayel, 1994). However, stereoselective effects again become apparent when 5-HT$_2$ antagonists are administered to mice prior to racemic or $S(+)$-MDMA. Although ketanserin and M100907 both attenuated the hyperthermic effects of racemic MDMA in the mouse at doses that were not hypothermic on their own, neither compound altered the effects of $S(+)$-MDMA on core temperature at such doses (Fantegrossi et al., 2003). Likewise, both antagonists reduced the locomotor stimulant effects of racemic MDMA in the mouse, but *potentiated* the hyperactivity elicited by $S(+)$-MDMA (Fantegrossi et al., 2003).

Behavioral effects in laboratory animals

High doses of serotonin agonists elicit a characteristic set of unconditioned behaviors that are consistent with what has come to be known as "the serotonin syndrome" in rodents (Hiramatsu, Nabeshima, Kameyama, Maeda, & Cho, 1989; Spanos & Yamamoto, 1989) and primates (Slikker et al., 1989). This behavioral complex is characterized by increasingly severe symptoms (dependent on dose) such as stimulated locomotor activity, reciprocal forepaw treading, head twitching, tail flicking, piloerection, hind limb abduction, proptosis, ataxia and low body posture, and convulsions leading to death. The elements of this syndrome most likely to be observed following MDMA administration are low body posture, forepaw treading, and increased tail flicks (Geyer & Callaway, 1994). Although both $S(+)$- and $R(-)$-MDMA elicit head twitch behavior to a similar extent, the racemate does not induce this behavior at any dose (Fantegrossi et al., 2004a). These findings, as well as many of those mentioned above, recapitulate the "disconcerting absence of additivity between the component isomers in comparison with the activity of the racemate" previously noted in studies of MDMA and its enantiomers in rabbit thermoregulation and human intoxication (Anderson, Braun, Braun, Nichols, & Shulgin, 1978).

The locomotor hyperactivity engendered by MDMA administration adds to the compound's unique behavioral profile. Gold, Koob, and Geyer (1988) noted that MDMA fails to induce motor stereotypy, even at high doses. Additionally, doses of MDMA that produce hyperactivity also suppress rearing and exploratory responses (Geyer, 1996). Finally, the pattern of ambulatory activity observed following administration of MDMA reveals increased locomotor behavior around the perimeter of the activity chamber along an exceptionally straight course (Callaway, Johnson, Gold, Nichols, & Geyer, 1991). This unique cluster of locomotor activating effects further distinguishes MDMA from both the classical psychostimulants and the traditional hallucinogens (Geyer and Callaway, 1994).

Despite the widespread recreational use of MDMA, the reinforcing effects of ring-substituted amphetamine derivatives have not been extensively characterized in laboratory animals. However, MDMA has been shown to elicit conditioned place preference (Bilsky, Hui, Hubbell, & Reid, 1990; Marona-Lewicka, Rhee, Sprague, & Nichols, 1996) in rats. Additionally, brain stimulation studies have shown a decrease in the threshold current required to maintain behavior in rats following MDMA administration

(Hubner, Bird, Rassnick, & Kornetsky, 1988). Finally, racemic MDMA has been shown to act as a reinforcer in intravenous self-administration paradigms in primates (Beardsley, Balster, & Harris, 1986; Lamb & Griffiths, 1987; Fantegrossi et al., 2002), and both enantiomers also maintain self-administration behavior in the rhesus monkey (Fantegrossi et al., 2002). In addition to MDMA, several structural analogues also maintain self-administration behavior in primates, most notably N-ethyl-3,4-methylenedioxyamphetamine (MDE) (Sannerud, Kaminski, & Griffiths, 1996) and MDA (Griffiths, Winger, Brady, & Snell, 1976). This is an important point to consider, as the traditional hallucinogens of phenylisopropylamine and indolealkylamine structures have long stood out as drugs that are abused by humans but fail to engender reliable self-administration behavior in laboratory animals (Fantegrossi, Woods & Winger, 2004; Poling & Bryceland, 1979).

Neurotoxicity

The neurotoxic effects of amphetamine analogues upon the serotonin system were first described by Pletscher et al. (1963, 1964) in reports demonstrating sustained depletions of 5-HT and its metabolite 5-hydroxyindoleacetic acid (5-HIAA) following treatment with *para*-chloroamphetamine (PCA). In subsequent studies, Fuller and colleagues established structure–activity relationships for the amphetamine analogues that allowed the prediction of neurotoxic potential and demonstrated that PCA was most potent in inducing 5-HT depletion (Fuller, Snoddy, Roush, & Molloy, 1973). The neurotoxic effects of PCA were extended by studies reporting inhibition of 5-HT synthesis and uptake (Sanders-Bush & Sulser, 1970), as well as persistent anatomical changes (Harvey, McMaster, & Yunger, 1975) following a single administration of the drug. Study of the neurotoxic effects of other amphetamine analogues soon followed.

Gibb and colleagues examined the neurotoxic effects of the structurally related psychostimulant methamphetamine (METH) in great detail, and described various effects on the dopamine system. For example, these investigators reported a long-lasting inhibition of tyrosine hydroxylase (the rate-limiting enzyme in dopamine synthesis) activity following repeated high doses of METH in the rat, as well as a concomitant depletion of dopamine and its metabolites dihydroxyphenylacetic acid (DOPAC) and homovanillic acid (HVA) (Gibb, Johnson, Stone, & Hanson, 1990). All of these effects are detectable 12–18 hours post-METH (Gibb, Hanson, & Johnson, 1994) in the rat, and similar effects have been documented in the monkey (Seiden, Fischman, & Schuster, 1976).

The effects of METH proved to be even more pronounced on the 5-HT system. Following administration of large doses of METH, an enormous (> 90%) long-lasting inhibition of tryptophan hydroxylase (TPH, the rate-limiting enzyme in 5-HT synthesis) activity was observed, and, similar to

PCA, METH also produced a decrease in 5-HT and 5-HIAA content (Gibb et al., 1994). These effects were readily differentiated from those on the dopamine system not only in terms of magnitude, but also by their rapid time course, as the 5-HT effects could be detected in as little as 20 minutes post-METH (Bakhit & Gibb, 1981) in the rat. Curiously, these toxic effects appear to be restricted to the dopamine and 5-HT systems. Levels of choline acetyltransferase (ChAT, the rate-limiting enzyme in acetylcholine synthesis) and glutamate decarboxylase (GAD, the rate-limiting enzyme in γ-aminobutyric acid [GABA] synthesis) were not altered following METH administration, and although several changes were observed in various neuropeptide systems, levels returned to baseline within 2–3 days post-METH (Gibb et al., 1994). Why the previously described actions of METH should be limited to dopamine and 5-HT remains unknown.

Studies of the toxic effects of MDMA present a complex picture, but its actions on the 5-HT system are thought to be more selective and more potent than those of METH. In rats, MDMA transiently inhibits TPH activity and depletes 5-HT and 5-HIAA after a single dose, and these effects gradually return to baseline within approximately 2 weeks post-MDMA (Gibb et al., 1990). Administration of a single large dose, or multiple moderate doses, of MDMA produces similar effects, although they are increased in both magnitude and duration, prompting speculation that the short- and long-term neurochemical effects of MDMA may be separable phenomena (Gibb et al., 1990). These toxic effects are specific to the 5-HT system, as MDMA administration has not been shown to affect levels of HVA, 3-methoxy-4-hydroxyphenylethyleneglycol (MHPG, a major metabolite of norepinephrine), dopamine, or norepinephrine in rats (De Souza, Battaglia, & Insel, 1990). A single report demonstrating dopamine depletion following MDMA administration in squirrel monkeys and baboons (Ricaurte, Yuan, Hatzidimitriou, Cord, & McCann, 2002) was later retracted (Ricaurte, Yuan, Hatzidimitriou, Cord, & McCann, 2003) due to methodological flaws. Interestingly, in the mouse, the toxic effects of MDMA, like those of METH, are largely manifested in dopaminergic systems ((Miller & O'Callaghan, 1994; O'Callaghan & Miller, 1994). The explanation for this species difference remains an area of active research.

The MDMA dose regimens used to induce the previously described neurochemical depletions also result in anatomical changes. Using 5-HT immunocytochemistry, a pronounced MDMA-induced denervation has been visualized throughout the neocortex, striatum, and thalamus, while lesser damage was observed in the hippocampus, hypothalamus, and basal forebrain in rats (Molliver et al., 1990). Further work has revealed heterogeneous vulnerability to MDMA-induced degeneration within the 5-HT system. Fine axon terminals (with cell bodies originating in the dorsal raphe nucleus) seem to be especially susceptible to MDMA-induced damage, while axons with large round varicosities (so-called "beaded axons" originating in the median raphe nucleus) are typically spared – a relationship that also holds true for

PCA-induced neurotoxicity (Molliver et al., 1990). Although the anatomic distribution of these distinct populations of 5-HT neurons differs somewhat between rats and primates, the differential vulnerability to MDMA-induced neurotoxicity is retained across species (Wilson, Ricaurte, & Molliver, 1989). The significance of this selective neurotoxic effect on fine axons is poorly understood.

Attempts to identify the potential mechanisms of MDMA-induced toxicity and neurodegeneration have been complicated by the observation that these effects appear to be tightly interwoven with MDMA-induced hyperthermia (Broening, Bowyer, & Slikker, 1995). The hyperthermic effects of MDMA in rodents were first described by Nash, Meltzer, and Gudelsky (1988), and the protective effects of several compounds against MDMA-induced neurodegeneration have been attributed solely to their effectiveness in inducing hypothermia on their own (Farfel & Seiden, 1995; Malberg, Sabol, & Seiden, 1996) or in blocking MDMA-induced hyperthermia (Colado, Granados, O'Shea, Esteban, & Green, 1998). Further studies have also demonstrated protection against MDMA-induced neurotoxicity by lowering core temperature via nonpharmacological means, including restraint stress (e.g., Miller & O'Callaghan, 1994) and manipulation of the ambient temperature (e.g., Malberg & Seiden, 1998). Curiously, cooling the ambient temperature reduces the lethal effects of racemic MDMA in singly-housed mice, but does not protect against lethality induced by either isomer (Fantegrossi et al., 2003). However, in group-housed mice (a manipulation which potentiates the lethal effects of many drugs), a cool ambient environment profoundly attenuates the lethal effects of racemic and $S(+)$-MDMA, but does not protect against $R(-)$-MDMA-induced lethality (Fantegrossi et al., 2003). These studies suggest that the toxic effects of MDMA depend not only on pharmacodynamics, but also on complex environmental variables.

Despite this widespread interest in the relationship between temperature and MDMA-induced neurodegeneration and lethality, no widely accepted mechanism for the hyperthermic effects of MDMA has yet been described. However, the structurally similar selective 5-HT$_{2A/2C}$ agonist 1-(4-iodo-2,5-dimethoxyphenyl)-2-aminopropane (DOI) and the selective 5-HT$_{2C}$ agonist m-chlorophenylpiperazine (m-CPP) have both been shown to induce hyperthermia (Mazzola-Pomietto, Aulakh, Tolliver, & Murphy, 1997) in rats, and MDMA has also been shown to act as an agonist at these receptors (Nash, Roth, Brodkin, Nichols, & Gudelsky, 1994). However, in the mouse, DOI failed to induce hyperthermia at doses up to 30 times higher than those required to elicit significant head twitch behavior (Fantegrossi et al., 2004a), and m-CPP also did not elicit hyperthermia in this species (unpublished results). In the rabbit, it has been previously demonstrated that cutaneous vasoconstriction contributes to MDMA-induced hyperthermia (Pedersen & Blessing, 2001), and these vascular effects of MDMA are predominantly mediated by α_1-adrenergic receptors (McDaid & Docherty, 2001). Similarly, in the mouse, the α_1-adrenergic receptor antagonist prazosin blocked the induction of MDMA-induced hyperthermia (Fantegrossi et al., 2004a). The hyperthermic effects of MDMA are clearly complex.

MDMA has been shown to deplete 5-HT and 5-HIAA more potently in monkeys than it does in rats, although the drug's effects on 5-HT uptake sites are comparable across these two species (De Souza et al., 1990). The threshold neurotoxic dose of MDMA in rats is 20 mg/kg, but only 5 mg/kg MDMA is required to produce neurotoxicity in the monkey (Ricaurte, Yuan, & McCann, 2000). This increased sensitivity of primate brains to MDMA-induced toxicity has been suggested to imply that humans may be especially susceptible to these neurotoxic effects, but the high doses and increased frequencies of administration utilized in these studies have caused some to question their relevance to humans (Kish, 2002; Saunders, 1995). Nonetheless, application of some formulae for interspecies scaling places some of these experimental animal doses within the range of those commonly administered by humans in recreational settings (Morgan, 2000), implying that there may be no significant margin of safety between neurotoxic and recreational doses in humans (but see Vollenweider, Jones, & Baggott, 2001, for a critique of allometric interspecies scaling).

Although multiple measures of serotonergic neurotoxicity have been employed to yield evidence of MDMA-induced neurochemical and neuroanatomical changes in laboratory animals, only rarely have these effects been correlated with functional deficits. Despite demonstrated MDMA-induced decreases in levels of 5-HT, 5-HIAA, 5-HT transporters, vesicular monoamine transporters (VMAT), measures of anterograde transport, and TPH activity, as well as histological evidence of 5-HT axon degeneration and the concomitant "pruning effect" (Ricaurte et al., 2000), the behavioral correlates of such changes are much more subtle and less well described (Winsauer et al., 2002). However, alterations in both the startle response (Schmidt & Kehne, 1990) and rates of isolation calling (Winslow & Insel, 1991), increased responsiveness to morphine analgesia (Nencini, Woolverton, & Seiden, 1988), and impaired thermoregulation (Miller & O'Callaghan, 1995) have been observed following a neurotoxic regimen of MDMA in laboratory animals. However, none of these effects have proven especially robust. This incongruity, along with the general lack of demonstrated reactive gliosis following MDMA administration (Kish, 2002), has served to maintain a continued debate regarding the appropriateness of the term "neurotoxicity" when applied to the neurochemical changes induced by MDMA (e.g. Kalia, 2000).

In this regard, there are at least three validated morphological criteria that are generally agreed to indicate incontrovertable neural damage: frank cell loss, argyrophilia (silver staining), and reactive gliosis. With regard to the latter measure, immunocytochemistry techniques have traditionally been used to quantify glial fibrilliary acidic protein (GFAP), the major protein of astrocyte intermediate filaments, in various brain preparations following application of some suspected toxicant (O'Callaghan & Miller, 1993). Argyrophilia indicative of degenerated axon terminals and cell bodies was visualized by Commins et al. (1987) in rats using the Fink-Heimer method following a particularly extreme MDMA dose regimen (80 mg/kg, twice daily, for two days). Similarly, the anionic xanthene dye Fluoro-Jade B has been developed as a simple and reliable marker of neuronal degeneration, and was used to localize MDMA-induced toxicity in the rat forebrain and mouse hippocampus (Fornai et al., 2004). While this agent is a reasonably selective stain for degenerated neurons in the rodent, Fluoro-Jade appears to be a more ubiquitous labeling agent in the primate (Colombo & Puissant, 2002). Recently, binding of the peripheral benzodiazepine receptor (PBR) ligand [^{3}H]PK11195 has been employed as an index of microglial activation. As the name implies, PBRs are expressed in the periphery, but are also located centrally in glial cells, primarily in astrocytes and microglia (Park, Carboni, Wood, & Gee, 1996). Multiple studies have reported that the density of PBRs increases concomitantly with glial activation following neural injury induced by various insults, including inflammation, metabolic stress, trauma, transient global forebrain ischemia, and chemically-induced brain injury (Casellas, Galiegue, & Basile, 2002). In some cases of central nervous system injury, microgliosis can occur rapidly after the insult (Stephenson et al., 1995; Streit & Graeber, 1993), leading some to speculate that this early increase in PBR density may be an index of microglial activation which could be used as an indirect marker of neuronal damage (Benavides, Fage, Carter, & Scatton, 1987; Escubedo et al., 1998). Most germane to the present topic, microglial activation has recently been described as a pharmacologically specific marker for the neurotoxic amphetamines in mice, and may represent one of the earliest components of the neurotoxic process induced by particular dose regimens of these drugs (Thomas et al., 2004).

Recently, *ex vivo* [^{3}H]PK11195 binding in the rat brain has been used to compare and contrast the neurotoxic effects of METH and MDMA (Pubill et al., 2003). In this study, increased PBR binding was noted in the striatum and cortex following METH administration, but not following MDMA administration, leading the authors to conclude that "there are differences between the brain responses to the neurotoxicity induced by METH and MDMA as far as glial activation is concerned." Based upon these data, however, it seems difficult to determine whether this conclusion truly represents a real difference between the neurotoxic potentials of MDMA and METH, or simply reflects the methodological peculiarities of this particular study. In this regard, two points seem especially relevant: the specific dosing regimens employed, and the species in which these effects were studied. Firstly, data were obtained from a single regimen of each drug: 10 mg/kg METH subcutaneously (s.c.) every 2 hours for four total doses, and 20 mg/kg MDMA sc twice per day (at 7-hour intervals) for 4 days. Thus, METH-exposed animals were dosed much more frequently than were MDMA-exposed animals, potentially leading to very different pharmacokinetics across these two drug regimens. Additionally, the neurochemical effects of METH are distributed across dopaminergic and serotonergic systems in the rat (Gibb et al., 1990,

1994), while MDMA exerts selective serotonergic effects in this species (De Souza et al., 1990; Gibb et al., 1990). Thus, it may be the case that [^{3}H]PK11195 binding is simply more sensitive to DA manipulation than to 5-HT manipulation. Indeed, the effects of 5-HT selective neurotoxicants such as PCA on PBR binding potential have not been previously described. These factors illustrate the difficulty and complexity behind an issue as seemingly straightforward as determining whether or not a drug truly is neurotoxic, particularly as methods to answer this question continue to evolve.

Human studies

Given that MDMA administration is associated with neurotoxicity in preclinical models, it is reasonable to infer that the same consequences also would be observed in human users; however, several methodological difficulties have hindered researchers' efforts to study this phenomenon in human users. For example, because it has been argued that administration of repeated doses of MDMA to human subjects in double-blind, placebo-controlled experiments would be unethical (Parrott, 2000), researchers must instead rely on indirect evidence gathered from retrospective surveys of drug use to gauge the extent of drug exposure in their subjects. Attempts are then typically made to correlate these survey data with markers of serotonergic function, performance on various cognitive and behavioral tasks, or psychiatric morbidity (Curran, 2000). In this regard, significant changes have been noted in sleep patterns, mood, anxiety, impulsiveness, hostility, memory, and attention in long-term MDMA users (Morgan, 2000).

Surprisingly, forensic drug analysis to confirm the use of MDMA by experimental subjects has been performed only rarely, and has regularly utilized measures inadequate to determine both the length of drug use and the extent of co-use of other nonamphetamine drugs of abuse (Kish, 2002). This latter point may be particularly relevant given the inability of most researchers to exclude polydrug users from their experimental "ecstasy group." In this regard, Schifano, Di Furia, Forza, Minicuci, and Bricolo (1998) have argued that almost all ecstasy users abuse other drugs as well, many of which have effects on behavior and cognition that overlap those assayed by researchers. A combination of the two complications outlined above is illustrated in the SPECT imaging study conducted by Semple, Ebmeier, Glabus, O'Carroll, and Johnstone (1999), where three subjects testing negative for MDMA in hair analysis were nonetheless included in the experimental MDMA group based solely upon their self-report data. However, MDMA toxicity, like all polydrug toxicity, is likely to be cumulative with increased dose. Thus, verification that someone was actually exposed to MDMA during a defined period – in the absence of determination as to *how much* MDMA that individual was exposed to – is probably of limited utility in quantifying accumulated toxicity. Therefore, forensic confirmation of MDMA use seems critical only in studies requiring verification of abstinence for a long period of time. In such studies, a positive test should be used as an exclusion criterion. Furthermore, subject self-report of drug ingestion is the foundation of the great majority of published drug abuse literature in humans, and the consistency of findings in this field, even in the absence of forensic confirmation, probably relates to the fact that drug users can discriminate whether or not a given dose of drug induces their desired subjective effects.

A further criticism of the few studies assessing neurotoxicity in human ecstasy users is that the majority of these reports assess only a single marker of brain 5-HT terminal density. In studies of dopamine neurotoxicity, multiple targets are available for measure in living brain, including dopamine transporter (DAT), vesicular monoamine transporters (VMAT) in dopamine-rich areas, and dopa decarboxylase activity (Kish, 2002). However, thus far the only available selective marker of 5-HT neuron density in living human brain is 5-HT transporter (SERT) (Kish, 2002), and anatomical and functional evidence has shown that SERT is not exclusively expressed on synaptic 5-HT membranes. In fact, SERT has been localized on 5-HT axons distal from the synapse (Zhou, Tao-Cheng, Segu, Patel, & Wang, 1998), suggesting that it may not be a particularly selective marker of 5-HT terminal fields. Additionally, analogous changes in the levels of DAT have been shown to occur without corresponding changes in dopamine neuron number in cocaine users (Wilson et al., 1996). Further, depleted DAT levels in methamphetamine users have been shown to recover with prolonged abstinence (Volkow et al., 2001). These findings suggest that SERT may be susceptible to comparable compensatory mechanisms following drug exposure, and evidence that may support this assertion has been obtained in postmortem (Mash, Staley, Izenwasser, Basile, & Ruttenber, 2000) and SPECT imaging studies (Jacobsen et al., 2000) of cocaine users.

Importantly, the fact that all previous experiments regarding the neurotoxic effects of MDMA in laboratory animals have relied on noncontingent MDMA administration begs the question of whether or not these effects would be obtained via self-administration of the drug. In other words, do the effects of experimenter-administered MDMA differ from the effects of self-administered MDMA? Several cases from diverse pharmacological classes serve to illustrate the point that response-dependent drug administration can have vastly different effects than one may expect based upon noncontingent drug administration. For example, self-administration of morphine produces more severe withdrawal symptoms than does noncontingent morphine administration (Siegel, 1988). Finally, there is evidence that the contingencies governing drug administration can even affect neurochemical measures, as experiments have demonstrated significantly increased extracellular dopamine concentrations in the nucleus accumbens, despite equivalent brain concentrations of drug, in rats self-administering cocaine compared to a yoked-control group (Hemby, Co, Koves, Smith, & Dworkin, 1997).

Corresponding experiments directly comparing the effects of contingent and noncontingent MDMA have not yet been conducted, however the effects of self-administered MDMA on monoamines and VMAT binding have been studied in rhesus monkeys (Fantegrossi et al., 2004b). The initial finding was that it was difficult to replicate MDMA dose–response curves in monkeys that had been taking the drug consistently for some time. Subjects were then exposed to the opportunity to self-administer MDMA over an 18-month period. All subjects initially self-administered MDMA, but there was a general decrease in rates of responding maintained by a range of doses of MDMA over the duration of the experiment, whereas no change was observed in the effectiveness of cocaine as a reinforcer in these animals. The possibility that this change in the reinforcing effectiveness of MDMA might reflect neural changes suggestive of neurotoxicity was explored by positron emission tomography (PET) analysis at least 2 months after the last MDMA exposure, using labeled dihydrotetrabenazine (DTBZ) to quantify levels of VMAT. No significant differences were found between VMAT levels in monkeys that had an extensive history of MDMA self-administration and those that had no such history. Postmortem histological study of multiple brain regions from these MDMA-exposed monkeys revealed some potentially interesting trends in serotonergic changes that might be consistent with neurotoxicity, but no statistically significant effects were obtained in any brain regions assayed. These data are in conflict with essentially all previous neurotoxicological findings in nonhuman primates, indicating that noncontingent administration of large doses of MDMA produces pronounced reductions in 5-HT, its metabolites, and VMAT density in multiple brain regions (Ricaurte et al., 2000), and suggests that the contingencies surrounding MDMA administration might be important variables in the neurochemical effects observed following its administration. Thus, the relationship of animal neurotoxicity studies relying on noncontingent MDMA administration to the human experience remains unknown. However, recent data (Bowyer et al., 2003) suggest that the noncontingent doses typically used to study the persistent neurochemical effects of MDMA in nonhuman primates produce blood levels up to tenfold higher than those measured in humans administered a typical recreational dose of the drug. Allowing animals to regulate their own drug intakes thus eliminates the need to rely on controversial models of allometric interspecies dose scaling and can result in MDMA intakes quite similar to those estimated in human users (Fantegrossi et al., 2004b). The further use of nonhuman primate self-administration paradigms to study the persistent neurochemical effects of MDMA may therefore represent a powerful means of bridging the often cavernous divide between data gathered from studies in laboratory animals and the clinical realities of human MDMA users.

These limitations notwithstanding, the available research using human study participants provides researchers with a foundation for making statements regarding MDMA-associated central nervous system abnormalities. As such, the next two sections focus on human studies of MDMA-associated neurotoxicity. The first section will include studies that utilized neuroimaging to characterize these deficits. The second will focus on studies that utilized neuropsychological assessment to examine the consequences of MDMA use.

This review includes studies of original research using various neuroimaging modalities to evaluate the chronic effects of MDMA exposure in human MDMA users. Studies were included if they appeared to contain unique subject cohorts; preliminary reports were included if they were not superseded by a subsequent follow-up report.

Neuroimaging studies in human MDMA users

Serotonin transporter (SERT) in human MDMA users

The serotonin reuptake transporter (SERT) is located at serotonin release sites along serotonergic axons (REF); therefore, noncompensated loss of serotonergic axons would predict a reduction in levels of SERT. Several investigators have examined SERT levels in MDMA users by employing PET using the ligand $^{11}C(+)McN5652$ and single photon emission tomography (SPECT) using the ligand $[^{123}I]beta$-CIT. The sensitivity and specificity of both ligands are not ideal, however reasonably solid arguments can be made for interpreting cortical reductions in binding to loss of SERT binding sites.

Overall, multiple groups of investigators using $^{11}C(+)McN5652$ PET (Buchert et al., 2004; McCann, Szabo, Scheffel, Dannals, & Ricaurte, 1998) or using $[^{123}I]beta$-CIT SPECT (Reneman, Majoie, Habraken, & den Heeten, 2001; Semple et al., 1999) have found global or regional reductions in SERT binding in MDMA users when compared to controls. Two of these studies reported greater reductions in SERT binding in female MMDA users and also reported "recovery" of SERT binding with prolonged abstinence (Buchert et al., 2004; Reneman et al., 2001). Among issues requiring clarification are whether SERT levels actually recover (or whether current ligands lack sensitivity to detect residual differences), whether axon sprouting (functional or nonfunctional) may contribute to apparent recovery of SERT levels found in two studies, and whether decreased SERT levels correspond to actual loss of axons or whether SERT may be chronically downregulated in MDMA users (Horschitz, Hummerich, & Schloss, 2001).

Serotonin receptors in MDMA users

Because many brain neurotransmitter receptors undergo agonist-induced downregulation and antagonist induced or denervation-induced upregulation, the status of (primarily) postsynaptic 5-HT receptors has been investigated in human MDMA users. Since MDMA exposure produces an acute release of large amounts of 5-HT at the synapse, postsynaptic receptors would be expected to undergo agonist-induced downregulation immediately following MDMA exposure. In the face of MDMA-induced serotonergic axotomy, postsynaptic 5-HT receptors would be predicted to increase in numbers due to loss of agonist. Reneman et al. (2002) used [^{123}I]R91150 SPECT to examine cortical binding ratios of (largely) 5-HT$_{2A}$ receptors. As predicted by agonist-induced regulation effects, recent MDMA users had reduced 5-HT$_{2A}$ receptor binding in frontal, parietal, and occipital cortex versus controls, whereas long-abstinent MDMA users showed numerically increased receptor binding in frontal and parietal regions with a statistically significant increase over controls in occipital cortex.

Brain gray matter in MDMA users

Animal studies to date have not strongly suggested that MDMA causes direct neuronal cell body or glial loss. Instead, MDMA toxicity appears to be largely confined to fine-diameter serotonergic axons in most species. However, 5-HT release is known to stimulate neurotrophic factors such as brain-derived nerve growth factor, and 5-HT-coupled alterations in growth factor release are hypothesized to play a role in depression and other illnesses (Mattson, Maudsley, & Martin, 2004). Cowan et al. (2003) hypothesized that MDMA users might show evidence of reduced brain gray matter due to loss of 5-HT-coupled growth factors. Using voxel-based morphometry (VBM), we examined brain gray matter concentration in a group of MDMA polydrug users compared to a group of non-MDMA users. Overall, MDMA users had multiple regions of reduced brain gray matter concentration in areas of neocortex, brainstem, and cerebellum. However, polydrug exposure or preexisting differences in brain structure could not be ruled out as the origin of these findings. Further, it was not possible to link altered gray matter specifically to changes in serotonin function. In a study of cerebral blood flow (reviewed below) in MDMA users (and therefore not specifically designed to assay for regional volumetric effects), Chang et al. (2000) reported a significant negative correlation between age-adjusted duration of MDMA use and global brain volume, but did not specifically report on gray matter *per se*.

Brain metabolites in MDMA users

Several magnetic resonance spectroscopy (MRS) studies have investigated regional brain metabolite concentrations of a putative neuronal marker (*N*-acetylaspartate, NAA) and/or a putative glial marker (myoinositol). Chang, Ernst, Grob, and Poland (1999) and Reneman et al. (2002) examined NAA and myoinositol in frontal and occipital gray matter plus temporoparietal white matter in MDMA users versus controls. Chang and colleagues found no differences between NAA (expressed as NAA/Creatine (Cr) ratios) in all regions studied but detected increased myoinositol (expressed as MI/Cr) in temporoparietal white matter but not other regions. Additionally, myoinositol in temporoparietal white matter and occipital cortex was positively correlated with lifetime MDMA dose. Conversely, in a group of heavy MDMA users, Reneman et al. (2002) found decreased NAA in frontal cortex but unchanged NAA in other cortical regions and no differences in myoinositol in all regions studied. In an earlier preliminary report, Reneman et al. (2001) demonstrated a negative association between delayed verbal memory recall and prefrontal NAA/Cr, but there was no association with memory performance in temporoparietal white matter or mid-occipital gray matter. In a small sample study using magnetic resonance spectroscopic imaging (MRSI) to assay hippocampal NAA, Obergriesser, Ende, Braus, and Henn (2001) reported no differences in NAA between MDMA users and control subjects. Similarly, Daumann, Fischermann, Pilatus, Thron, Moeller-Hartmann, and Gouzoulis-Mayfrank (2004), using proton MRS, reported no significant differences in neocortical (midline midfrontal and midoccipital regions) or left (right hippocampus was not assayed) hippocampal NAA/Cr ratios in a comparison of MDMA users and controls (but reported a nonsignificant trend for lower left hippocampal NAA/Cr ratios in MDMA users). In sum, there are no consistent data to support changes in myoinositol or NAA in MDMA users.

Axonal integrity in MDMA users

In a preliminary report applying diffusion and perfusion MRI to analyze fiber tract (axon) integrity in MDMA users, Reneman et al. (2001) found significant increases in both relative cerebral blood volume ratios (rCBV) and apparent diffusion coefficients (ADC) in the globus pallidi of MDMA users. The ADC method is thought to reflect the integrity of brain structures, such as fiber tracts, that limit the diffusion of water. Thus, Reneman and colleagues speculated that loss of serotonergic axons in the globus pallidi of MDMA users might account for an increased ADC due to less restriction of water movement. The increased rCBV is discussed below.

Cerebral vasculature in MDMA users

Serotonin innervates cerebral arterioles where it appears to have a complex but largely vasoconstrictive action; however, serotonin release can also function indirectly as a vasodilator in some brain regions (Cohen, 1996). If MDMA induces axotomy in serotonergic fibers, loss of serotonergic innervation might therefore lead to a relative vasodilation. As mentioned above, Reneman et al. (2001) investigated rCBV ratios in MDMA users and found increased rCBV relative to controls in globus pallidus, consistent with their predictions of the effects of serotonergic axotomy-induced vasodilation. Chang et al. (2000) investigated both the chronic and acute effects of MDMA on cerebral blood flow using SPECT. With regard to chronic effects, MDMA users showed a numerically small (2.3%) decrease in global regional cerebral blood flow but no significant differences in ^{133}xenon and ^{99m}technetium

SPECT-assayed regional cerebral blood flow when compared to control subjects.

Resting metabolism in MDMA users

Obrocki and colleagues (2002) examined resting brain metabolism in MDMA users and controls using [^{18}F]fluorodeoxyglucose (FDG) PET. Versus controls, MDMA users had multiple areas of reduced glucose utilization at rest. Notably, caudate and putamen showed bilateral significant reductions in metabolism. The left amygdala also had significant reductions in glucose uptake, with a similar, but nonspecific trend in right amygdala.

Task-evoked functional neuroimaging in MDMA users

For the purposes of this review, functional neuroimaging studies include those using PET or functional magnetic resonance imaging (fMRI) studies to examine task-evoked brain activity. Tasks are defined as measures of neurocognition, including attention, working memory, and episodic memory.

Attention

Gamma, Buck, Berthold, and Vollenweider (2001) examined regional brain activation in MDMA users and controls using $H_2^{15}O$ PET during an attentional task. Using a computerized version of a continuous performance task (CPT), Gamma and colleagues found (common to both groups) task-related regional brain activation in right medial occipital lobe, left precentral area, right postcentral area, and right superior frontal lobe. Task-related regional brain deactivations were seen in bilateral medial and superior temporal lobe and right precuneus. When MDMA users were directly compared to controls on measures of regional brain activation, there were no significant regional cerebral blood flow differences between the groups. Further, there were no significant associations between MDMA/polydrug exposure and outcome variables.

Working memory

Jacobsen, Mencl, Pugh, Skudlarski, and Krystal (2004) used fMRI BOLD to examine hippocampal activation during working memory in a small cohort of adolescents who were enrolled in a study of adolescent tobacco use. Subjects were also assessed using psychological testing for divided attention and working memory performance. Jacobsen and colleagues assessed sustained, divided, and auditory and visual select attention outside the fMRI. An fMRI task was employed to assess hippocampal activation during a working memory and selective attention task. The fMRI task consisted of an auditory *n*-back task that had two levels of working memory and two levels of selective attention. When compared to control subjects, MDMA-using adolescents had increased reaction times for some attention tasks and higher levels of hippocampal activation (assayed as reduced hippocampal deactivation) during a working memory task that strongly taxed verbal working memory.

Daumann and colleagues used BOLD fMRI to assay working memory task in controls and moderate and heavy MDMA users (Daumann et al., 2003a), as well as a group of "pure" MDMA users who had minimal polydrug exposure within the last two years (Daumann et al., 2003b). Subjects underwent neuroimaging during performance of various n-back tasks having different levels of working memory load. The n-back tasks activated regions of frontal, parietal, occipital, and cingulate cortex. For the three-group comparison study (Daumann et al., 2003a) fMRI data were analyzed using a conservative p value (less than 0.05 corrected for multiple whole brain comparisons) and there were no significant group differences. A more liberal statistical criterion ($p<0.01$, uncorrected) revealed significantly greater right parietal activation in moderate and heavy MDMA users versus controls, whereas an intermediate statistical threshold ($p<0.001$, uncorrected) found differences between moderate (but not heavy) users and controls.

In the comparison examining controls, MDMA polydrug, and "pure" MDMA users (many of whom overlapped with the Daumann et al., 2003a, study), the "pure" MDMA users had increased or decreased regional brain activation in multiple brain regions in relation to MDMA polydrug users or control subjects during performance of a 1-back or 2-back task. There was no consistently discernible pattern of BOLD signal alterations and there were no differences in task performance between the groups. There were no differences in n-back task performance between the two groups of subjects at the baseline assessment or at the 18-month follow-up study.

Daumann and colleagues also employed an n-back task (Daumann et al., 2004) to examine working memory performance after an 18-month follow-up period in MDMA users who either continued or refrained from ongoing MDMA and amphetamine exposure. There were no task performance or regional brain BOLD signal differences in the two groups at the baseline assessment. Despite similar task performance between the two groups at the 18-month follow-up, subjects who continued MDMA or amphetamine use had increased midline and right hemisphere parietal activation (compared to their baseline), whereas those who did not have interim MDMA exposure showed no differences from their baseline scans. Further, parietal activation in the group with continued MDMA use positively correlated with self-report of average one-night MDMA dose.

Moeller and colleagues (2004) studied working memory performance in MDMA users and controls by comparing task-elicited fMRI BOLD activation. The working memory task consisted of an Immediate Memory Task and a Delayed Memory Task (DMT). Working memory demands were varied by task complexity and delay interval between target and probe stimuli. Day-of-study urine drug screens were positive in 10 of 15 MDMA users but were negative for all controls. The researchers attempted to control for the effects of other drug use and the presence of positive urine drug screens. Overall, Moeller and colleagues found (despite largely normal performance on the DMT) increased BOLD signal activation in prefrontal cortical regions, hippocampus, thalamus, and basal ganglia in MDMA users when compared to controls.

Episodic memory

Daumann and colleagues (2004) examined hippocampal activation during an fMRI episodic memory task (consisting of an encoding condition and a recall/retrieval task) in MDMA users and controls. Pilot experiments in the investigator's laboratory had revealed that hippocampal activation was associated only with the retrieval task in control subjects, therefore these investigators examined only the retrieval phase in this study. Overall, the MDMA-using group had reduced left hippocampal activation in a single cluster (10 voxels) compared to the non-MDMA-using controls in a small region of hippocampus. However, there were no differences in performance between the groups.

Summary of functional neuroimaging studies

In general, extant neuroimaging studies in MDMA users have employed noncomparable tasks in relatively small sample sizes of MDMA users having differing levels of MDMA and polydrug exposure, therefore the conclusions from these studies are best characterized as preliminary. Overall, functional neuroimaging studies have found relatively slight or inconsistent differences between MDMA users and various control groups. The divergence in brain regions probed by various tasks, differences in polydrug use histories, differences in levels of MDMA exposure and duration of abstinence, and the residual effects of other drugs probably contribute, at least partially, to group differences. To advance our understanding of MDMA effects using functional neuroimaging, aside from using larger, relatively homogenous samples and multiple assessments of study participants, future studies will need to focus on integrating region-specific neural circuitry and the known physiological effects of serotonin to more specifically test hypotheses regarding serotonergic effects.

Neuropsychological consequences of MDMA exposure

Given the findings from the preclinical pharmacology and neuroimaging studies, which collectively showed that MDMA exposure resulted in neurotoxicity, it is reasonable to expect that MDMA exposure would result in neuropsychological deficits. In this section of the chapter, we review studies that examined whether MDMA exposure is associated with residual neuropsychological consequences. Moreover, we examine whether there are factors that moderate this association.

Inclusion of studies for review of neurocognitive consequences

The relevant studies for this review, which are listed in Table 6.1, were retrieved using an on-line computer search of *PsycInfo* and *Medline*. The search terms utilized in the computer search, *MDMA, neurocognition, neuropsychology,* and *cognition*, provided an initial bibliography of 61 papers. Studies were included in this review if they met the following criteria:

(1) The study included measures of neurocognition.
(2) The study included matched controls.
(3) The matched controls were similar to the MDMA users in terms of age, education, and/or estimated level of premorbid intellectual functioning.
(4) The MDMA users were abstinent at the time of the assessment.

Based on the literature searches and the review criteria, seven studies were included for the review (Bhattachary & Powell, 2001; Daumann et al., 2003a; Hanson & Luciana, 2004; McCardle, Luebbers, Carter, Croft, & Stough, 2004; Parrott, Lees, Garnham, Jones, & Wesnes, 1998; Thomasius et al., 2003; Verkes et al., 2001). For the purpose of this review, the following neurocognitive domains will be evaluated: attention/concentration, visuospatial skills, verbal learning and memory, nonverbal learning and memory, motor/psychomotor speed, and executive systems functioning. Because the studies included in this review matched study participants according to education and/or intellectual functioning, performance on measures of intellectual functioning and language was not reviewed here. Incidentally, with the exception of the study by Hanson and Luciana, the study participants were recreational users of MDMA whose level of use was not severe enough to be classified as abuse.

Table 6.1 Description of the studies included in the review

Study Author(s)	Year Published	Sample Size[1]	
		Controls	MDMA Users
Bhattachary & Powell	2001	11m/9f	10m/6f
Daumann et al.	2003a	8m/3f	8m/3f
Hanson & Luciana	2004	14m/12f	14m/12f
McCardle et al.	2004	13m/2f	13m/4f
Parrott et al.	1998	4m/6f	8m/2f
Thomasius et al.	2003	15m/15f	16m/15f
Verkes et al.	2001	20m	21m

[1] m = male/f = female

Attention/concentration

A review of the four studies that included measures of attention/concentration revealed mixed findings. For example, MDMA exposure was associated with poorer repetition of a series of numbers (Digit Span – Forward) in one study (McCardle et al., 2004), but not in another (Hanson & Luciana, 2004); in contrast, on Digit Span – Backward, a more difficult version of the test, MDMA exposure did not affect the task (Hanson & Luciana, 2004; McCardle et al., 2004). On a letter-cancellation task, speed of performance was unaffected across groups whereas MDMA users tended to make more errors of omission (i.e., did not "cancel" specified stimuli) (Hanson & Luciana, 2004). On a test of sustained attention, reaction time and number of correct responses did not differ across MDMA users and matched controls (Parrott et al., 1998). MDMA users and matched controls did not differ with respect to performance on the Trailmaking Test – Part A (McCardle et al., 2004).

Visuospatial functioning

None of the studies included in this review assessed visuospatial functioning.

Verbal learning and memory

Six of the seven studies included in this review examined the effects of MDMA exposure on memory (Bhattachary & Powell, 2001; McCardle et al., 2004; Parrott et al., 1998; Thomasius et al., 2003; Verkes et al., 2001). On measures of verbal learning and memory, MDMA exposure was associated with poorer performance on the delayed free recall section of list-learning tasks in three of the six studies that used this type of measure (McCardle et al., 2004; Parrott et al., 1998; Thomasius et al., 2003). Similarly, MDMA exposure was associated with poorer performance on the delayed free recall of detailed paragraphs in the three studies that used this type of measure (Bhattachary & Powell, 2001; Hanson & Luciana, 2004; Thomasius et al., 2003). Recognition of words was poorer for MDMA users on one of two tasks that assessed this domain (Verkes et al., 2001).

Nonverbal learning and memory

Nonverbal learning and memory was assessed in two of the seven studies. With respect to delayed free recall, MDMA users and matched controls' performance was similar on the Rey-Osterrieth Complex Figure Test (Bhattachary & Powell, 2001). MDMA users' capacity to recognize nonverbal material was worse than matched controls on one of two tests (Verkes et al., 2001).

Motor/psychomotor speed

Motor/psychomotor speed was assessed in five of the seven articles included in the review (Daumann et al., 2003a; Hanson & Luciana, 2004; McCardle et al., 2004; Parrott et al., 1998; Verkes et al., 2001). Two of the studies used traditional measures of motor/psychomotor speed. In those studies, MDMA users performed poorly relative to matched controls on the Finger Tapping Test (Hanson & Luciana, 2004); however, the groups did not differ with respect to performance on the Grooved Pegboard test (Hanson & Luciana, 2004) and the Digit Symbol test (McCardle et al., 2004).

Three of the seven articles used computerized measures of psychomotor speed (simple reaction time) (Daumann et al., 2003a; Parrott et al., 1998; Verkes et al., 2001). For studies that utilized visual stimuli to signal participants' response, differences were observed in one study (Verkes et al., 2001), but not the other two (Daumann et al., 2003b; Parrott et al., 1998). In the one study that utilized auditory stimuli to signal participant response (Verkes et al., 2001), MDMA users demonstrated a slower response time relative to matched controls.

Executive system functioning (frontal lobe functioning)

Each of the seven studies included measures of executive system functioning. Four of the studies used traditional measures of motor/psychomotor speed. In those studies, MDMA users performed poorly relative to matched controls on a verbal fluency test (Bhattachary & Powell, 2001); in contrast, the groups performed similarly on the Wisconsin Card Sorting Test (Thomasius et al., 2003), a verbal fluency test (Hanson & Luciana, 2004), and the Trailmaking Test – Part B (McCardle et al., 2004).

Four of the seven articles used computerized measures of complex reaction time to assess executive system functioning. Performance on measures of choice reaction time was associated with MDMA exposure in one study (Verkes et al., 2001), but not in another (Parrott et al., 1998). The n-back tests, which were used in one study, were relatively insensitive to MDMA-associated frontal lobe deficits (Daumann et al., 2003a). MDMA user performance was poorer than matched controls on a computerized version of the Corsi block tapping test (Verkes et al., 2001). The performance of MDMA users and matched controls generally did not differ using a set of novel working memory tests (Hanson & Luciana, 2004).

Mood/emotional functioning

Of the seven studies reviewed, four evaluated the association between MDMA use and mood/emotional functioning (Hanson & Luciana, 2004; McCardle et al., 2004; Thomasius et al., 2003; Verkes et al., 2001). Three of the four studies found that MDMA users reported greater levels of depressive symptomatology, as indexed using the Beck Depression Inventory (BDI) (Hanson & Luciana, 2004; McCardle et al., 2004; Thomasius et al., 2003); however, in these studies, ex-MDMA users generally reported minimal levels of depressive symptomatology (i.e., BDI score ≤ 10) (Verkes et al., 2001). The fourth study also reported that ex-MDMA users reported greater levels of depressive symptomatology than matched controls, but did not specify the test scores (Verkes et al., 2001).

Factors that moderate neuropsychological functioning

Two of the seven studies examined the association between patterns of MDMA and neuropsychological functioning, though neither study looked at the association in the subset of the MDMA users who were abstinent (Bhattachary & Powell, 2001; Hanson & Luciana, 2004). Self-reported level of depressive symptomatology was not associated with cognitive functioning in the one study that tested this association (Hanson & Luciana, 2004). None of the studies determined whether recreational MDMA users demonstrated recovery of function with sustained abstinence.

Summary of neuropsychological assessment

In the seven studies selected for the review, the study participants were recreational users. Each of the studies utilized a different battery to assess neuropsychological functioning. Although the studies did not include individuals who abused MDMA, the findings collectively indicate that recreational MDMA use is associated with deficits in the following neurocognitive domains: attention/concentration, learning and memory, motor/psychomotor speed, executive system functioning. In order to determine more definitively the magnitude of these associations, it is recommended that these studies be included in a quantitative review (meta-analysis).

Clinical applications of MDMA

Based on the findings from the preclinical studies, MDMA administration is clearly associated with neurotoxicity. The findings from the studies that used functional neuroimaging and neuropsychological assessment techniques are less definitive; however, they are consistent with the findings from the preclinical studies. These findings notwithstanding, it is periodically suggested that MDMA be administered as an adjunct to psychotherapy in individuals with various anxiety disorders (e.g., social phobia, post-traumatic stress disorder) for the purpose of enhancing the probability of a positive treatment outcome. In this final section, we review the extant literature on the topic.

Sometime after the publication of this study (Hardman et al., 1973), an indeterminate number of psychiatrists on the West Coast began using MDMA as a psychotherapeutic agent with their patients. The first such sessions seem to have been conducted in 1976 by Zeff, a clinical psychologist with previous experience performing therapy sessions involving lysergic acid diethylamide (LSD) administration (Greer & Tolbert, 1990). It is claimed that Zeff "... had conducted hundreds of MDMA sessions and had achieved dramatic results without complications" (Greer & Tolbert, 1990); however, these results do not seem to have been published in any peer-reviewed journals. Subsequent efforts were made by others to more rigorously document and codify the putative efficacy of MDMA-assisted therapy, but few such reports seem to have made it into the scientific literature. Greer and Tolbert's account detailing the clinical experiences of their patients with MDMA (1986) appears to be one of the only peer-reviewed articles published on this topic, yet the authors later described this report as "more in the spirit of a descriptive 'medical anthropology' study than a rigorously controlled experiment" (Greer & Tolbert, 1990). Thus, the assertion that MDMA was widely used in psychotherapy and is highly efficacious in treating a range of emotional disorders seems to have little empirical support.

In 1984, representatives from the World Health Organization (WHO) submitted a formal request to the Food and Drug Administration (FDA) concerning information on the abuse potential, observed abuse patterns, and possible therapeutic value of 28 new psychotropic compounds, including MDMA (Randolph, 1984). Within days, amidst reports of increasing recreational popularity and neurotoxic effects in laboratory animals (Ricaurte, Bryan, Strauss, Seiden, & Schuster, 1985), the Drug Enforcement Administration (DEA) officially stated their intent to place MDMA into Schedule I of the Controlled Substances Act (Mullen, 1984). Much debate and controversy surrounded the subsequent scheduling hearings, sparked by the DEA's provocative decision to invoke the Emergency Scheduling Act just days before the initial proceedings, resulting in the temporary placement of MDMA into the maximally restrictive Schedule I (Shulgin, 1986). The outcome of the scheduling hearings was no less controversial. The judicial recommendation was that, based on the testimony of several therapists, MDMA appeared to have potential therapeutic benefit and should therefore be placed into the less restrictive Schedule III. The DEA, however, disagreed, and extended the temporary emergency status of MDMA, prolonging its placement in Schedule I (Beck & Rosenbaum, 1994). Finally, in a move of questionable legality, the DEA made this Schedule I placement permanent in November of 1986, despite the result of the earlier hearings (Shulgin, 1990). This course of action was appealed in 1987, and the DEA was instructed to remove MDMA from Schedule I until more data regarding the compound's putative therapeutic effects could be collected (Beck & Rosenbaum, 1994). Although the DEA initially complied, they reversed their decision within a matter of months, and MDMA was again returned to Schedule I where it has remained ever since (Shulgin, 1990).

References

Acquas, E., Marrocu, P., Pisanu, A., Cadoni, C., Zernig, G., Saria, A., et al. (2001). Intravenous administration of ecstasy (3,4-methylendioxymethamphetamine) enhances cortical and striatal acetylcholine release in vivo. *European Journal of Pharmacology, 418*, 207–211.

Anderson, G. M., III, Braun, G., Braun, U., Nichols, D. E., & Shulgin, A. T. (1978). Absolute configuration and psychotomimetic activity. *NIDA Research Monograph, 22*, 8–15.

Bakhit, C., & Gibb, J. W. (1981). Methamphetamine-induced depression of tryptophan hydroxylase: Recovery following acute treatment. *European Journal of Pharmacology, 76*, 229–233.

Battaglia, G., Brooks, B. P., Kulsakdinun, C., & De Souza, E. B. (1988). Pharmacologic profile of MDMA (3,4-methylenedioxymethamphetamine) at various brain recognition sites. *European Journal of Pharmacology, 149*, 159–163.

Battaglia, G., & De Souza, E. B. (1989). Pharmacologic profile of amphetamine derivatives at various brain recognition sites: Selective effects on serotonergic systems. *NIDA Research Monograph, 94*, 240–258.

Beardsley, P. M., Balster, R. L., & Harris, L. S. (1986). Self-administration of methylenedioxymethamphetamine (MDMA) by rhesus monkeys. *Drug and Alcohol Dependence, 18*, 149–157.

Beck, J., & Rosenbaum, M. (1994). *Pursuit of ecstasy: The MDMA experience.* Albany: State University of New York Press.

Benavides, J., Fage, D., Carter, C., & Scatton, B. (1987). Peripheral type benzodiazepine binding sites are a sensitive indirect index of neuronal damage. *Brain Research, 421*, 167–172.

Bhattachary, S., & Powell, J. H. (2001). Recreational use of 3,4-methylenedioxymethamphetamine (MDMA) or "ecstasy": Evidence for cognitive impairment. *Psychological Medicine, 31*, 647–658.

Bilsky, E. J., Hui, Y. Z., Hubbell, C. L., & Reid, L. D. (1990). Methylenedioxymethamphetamine's capacity to establish place preferences and modify intake of an alcoholic beverage. *Pharmacology, Biochemistry and Behavior, 37*, 633–638.

Bowyer, J. F., Young, J. F., Slikker, W., Itzak, Y., Mayorga, A. J., Newport, G. D., et al. (2003). Plasma levels of parent compound and metabolites after doses of either d-fenfluramine or d-3,4-methylenedioxymethamphetamine (MDMA) that produce long-term serotonergic alterations. *Neurotoxicology, 24*, 379–390.

Broening, H. W., Bowyer, J. F., & Slikker, W., Jr. (1995). Age-dependent sensitivity of rats to the long-term effects of the serotonergic neurotoxicant (+/−)-3,4-methylenedioxymethamphetamine (MDMA) correlates with the magnitude of the MDMA-induced thermal response. *Journal of Pharmacology and Experimental Therapeutics, 275*, 325–333.

Buchert, R., Thomasius, R., Wilke, F., Petersen, K., Nebeling, B., Obrocki, J., et al. (2004). A voxel-based PET investigation of the long-term effects of "ecstasy" consumption on brain serotonin transporters. *American Journal of Psychiatry, 161*, 1181–1189.

Bunzow, J. R., Sonders, M. S., Arttamangkul, S., Harrison, L. M., Zhang, G., Quigley, D. I., et al. (2001). Amphetamine, 3,4-methylenedioxymethamphetamine, lysergic acid diethylamide, and metabolites of the catecholamine neurotransmitters are agonists of a rat trace amine receptor. *Molecular Pharmacology, 60*, 1181–1188.

Callaway, C. W., Johnson, M. P., Gold, L. H., Nichols, D. E., & Geyer, M. A. (1991). Amphetamine derivatives induce locomotor hyperactivity by acting as indirect serotonin agonists. *Psychopharmacology (Berlin)*, *104*, 293–301.

Callaway, C. W., Wing, L. L., & Geyer, M. A. (1990). Serotonin release contributes to the locomotor stimulant effects of 3,4-methylenedioxymethamphetamine in rats. *Journal of Pharmacology and Experimental Therapeutics*, *254*, 456–464.

Casellas, P., Galiegue, S., & Basile, A. S. (2002). Peripheral benzodiazepine receptors and mitochondrial function. *Neurochemistry International*, *40*, 475–486.

Chang, L., Ernst, T., Grob, C. S., & Poland, R. E. (1999). Cerebral (1)h MRS alterations in recreational 3,4-methylenedioxymethamphetamine (MDMA, "ecstasy") users. *Journal of Magnetic Resonance Imaging*, *10*, 521–526.

Chang, L., Grob, C. S., Ernst, T., Itti, L., Mishkin, F. S., Jose-Melchor, R., et al. (2000). Effect of ecstasy [3,4-methylenedioxymethamphetamine (MDMA)] on cerebral blood flow: A co-registered SPECT and MRI study. *Psychiatry Research*, *98*, 15–28.

Cohen, R. S. (1996). Adverse symptomatology and suicide associated with the use of methylenedioxymethamphetamine (MDMA; "ecstasy"). *Biological Psychiatry*, *39*, 819–820.

Colado, M. I., Granados, R., O'Shea, E., Esteban, B., & Green, A. R. (1998). Role of hyperthermia in the protective action of clomethiazole against MDMA ("ecstasy")-induced neurodegeneration, comparison with the novel NMDA channel blocker AR-R15896AR. *British Journal of Pharmacology*, *124*, 479–484.

Colombo, J. A., & Puissant, V. I. (2002). Fluoro Jade stains early and reactive astroglia in the primate cerebral cortex. *Journal of Histochemistry and Cytochemistry*, *50*, 1135–1137.

Commins, D. L., Vosmer, G., Virus, R. M., Woolverton, W. L., Schuster, C. R., & Seiden, L. S. (1987). Biochemical and histological evidence that methylenedioxymethylamphetamine (MDMA) is toxic to neurons in the rat brain. *Journal of Pharmacology and Experimental Therapeutics*, *241*, 338–345.

Cowan, R. L., Lyoo, I. K., Sung, S. M., Ahn, K. H., Kim, M. J., Hwang, J., et al. (2003). Reduced cortical gray matter density in human MDMA (ecstasy) users: A voxel-based morphometry study. *Drug and Alcohol Dependence*, *72*, 225–235.

Curran, H. V. (2000). Is MDMA ("ecstasy") neurotoxic in humans? An overview of evidence and of methodological problems in research. *Neuropsychobiology*, *42*, 34–41.

Daumann, J., Fimm, B., Willmes, K., Thron, A., & Gouzoulis-Mayfrank, E. (2003a). Cerebral activation in abstinent ecstasy (MDMA) users during a working memory task: A functional magnetic resonance imaging (FMRI) study. *Brain Research and Cognitive Brain Research*, *16*, 479–487.

Daumann, J., Fischermann, T., Pilatus, U., Thron, A., Moeller-Hartmann, W., & Gouzoulis-Mayfrank, E. (2004). Proton magnetic resonance spectroscopy in ecstasy (MDMA) users. *Neuroscience Letters*, *362*, 113–116.

Daumann, J., Schnitker, R., Weidemann, J., Schnell, K., Thron, A., & Gouzoulis-Mayfrank, E. (2003b). Neural correlates of working memory in pure and polyvalent ecstasy (MDMA) users. *Neuroreport*, *14*, 1983–1987.

De Souza, E. B., Battaglia, G., & Insel, T. R. (1990). Neurotoxic effect of MDMA on brain serotonin neurons: Evidence from neurochemical and radioligand binding studies. *Annals of the New York Academy of Sciences*, *600*, 682–688.

Escubedo, E., Guitart, L., Sureda, F. X., Jimenez, A., Pubill, D., Pallas, M., et al.

(1998). Microgliosis and down-regulation of adenosine transporter induced by methamphetamine in rats. *Brain Research, 814*, 120–126.

Fantegrossi, W. E., Godlewski, T., Karabenick, R. L., Stephens, J. M., Ullrich, T., Rice, K. C., et al. (2003). Pharmacological characterization of the effects of 3,4-methylenedioxymethamphetamine ("ecstasy") and its enantiomers on lethality, core temperature, and locomotor activity in singly housed and crowded mice. *Psychopharmacology (Berlin), 166*, 202–211.

Fantegrossi, W. E., Kiessel, C. L., Leach, P. T., Van Martin, C., Karabenick, R. L., Chen, X., et al. (2004a). Nantenine: An antagonist of the behavioral and physiological effects of MDMA in mice. *Psychopharmacology (Berlin), 173*, 270–277.

Fantegrossi, W. E., Ullrich, T., Rice, K. C., Woods, J. H., & Winger, G. (2002). 3,4-Methylenedioxymethamphetamine (MDMA, "ecstasy") and its stereoisomers as reinforcers in rhesus monkeys: Serotonergic involvement. *Psychopharmacology (Berlin), 161*, 356–364.

Fantegrossi, W. E., Woods, J. H., & Winger, G. (2004). Transient reinforcing effects of phenylisopropylamine and indolealkylamine hallucinogens in rhesus monkeys. *Behavioral Pharmacology, 15*, 149–157.

Fantegrossi, W. E., Woolverton, W. L., Kilbourn, M., Sherman, P., Yuan, J., Hatzidimitriou, G., et al. (2004b). Behavioral and neurochemical consequences of long-term intravenous self-administration of MDMA and its enantiomers by rhesus monkeys. *Neuropsychopharmacology, 29*, 1270–1281.

Farfel, G. M., & Seiden, L. S. (1995). Role of hypothermia in the mechanism of protection against serotonergic toxicity. I. Experiments using 3,4-methylenedioxymethamphetamine, dizocilpine, CGS 19755 and NBQX. *Journal of Pharmacology and Experimental Therapeutics, 272*, 860–867.

Fischer, H. S., Zernig, G., Schatz, D. S., Humpel, C., & Saria, A. (2000). MDMA ("ecstasy") enhances basal acetylcholine release in brain slices of the rat striatum. *European Journal of Neuroscience, 12*, 1385–1390.

Fornai, F., Gesi, M., Lenzi, P., Ferrucci, M., Lazzeri, G., Pizzanelli, C., et al. (2004). Effects of repeated low doses of MDMA on EEG activity and Fluoro-Jade B histochemistry. *Annals of the New York Academy of Sciences, 1025*, 181–188.

Fuller, R. W., Snoddy, H. D., Roush, B. W., & Molloy, B. B. (1973). Further structure–activity studies on the lowering of brain 5-hydroxyindoles by 4-chloramphetamine. *Neuropharmacology, 12*, 33–42.

Gamma, A., Buck, A., Berthold, T., & Vollenweider, F. X. (2001). No difference in brain activation during cognitive performance between ecstasy (3,4-methylenedioxymethamphetamine) users and control subjects: A [$H_2^{15}O$]-positron emission tomography study. *Journal of Psychopharmacology, 21*, 66–71.

Geyer, M. A. (1996). Serotonergic functions in arousal and motor activity. *Behavioral Brain Research, 73*, 31–35.

Geyer, M., & Callaway, C. (1994). Behavioral pharmacology of ring-substituted amphetamine analogues. In A. K. Cho & D. S. Segal (Eds.), *Amphetamine and its analogues: Psychopharmacology, toxicity, and abuse* (pp. 177–208). San Diego, CA: Academic Press.

Gibb, J., Hanson, G., & Johnson, M. (1994). Neurochemical mechanisms of toxicity. In A. K. Cho & D. S. Segal (Eds.), *Amphetamine and its analogues: Psychopharmacology, toxicity, and abuse* (pp. 269–295). San Diego, CA: Academic Press.

Gibb, J. W., Johnson, M., Stone, D., & Hanson, G. R. (1990). MDMA: Historical perspectives. *Annals of the New York Academy of Sciences, 600*, 601–620.

Glennon, R. A. (1989). Stimulus properties of hallucinogenic phenalkylamines and related designer drugs: Formulation of structure–activity relationships. *NIDA Research Monograph, 94*, 43–67.

Glennon, R. A., Young, R., & Rosecrans, J. A. (1983). Antagonism of the effects of the hallucinogen DOM and the purported 5-HT agonist quipazine by 5-HT$_2$ antagonists. *European Journal of Pharmacology, 91*, 189–196.

Gold, L. H., Koob, G. F., & Geyer, M. A. (1988). Stimulant and hallucinogenic behavioral profiles of 3,4-methylenedioxymethamphetamine and N-ethyl-3,4-methylenedioxyamphetamine in rats. *Journal of Pharmacology and Experimental Therapeutics, 247*, 547–555.

Greer, G. R., & Tolbert, R. (1990). The therapeutic use of MDMA. In S. J. Peroutka (Ed.), *Ecstasy: the clinical, pharmacological and neurotoxicological effects of the drug MDMA* (pp. 21–36). Boston: Kluwer Academic.

Griffith, J. D., Nutt, J. G., & Jasinski, D. R. (1975). A comparison of fenfluramine and amphetamine in man. *Clinical Pharmacology and Therapeutics, 18*, 563–570.

Griffiths, R. R., Winger, G., Brady, J. V., & Snell, J. D. (1976). Comparison of behavior maintained by infusions of eight phenylethylamines in baboons. *Psychopharmacology (Berlin), 50*, 251–258.

Gudelsky, G. A., Yamamoto, B. K., & Nash, J. F. (1994). Potentiation of 3,4-methylenedioxymethamphetamine-induced dopamine release and serotonin neurotoxicity by 5-HT$_2$ receptor agonists. *European Journal of Pharmacology, 264*, 325–330.

Hanson, K. L., & Luciana, M. (2004). Neurocognitive function in users of MDMA: The importance of clinically significant patterns of use. *Psychological Medicine, 34*, 229–246.

Hardman, H. F., Haavik, C. O., & Seevers, M. H. (1973). Relationship of the structure of mescaline and seven analogs to toxicity and behavior in five species of laboratory animals. *Toxicology and Applied Pharmacology, 25*, 299–309.

Harvey, J. A., McMaster, S. E., & Yunger, L. M. (1975). *p*-Chloramphetamine: Selective neurotoxic action in brain. *Science, 187*, 841–843.

Hemby, S. E., Co, C., Koves, T. R., Smith, J. E., & Dworkin, S. I. (1997). Differences in extracellular dopamine concentrations in the nucleus accumbens during response-dependent and response-independent cocaine administration in the rat. *Psychopharmacology (Berlin), 133*, 7–16.

Hiramatsu, M., Nabeshima, T., Kameyama, T., Maeda, Y., & Cho, A. K. (1989). The effect of optical isomers of 3,4-methylenedioxymethamphetamine (MDMA) on stereotyped behavior in rats. *Pharmacology, Biochemistry and Behavior, 33*, 343–347.

Horschitz, S., Hummerich, R., & Schloss, P. (2001). Down-regulation of the rat serotonin transporter upon exposure to a selective serotonin reuptake inhibitor. *Neuroreport, 12*, 2181–2184.

Hubner, C. B., Bird, M., Rassnick, S., & Kornetsky, C. (1988). The threshold lowering effects of MDMA (ecstasy) on brain-stimulation reward. *Psychopharmacology (Berlin), 95*, 49–51.

Jacobsen, L. K., Mencl, W. E., Pugh, K. R., Skudlarski, P., & Krystal, J. H. (2004). Preliminary evidence of hippocampal dysfunction in adolescent MDMA ("ecstasy") users: Possible relationship to neurotoxic effects. *Psychopharmacology (Berlin), 173*, 383–390.

Jacobsen, L. K., Staley, J. K., Malison, R. T., Zoghbi, S. S., Seibyl, J. P., Kosten, T. R., et al. (2000). Elevated central serotonin transporter binding availability in acutely abstinent cocaine-dependent patients. *American Journal of Psychiatry, 157*, 1134–1140.

Kalia, M. (2000). Do validated biological measures of neurotoxicity really support the claim that MDMA is neurotoxic to man? *Neuropsychobiology, 42*, 45.

Kehne, J. H., Ketteler, H. J., McCloskey, T. C., Sullivan, C. K., Dudley, M. W., & Schmidt, C. J. (1996). Effects of the selective 5-HT$_{2a}$ receptor antagonist MDL 100,907 on MDMA-induced locomotor stimulation in rats. *Neuropsychopharmacology, 15*, 116–124.

Kish, S. J. (2002). How strong is the evidence that brain serotonin neurons are damaged in human users of ecstasy? *Pharmacology, Biochemistry and Behavior, 71*, 845–855.

Lamb, R. J., & Griffiths, R. R. (1987). Self-injection of d,1-3,4-methylenedioxymethamphetamine (MDMA) in the baboon. *Psychopharmacology (Berlin), 91*, 268–272.

Liechti, M. E., Geyer, M. A., Hell, D., & Vollenweider, F. X. (2001). Effects of MDMA (ecstasy) on prepulse inhibition and habituation of startle in humans after pretreatment with citalopram, haloperidol, or ketanserin. *Neuropsychopharmacology, 24*, 240–252.

Liechti, M. E., Saur, M. R., Gamma, A., Hell, D., & Vollenweider, F. X. (2000). Psychological and physiological effects of MDMA ("ecstasy") after pretreatment with the 5-HT(2) antagonist ketanserin in healthy humans. *Neuropsychopharmacology, 23*, 396–404.

Liechti, M. E., & Vollenweider, F. X. (2000). The serotonin uptake inhibitor citalopram reduces acute cardiovascular and vegetative effects of 3,4-methylenedioxymethamphetamine ("ecstasy'") in healthy volunteers. *Journal of Psychopharmacology, 14*, 269–274.

Malberg, J. E., Sabol, K. E., & Seiden, L. S. (1996). Co-administration of MDMA with drugs that protect against MDMA neurotoxicity produces different effects on body temperature in the rat. *Journal of Pharmacology and Experimental Therapeutics, 278*, 258–267.

Malberg, J. E., & Seiden, L. S. (1998). Small changes in ambient temperature cause large changes in 3,4-methylenedioxymethamphetamine (MDMA)-induced serotonin neurotoxicity and core body temperature in the rat. *Journal of Neuroscience, 18*, 5086–5094.

Marona-Lewicka, D., Rhee, G. S., Sprague, J. E., & Nichols, D. E. (1996). Reinforcing effects of certain serotonin-releasing amphetamine derivatives. *Pharmacology, Biochemistry and Behavior, 53*, 99–105.

Mash, D. C., Staley, J. K., Izenwasser, S., Basile, M., & Ruttenber, A. J. (2000). Serotonin transporters upregulate with chronic cocaine use. *Journal of Chemical Neuroanatomy, 20*, 271–280.

Mattson, M. P., Maudsley, S., & Martin, B. (2004). BDNF and 5-HT: A dynamic duo in age-related neuronal plasticity and neurodegenerative disorders. *Trends in Neuroscience, 27*, 589–594.

Mazzola-Pomietto, P., Aulakh, C. S., Tolliver, T., & Murphy, D. L. (1997). Functional subsensitivity of 5-HT$_{2a}$ and 5-HT$_{2c}$ receptors mediating hyperthermia following acute and chronic treatment with 5-HT$_{2a/2c}$ receptor antagonists. *Psychopharmacology (Berlin), 130*, 144–151.

McCann, U. D., Szabo, Z., Scheffel, U., Dannals, R. F., & Ricaurte, G. A. (1998).

Positron emission tomographic evidence of toxic effect of MDMA ("ecstasy") on brain serotonin neurons in human beings. *Lancet, 352*, 1433–1437.

McCardle, K., Luebbers, S., Carter, J. D., Croft, R. J., & Stough, C. (2004). Chronic MDMA (ecstasy) use, cognition and mood. *Psychopharmacology (Berlin), 173*, 434–439.

McDaid, J., & Docherty, J. R. (2001). Vascular actions of MDMA involve alpha1 and alpha2-adrenoceptors in the anaesthetized rat. *British Journal of Pharmacology, 133*, 429–437.

Miller, D. B., & O'Callaghan, J. P. (1994). Environment-, drug- and stress-induced alterations in body temperature affect the neurotoxicity of substituted amphetamines in the C57BL/6J mouse. *Journal of Pharmacology and Experimental Therapeutics, 270*, 752–760.

Miller, D. B., & O'Callaghan, J. P. (1995). The role of temperature, stress, and other factors in the neurotoxicity of the substituted amphetamines 3,4-methylenedioxymethamphetamine and fenfluramine. *Molecular Neurobiology, 11*, 177–192.

Millman, R., & Breeder, A. (1994). The new psychedelic culture: LSD, ecstasy, rave parties, and the Grateful Dead. *Psychiatric Annals, 24*, 148–150.

Moeller, F. G., Steinberg, J. L., Dougherty, D. M., Narayana, P. A., Kramer, L. A., & Renshaw, P. F. (2004). Functional MRI study of working memory in MDMA users. *Psychopharmacology (Berlin), 177*, 185–194.

Mokler, D. J., Commissaris, R. L., Warner, M. R., & Rech, R. H. (1983). Blockade of the behavioral effects of lysergic acid diethylamide, 2,5-dimethoxy-4-methylamphetamine, quipazine and lisuride by 5-hydroxytryptamine antagonists. *Journal of Pharmacology and Experimental Therapeutics, 227*, 557–562.

Molliver, M. E., Berger, U. V., Mamounas, L. A., Molliver, D. C., O'Hearn, E., & Wilson, M. A. (1990). Neurotoxicity of MDMA and related compounds: Anatomic studies. *Annals of the New York Academy of Sciences, 600*, 649–661.

Morgan, M. J. (2000). Ecstasy (MDMA): A review of its possible persistent psychological effects. *Psychopharmacology (Berlin), 152*, 230–248.

Mullen, F. M. (1984). Schedules of controlled substances. Proposed placement of 3,4-methylenedioxymethamphetamine into Schedule I. *Federal Register, 49*, 30210–30211.

Naranjo, C., Shulgin, A. T., & Sargent, T. (1967). Evaluation of 3,4-methylenedioxyamphetamine (MDA) as an adjunct to psychotherapy. *Medicina et Pharmacologia Experimentalis, 17*, 359–364.

Nash, J. F., Jr., Meltzer, H. Y., & Gudelsky, G. A. (1988). Elevation of serum prolactin and corticosterone concentrations in the rat after the administration of 3,4-methylenedioxymethamphetamine. *Journal of Pharmacology and Experimental Therapeutics, 245*, 873–879.

Nash, J. F., Roth, B. L., Brodkin, J. D., Nichols, D. E., & Gudelsky, G. A. (1994). Effect of the R(–) and S(+) isomers of MDA and MDMA on phosphatidyl inositol turnover in cultured cells expressing 5-HT_{2a} or 5-HT_{2c} receptors. *Neuroscience Letters, 177*, 111–115.

Nencini, P., Woolverton, W. L., & Seiden, L. S. (1988). Enhancement of morphine-induced analgesia after repeated injections of methylenedioxymethamphetamine. *Brain Research, 457*, 136–142.

Nichols, D. E. (1986). Differences between the mechanism of action of MDMA, MBDB, and the classic hallucinogens. Identification of a new therapeutic class: Entactogens. *Journal of Psychoactive Drugs, 18*, 305–313.

Nichols, D. E., & Glennon, R. A. (1984). Medicinal chemistry and structure – activity relationships of hallucinogens. In B. L. Jacobs (Ed.), *Hallucinogens: Neurochemical, behavioral, and clinical perspectives* (pp. 95–142). New York: Raven Press.

Nichols, D. E., Lloyd, D. H., Hoffman, A. J., Nichols, M. B., & Yim, G. K. (1982). Effects of certain hallucinogenic amphetamine analogues on the release of [^{3}H]serotonin from rat brain synaptosomes. *Journal of Medical Chemistry, 25*, 530–535.

Obergriesser, T., Ende, G., Braus, D. F., & Henn, F. A. (2001). Hippocampal ^{1}H-MRSI in ecstasy users. *European Archives of Psychiatry and Clinical Neuroscience, 251*, 114–116.

Obrocki, J., Schmoldt, A., Buchert, R., Andresen, B., Petersen, K., & Thomasius, R. (2002). Specific neurotoxicity of chronic use of ecstasy. *Toxicology Letters, 127*, 285–297.

O'Callaghan, J. P., & Miller, D. B. (1993). Quantification of reactive gliosis as an approach to neurotoxicity assessment. *NIDA Research Monograph, 136*, 188–212.

O'Callaghan, J. P., & Miller, D. B. (1994). Neurotoxicity profiles of substituted amphetamines in the C57BL/6J mouse. *Journal of Pharmacology and Experimental Therapeutics, 270*, 741–751.

Park, C. H., Carboni, E., Wood, P. L., & Gee, K. W. (1996). Characterization of peripheral benzodiazepine type sites in a cultured murine BV-2 microglial cell line. *Glia, 16*, 65–70.

Parrott, A. C. (2000). Human research on MDMA (3,4-methylenedioxymethamphetamine) neurotoxicity: Cognitive and behavioural indices of change. *Neuropsychobiology, 42*, 17–24.

Parrott, A. C. (2001). Human psychopharmacology of ecstasy (MDMA): A review of 15 years of empirical research. *Human Psychopharmacology, 16*, 557–577.

Parrott, A. C., Lees, A., Garnham, N. J., Jones, M., & Wesnes, K. (1998). Cognitive performance in recreational users of MDMA of "ecstasy": Evidence for memory deficits. *Journal of Psychopharmacology, 12*, 79–83.

Parrott, A. C., & Yeomans, M. (1995). Wobble, rave, inhale or crave: Psychoactive drugs of abuse symposium. *Psychologist, July*, 305.

Pedersen, N. P., & Blessing, W. W. (2001). Cutaneous vasoconstriction contributes to hyperthermia induced by 3,4-methylenedioxymethamphetamine (ecstasy) in conscious rabbits. *Journal of Neuroscience, 21*, 8648–8654.

Pletscher, A., Bartholini, G., Bruderer, H., Burkard, W. P., & Gey, K. F. (1964). Chlorinated arylalkylamines affecting the cerebral metabolism of 5-hydroxytryptamine. *Journal of Pharmacology and Experimental Therapeutics, 145*, 344–350.

Pletscher, A., Burkard, W. P., Bruderer, H., & Gey, K. F. (1963). Decrease of cerebral 5-hydroxytryptamine and 5-hydroxyindolacetic acid by an arylalkylamine. *Life Sciences, 11*, 828–833.

Poling, A., & Bryceland, J. (1979). Voluntary drug self-administration by nonhumans: A review. *Journal of Psychedelic Drugs, 11*, 185–190.

Pubill, D., Canudas, A. M., Pallas, M., Camins, A., Camarasa, J., & Escubedo, E. (2003). Different glial response to methamphetamine- and methylenedioxymethamphetamine-induced neurotoxicity. *Naunyn Schmiedeberg's Archives of Pharmacology, 367*, 490–499.

Randolph, W. F. (1984). International drug scheduling; conventions on psychotropic substances; stimulant and/or hallucinogenic drugs. *Federal Register, 49*, 29273–29274.

Reneman, L., Booij, J., Habraken, J. B., De Bruin, K., Hatzidimitriou, G., Den

Heeten, G. J., et al. (2002). Validity of [^{123}I]beta-CIT SPECT in detecting MDMA-induced serotonergic neurotoxicity. *Synapse, 46*, 199–205.

Reneman, L., Majoie, C. B., Habraken, J. B., & den Heeten, G. J. (2001). Effects of ecstasy (MDMA) on the brain in abstinent users: Initial observations with diffusion and perfusion mr imaging. *Radiology, 220*, 611–617.

Ricaurte, G., Bryan, G., Strauss, L., Seiden, L., & Schuster, C. (1985). Hallucinogenic amphetamine selectively destroys brain serotonin nerve terminals. *Science, 229*, 986–988.

Ricaurte, G. A., Yuan, J., Hatzidimitriou, G., Cord, B. J., & McCann, U. D. (2002). Severe dopaminergic neurotoxicity in primates after a common recreational dose regimen of MDMA ("ecstasy"). *Science, 297*, 2260–2263.

Ricaurte, G. A., Yuan, J., Hatzidimitriou, G., Cord, B. J., & McCann, U. D. (2003). Retraction. *Science, 301*, 1479.

Ricaurte, G. A., Yuan, J., & McCann, U. D. (2000). (+/−)3,4-Methylenedioxymethamphetamine ("ecstasy")-induced serotonin neurotoxicity: Studies in animals. *Neuropsychobiology, 42*, 5–10.

Rothman, R. B., Baumann, M. H., Dersch, C. M., Romero, D. V., Rice, K. C., Carroll, F. I., et al. (2001). Amphetamine-type central nervous system stimulants release norepinephrine more potently than they release dopamine and serotonin. *Synapse, 39*, 32–41.

Rudnick, G., & Wall, S. C. (1992). The molecular mechanism of "ecstasy" [3,4-methylenedioxy-methamphetamine (MDMA)]: Serotonin transporters are targets for MDMA-induced serotonin release. *Proceedings of the National Academy of Sciences of the United States of America, 89*, 1817–1821.

Sabol, K. E., & Seiden, L. S. (1998). Reserpine attenuates *d*-amphetamine and MDMA-induced transmitter release in vivo: A consideration of dose, core temperature and dopamine synthesis. *Brain Research, 806*, 69–78.

Sadzot, B., Baraban, J. M., Glennon, R. A., Lyon, R. A., Leonhardt, S., Jan, C. R., et al. (1989). Hallucinogenic drug interactions at human brain 5-HT$_2$ receptors: Implications for treating LSD-induced hallucinogenesis. *Psychopharmacology (Berlin), 98*, 495–499.

Sanchez, V., Camarero, J., Esteban, B., Peter, M. J., Green, A. R., & Colado, M. I. (2001). The mechanisms involved in the long-lasting neuroprotective effect of fluoxetine against MDMA ("ecstasy")-induced degeneration of 5-HT nerve endings in rat brain. *British Journal of Pharmacology, 134*, 46–57.

Sanders-Bush, E., & Sulser, F. (1970). *p*-Chloroamphetamine: In vivo investigations on the mechanism of action of the selective depletion of cerebral serotonin. *Journal of Pharmacology and Experimental Therapeutics, 175*, 419–426.

Sannerud, C. A., Kaminski, B. J., & Griffiths, R. R. (1996). Intravenous self-injection of four novel phenethylamines in baboons. *Behavioral Pharmacology, 7*, 315–323.

Saunders, N. (1995). *Ecstasy and dance culture*. London: Neal's Yard Desktop Publishing.

Schifano, F., Di Furia, L., Forza, G., Minicuci, N., & Bricolo, R. (1998). MDMA ("ecstasy") consumption in the context of polydrug abuse: A report on 150 patients. *Drug and Alcohol Dependence, 52*, 85–90.

Schmidt, C. J., & Kehne, J. H. (1990). Neurotoxicity of MDMA: Neurochemical effects. *Annals of the New York Academy of Sciences, 600*, 665–681.

Schmidt, C. J., Sullivan, C. K., & Fadayel, G. M. (1994). Blockade of striatal 5-hydroxytryptamine$_2$ receptors reduces the increase in extracellular concentrations of dopamine produced by the amphetamine analogue 3,4-methylenedioxymethamphetamine. *Journal of Neurochemistry, 62*, 1382–1389.

Schmidt, C. J., & Taylor, V. L. (1987). Depression of rat brain tryptophan hydroxylase activity following the acute administration of methylenedioxymethamphetamine. *Biochemistry and Pharmacology, 36*, 4095–4102.

Seiden, L. S., Fischman, M. W., & Schuster, C. R. (1976). Long-term methamphetamine induced changes in brain catecholamines in tolerant rhesus monkeys. *Drug and Alcohol Dependence, 1*, 215–219.

Semple, D. M., Ebmeier, K. P., Glabus, M. F., O'Carroll, R. E., & Johnstone, E. C. (1999). Reduced in vivo binding to the serotonin transporter in the cerebral cortex of MDMA ("ecstasy") users. *British Journal of Psychiatry, 175*, 63–69.

Shulgin, A. T. (1973). Stereospecific requirements for hallucinogenesis. *Journal of Pharmacy and Pharmacology, 25*, 271–272.

Shulgin, A. T. (1978). Psychotomimetic drugs: Structure activity relationships. In L. L. Iversen, S. D. Iversen, & S. H. Snyder (Eds.), *Handbook of psychopharmacology* (Vol. 11, pp. 243–333). New York: Plenum Press.

Shulgin, A. T. (1986). The background and chemistry of MDMA. *Journal of Psychoactive Drugs, 18*, 291–304.

Shulgin, A. T. (1990). History of MDMA. In S. J. Peroutka (Ed.), *Ecstasy: The clinical, pharmacological and neurotoxicological effects of the drug MDMA* (pp. 1–20). Boston: Kluwer Academic.

Siegel, S. (1988). Drug anticipation and drug tolerance. In M. Lader (Ed.), *The psychopharmacology of addiction* (pp. 73–96). New York: Oxford University Press.

Slikker, W., Jr., Holson, R. R., Ali, S. F., Kolta, M. G., Paule, M. G., Scallet, A. C., et al. (1989). Behavioral and neurochemical effects of orally administered MDMA in the rodent and nonhuman primate. *Neurotoxicology, 10*, 529–542.

Spanos, L. J., & Yamamoto, B. K. (1989). Acute and subchronic effects of methylenedioxymethamphetamine [(+/−)MDMA] on locomotion and serotonin syndrome behavior in the rat. *Pharmacology, Biochemistry and Behavior, 32*, 835–840.

Stephenson, D. T., Schober, D. A., Smalstig, E. B., Mincy, R. E., Gehlert, D. R., & Clemens, J. A. (1995). Peripheral benzodiazepine receptors are colocalized with activated microglia following transient global forebrain ischemia in the rat. *Journal of Neuroscience, 15*, 5263–5274.

Streit, W. J., & Graeber, M. B. (1993). Heterogeneity of microglial and perivascular cell populations: Insights gained from the facial nucleus paradigm. *Glia, 7*, 68–74.

Thomas, D. M., Dowgiert, J., Geddes, T. J., Francescutti-Verbeem, D., Liu, X., & Kuhn, D. M. (2004). Microglial activation is a pharmacologically specific marker for the neurotoxic amphetamines. *Neuroscience Letters, 367*, 349–354.

Thomasius, R., Petersen, K., Buchert, R., Andresen, B., Zapletalova, P., Wartberg, L., et al. (2003). Mood, cognition and serotonin transporter availability in current and former ecstasy (MDMA) users. *Psychopharmacology (Berlin), 167*, 85–96.

Verkes, R. J., Gijsman, H. J., Pieters, M. S., Schoemaker, R. C., de Visser, S., Kuijpers, M., et al. (2001). Cognitive performance and serotonergic function in users of ecstasy. *Psychopharmacology (Berlin), 153*, 196–202.

Volkow, N. D., Chang, L., Wang, G. J., Fowler, J. S., Franceschi, D., Sedler, M., et al. (2001). Loss of dopamine transporters in methamphetamine abusers recovers with protracted abstinence. *Journal of Neuroscience, 21*, 9414–9418.

Vollenweider, F. X., Jones, R. T., & Baggott, M. J. (2001). Caveat emptor: Editors beware. *Neuropsychopharmacology, 24*, 461–463.

Wilson, J. M., Levey, A. I., Bergeron, C., Kalasinsky, K., Ang, L., Peretti, F., et al. (1996). Striatal dopamine, dopamine transporter, and vesicular monoamine transporter in chronic cocaine users. *Annals of Neurology, 40,* 428–439.

Wilson, M. A., Ricaurte, G. A., & Molliver, M. E. (1989). Distinct morphologic classes of serotonergic axons in primates exhibit differential vulnerability to the psychotropic drug 3,4-methylenedioxymethamphetamine. *Neuroscience, 28,* 121–137.

Winsauer, P. J., McCann, U. D., Yuan, J., Delatte, M. S., Stevenson, M. W., Ricaurte, G. A., et al. (2002). Effects of fenfluramine, *m*-CPP and triazolam on repeated-acquisition in squirrel monkeys before and after neurotoxic MDMA administration. *Psychopharmacology (Berlin), 159,* 388–396.

Winslow, J. T., & Insel, T. R. (1991). Serotonergic modulation of the rat pup ultrasonic isolation call: Studies with $5HT_1$ and $5HT_2$ subtype-selective agonists and antagonists. *Psychopharmacology (Berlin), 105,* 513–520.

Zhou, F. C., Tao-Cheng, J. H., Segu, L., Patel, T., & Wang, Y. (1998). Serotonin transporters are located on the axons beyond the synaptic junctions: Anatomical and functional evidence. *Brain Research, 805,* 241–254.

7 Methamphetamine (crystal meth)

Ari Kalechstein and Thomas F. Newton

Introduction

Methamphetamine use in the United States has increased dramatically in recent years, and the user population has broadened in nature and in regional distribution. Moreover, the scope of the problem is becoming worldwide. For example, according to the World Health Organization, there are more than 35 million regular users of amphetamine/methamphetamine worldwide, which makes methamphetamine the most commonly used illicit drug after cannabis.

Amphetamine (the N-demethylated form of methamphetamine, which produces similar effects) was initially synthesized in the late 19th century (Anglin, Kalechstein, Maglione, Annon, & Fiorentine, 1997). As the stimulant properties of the drug became evident, it was increasingly utilized for its performance-enhancing effects. For example, during World War II, Axis power fighter pilots used methamphetamine to stay awake for extended periods of time.

In the 1950s and 1960s in the United States, methamphetamine was viewed as a "utilitarian drug" that was used by isolated pockets of individuals (Anglin, Burke, Perrochet, Stamper, & Dawud-Noursi, 2000). For example, methamphetamine was used as an anorectic or as a stimulant that enabled truck drivers to drive for extended periods of time without sleeping. Over time, due in part to the ease of production and the easy availability of low-cost ingredients, methamphetamine production escalated to the current levels.

The upswing in methamphetamine use is particularly troubling, as the drug produces long-lasting and negative changes in brain structure and function. These changes are the focus on this chapter. In the first section, we briefly review the pathophysiology of methamphetamine use. We then describe the effects of intoxication and withdrawal. Finally, we address the residual neuropsychological consequences of methamphetamine use.

Pathophysiology

In this section, we review the findings from studies on methamphetamine-associated neurotoxicity using animal models, postmortem studies in humans, studies on cerebrovascular accidents in humans, and neuroimaging studies that utilized human subjects.

Animal models

There are literally thousands of studies utilizing rodents and primates as subjects that document methamphetamine-associated neurotoxicity. Here we present a succinct review of the salient findings from these studies.

Seiden and colleagues conducted the pioneering studies that elucidated the neurophysiological consequences of methamphetamine dependence in rodents (Seiden, Fischman, & Schuster, 1976, 1977). They demonstrated that exposure to a high-dose regimen of methamphetamine resulted in a significant reduction in monoamine levels, particularly involving dopamine and serotonin, lasting three to six months after the last dose was administered. These findings were replicated in other studies (Ricaurte, Schuster, & Seiden, 1980), and studies utilizing primates documented similar changes lasting at least four years after the last methamphetamine administration (Woolverton, Ricaurte, Forno, & Seiden, 1989).

While the findings from these and other studies were compelling, they were criticized on the basis of the large doses of methamphetamine and intensive dosing patterns used. Questions were raised as to whether the results from those studies could be generalized to the patterns of use that have been reported by methamphetamine addicts; however, the findings from more recent investigations reveal that a relatively small number of low-dose administrations of methamphetamine also cause relatively long-lasting neurophysiological changes. For example, binding of 11C35,428-WIN-PET, a marker for presynaptic dopamine levels, was reduced by 85% following administration of two modest doses of methamphetamine spaced one week apart (Melega et al., 1996; Villemagne et al., 1998). In another study, administration of increasing doses of methamphetamine was associated with up to 95% reduction in striatal dopamine concentrations for up to six weeks following administration (Melega et al., 1996).

A series of studies by Castner and colleagues complement the previous studies. They demonstrated that low-dose methamphetamine administration produced significant changes in presynaptic dopamine functioning, imaged by ^{123}I IBZM uptake using single proton emission computed tomography (SPECT), even six months after the cessation of amphetamine administration. More importantly, they established an association between methamphetamine dependence, alterations in neurochemistry, and subsequent behavioral changes (Castner & Goldman, 1999; Castner & Goldman-Rakic, 1999; Castner et al., 2000).

Postmortem studies in humans

A search of the National Library of Medicine revealed that a number of studies utilized postmortem techniques to study the neurotoxic effects of methamphetamine (e.g., Karch, Stephens, & Ho, 1999; Siegal et al., 2004; Wilson et al., 1996). In the first study, Wilson and colleagues found reduced levels of three dopamine nerve terminal markers (dopamine, tyrosine hydroxylase, and the dopamine transporter) in postmortem striatum (nucleus accumbens, caudate, putamen) of chronic methamphetamine users; in contrast, levels of dopa decarboxylase and the vesicular monoamine transporter (VMAT), known to be reduced in Parkinson's disease, were normal. Because the VMAT is localized to neuronal terminals, Wilson et al. suggested that chronic methamphetamine use is not associated with permanent degeneration of striatal dopamine nerve terminals, but rather with long-lasting changes in phenotype and function.

In a separate study, Siegal and colleagues examined concentrations of vesicular acetylcholine transporter, which is considered to be a "stable" marker of cholinergic neurons, in the caudate and hippocampus of chronic users of methamphetamine users (Siegal et al., 2004). The comparison groups included assays of the brains of users of cocaine, heroin, and matched controls. While differences were not observed in the hippocampal regions, marked differences were observed in the caudate of the methamphetamine users. Based on these findings, the authors did not infer that methamphetamine use caused a loss of striatal cholinergic neurons; rather, they suggested that striatal cholinergic activity could be disrupted as a result of methamphetamine use.

The study by Karch and colleagues examined the cause of death in 413 decedents in which drug use was relevant versus 114 cases in which the decedents were "drug free" (Karch et al., 1999). The study found that methamphetamine use was associated with an increased risk for experiencing intracranial hemorrhage and that methamphetamine toxicity partially contributed to 65% of the deaths. The latter statement, while provocative, was probably difficult to substantiate.

Another subset of studies examined the association between methamphetamine use and onset of cerebrovascular accidents (Ohta, Mori, Yoritaka, Okamoto, & Kishida, 2005; Perez, Arsura, & Strategos, 1999; Rothrock, Rubenstein, & Lyden, 1988; Sachdeva & Woodward, 1989; Yen et al., 1994). Each publication utilized a case study approach. The five articles include 14 patients, each of whom experienced a cerebrovascular accident (CVA) following methamphetamine exposure. Given the approach used in each paper, the authors were circumspect in terms offering conclusions regarding the mechanism of action that underlied the onset of a CVA following methamphetamine exposure. They acknowledged that the mechanism underlying the onset of methamphetamine-associated CVAs has not been identified; however, the authors speculated that methamphetamine-associated CVAs might have occurred as a result of the following factors: increased blood pressure, vasculitis that occurred as a result of chronic methamphetamine use, and/or the direct, toxic effects of methamphetamine on cerebral vasculature.

The risk for the onset of CVAs may be related to methamphetamine-associated cardiac abnormalities (He, Matoba, Fujitani, Sodesaki, & Onishi, 1996; Hong, Matsuyama, & Nur, 1991; Wijetunga, Seto, Lindsay, & Schatz, 2003). For example, in one study of methamphetamine addicts, echocardiograms revealed the presence of cardiomyopathy in 19 of 21 users (Wijetunga et al., 2003). Similarly, a 56-day trial of methamphetamine exposure revealed marked damage to the hearts of rodents (He et al., 1996). He and colleagues commented that the damage to the hearts of the rats was consistent with the type and severity of the damage observed in human methamphetamine addicts.

Neuroimaging and electrophysiological studies in humans

In the last ten years, a growing body of literature has documented methamphetamine-associated neurotoxicity using various neuroimaging (Chang et al., 2002; Ernst, Chang, Leonido-Yee, & Speck, 2000; McCann et al., 1998; Paulus et al., 2002; Thompson et al., 2004; Volkow et al., 2001a, 2001b, 2001c) and electrophysiological (Newton, Cook, Kalechstein, Duran, Monroy, Ling, & Leuchter, 2003) techniques. The neuroimaging studies revealed that the following neurotoxic effects were associated with chronic methamphetamine exposure: reduced striatal dopamine transporter density (McCann et al., 1998; Volkow, et al., 2001a, 2001c), frontal lobe dysfunction, most evident in dorsolateral prefrontal and orbitofrontal regions (Paulus et al., 2002), alterations in cerebral metabolism (Volkow et al., 2001b), neuronal damage in the frontal lobes and the basal ganglia (Ernst et al., 2000), reductions in hippocampal volume (Thompson et al., 2004), and marked reductions in cerebral blood flow (Chang et al., 2002).

To our knowledge, one study has documented the electrophysiological changes associated with chronic methamphetamine users. In that study, Newton and colleagues evaluated methamphetamine-dependent volunteers with four days of abstinence and compared them to matched controls. Methamphetamine-dependent individuals, in comparison to matched controls, demonstrated increased electroencephalogram (EEG) power in the delta and theta bands while power in the alpha and beta bands did not differ between the groups. Within the methamphetamine-dependent group, 64% of the conventional EEGs were abnormal compared to 18% in the nonmethamphetamine-using group. These EEG changes correlated with changes in cognition as well (Newton, Kalechstein, Hardy et al., 2004b).

Within the last five years, several studies have also addressed the question of whether the methamphetamine-associated neurobiological changes observed during the initial phases of abstinence are permanent or whether they are reversible with sustained abstinence (Nordahl et al., 2005; Volkow et al.,

2001a, 2001c). One study showed that metabolite abnormalities were evident in the anterior cingulate, even three years after the initiation of abstinence (Nordahl et al., 2005). Another series of studies, which focused on recovery of dopamine transporter levels, demonstrated that partial recovery may occur as a result of sustained abstinence (Volkow et al., 2001a, 2001c).

Summary of pathophysiology of methamphetamine

The findings from the preclinical studies collectively reveal that chronic methamphetamine exposure is associated with abnormalities in brain structure and function. These abnormalities were consistently observed in preclinical studies using animal models, human postmortem studies, and human neuroimaging studies. Frontal-subcortical abnormalities tended to predominate. Interestingly, the neurotoxicity might not be permanent.

Human models of methamphetamine-associated neurotoxicity

Given the findings from studies of methamphetamine-associated neurotoxicity, it is reasonable to infer that similar findings would be observed in clinical studies of chronic methamphetamine users. In this section, we review the findings from studies that:

(1) characterized the effects of methamphetamine on cognition and/or emotional functioning during intoxication or withdrawal;
(2) characterized the residual effects of methamphetamine following intoxication and withdrawal;
(3) examined the association between neuroimaging and cognition or emotional functioning in human study participants.
(4) evaluated the relationship between neural functioning and treatment outcome.

Intoxication/withdrawal

Effects of methamphetamine on cognition

To our knowledge, there are no peer-reviewed studies that have characterized the acute effects of methamphetamine on cognition in methamphetamine-dependent individuals; however, preliminary data from our laboratory, which were presented at the College of Problems on Drug Dependence in 2005, offer an initial answer to this question. We present those data here.

Participants included 13 nontreatment-seeking, methamphetamine-dependent individuals recruited from the community through advertisements in local newspapers and provided with informed consent before participating in the study.

In brief, study participants detoxified in a controlled clinical environment.

On day 4 of the study, study participants received a dose of saline (placebo) intravenously (i.v.). Five days later (day 9 of the study), study participants received a 30 mg dose of methamphetamine i.v.

On days 4 and 9, the study participants were administered a battery of reaction time tests. The tests administered included: Simple Reaction Time – Part 1, the 1- and 2-back tests (measures of working memory and information processing speed), and Simple Reaction Time – Part 2. The measures were selected because of their demonstrated sensitivity to methamphetamine-associated neurotoxicity (Newton et al., 2004b).

Preliminary analyses revealed that age was associated with slower reaction time and reduced accuracy of decision-making on the 1-back test; therefore, it was included as a covariate for the analysis of performance on these tests. None of the other reaction indices were associated with demographic variables, such as age, education, estimated premorbid IQ, or self-reported level of depression, indexed using the Beck Depression Inventory (BDI; Beck, Ward, Mendelson, Mock, & Erbaugh, 1968).

On measures of speed of information processing (Simple Reaction Time; Figure 7.1A), subjects exhibited a trend toward slower response times and demonstrated greater susceptibility to fatigue on the day in which they received methamphetamine ($F(1,11) = 2.58$, $p < .15$, $\eta^2 = .18$). On a relatively difficult decision-making test (2-back; Figure 7.1B), study participants responded more quickly but less accurately ($F(1,11) = 5.57$, $p < .05$, $\eta^2 = .32$). In addition, methamphetamine administration was associated with performance decrements on two indices of decision-making accuracy (Figure 7.1C), the 1-back test ($F(2,10) = 2.52$, $p < .15$, $\eta^2 = .21$) and the 2-back test ($F(1,11) = 3.75$, $p < .10$, $\eta^2 = .24$). It is noteworthy that participants' decision-making accuracy declined even though they had been exposed to the tests four days earlier.

These preliminary data support the validity of some longstanding beliefs regarding the effects of methamphetamine and raised questions about the validity of others. For example, and consistent with what would be expected regarding the effects of methamphetamine, the study participants demonstrated poorer decision-making ability after taking methamphetamine. Unexpectedly, study participants demonstrated slower performance over time on the Simple Reaction Time task. Although most of the statistical comparisons did not reach significance using traditional p values, it is important to note that the findings were in the predicted direction and that the effects sizes, calculated using η^2, were moderate to large.

A review of the literature also revealed that several studies examined the effects of methamphetamine in nondrug-using controls e.g., (Mewaldt & Ghoneim, 1979; Mohs, Tinklenberg, Roth, & Kopell, 1978; Talland & Quarton, 1965; Ward, Kelly, Foltin, & Fischman, 1997). In contrast to the findings from our pilot study, in which methamphetamine exposure was associated with performance decrements on measures of motor/psychomotor speed and accuracy of decision-making, these studies reported that methamphetamine

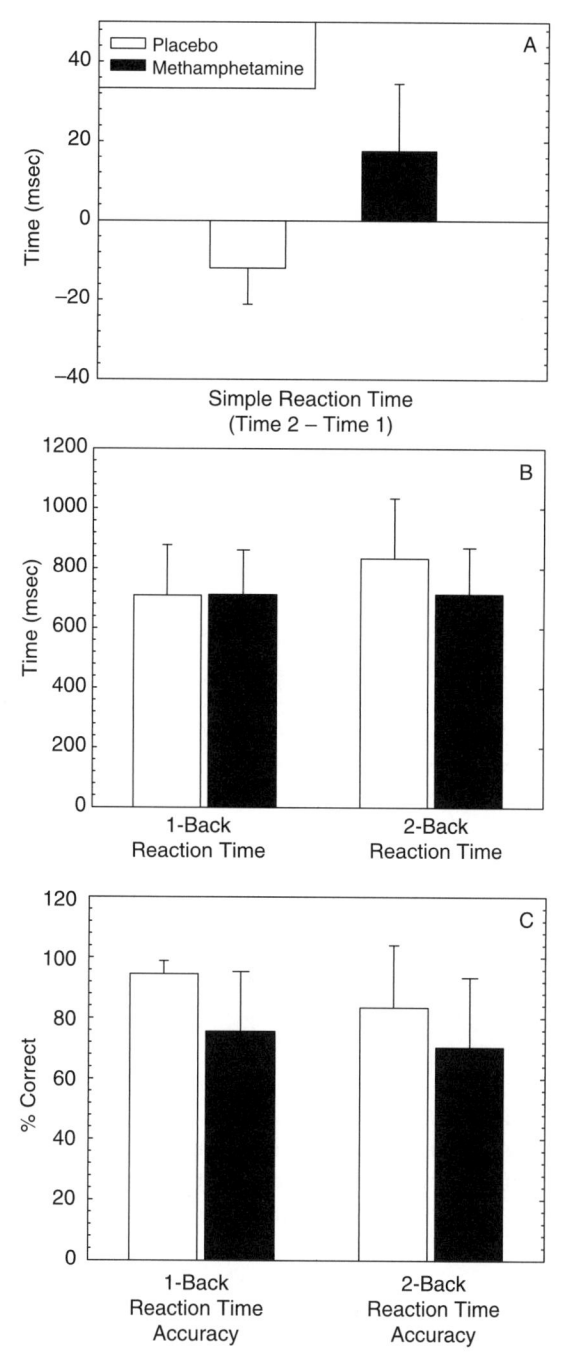

Figure 7.1 Response to acute methamphetamine administration.

administration was associated with enhanced performance on measures of motor/psychomotor speed. This suggests that methamphetamine-associated neurotoxicity/neuroadaptation alters the effects of the drug in chronic users.

Effects of methamphetamine on emotional/psychological profile

This subsection will focus on the presence of mood and psychotic symptoms during intoxication and/or withdrawal. With respect to the former, several articles have sought to characterize onset and resolution of mood symptom following the cessation of use (Newton et al., 2004a; Srisurapanont, Jarusuraisin, & Jittiwutikan, 1999a, 1999b). The work from Srisurapanont and colleagues focused on the development of a questionnaire for assessing withdrawal symptoms based on the criteria listed in DSM-IV (American Psychiatric Association, 1994). They recruited only those patients who were experiencing withdrawal symptoms and did not include threshold criteria for determining the severity of mood-related symptoms; in contrast, the study by Newton et al. (2004a) specifically addressed this point. Presence or absence of withdrawal symptoms was not a factor in determining whether participants would be included in the study. Upon enrollment, 21 participants were hospitalized in the General Clinical Research Center (GCRC). Urine toxicology screens revealed that study participants tested positive for methamphetamine at the time of study entry, did not test positive for other drugs, and remained abstinent during the course of the study. Mood symptoms were assessed using the BDI (Beck et al., 1968).

The results revealed that study participants tended to report mild levels of depressive symptoms on day 1 ($M = 14.5$) and day 2 of the study ($M = 11.4$). On day 3 of the study, the level of depressive symptoms decreased from mild to minimal ($M = 7.3$). The symptoms most frequently reported by the study participants included depressed mood, anhedonia, change in appetite, sleep disturbance, psychomotor agitation or retardation, fatigue, guilt, poor concentration, and thoughts of death. Depressed mood was reported less frequently than anhedonia, lack of energy, irritability, and poor concentration, all symptoms that characterize *apathy*, a syndrome commonly seen in the context of several neuropsychiatric disorders, such as Parkinson's disease or Huntington's disease (Levy et al., 1998).

The data in Figure 7.2 provide additional information regarding the nature of mood symptoms following the cessation of methamphetamine use. These preliminary data suggest that, following cessation of methamphetamine use, individuals will fall roughly into one of three subgroups. In the first subgroup, there are individuals who never experienced clinically significant levels of self-reported mood symptoms. In the second subgroup, there are individuals who initially experienced clinically significant levels of self-reported mood symptoms that resolved by day 3. In the third subgroup, the self-reported level of symptoms did not resolve by day 3. Factors that underlying this variability in response following initiation of methamphetamine

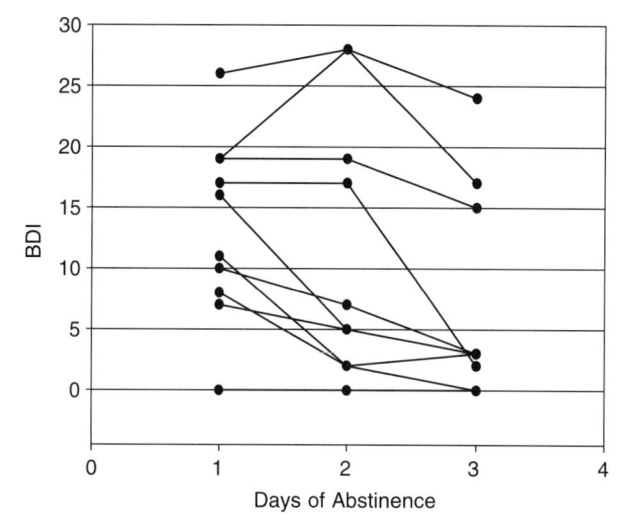

Figure 7.2 Beck Depression Inventory responses over time.

abstinence are unknown, but identification of these factors would clearly facilitate the development of treatments for dependence.

The development of psychosis following methamphetamine exposure was studied extensively during the 1960s and 1970s (Angrist, Sathananthan, Wilk, & Gershon, 1974; Bell, 1965, 1973; Hall, Hando, Darke, & Ross, 1996; Jonsson, Anggard, & Gunne, 1971; Kramer, Fischman, & Littlefield, 1967). These studies revealed that study participants tended to experience paranoid delusions, disordered thoughts, and auditory, visual, or tactile hallucinations following administration of doses that ranged from 15 to 1000 mg/day (Table 7.1). The episodes typically ended within several days of last use, but potentially lasted as long as ten days. Again, factors contributing risk for or protection from the development of psychosis following methamphetamine exposure are unknown.

Residual consequences of methamphetamine dependence

Cognition

In the last ten years, an emerging body of literature has documented the neurocognitive consequences of methamphetamine dependence (Chang et al., 2002; Kalechstein, Newton, & Green, 2003; Monterosso et al., 2005; Newton et al., 2004b; Paulus et al., 2002; Rogers et al., 1999; Thompson et al., 2004; Trites, 1975; Volkow et al., 2001c). These studies, with the exception of Trites, administered batteries that focused on cognitive domains that are mediated by frontal-subcortical functioning, including attention/speed of information processing, learning and memory, and executive system functioning. Each of the studies found that methamphetamine-dependent individuals showed

Table 7.1 Profile of methamphetamine-induced psychosis

Author	Number of study subjects	Methamphetamine indices		Psychotic symptoms						Disordered thoughts	Length of episode
		Dose (mg/day)	Route of intake	Delusions		Hallucinations					
				Paranoid	Grandiose	Somatic	Auditory	Visual			
Kramer et al. (1967)	Review	100–300	i.v.	a	b	b	a	a		a	b
Bell (1965)	7	b	b	7/7	b	b	7/7	4/7		b	7–10 days
Jonnson et al. (1971)	12	b	b	12/12	b	12/12 (not specified)				11/12	0–3 days
Bell (1973)	16	15–1000	i.v.	12/14	b	b	10/14	6/14		Not present	0–6 days
Angrist et al. (1974)	8	b	b	a	a	(Present, types not specified)				a	b
Hall et al. (1996)	301	b	i.v., oral	198/301	b	b	120/301	33/301		b	0–2 hours

a Not quantitated.
b Not reported.

poorer performance on a variety of measures of neurocognition. Some of the papers utilized traditional measures of cognitive function (e.g., Kalechstein et al., 2003; Volkow et al., 2001c). Others used reaction time measures sensitive to speed of information processing and decision-making accuracy that enabled the authors to determine more precisely the neurocognitive functions that were adversely affected as a result of methamphetamine exposure (e.g., Newton et al., 2004b; Salo et al., 2005). Still others utilized novel decision-making tasks that are presumed to assess the intactness of orbitofrontal cortex (Monterosso et al., 2005; Rogers et al., 1999).

The degree to which neurocognition recovers following cessation of use has received limited attention in the extant literature. Because preclinical research has shown that methamphetamine exposure, even relatively small doses, is associated with residual impairment, it is reasonable to hypothesize that neurocognitive deficits will be observed. For example, in a study from our laboratory, we sought to determine the prevalence rates of impairment for particular neurocognitive domains in the first two weeks following cessation of methamphetamine use (Kalechstein et al., 2003). An individual was characterized as impaired if a test score in a particular domain was at or below the 8th percentile in comparison to a relevant normative sample.

As shown in Figure 7.3, methamphetamine-dependent individuals were

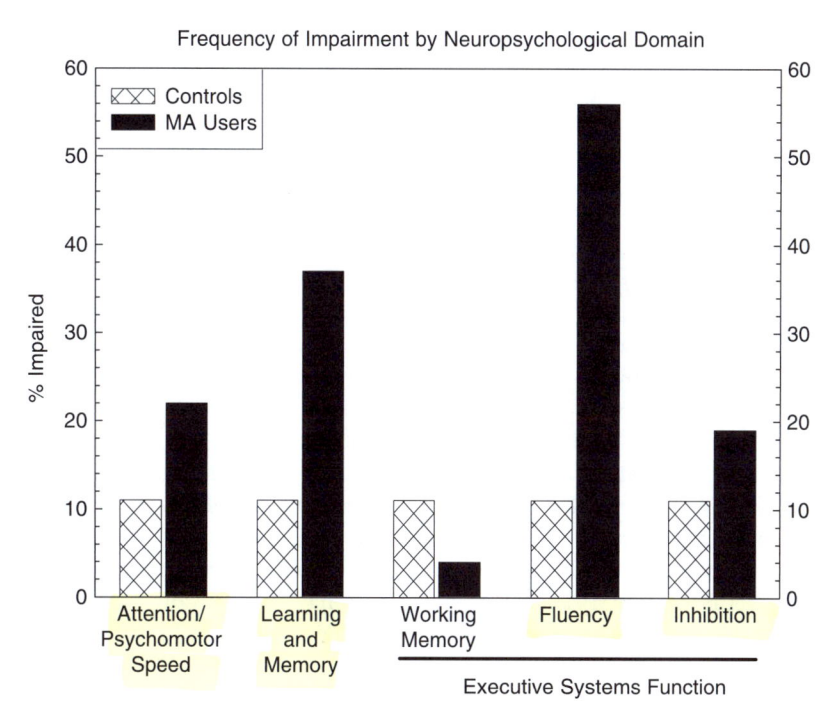

Figure 7.3 Rate of neurocognitive impairment by domain.

much more likely to demonstrate impairment than matched controls, particularly on measures of learning and memory and fluency, an executive function. To our knowledge, this level of impairment has not been observed in users of other stimulants.

At present, two studies from the same group examined the long-term consequences of methamphetamine dependence (Volkow et al., 2001a; Wang et al., 2004). In one study (Volkow et al., 2001a), five methamphetamine-dependent individuals were evaluated within six months of initiating abstinence and then after 12–17 months of abstinence. The data revealed that the neurocognitive impairments did not resolve after at least one year of abstinence. In the follow-up study (Wang et al., 2004), which included the same sample of methamphetamine users and two additional comparison groups, it was suggested that the methamphetamine-associated neurocognitive impairments resolved, at least to some degree. These data, while preliminary, raise the question of whether permanent neurocognitive impairment might occur as a result of chronic methamphetamine exposure.

It is noteworthy that a subset of these studies has linked neurocognitive impairments to neuroimaging and electrophysiological abnormalities during the early phases of abstinence (Chang et al., 2002, 2005; Newton et al., 2004b; Paulus et al., 2002; Volkow et al., 2001c). These studies have consistently shown that methamphetamine-associated neuroimaging abnormalities are linked to neurocognitive impairments. For example, Volkow and colleagues demonstrated that reduced levels of dopamine transporter were associated with poorer performance on measures of psychomotor and episodic memory. Moreover, Paulus et al., using functional MRI (fMRI), found that for methamphetamine addicts frontal lobe activation was reduced when they attempted a decision-making task. Furthermore, Chang and colleagues showed that alterations in cerebral blood flow were associated with poorer performance on a computerized working memory task. Finally, Newton et al. demonstrated that slow-wave abnormalities, indexed using quantitative electroencephalography (QEEG), were associated with slower reaction times and poorer working memory using simple reaction time and n-back tasks (Newton et al., 2004b).

A recent study by Chang and colleagues revealed a more complex association between neuroimaging and neurocognition (Chang et al., 2005). In this study, neurocognitive impairment was observed only in methamphetamine users who had smaller striatal structures, including the globus pallidus and putamen. The authors did not observe the presence of sex by morphometry differences, which was a primary interest of the study. They reported that individuals with larger striatal structures used less methamphetamine. Chang et al. theorized that the striatal structures may have become enlarged to compensate for methamphetamine exposure and the central nervous system injuries that occurred as a result of methamphetamine use.

Emotional/psychological functioning

Within the last five years, researchers have sought to determine if methamphetamine-dependent individuals are prone to experiencing mental health disorders following the cessation of use. For example, a subset of studies have evaluated addicts in inpatient settings (London et al., 2004) or ensured that patients remained abstinent as outpatients using urine analysis to ensure abstinence (Newton et al., 2004a). The study conducted by London and colleagues showed that methamphetamine-dependent individuals experienced minimal levels of symptoms, assessed using the BDI, 4–7 days after the cessation of use. Similarly, Newton et al. showed that methamphetamine-dependent individuals enrolled in an outpatient study whose drug usage was monitored using urine toxicology reported minimal levels of symptoms approximately 12–14 days following cessation of substance use.

As clinicians, we are often asked whether methamphetamine-dependent individuals use methamphetamine as a form of self-medication for the depression and cognitive impairment associated with dependence. The question is based on the presumption that methamphetamine users take the stimulant to self-medicate depressive symptoms, and if the methamphetamine use is discontinued then the addicts will experience the onset of depressive symptoms. The data from the aforementioned studies do not support this contention.

Retrospective and long-term follow-up studies suggest that methamphetamine misuse is actually a risk factor for the onset of depressive symptoms. For example, in a retrospective study that evaluated 1580 forensic detainees, methamphetamine dependence was identified as a risk factor for the onset of depressive symptoms, even after controlling for the demographic profile and use of other drugs (Kalechstein et al., 2000). Furthermore, prospective studies, in which addicts were evaluated following the completion of treatment, suggest that treatment is associated with positive outcomes. For example, for 114 methamphetamine addicts evaluated 2–5 years after treatment, the follow-up status of the sample was much improved as compared to before treatment, though the prevalence of depressive symptoms at the time of the interview was similar to that treatment admission.

To our knowledge, one study has examined the association between mood symptoms (London et al., 2004). In that study, reduced regional cerebral metabolism in frontal-subcortical regions was associated with higher levels of self-reported depressive symptoms in study participants who tended to be minimally depressed. It is possible that the magnitude of the association would increase if the sample included patients who were experiencing mild, moderate, and/or severe levels of self-reported depressive symptoms.

Another subset of studies have focused on identifying neurobiological risk factors of methamphetamine-associated psychosis and other psychiatric symptoms (Iyo, Sekine, & Mori, 2004; Iyo et al., 1993; Sekine et al., 2001, 2002, 2003). Four of the five studies utilized radioligands to demonstrate that striatal dysfunction, particularly reduced levels of dopamine transporter, were associated with the onset of psychosis (Iyo et al., 1993, 2004; Sekine et al., 2002, 2003). A complementary study showed that metabolite alterations in the basal ganglia were associated with increased likelihood of methamphetamine-related psychiatric symptoms (Sekine et al., 2002).

Relapse

To our knowledge, only one study has linked methamphetamine-associated neurobiological changes to relapse. In that study, fMRI and performance on a decision-making task were utilized to predict time to relapse in a sample of 18 methamphetamine-dependent individuals (Paulus, Tapert, & Schuckit, 2005). The authors showed that reduced activation in the dorsolateral prefrontal cortex (including the anterior cingulate) and the temporal cortex was associated with time to relapse.

Summary

Taken together, the available research supports the supposition that methamphetamine has damaging effects on the nervous system. Preclinical studies, neuroimaging studies, emergency room data, autopsy data, and neuropsychological assessments all confirm this. The findings were consistent; very few studies, to our knowledge, reported negative findings.

The literature on the neurotoxic effects of methamphetamine can serve as a foundation for future studies. One subset of studies might focus on elucidating the chronicity of the neurotoxic effects of methamphetamine. While animal models of methamphetamine exposure revealed that the neurotoxicity was present even three years after the cessation of administration, the degree to which this has been assessed in humans has been evaluated in studies of only a few subjects. It is likely that this issue will be addressed over the next several years.

It is worth pointing out that chronic methamphetamine exposure is a *risk factor* for neuropsychological impairment; however, not all users become impaired. Further research is needed to elucidate risk factors for impairment. Likely candidates include increased age, limited education, duration of use and amount used, and possibly patterns of use. There may be genetic or other personal factors as well.

The mechanisms that underlie methamphetamine-associated neuropsychological impairment represent a burgeoning area of research. Based on the results of studies using rodents and primates, recent studies have demonstrated a linkage between alterations in presynaptic dopaminergic function and neurocognition. Future studies might attempt to refine these initial findings and determine the specific elements of presynaptic dopamine function that are affected as a result of chronic methamphetamine exposure. Others might utilize animal models of methamphetamine-associated neurotoxicity to determine whether alterations in the function of other monoamines contribute to neurocognitive impairment.

Another question that has yet to be addressed is the relationship between neurocognition and functional outcomes. The recent publication by Paulus and colleagues highlights the innovative manner in which neuroimaging can be used to assist treatment providers in identifying those individuals who are at risk of relapse (Paulus et al., 2005). One limitation of neuroimaging is the cost associated with study and the availability of fMRI laboratories. A more feasible and cost-effective approach would be to identify neurocognitive tests that are associated with brain abnormalities, as defined by fMRI, *and* time to relapse. For example, it is much easier to obtain access to neuropsychological testing than fMRI. Furthermore, the cost of neuropsychological assessment is likely to be less than the cost of conducting an fMRI.

It is likely that the severity of the neurocognitive impairment observed in this sample is associated with other functional outcomes, including poorer vocational functioning and possibly increased risk for relapse to dependence. Although the association between neurocognition and functional outcomes has not been examined in methamphetamine-dependent individuals, it has been documented in other disorders (Green, 1998; Kalechstein, Newton, & van Gorp, 2003) and other drugs (e.g., Aharonovich, Nunes, & Hasin, 2003). Neurocognitive impairment may undermine the effectiveness of psychosocial treatments for methamphetamine dependence as well, suggesting an important area of study.

Given that methamphetamine dependence is a risk factor for neurocognitive impairment, it would seem reasonable to utilize these measures as markers of neurotoxicity. If neurocognitive measures are sensitive to the neurotoxic effects of methamphetamine, then it is also reasonable to consider that these measures are sensitive to the effects of medications aimed at reversing the neurotoxic effects. As previously noted, because impaired neurocognitive functioning is associated with poorer functional outcomes (e.g., employment status, treatment outcome), reversal of these impairments could enhance the quality of treatments for methamphetamine dependence. While this issue has not been the subject of peer review publications, our laboratory is presently investigating this topic. We expect that the data generated from this study will eventually provide valuable insights into the neurobiological mechanisms that underlie methamphetamine-associated neurocognitive impairments and that the findings from these studies can be rapidly and practically integrated into current treatment models.

As previously reported, methamphetamine is the second most frequently used drug based on worldwide epidemiological studies. This finding is particularly problematic because, not only is methamphetamine misuse associated with a variety of public health issues, but misuse of the drug is a risk factor for the onset of brain damage. The limited numbers of studies that have been published on methamphetamine-associated neurotoxicity consistently report the presence of changes in brain structure and function. Based on these findings, it is hoped that future studies will focus on identifying risk factors for the onset of methamphetamine-associated neuropsychological impairment and developing treatments aimed at reversing and/or circumventing these impairments.

References

Aharonovich, E., Nunes, E., & Hasin, D. (2003). Cognitive impairment, retention and abstinence among cocaine abusers in cognitive-behavioral treatment. *Drug and Alcohol Dependence, 71*, 207–211.

American Psychiatric Association (1994). *Diagnostic and Statistical Manual* (4th ed., DSM-IV). Washington, DC: American Psychiatric Association.

Anglin, M., Burke, C., Perrochet, B., Stamper, E., & Dawud-Noursi, S. (2000). History of the methamphetamine problem. *Journal of Psychoactive Drugs, 32*, 137–141.

Anglin, M., Kalechstein, A. D., Maglione, M. M., Annon, J., & Fiorentine, R. (1997). *Epidemiology and treatment of methamphetamine abuse in California: A regional report*. Prepared for Center for Substance Abuse Treatment and the Robert Wood Johnson Substance Abuse Policy Research.

Angrist, B., Sathananthan, G., Wilk, S., & Gershon, S. (1974). Amphetamine psychosis: behavioral and biochemical aspects. *Journal of Psychiatric Research, 11*, 13–23.

Beck, A. T., Ward, C. H., Mendelson, J., Mock, J., & Erbaugh, J. (1968). The Beck Depression Inventory. *Archives of General Psychiatry, 4*, 561–571.

Bell, D. S. (1965). Comparison of amphetamine psychosis and schizophrenia. *British Journal of Psychiatry, 111*, 701–707.

Bell, D. S. (1973). The experimental reproduction of amphetamine psychosis. *Archives of General Psychiatry, 29*, 35–40.

Castner, S. A., Al-Tikriti, M. S., Baldwin, R. M., Seibyl, J. P., Innis, R. B., & Goldman-Rakic, P. S. (2000). Behavioral changes and [^{123}I]IBZM equilibrium SPECT measurement of amphetamine-induced dopamine release in rhesus monkeys exposed to subchronic amphetamine. *Neuropsychopharmacology, 22*, 4–13.

Castner, S. A., & Goldman, P. S. (1999). *Profound cognitive impairments in nonhuman primates exposed to amphetamine*. Paper presented at the Society for Neuroscience, New Orleans, LA.

Castner, S. A., & Goldman-Rakic, P. S. (1999). Long-lasting psychotomimetic consequences of repeated low-dose amphetamine exposure in rhesus monkeys. *Neuropsychopharmacology, 20*, 10–28.

Chang, L., Cloak, C., Patterson, K., Grob, C., Miller, E. N., & Ernst, T. (2005). Enlarged striatum in abstinent methamphetamine abusers: a possible compensatory response. *Biological Psychiatry, 57*, 967–974.

Chang, L., Ernst, T., Speck, O., Patel, H., DeSilva, M., Leonido-Yee, M., et al. (2002). Perfusion MRI and computerized cognitive test abnormalities in abstinent methamphetamine users. *Psychiatry Research, 114*, 65–79.

Ernst, T., Chang, L., Leonido-Yee, M., & Speck, O. (2000). Evidence for long-term neurotoxicity associated with methamphetamine abuse: A ^{1}H MRS study. *Neurology, 54*, 1344–1349.

Green, M. F. (1998). *Schizophrenia from a neurocognitive perspective: Probing the impenetrable darkness*. Needham Heights, MA: Allyn & Bacon.

Hall, W., Hando, J., Darke, S., & Ross, J. (1996). Psychological morbidity and route of administration among amphetamine users in Sydney, Australia. *Addiction, 91*, 81–87.

He, S. Y., Matoba, R., Fujitani, N., Sodesaki, K., & Onishi, S. (1996). Cardiac muscle lesions associated with chronic administration of methamphetamine in rats. *American Journal of Forensic Medical Pathology, 17*, 155–162.

Hong, R., Matsuyama, E., & Nur, K. (1991). Cardiomyopathy associated with the smoking of crystal methamphetamine. *Journal of the American Medical Association, 265*, 1152–1154.

Iyo, M., Nishio, M., Itoh, T., Fukuda, H., Suzuki, K., Yamasaki, T., et al. (1993). Dopamine D2 and serotonin S2 receptors in susceptibility to methamphetamine psychosis detected by positron emission tomography. *Psychiatry Research, 50*, 217–231.

Iyo, M., Sekine, Y., & Mori, N. (2004). Neuromechanism of developing methamphetamine psychosis: a neuroimaging study. *Annals of the New York Academy of Sciences, 1025*, 288–295.

Jonsson, L. E., Anggard, E., & Gunne, L. M. (1971). Blockade of intravenous amphetamine euphoria in man. *Clinical Pharmacology and Therapeutics, 12*, 889–896.

Kalechstein, A. D., Newton, T. F., & Green, M. (2003). Methamphetamine dependence is associated with neurocognitive impairment in the initial phases of abstinence. *Journal of Neuropsychiatry and Clinical Neuroscience, 15*, 215–220.

Kalechstein, A. D., Newton, T. F., Longshore, D., Anglin, M. D., van Gorp, W. G., & Gawin, F. H. (2000). Psychiatric comorbidity of methamphetamine dependence in a forensic sample. *Journal of Neuropsychiatry and Clinical Neuroscience, 12*, 480–484.

Kalechstein, A. D., Newton, T. F., & van Gorp, W. G. (2003). A meta-analytic review of the association between neuropsychological profile and vocational outcomes. *Journal of Clinical and Experimental Neuropsychology, 25*, 1186–1191.

Karch, S. B., Stephens, B. G., & Ho, C. H. (1999). Methamphetamine-related deaths in San Francisco: demographic, pathologic, and toxicologic profiles. *Journal of Forensic Science, 44*, 359–368.

Kramer, J. C., Fischman, V. S., & Littlefield, D. C. (1967). Amphetamine abuse. Pattern and effects of high doses taken intravenously. *Journal of the American Medical Association, 201*, 305–309.

Levy, M. L., Cummings, J. L., Fairbanks, L. A., Masterman, D., Miller, B. L., Craig, A. H., et al. (1998). Apathy is not depression. *Journal of Neuropsychiatry and Clinical Neuroscience, 10*, 314–319.

London, E. D., Simon, S. L., Berman, S. M., Mandelkern, M. A., Lichtman, A. M., Bramen, J., et al. (2004). Mood disturbances and regional cerebral metabolic abnormalities in recently abstinent methamphetamine abusers. *Archives of General Psychiatry, 61*, 73–84.

McCann, U. D., Wong, D. F., Yokoi, F., Villemagne, V., Dannals, R. F., & Ricaurte, G. A. (1998). Reduced striatal dopamine transporter density in abstinent methamphetamine and methcathinone users: Evidence from positron emission tomography studies with [^{11}C]WIN-35,428. *Journal of Neuroscience, 18*, 8417–8422.

Melega, W. P., Quintana, J., Raleigh, M. J., Stout, D. B., Yu, D. C., Lin, K. P., et al. (1996). 6-[^{18}F]fluoro-L-DOPA-PET studies show partial reversibility of long-term effects of chronic amphetamine in monkeys. *Synapse, 22*, 63–69.

Mewaldt, S. P., & Ghoneim, M. M. (1979). The effects and interactions of scopolamine, physostigmine and methamphetamine on human memory. *Pharmacology, Biochemistry and Behavior, 10,* 205–210.

Mohs, R. C., Tinklenberg, J. R., Roth, W. T., & Kopell, B. S. (1978). Methamphetamine and diphenhydramine effects on the rate of cognitive processing. *Psychopharmacology (Berlin), 59,* 13–19.

Monterosso, J. R., Aron, A. R., Cordova, X., Xu, J., & London, E. D. (2005). Deficits in response inhibition associated with chronic methamphetamine abuse. *Drug and Alcohol Dependence, 79,* 273–277.

Newton, T. F., Cook, I. A., Kalechstein, A. D., Duran, S. D., Monroy, F., Ling, W., & Leuchter, A. F. (2003). Quantitative EEG abnormalities in recently abstinent methamphetamine dependent individuals. *Clinical Neurophysiology, 114,* 410–415.

Newton, T. F., Kalechstein, A. D., Duran, S., Vansluis, N., & Ling, W. (2004a). Methamphetamine abstinence syndrome: Preliminary findings. *American Journal of Addiction, 13,* 248–255.

Newton, T. F., Kalechstein, A. D., Hardy, D. J., Cook, I. A., Nestor, L., Ling, W., et al. (2004b). Association between quantitative EEG and neurocognition in methamphetamine-dependent volunteers. *Clinical Neurophysiology, 115,* 194–198.

Nordahl, T. E., Salo, R., Natsuaki, Y., Galloway, G. P., Waters, C., Moore, C. D., et al. (2005). Methamphetamine users in sustained abstinence: A proton magnetic resonance spectroscopy study. *Archives of General Psychiatry, 62,* 444–452.

Ohta, K., Mori, M., Yoritaka, A., Okamoto, K., & Kishida, S. (2005). Delayed ischemic stroke associated with methamphetamine use. *Journal of Emergency Medicine, 28,* 165–167.

Paulus, M. P., Hozack, N. E., Zauscher, B. E., Frank, L., Brown, G. G., Braff, D. L., et al. (2002). Behavioral and functional neuroimaging evidence for prefrontal dysfunction in methamphetamine-dependent subjects. *Neuropsychopharmacology, 26,* 53–63.

Paulus, M. P., Tapert, S. F., & Schuckit, M. A. (2005). Neural activation patterns of methamphetamine-dependent subjects during decision making predict relapse. *Archives of General Psychiatry, 62,* 761–768.

Perez, J. A., Jr., Arsura, E. L., & Strategos, S. (1999). Methamphetamine-related stroke: four cases. *Journal of Emergency Medicine, 17,* 469–471.

Ricaurte, G. A., Schuster, C. R., & Seiden, L. S. (1980). Long-term effects of repeated methylamphetamine administration on dopamine and serotonin neurons in the rat brain: a regional study. *Brain Research, 193,* 153–163.

Rogers, R. D., Everitt, B. J., Baldacchino, A., Blackshaw, A. J., Swainson, R., Wynne, K., et al. (1999). Dissociable deficits in the decision-making cognition of chronic amphetamine abusers, opiate abusers, patients with focal damage to prefrontal cortex, and tryptophan-depleted normal volunteers: Evidence for monoaminergic mechanisms. *Neuropsychopharmacology, 20,* 322–339.

Rothrock, J. F., Rubenstein, R., & Lyden, P. D. (1988). Ischemic stroke associated with methamphetamine inhalation. *Neurology, 38,* 589–592.

Sachdeva, K., & Woodward, K. G. (1989). Caudal thalamic infarction following intranasal methamphetamine use. *Neurology, 39,* 305–306.

Salo, R., Nordahl, T. E., Moore, C., Waters, C., Natsuaki, Y., Galloway, G. P., et al. (2005). A dissociation in attentional control: evidence from methamphetamine dependence. *Biological Psychiatry, 57,* 310–313.

Seiden, L. S., Fischman, M. W., & Schuster, C. R. (1976). Long-term methamphetamine induced changes in brain catecholamines in tolerant rhesus monkeys. *Drug and Alcohol Dependence, 1*, 215–219.

Seiden, L. S., Fischman, M. W., & Schuster, C. R. (1977). Changes in brain catecholamines induced by long-term methamphetamine administration in rhesus monkeys. In E. H. Ellinwood, Jr., & M. M. Kilbey (Eds.), *Cocaine and other stimulants* (pp. 179–185). New York: Plenum Press.

Sekine, Y., Iyo, M., Ouchi, Y., Matsunaga, T., Tsukada, H., Okada, H., et al. (2001). Methamphetamine-related psychiatric symptoms and reduced brain dopamine transporters studied with PET. *American Journal of Psychiatry, 158*, 1206–1214.

Sekine, Y., Minabe, Y., Kawai, M., Suzuki, K., Iyo, M., Isoda, H., et al. (2002). Metabolite alterations in basal ganglia associated with methamphetamine-related psychiatric symptoms. A proton MRS study. *Neuropsychopharmacology, 27*, 453–461.

Sekine, Y., Minabe, Y., Ouchi, Y., Takei, N., Iyo, M., Nakamura, K., et al. (2003). Association of dopamine transporter loss in the orbitofrontal and dorsolateral prefrontal cortices with methamphetamine-related psychiatric symptoms. *American Journal of Psychiatry, 160*, 1699–1701.

Siegal, D., Erickson, J., Varoqui, H., Ang, L., Kalasinsky, K. S., Peretti, F. J., et al. (2004). Brain vesicular acetylcholine transporter in human users of drugs of abuse. *Synapse, 52*, 223–232.

Srisurapanont, M., Jarusuraisin, N., & Jittiwutikan, J. (1999a). Amphetamine withdrawal: I. Reliability, validity and factor structure of a measure. *Australian and New Zealand Journal of Psychiatry, 33*, 89–93.

Srisurapanont, M., Jarusuraisin, N., & Jittiwutikan, J. (1999b). Amphetamine withdrawal: II. A placebo-controlled, randomised, double-blind study of amineptine treatment. *Australian and New Zealand Journal of Psychiatry, 33*, 94–98.

Talland, G. A., & Quarton, G. C. (1965). Methamphetamine and pentobarbital effects on human motor performance. *Psychopharmacologia, 8*, 241–250.

Thompson, P. M., Hayashi, K. M., Simon, S. L., Geaga, J. A., Hong, M. S., Sui, Y., et al. (2004). Structural abnormalities in the brains of human subjects who use methamphetamine. *Journal of Neuroscience, 24*, 6028–6036.

Trites, R. (1975). Neuropsychological deficits in "primary" and "secondary" non-medical drug users. *Canadian Psychiatric Association Journal, 20*, 351–357.

Villemagne, V., Yuan, J., Wong, D. F., Dannals, R. F., Hatzidimitriou, G., Mathews, W. B., et al. (1998). Brain dopamine neurotoxicity in baboons treated with doses of methamphetamine comparable to those recreationally abused by humans: evidence from [^{11}C]WIN-35,428 positron emission tomography studies and direct in vitro determinations. *Journal of Neuroscience, 18*, 419–427.

Volkow, N. D., Chang, L., Wang, G. J., Fowler, J. S., Franceschi, D., Sedler, M., et al. (2001a). Loss of dopamine transporters in methamphetamine abusers recovers with protracted abstinence. *Journal of Neuroscience, 21*, 9414–9418.

Volkow, N. D., Chang, L., Wang, G. J., Fowler, J. S., Franceschi, D., Sedler, M. J., et al. (2001b). Higher cortical and lower subcortical metabolism in detoxified methamphetamine abusers. *American Journal of Psychiatry, 158*, 383–389.

Volkow, N. D., Chang, L., Wang, G. J., Fowler, J. S., Leonido-Yee, M., Franceschi, D., et al. (2001c). Association of dopamine transporter reduction with psychomotor impairment in methamphetamine abusers. *American Journal of Psychiatry, 158*, 377–382.

Wang, G. J., Volkow, N. D., Chang, L., Miller, E., Sedler, M., Hitzemann, R., et al. (2004). Partial recovery of brain metabolism in methamphetamine abusers after protracted abstinence. *American Journal of Psychiatry, 161*, 242–248.

Ward, A. S., Kelly, T. H., Foltin, R. W., & Fischman, M. W. (1997). Effects of d-amphetamine on task performance and social behavior of humans in a residential laboratory. *Experimental and Clinical Psychopharmacology, 5*, 130–136.

Wijetunga, M., Seto, T., Lindsay, J., & Schatz, I. (2003). Crystal methamphetamine-associated cardiomyopathy: tip of the iceberg? *Journal of Toxicology and Clinical Toxicology, 41*, 981–986.

Wilson, J. M., Kalasinsky, K. S., Levey, A. I., Bergeron, C., Reiber, G., Anthony, R. M., et al. (1996). Striatal dopamine nerve terminal markers in human, chronic methamphetamine users. *Nature Medicine, 2*, 699–703.

Woolverton, W. L., Ricaurte, G. A., Forno, L. S., & Seiden, L. S. (1989). Long-term effects of chronic methamphetamine administration in rhesus monkeys. *Brain Research, 486*, 73–78.

Yen, D. J., Wang, S. J., Ju, T. H., Chen, C. C., Liao, K. K., Fuh, J. L., et al. (1994). Stroke associated with methamphetamine inhalation. *European Neurology, 34*, 16–22.

8 Nicotine

Heather G. Belanger, Vani Simmons, and John Schinka

The 2000 United States National Household Survey on Drug Abuse estimated that 65.5 million Americans use a tobacco product, a figure which represents a 29.3% prevalence rate for the population inclusive of persons aged 12 and older (Substance Abuse and Mental Health Services Administration, 2001). Though there are more than 2000 compounds in cigarette smoke, nicotine alone has been shown to produce tolerance, dependence, and withdrawal symptoms in both animals and humans (Henningfield, Miyasato, & Jasinski, 1985). Lifetime prevalence of nicotine dependence, as defined by DSM-III-R criteria, is estimated at 24%, with dependence leading to increased risk of smoking persistence with an odds ratio of 2.2 (Breslau, Johnson, Hiripi, & Kessler, 2001).

Multiple factors appear to underlie the onset of smoking behavior. Recent reviews of this literature have concluded that genetic and environmental factors contribute equally to the risk of becoming a smoker (Hughes, 1986; Sullivan & Kendler, 1999). A recent meta-analysis (Li, Cheng, Ma, & Swan, 2003) of studies investigating heritability of smoking initiation and smoking persistence found that genetic factors play a more significant role for females in smoking initiation, whereas genetic influences play a more significant role for males in smoking persistence.

Smoking behavior is associated with a variety of comorbid disorders, including heavy drinking (Jensen et al., 2003), attention deficit/hyperactivity disorder (ADHD; Riggs, Mikulich, Whitmore, & Crowley, 1999), and other psychiatric disorders (Breslau, Davis, & Schultz, 2003; De Leon, Becona, Gurpegui, Gonzalez-Pinto, & Diaz, 2002; Isensee, Wittchen, Stein, Hofler, & Lieb, 2003; Upadhyaya, Brady, Wharton, & Liao, 2003). Other studies have consistently found an association between smoking and depression (e.g., Breslau, Peterson, Schultz, Chilcoat, & Andreski, 1998; Brown, Lewinsohn, Seeley, & Wagner, 1996; Kandel et al., 1997; van Gool, Kempen, Penninx, Deeg, Beekman, & van Eijk, 2003). The direction of the relationship between smoking and depression is unclear. Higher rates of smoking and major depression in the co-twins of monozygotic probands relative to dizygotic probands suggest that genetic factors may predispose individuals to both conditions (Kendler, Neale, MacLean, Heath, Eaves, & Kessler, 1993), though this may vary somewhat depending on depressive subtype and amount smoked (Dierker, Avenevoli, Stolar, & Merikangas, 2002).

To date, multiple review articles have summarized the results of studies pertaining to the effects of nicotine on cognitive performance (Cook, Gerkovich, Graham, Hoffman, & Peterson, 2003; Heishman, 1999; Heishman, Taylor, & Henningfield, 1994; Kassel, 1997; Newhouse, Potter, & Singh, 2004; Sherwood, 1993; US Department of Health and Human Services, 1988; Warburton, 1992). This chapter will extend the findings from these reviews and provide an overarching summary of the effects of nicotine on the brain, with an emphasis on: (1) the manner in which nicotine influences performance on neuropsychological and cognitive measures; (2) pharmacological, metabolic and structural changes associated with nicotine use; and (3) the factors that mediate or moderate these effects. The focus will be on cognitive effects of direct nicotine administration rather than on withdrawal effects. Finally, the application of these findings toward treating various neurological disorders will be discussed.

Effects of nicotine on cognition

Research suggests that nicotine can have both acute and chronic effects on cognition. Acute effects have been studied across a variety of cognitive domains, including attention/information processing speed, psychomotor functioning, executive functioning, and learning and memory. The most studied domains are attention and speed of processing. To the extent that nicotine impacts attention and processing speed, other domains are in turn likely to be affected, as most other domains require attention and/or speed. Emphasis in research on chronic effects has focused on individual differences, with less work done on individual cognitive domains. Methodological variation likely accounts for disparate findings and will be discussed in detail.

Acute effects

There is convincing evidence that nicotine improves performance on tasks of memory (Hale, Gentry, & Meliska, 1999; Krebs, Petros, & Beckwith, 1994; Rusted & Eaton-Williams, 1991), attention (Baker and Walsh, 1996; Kassel 1997; Landers, Crews, Boutcher, Skinner, & Gustafsen, 1992), executive function (Hasenfratz & Battig, 1992; Landers et al., 1992), processing speed (Edwards, Wesnes, Warbuton, & Gale, 1985; Wesnes & Warburton, 1984), and motor performance (Perkins et al., 1994, 1995; Sherwood, 1993, 1995); however, some studies did not find a facilitative effect (Dunne, MacDonald, & Hartley, 1986; Sakurai & Kanazawa, 2002). These conflicting findings are likely due in part to methodological difficulties and variation in procedural approach. One especially complicating factor may be the short-acting effect of nicotine. Sakurai and Kanazawa (2002), for example, found that blood levels of nicotine, after smoking two cigarettes, reduce to presmoking levels in only about 10 minutes. Other methodological issues of importance include the route of administration (i.e., smoking, nasal spray, or injection), the degree to which smokers are deprived prior to the study (and consequently may be experiencing withdrawal and, therefore, withdrawal relief during the experiment), varying amounts of nicotine in different brands of cigarettes, amount smoked prior to the experiment, whether a placebo control condition was included, and whether or not blood tests were used to determine nicotine blood levels. Furthermore, many of the studies that examined the cognitive effects of nicotine did not specifically address the extent to which effects are acute versus chronic. Many comparisons are made, for instance, using between-subject research designs (smokers versus nonsmokers) rather than utilizing a within-subject repeated measures approach (before smoking versus after smoking).

Withdrawal relief may account for some or all of the positive effects of nicotine on mood, arousal, and cognition. As nicotine withdrawal occurs rapidly and can be associated with effects on mood, arousal, and cognition, these experiments are necessarily confounded. Many studies utilize smokers who have been through a withdrawal period prior to the experiment (typically overnight); as a result, the effects of withdrawal confound the study and render it impossible to determine the unique, facilitative effects of nicotine (Heishman, Taylor, & Henningfield 1994).

While any review of this literature will suggest some positive effects of nicotine independent of withdrawal effects (e.g., Foulds, Stapleton, Swettenham, Bell, McSorley, & Russell, 1996; Mancuso, Warburton, Melen, Sherwood, & Tirelli, 1999; Warburton & Arnall, 1994; Wesnes & Warburton, 1984), it is unclear to what extent chronic smokers may develop tolerance to these withdrawal effects over time. In smokers, nicotine deprivation can lead to loss of cognitive performance, which can be reversed with nicotine administration (Bell, Taylor, Singleton, Henningfield, & Heishman, 1999; Parrott & Roberts, 1991; Snyder & Henningfield, 1989; Snyder, Davis, & Henningfield, 1989). Obviously, this reversal of cognitive deficit may facilitate dependence; however, most studies deprive participants for 24 hours or less. Cook et al. (2003) deprived their participants for 24–48 hours and found no facilitative effect of nicotine. While using nonsmokers may help to elucidate the cognitive effects of nicotine independent of withdrawal effects, nonsmokers often suffer side effects that make dose-related studies in particular quite difficult.

Nicotine also may exert an indirect effect on cognition by means of influence on arousal and mood (Waters & Sutton, 2000), both of which have been shown to affect cognitive and motor performance (Ashby, Isen, & Turken, 1999; Cahill & McGaugh, 1995; Noteboom, Fleshner, & Enoka, 2001; Robbins, 1997). Moreover, nicotine has a dose-related, stimulant-type effect on mood (Perkins et al., 1994; Pomerleau & Pomerleau, 1987; Pomerleau, Teuscher, Goeters, & Pomerleau, 1994; but see File, Dinnis, Heard, & Irvine, 2002; Heishman & Henningfield, 2000; Knott, Bosman, Mahoney, Ilivitsky, & Quirt, 1999; Newhouse et al., 1990). Nicotine also increases self-perceived vigor (Levin et al., 1998; Parrott, 1993; Stein et al., 1998), as well as electroencephalogram (EEG) and self-ratings of alertness (Griesar, Zajdel, & Oken, 2000). Furthermore, some experimental studies have demonstrated that nicotine reduces stress or anxiety and increases arousal (Kassel & Shiffman, 1997; Perkins, Grobe, Epstein, Caggiula, & Stiller, 1992; Pomerleau & Pomerleau, 1987; Pomerleau, Turk, & Fertig, 1984), though this is controversial (e.g., Fleming & Lombardo, 1987; Foulds, Stapleton, Swettenham, Jarvis, & Russell, 1997; Heishman & Henningfield, 2000; Herbert, Foulds, & Fife-Schaw, 2001; Meliska & Gilbert, 1991; Pomerleau & Pomerleau, 1991). Conversely, abstinence from nicotine in smokers leads to greater perceived stress, lower perceived arousal, and less pleasure (Parrott & Kaye, 1999). Stein et al. (1998) demonstrated the activation of brain areas associated with mood elevation and arousal after intravenous injection of nicotine in a functional magnetic resonance imaging (fMRI) study of smokers.

Attention/speed of processing findings

Nicotine generally enhances speed of processing/reaction time/psychomotor speed (Ernst, Heishman, Spurgeon, & London, 2001a; Kerr, Sherwood, & Hindmarch, 1991; Knott et al., 1999; Mancuso et al., 1999; Pritchard, Robinson, & Guy, 1992; Snyder & Henningfield, 1989; Warburton, Skinner, & Martin, 2001). Nicotine decreases decision time in deprived smokers (Bates, Mangan, Stough, & Corballis, 1995; Pineda, Herrera, Kang, & Sandler, 1998) and decreases reaction time in visual and auditory odd-ball tasks in 12-hour deprived smokers (Houlihan, Pritchard, & Robinson, 1996). Hindmarch, Kerr, and Sherwood (1990) found no effect of nicotine gum on choice reaction time in nonsmokers but a facilitative effect in nonabstinent smokers.

In nonsmokers, nicotine administration was associated with a reduced number of omission errors on the Continuous Performance Test (CPT), a neuropsychological measure frequently used to identify individuals with ADHD. In one study (Levin et al., 1998), low-dose transdermal nicotine was used (7 mg/day) and the reported effect on omission errors was not simply due to increased response rate. A reduction in hit reaction time variance was also noted. Nicotine did not significantly reduce commission errors. Other studies have similarly reported positive effects on tests of vigilance (Pritchard et al., 1992; Wesnes, Warburton, & Matz, 1983).

On the rapid visual information processing test, another test of vigilance or sustained attention, reaction time improved in terms of detecting three consecutive odd or even numbers in a series of numbers in abstinent smokers (Baldinger, Hasenfratz, & Battig, 1995; Edwards et al., 1985; Foulds et al., 1996; Gilbert, Estes, & Welser, 1997; Lawrence, Ross, & Stein, 2002; Parrott & Craig, 1992; Parrott & Winder, 1989; Wesnes & Warburton, 1983) but not in nonsmokers (Jones, Sahakian, Levy, Warburton, & Gray, 1992; Wesnes & Revell, 1984; Wesnes & Warburton, 1984; but see Foulds et al., 1996). Furthermore, improved performance, operationally defined as faster reaction time, was mediated by dose (Parrott & Winder, 1989) and was not confounded by a greater number of errors (Wesnes & Warburton, 1984). On a letter-searching task, nicotine facilitated performance (Parrott & Craig, 1992) and both cigarette and nicotine gum administration returned deprived smokers' performance to pre-deprivation levels (Bell et al., 1999; Snyder & Henningfield, 1989; but see Spilich, June, & Renner, 1992). In nonsmokers, however, nicotine has been shown to have either no effect or deleterious effects on measures such as letter searching time and accuracy (Heishman & Henningfield, 2000; Heishman, Snyder, & Henningfield, 1993; Provost & Woodward, 1991). Nicotine enhances performance on orienting of attention in space (Murphy & Klein, 1998; Witte, Davidson, & Marrocco, 1997), with the nicotine metabolite cotinine predicting this effect during abstinence. This effect has not been demonstrated in nonsmokers (Griesar et al., 2000). Finally, nicotine facilitates performance on measures requiring focused attention, or the ability to ignore distraction (Herning & Pickworth, 1985; Knott, 1986).

Psychomotor findings

Nicotine administration is generally associated with improved psychomotor functioning. For example, finger tapping performance improved following nicotine administration in nonsmokers and in smokers deprived of nicotine overnight (Jones et al., 1992; Perkins, Epstein, Stiller, Sexton, Debski, & Jacob, 1990; Perkins et al., 1994, 1995; West & Jarvis, 1986); in contrast, Foulds et al. (1996) did not observe this effect in nonsmokers. Furthermore, on a measure of gross hand–eye coordination, the circular lights test, Heishman and Henningfield (2000) found impaired performance with varying doses of nicotine administered via nicotine gum to nonsmokers.

Ecologically valid studies provided mixed results. For instance, Sherwood (1995) found decreased braking time and improved tracking in nondeprived smokers after smoking in a simulated driving test. On the other hand, Spilich et al. (1992) reported more rear-end collisions in smokers who had just smoked relative to nonsmokers when participants were asked to drive as long as possible without accident.

Executive function findings

While nicotine generally facilitates attention and speed, performance on measures of more complex executive functions is not generally mediated by nicotine administration. For example, on tasks requiring shifting of attention (e.g., the Flexibility of Attention Test), nicotine did not influence speed of information processing in deprived smokers (Mancuso et al., 1999; Sherwood, Kerr, & Hindmarch, 1992) or in nonabstinent smokers and nonsmokers (Hindmarch et al., 1990; Kerr et al., 1991). Nicotine administration also did not affect the accuracy of responses in these speed-of-processing tasks

(Ernst et al., 2001a; Le Houezec, Halliday, Benowitz, Callaway, Naylor, & Herzig, 1994; Mancuso et al., 1999; Snyder & Henningfield, 1989) unless the task required divided attention (Hindmarch et al., 1990; Kerr et al., 1991; Sherwood et al., 1992). In those studies, fewer errors were observed. Finally, nicotine administration did not facilitate problem-solving (Dunne et al., 1986), logical reasoning, or arithmetic (Ernst et al., 2001a; Foulds et al., 1996; Heishman & Henningfield, 2000; Heishman, Snyder, & Henningfield, 1993).

A commonly used measure of executive ability is the Stroop test. A frequent variant of the Stroop test involves naming color words (called the color condition) and then being asked to name the ink color of color words while ignoring the word itself (called the incongruent condition). The Stroop effect, a measure of interference, is the difference in total speed in the color condition relative to the incongruent condition. Results of nicotine administration on the Stroop performance have been mixed, with studies showing no positive effects on either the color condition or the Stroop effect (Foulds et al., 1996; Kos, Hasenfratz, & Battig, 1997; Levin et al., 1996; Parrot & Craig, 1992; Sutter, Buzzi, Woodson, & Battig, 1983; Wesnes & Revell, 1984), faster color naming but no effect or an adverse effect on the interference condition (Cook et al., 2003; Landers et al., 1992; Mancuso et al., 1999; Pomerleau et al., 1994; Provost & Woodward, 1991), or positive effects on both speed of color naming and the Stroop effect (Hasenfratz & Battig, 1992).

One explanation for these findings is that nicotine facilitates performance on easy, but not difficult, tasks (Spilich et al., 1992). For instance, Mancuso et al. (1999) found that nicotine administered via a patch facilitated performance on speed of number generation and the speed of processing on the control and interference conditions of the Stroop, but did not improve performance on attentional switching or the Stroop effect. These authors contended that nicotine primarily improves the intensity feature of attention, rather than the selectivity feature. Indeed, in their review of the literature, Heishman et al. (1994) found that nicotine generally did not improve performance on tasks requiring divided or selective attention. While intensity is needed to sustain attention, selectivity is needed in focused attention tasks which involve excluding competing information (e.g., Stroop effect) or divided attention tasks.

Performance on working memory tasks such as the *n*-back is facilitated by nicotine to some extent. Ernst et al. (2001b), on a 2-back test, found that while nicotine gum did not improve reaction time or accuracy compared to placebo, for ex-smokers, the variability of reaction time to all stimuli was reduced and the number of errors decreased. Kumari et al. (2003), in a sample of nonsmoking males, found that nicotine produced increased response accuracy in 0-back, 1-back, 2-back, and 3-back conditions and shorter latencies on the 3-back test. Findings were associated with frontoparietal activation across all levels of working memory. On other measures of working memory, such as the digit recall task, nicotine gum administered to nonsmokers decreased reaction time but impaired accuracy (Heishman &

Henningfield, 2000). Indeed, Foulds et al. (1997) replicated these findings in nonsmokers when nicotine was administered intravenously. Deleterious effects have also been found in spatial working memory tasks using young smokers (Park, Knopick, McGurk, & Meltzer, 2000).

Learning and memory findings

Fewer studies have examined the association between nicotine exposure and declarative memory. The results are mixed and moderated by methodology. For example, the recall of prose passages was facilitated by nicotine administration in deprived smokers (Krebs et al., 1994; Warburton, Rusted, & Fowler, 1992), although there may have been a placebo effect as well. In contrast, Spilich, June, and Renner (1992) reported that nicotine administration was associated with deleterious effects on story recall. Additionally, nonsmokers did not benefit from nicotine administration on tests of immediate and delayed recall (Hindmarch, Kerr, & Sherwood, 1990; Jones et al., 1992) and in one study performed less well (Dunne et al., 1986).

On list-learning tasks, immediate recall was facilitated by nicotine in abstinent smokers (Peeke & Peeke, 1984; Warburton, Rusted, & Muller, 1992; Warburton, Wesnes, Shergold, & James, 1986), but was hindered in nonabstinent smokers and nonsmokers after smoking two cigarettes (Sakurai & Kanazawa, 2002). Nicotine may improve performance more on delayed recall relative to immediate memory (Mangan, 1983). With regard to recognition memory, nicotine has a facilitative effect in deprived smokers (Foulds et al., 1996; Perkins et al., 1994; Warburton et al., 1986) and in nonsmokers (Perkins et al.,1994; but see Dunne et al., 1986).

In terms of temporal effects, smoking before and after list presentation enhanced list recall (Rusted, Graupner, & Warburton, 1995; Rusted & Warburton, 1992; Warburton et al., 1986), though this effect disappeared when participants were distracted with an intervening task. This finding suggests that proactive interference and/or the attentional function(s) that influence recall are not affected by nicotine administration (Warburton et al., 1986). In addition, nicotine seems to facilitate the rate of memory search in smokers, with facilitative effects found on search rate in Sternberg's memory search task (West & Hack, 1991). On the other hand, Spilich et al. (1992), who used larger set sizes and included smokers, deprived smokers, and nonsmokers, found a detrimental effect on this task when nicotine was administered via cigarette smoking.

Finally, it has been demonstrated that in deprived smokers nicotine administration facilitates learning nonsense syllables (Andersson & Post, 1974) and consolidation of word pairs over one week delay (Colrain, Mangan, Pellett, & Bates, 1992). Additional work is needed to investigate the effect of nicotine administration on more specific subcomponents of memory performance and on memory performance patterns. Examples include the potentially facilitative effect of nicotine on memory depending on associative strength (e.g., Rusted, Graupner, Tennant, & Warburton, 1998; Rusted et al., 1995; Warburton, Skinner, & Martin, 2001) and nicotine's facilitation of primacy and recency effects (Pineda et al., 1998; Warburton et al., 1992). Such studies may help to illuminate the mechanisms associated with varying degrees of facilitation following nicotine administration.

Chronic effects

Aspects of cognition affected

Fewer studies have focused on the residual neurocognitive effects of nicotine relative to acute effects. The extant literature on this topic reveals that lifetime smokers generally perform poorly on cognitive tasks relative to nonsmokers (Cervilla, Prince, Joels, Lovestone, & Mann, 2000; Deary, Pattie, Taylor, Whiteman, Starr, & Whalley, 2003; Elwood et al., 1999; Schinka, Vanderploeg, Rogish, & Ordorica, 2002b) and linear modeling suggests that smoking has independent effects on cognitive decline from age 11 to age 80 (Deary et al., 2003). The magnitude of these effects apeears to be modest, however. For example, Schinka et al. found a deleterious effect of smoking in middle-aged smokers, with pack-years accounting for only 0.2% of the variance in a measure of global cognitive functioning.

Whereas smoking acutely facilitates cognition, it appears to be associated with long-term decrements on speed of processing (Carmelli, Swan, Reed, Schellenberg, & Christian, 1999; Cerhan et al., 1998; Kalmijn, van Boxtel, Verschuren, Jolles, & Launer, 2002; Richards, Jarvis, Thompson, & Wadsworth, 2003) or no effect at all (Elwood et al., 1999; Howe & Price, 2001). Smoking is also associated with poorer performance and/or faster declines in verbal memory in middle age (Cerhan et al., 1998; Richards et al., 2003). In addition, chronic, low-dose nicotine administration is associated with poor object learning and delayed recall (Howe & Price, 2001).

Other findings relate more specifically to frontal/executive functioning; for example, smokers do not perform as well as nonsmokers on tests of working memory (Ernst et al., 2001a; Spilich et al., 1992). Furthermore, deficits on measures of orbitofrontal functioning in regular smokers (aged 17–25) relative to nonsmokers have recently been reported (Dinn, Aycicegi, & Harris, 2004). In this study, smokers reported more behaviors associated with frontal lobe syndromes (i.e., apathy, dysexecutive symptoms, and behavioral disinhibition) and were more impaired on the Object Alternation Task relative to nonsmokers.

Individual difference variables

Age

Epidemiological studies of smoking behavior have suggested that smoking is related to reduced performance on cognitive measures in middle-aged and older adults, particularly on tests of psychomotor speed (Carmelli et al., 1999; Elwood et al., 1999; Galanis, Petrovitch, Launer, Harris, Foley, & White, 1997; Hill, Nilsson, Nyberg, & Backman, 2003; Kilander, Nyman, Boberg, & Lithell, 1997; Zhou, Deng, Li, Wang, Zhang, & He, 2003), with some studies reporting a dose-dependent effect (Berkman et al., 1993; Kalmijn et al., 2002). Other studies have suggested the possibility that cigarette smokers perform more poorly on difficult (e.g., Block Design and free recall) as opposed to simple (e.g., general knowledge and word comprehension) cognitive tasks, irrespective of age (Hill et al., 2003). Because smoking is a risk factor for stroke and is associated with vascular dementia (Higa & Davanipour, 1991; Shinton & Beevers, 1989), it is possible that vascular changes underlie the decline in cognitive performance in smokers with age. For example, Kalmijn et al. found a relationship between current smoking in middle-aged participants and measures of psychomotor speed and cognitive flexibility; in contrast, Chen, Wang, Wang, Fuh, Lin, and Liu (2003), using a prospective study design that sampled nondemented elderly individuals, found that cigarette smoking and lifetime cigarette exposure were not associated with cognitive performance at baseline or 3 years later after controlling for age, education, hypertension, diabetes, and vascular events. In another prospective study, Edelstein, Kritz-Silverstein, and Barrett-Connor (1998) found that overall cognitive test scores did not differ from baseline scores obtained 13–18 years previously by smoking history. In women, however, scores on a long-term recall test for words and a measure of general cognitive function had declined in smokers, whereas measures of nonverbal memory, fluency, and cognitive flexibility did not differentially decline by smoking status.

Most of the aforementioned studies do not control for alcohol consumption. One exception (i.e., Schinka, Vanderploeg, Rogish, Graves, Mortimer, & Ordorica, 2002a) found no detrimental effect of smoking; nor was there any evidence of an interaction between alcohol and cigarette use on any cognitive measure after controlling for other potential cognitive risk factors such as diabetes, hypertension, and vascular disease.

Gender

Few studies have reported gender effects with regard to the cognitive effects of smoking and few have specifically examined this issue in an experimental fashion. Many of the epidemiological studies of lifetime smokers exclusively sample men or do not examine gender. As there are gender differences in nicotine sensitivity and metabolism (Grunberg, Winders, & Wewers, 1991; Staley et al., 2001), it would not be surprising to find differential cognitive effects as well; however, Deary et al. (2003), in a study of smokers and nonsmokers from age 11 to age 80, found that gender does not interact with smoking history to affect overall cognitive performance. Similarly, other epidemiological studies have failed to show a relationship between smoking history and gender (Schinka, Belanger, Mortimer, & Graves, 2003; Schinka et al., 2002a). On the other hand, Edelstein et al. (1998) found a gender difference in their prospective study of middle-aged adults such that female smokers tended to show declines on measures of verbal long-term recall and general cognitive function, whereas male smokers showed no differential change over the 13–18-year study.

Race

The association of white matter lesions in the brain with smoking and alcohol intake is greater in African Americans than in European Americans (Liao et al., 1997), suggesting the importance of studying the cognitive effects of chronic smoking in this subpopulation. In examining the influence of lifetime cumulative doses of cigarettes in current and ex-users, we found that smoking had a small impact on memory performance, as measured by the Hopkins Verbal Learning test (as a standardized summed score of three learning trials and free and cued recall) in a sample of 230 community-dwelling African American adults aged 60–84 (Schinka et al., 2003). While the effect of smoking itself was minimal, the combination of smoking and drinking was found to have a modest (i.e., 3% of the variance) deleterious effect on general cognitive ability after controlling for age, education, diabetes, and hypertension.

Ex-smokers versus current smokers

The results of studies examining the effects of smoking history on cognition are inconsistent. This outcome is not surprising given that these studies vary with respect to important methodological factors, such as participant sampling, measures of cognition, and range and type of consumption. Several of these variables appear to be especially critical. Because alcohol and cigarette consumption are related to education (Slater, Basil, & Maibach, 1999), and education is an especially strong predictor of cognitive ability (e.g., Vanderploeg & Schinka, 1995), statistical control of years of education is critical. Other variables that potentially confound comparisons between abstainers and users because of their association with use of alcohol and/or cigarettes and their impact on cognitive function include history of vascular disease, diabetes, and hypertension (Haan, Shemanski, Jagust, Manolio, & Kuller, 1999). A comprehensive analysis of the impact of drinking and smoking on cognition should also include analyses not only by category of use (abstainer, user, ex-user), but also of lifetime consumption. In one report (Page & Cleveland, 1987), for example, significant results were obtained for comparisons of groups based on category of smoking use, but not for analyses based on pack-year history. Finally, adequate measurement of cognitive function should include more sensitive measures of global function, as well as measures of important domains of cognition. As discussed previously, there are few studies that have examined the potential interactive effect of both smoking and drinking on cognition, despite the high frequency of their concordant use (DiFranza & Guerrera, 1990), their common genetic factors (Swan, Carmelli, & Cardon, 1996), and their contribution as risk factors to overall health status.

Smoking history is inconsistently associated with poorer cognitive function (Carmelli et al., 1999; Cerhan et al., 1998; Galanis et al., 1997; Kilander, Nyman, & Lithell, 1997; Launer, Feskens, Kalmijn, & Kromhout, 1996; Schinka et al., 2002b), but representative studies generally do not control for the impact of drinking. Notably, there are a number of reports failing to find a detrimental effect on cognition in smokers or ex-smokers (Carmelli, Swan, LaRue, & Eslinger, 1997; Cervilla et al., 2000; Elwood et al., 1999; Herbert et al., 1993). The Schinka et al. study (2002b), which did control for drinking, found a reliable, but small decrement in performance on a measure of general cognition associated with smoking in middle-aged participants.

Summary of cognitive effects of nicotine

In summary, nicotine seems to acutely facilitate speed of processing and attention in particular. Facilitative effects are more consistently demonstrated in deprived smokers. Inconsistent methodology makes drawing more specific conclusions difficult. In terms of studying the acute effects of nicotine on cognition, the absence of placebo controls, double-blind conditions, and imprecise methods of nicotine administration (e.g., ad lib cigarette smoking) are particularly problematic. When effects of nicotine on cognition are found, they tend to be small to medium in size and beg the question of clinical meaningfulness (Henningfield, 1994). Cook et al. (2003), for example, found an effect size of $d = .47$ for reaction time on a math processing task but a negative effect of $d = -.36$ for reaction time on a grammatical reasoning task. In general, more complicated tasks are associated with even smaller effects. So, for example, Dinn et al. (2004) found an effect size on a design fluency task of approximately $d = .01$ and similarly Cook et al. (2003) found an effect of $d = .04$ on a task of cognitive inhibition (Stroop interference condition). Nonetheless, additional work is needed to tease apart nicotine's effects with regard to specific components of tasks and determining potential dose–response relationships via nicotine plasma monitoring (Heishman, 1999).

In terms of the chronic effects of nicotine on cognition, nicotine appears to have a modest deleterious effect on cognition. One obvious methodological difficulty with these studies, however, is that associations between smoking history and cognitive decline may be confounded by a selection bias; namely, smokers have a shorter lifespan than nonsmokers (Peto, Lopez, Boreham, Thun, & Heath, 1992). Nonetheless, studies in middle-aged smokers reveal deleterious effects as well (Kalmijn et al., 2002; Richards et al., 2003; Schinka et al., 2002b). Again, the effects are modest, accounting for less than 5% of the variance. It is important to note that most of the studies reviewed in this section were large, epidemiological studies that used generalized, crude measures of cognition. Interestingly, it has been found that working memory performance on an *n*-back task varies with smoking history, independent of acute nicotine administration (Ernst et al., 2001a). Specifically, reaction time was fastest in nonsmokers, followed by ex-smokers, and slowest in smokers. This suggests a dose-dependent effect of nicotine exposure on working memory. Further research focusing on more specific cognitive subcomponents is needed.

Mechanisms of action

Animal models

Physiological

Animal models have been useful for the study of cognitive changes secondary to nicotine administration, as well as for understanding the mechanisms responsible for it. Most work has focused on addiction with implication of the mesolimbic dopamine pathway in nicotine-mediated reward (see Rose & Corrigall, 1997). Nicotine binds to the nicotinic receptors (nicotinic acetylcholine receptors, nAChRs) which are widely distributed in the brains of many species, including humans (see Paterson & Nordberg, 2000). Due to the wide distribution of nAChRs, chronic administration of nicotine probably affects most, if not all, brain regions. Interestingly, although many other receptors are downregulated following chronic administration of an agonist, nAChRs are upregulated after chronic nicotine administration (see Wonnacott, 1990 for a review). Nicotine binding sites increase after chronic administration in rodents (Pauly, Marks, Gross, & Collins, 1991; Pauly, Marks, Robinson, van de Kamp, & Collins, 1996) and humans (Court et al., 1998). Increases in nicotine binding sites with multiple injections of nicotine have generally been found in the cortex, the striatum, and the hippocampus (e.g., Ksir, Hakan, & Kellar, 1987; Romanelli, Ohman, Adem, & Nordberg, 1988; Wall, Gong, Johnson, Meyerson, & Zhang, 2000). As this upregulation of nAChR is accompanied by locomotor activity and enhanced cognitive performance, the upregulation may be related to the behavioral sensitization that occurs during chronic nicotine use exposure (e.g., Abdulla et al., 1996), the intensity of early withdrawal symptoms (Mathieu-Kia, Kellogg, Butelman, & Kreek, 2002), and the facilitative effects of nicotine on cognitive performance.

The hippocampus is a primary structure in attention and memory (Jarrard, 1995) and has a high concentration of nicotinic receptors (Martin & Aceto, 1981). Nicotine facilitates hippocampal synaptic activity (Gray, Rajan, Radcliffe, Yakehiro, & Dani, 1996) and increases hippocampal long-term potentiation (Hamid, Dawe, Gray, & Stephenson, 1997), which is thought to underlie learning and memory. The highest concentration of nicotinic receptors, however, is in the thalamus, caudate, and substantia nigra (Paterson & Nordberg, 2000), which may have implications for the acute effects of nicotine on attention, psychomotor speed, and executive functioning.

Psychopharmacology/pharmacokinetics

Nicotine binds to nicotinic receptors in the brain, augmenting the release of various neurotransmitters, including dopamine, serotonin, norepinephrine, acetylcholine, glutamate, and gamma-aminobutyric acid. Nicotine also inhibits monoamine oxidase, which is an enzyme responsible for the breakdown of norepinephrine, serotonin, and dopamine in the brain.

Nicotine reaches the brain within a few seconds through pulmonary and arterial absorption. This rate of absorption is consistent with other drugs that have high abuse potential (Quinn, Wodak, & Day, 1997). It is thought that the rapid arterial nicotine increase that occurs after each puff (10 ng/ml increase after 10 seconds; Rose, Behm, Westman, & Coleman, 1999) contributes to the greater reinforcing properties of cigarette smoking relative to other forms of administration (i.e., gum, patch, or nasal spray; Schneider, Lunell, Olmstead, & Fagerstrom, 1996). Circulating nicotine is oxidized into cotinine, a major metabolite eliminated in urine. In rodent models, nicotine levels in the blood rapidly increase and then decline. The overall half-life in the brain is slightly longer than in the blood itself and brain levels are typically two to three times higher than blood levels (Donny et al., 2000; Rowell & Li, 1997; Sastry, Chance, Singh, Horn, & Janson, 1995). In humans, the half-life of nicotine in the blood is estimated to be about 4–10 minutes, while the elimination half-life is about 2 hours (Perez-Stable, Herrera, Jacob, & Benowitz, 1998). As in rodent models, after a cigarette is smoked, the level of nicotine rapidly increases and then falls, creating a spike pattern throughout the day. Superimposed on this spike pattern is an overall increase in nicotine levels during the day with a gradual decrease at night (Benowitz, Kuyt, & Jacob, 1982).

Behavioral

The radial arm maze is typically used to test cognition in animals, particularly rodents. The radial arm maze has 8 or 16 arms which are variably baited with food to test an animal's memory. Both working memory, which is the ability to keep information "on line", as well as reference memory, which is the ability to store information, can be studied with the radial arm maze. Specifically, errors of reentry into initially-baited arms are classified as working memory errors, while entries into never-baited arms are classified as reference memory errors.

Acutely, it has been repeatedly demonstrated that nicotine or nicotine agonists improve working memory performance in the radial arm maze in rats (Decker, Brioni, Bannon, & Arneric, 1995; Levin, Kaplan, & Boardman, 1997; Levin & Simon, 1998) and in the delayed matching-to-sample task in monkeys (Elrod, Buccafusco, & Jackson, 1988). For instance, Levin et al. (1997), after training rats in the 16-arm radial arm maze, injected either saline or 0.2 mg/kg nicotine 20 minutes before testing and found that choice accuracy (i.e., the so-called "entries to repeat" or the number of correct entries into the arms until an error is made) was significantly increased following nicotine injection.

Similar experiments demonstrated that nicotine affects working memory chronically as well as acutely, though higher doses may be needed to maintain the effect after a 2-week period of no nicotine administration (Levin and Torry, 1996; Levin et al., 1990). Experiments conducted to investigate both acute and chronic effects have generally found that working memory, but not reference memory, is facilitated following nicotine administration in rats (Attaway, Compton, & Turner, 1999; Levin, Kim, & Meray, 1996; Levin et al., 1997; Rezvani & Levin, 2001), although there is some evidence that administering the nicotine after training trials rather than before training may lead to acute facilitation of reference memory as well (Brown, Beale, & Jay Frye, 2002).

Nicotine may have facilitative effects on "higher-order" executive and "social" functions in rats. Granon, Faure, and Changeux (2003) demonstrated that a nicotinic agonist facilitated performance on tasks requiring behavioral adaptation to changing external stimuli, more effective spatiotemporal exploration of their environment, and a higher rate of approach-related behaviors with another rat. These results conflict with the negative findings on cognitive flexibility in humans (Mancuso et al., 1999), although direct comparison of tasks is obviously limited.

Finally, the facilitative effects on attention found in humans have also been demonstrated in rats and monkeys. Specifically, nicotine facilitates performance on sustained attention (Gill, Sarter, & Givens, 2000; Mirza & Stolerman, 1998), divided attention (Turchi & Sarter, 1997), and attention orienting (Witte et al., 1997). Nicotine or nicotinic agonists also enhance psychomotor behavior in rats (Grottick, Wyler, & Higgins, 2000; Museo & Wise, 1990; Shim et al., 2001).

fMRI and PET studies

To elucidate the neuroanatomical substrates of the effects of nicotine on cognition, neuroimaging technology is critical. Nicotine is associated with dose-dependent increases in neuronal activation in several brain areas, including the frontal lobes, the anterior cingulate bilaterally, the nucleus accumbens, and amygdala. Activation in these structures may explain nicotine's behavior-arousing, behavior-reinforcing, and cognitive-enhancing properties (Stein et al., 1998).

Although investigators have used neuroimaging technology to study the brain mechanisms involved in nicotine's addictive properties (e.g., Due, Huettel, Hall, & Rubin, 2002; Rose et al., 2003), few have used it to specifically study cognitive aspects of nicotine use. In a positron emission tomography (PET) study, Ernst et al. (2001b) found that nicotine gum decreased activation during the 2-back task for smokers, but increased activation for ex-smokers. This discrepancy may be due to the need for a larger dose to maintain homeostasis in ex-smokers. Interestingly, brain activation during the 2-back task was not associated with actual performance for smokers following nicotine administration. For ex-smokers, however, there was a positive correlation between accuracy and right anterior cingulate activation and a negative correlation between reaction time and prefrontal and right inferior parietal regions. In both ex-smokers and current smokers, cingulate activity decreased significantly during nicotine administration. This decreased activation in the anterior cingulate during tasks requiring attention has been reported previously (Ghatan et al., 1998) and likely reflects the widely reported effects of nicotine on the attentional system.

Lawrence et al. (2002), in an fMRI study, found that performance on the rapid visual information-processing task, a task of visual vigilance, was associated with activation in a frontoparietal-thalamic network in both smokers and nonsmokers. Abstinent smokers showed less task-induced brain activation in the parietal cortex and caudate than did nonsmokers, which might explain why abstinent smokers report decrements in cognition. Transdermal nicotine administration improved task performance and increased brain activation in the parietal and occipital cortices, thalamus, and caudate. This study suggests that the improved attention induced by nicotine administration is mediated by enhanced activation in these brain areas. Finally, in an fMRI study of working memory, Kumari et al. (2003) reported increased activation in the anterior cingulate, superior frontal cortex, and superior parietal cortex in nonsmoking males performing an *n*-back task after nicotine administration. While participants were active, activation was also increased in the midbrain tectum. These patterns of activation suggest a nicotine-induced activation of an online task monitoring, attention, and arousal system in the brain that is associated with improved performance on working memory tasks.

Physiological changes

White matter changes

White matter hyperintensities (WMH), visible on MRI scans, are thought to reflect small vessel disease. Several researchers have reported that smoking history is associated with atrophy and WMH severity (Fukuda & Kitani, 1996; Liao et al., 1997; Longstreth et al., 2000; Roman, 1987; Swan, DeCarli, Miller, Reed, Wolf, & Carmelli, 2000; Tsushima, Tanizaki, Aoki, & Endo, 2002). This effect seems to be independent of other risk factors for WMH (e.g., age, hypertension, sex, ethnicity). There are a few negative findings, however (Yamashita, Kobayashi, Yamaguchi, & Koide, 1996; Yetkin, Fischer, Papke, & Haughton, 1993), which may be attributable to sample size.

Laterality changes

Gilbert (1995, 1997) proposed that the reinforcing properties of nicotine may be due to its lateralizing effect on cortical arousal. As there is evidence for lateralization of neurotransmitter systems (Tucker & Williamson, 1984; Wittling, 1995) and lateralization of mood and arousal (e.g., Heller, Etienne, & Miller, 1995), this hypothesis is tenable to the extent that nicotine impacts these systems. Gilbert proposed that nicotine facilitates left frontal activation, which has been associated with approach-related behaviors and emotions, controlled (vs. automatic) processing, and positive affect. Evidence for this hypothesis is drawn from studies demonstrating that nicotine seems to facilitate performance on primarily so-called left-hemisphere tasks and hinder performance on right-hemisphere tasks (McClernon, Gilbert, & Radtke, 2003). The difficulty inherent in this hypothesis is of course that most tasks are not mediated solely by one hemisphere, making conclusions tenuous at best.

A recent PET study (Rose et al., 2003) found that nicotine increased blood flow in left frontal regions, which adds further support to Gilbert's hypothesized lateralizing effect of nicotine. Interestingly, decreased blood flow was noted in the left amygdala, which may explain some of the anxiolytic effects associated with nicotine administration. In another PET study, Ernst et al. (2001b) found lateralized performance on a 2-back working memory task as a function of nicotine dependence such that ex-smokers predominantly activated the left hemisphere whereas smokers predominantly activated the right hemisphere. These authors contend that ex-smokers utilized a phonological strategy on this task whereas current smokers utilized a more visual strategy. Activation of right parietal cortex in only the smokers lends credence to this hypothesis, although further research is needed to clarify these findings. When stimuli are presented to one visual field or another (and, hence, to one hemisphere first), there is no difference in reaction time to visual cues by smoking status (Shirtcliff & Marrocco, 2003).

Other structural changes

Cigarette use, as measured by pack-year history, is associated with brain atrophy (Longstreth, Diehr, Manolio, Beauchamp, Jungreis, & Lefkowitz, 2001; Swan et al., 2000) and increased sulcal and ventricular size (Longstreth et al., 2000) in the elderly. In a sample of middle-aged adults, it was found that smokers have smaller gray matter volumes and lower gray matter densities than nonsmokers in prefrontal cortex bilaterally, as well as smaller volumes in the left dorsal anterior cingulate and lower gray matter densities in the right cerebellum (Brody et al., 2004). Nicotine administration increases cerebral blood flow an average of 16% (Skinhoj, Olesen, & Paulson, 1973), although decreases in specific brain regions have been reported (Ghatan et al., 1998). Finally, fMRI and PET studies demonstrate that smoking increases activation in the prefrontal cortex (Stein et al., 1998), ventral striatum (Nakamura, Tanaka, Nomoto, Ueno, & Nakayama, 2000; Stein et al., 1998), and thalamus (Domino, Ni, Xu, Koeppe, Guthrie, & Zubieta, 2004; Domino et al., 2000; Nakamura et al., 2000; Rose et al., 2003; Stein et al., 1998; Zubieta et al., 2001).

Summary of mechanisms of action

In summary, nicotine acts on the brain through a variety of mechanisms to affect cognition. Animal studies have demonstrated high concentrations of nicotinic receptors in the hippocampus, thalamus, caudate, and substantia nigra, which has obvious implications for most cognitive functions. Indeed, studies with animals suggest that nicotine facilitates performance on working memory tasks following both acute and chronic administration of nicotine. Other cognitive domains are less well studied in animals but are also suggestive of facilitative effects. Nicotine also seems to "activate" the brain, as demonstrated by neuroimaging studies which suggest activation-induced facilitation on attention and executive tasks in frontal, parietal, and possibly cingulate cortex.

Laterality research suggests the possibility that nicotine preferentially facilitates performance on tasks mediated largely by the left hemisphere, although more research is needed and this theory needs to be reconciled with other data suggesting the possibility of greater right-hemisphere activation via attention models (e.g., Heilman & Van Den Abell, 1980). Nicotine also negatively impacts the brain, as evidenced by structural changes such as increased WMH and atrophy.

Nicotine as a treatment for cognitive impairment

Alzheimer's disease/dementia

While Alzheimer's disease is primarily treated with acetylcholinesterase (AChE) inhibitors like tacrine and donepezil, there is evidence that activation of neuronal nAChRs in the brain may also be an effective treatment option. This is presumably due to the loss of nicotinic binding sites in patients with Alzheimer's disease, particularly in the cortex and hippocampus (Quirion et al., 1986; Shimohama, Taniguchi, Fujiwara, & Kameyama, 1986). Indeed, White and Levin (1999) found that nicotine administration, via transdermal patch, significantly improved performance on the Continuous Performance Task (CPT), a task which requires primarily vigilance and sustained attention. This was a double-blind, placebo-controlled, crossover study which consisted of two, 4-week periods separated by a washout period of 2 weeks. Nicotine reduced errors of omission and the response accuracy improved markedly (5–80%). While the attentional improvement persisted for 4 weeks (White & Levin, 1999), nicotine did not improve performance on other measures such as motor or memory tasks. Similarly, patients with age-associated memory impairment, thought to be a precursor to Alzheimer's disease in many cases, improved performance on the CPT after nicotine administration but not memory or motor performance (White & Levin, 2004). Finally, smoking in "at risk" elderly is associated with a decreased risk for decline on measures of attention and visuospatial ability (Leibovici, Ritchie, Ledesert, & Touchon, 1999).

Other studies have further demonstrated that nicotine administration in AD patients has facilitative effects on attention (Jones et al., 1992; Sahakian & Jones, 1991; Sahakian, Jones, Levy, Gray, & Warburton, 1989), as well as on learning (White & Levin, 1999) and memory (Newhouse et al., 1988; Parks et al., 1996), though these findings are not ubiquitous (see Snaedal, Johannesson, Jonsson, & Gylfadottir, 1996; Wilson et al., 1995). Small sample size and various methods of assessing cognitive functions may account for different findings. Nonetheless, given the multifactorial nature of the disease process, the treatment of Alzheimer's disease may include nicotine as an adjunctive treatment in the future. Certainly, preliminary findings provide optimism, at least with regard to improving attention. Recent work with animal models suggests that use of nicotine ligands, rather than nicotine itself, may be more efficacious and produce fewer side effects (Bontempi, Whelan, Risbrough, Lloyd, & Menzaghi, 2003). The use of nicotine metabolite, cotinine, as a treatment has also been suggested due to its longer half-life and facilitative effects on working memory (Buccafusco & Terry, 2003).

Schizophrenia

People diagnosed with schizophrenia have fewer nicotinic receptors, particularly in the hippocampus (Freedman, Hall, Adler, & Leonard, 1995). It is hypothesized that they smoke at a much higher rate than other psychiatric patients (Hughes, Hatsukami, Mitchell, & Dahlgren, 1996) in an attempt to compensate for a cognitive impairment, particularly with regard to verbal learning and memory and working memory impairments. Indeed, it has been found that schizophrenics have impaired sensory gating and nicotine seems to ameliorate this impairment (Adler, Hoffer, Wiser, & Freedman, 1993).

Several double-blind, placebo-controlled studies conducted with schizophrenics suggest beneficial effects of nicotine on cognition. One study (Levin, Wilson, Rose, & McEvoy, 1996), for instance, was conducted in which smoking schizophrenics who were also taking an antipsychotic, haloperidol, were administered varying levels of nicotine via transdermal patch. Three hours after administration of nicotine, variability of response speed on the CPT was significantly reduced in these patients. This effect was dose-dependent. Nicotine also reduced some of the adverse effects of haloperidol on working memory in schizophrenics. Another study, using transdermal patches to administer nicotine (Depatie et al., 2002), revealed that study participants demonstrated improved performance on the CPT in terms of overall hits, as well as facilitated performance on an oculomotor task. Finally, in a placebo-controlled, crossover study using high nicotine or nasal spray with daily pre- and postdrug evaluations in abstinent smokers (Smith, Singh, Infante, Khandat, & Kloos, 2002), it was found that the nasal spray had a positive effect on verbal memory and reaction time and both the nasal spray and cigarettes facilitated performance on a spatial organization task. Interestingly, high-nicotine cigarettes tended to decrease negative symptoms.

ADHD

Given the aforementioned facilitative effects of nicotine on attention, it follows that nicotine may remediate symptoms of ADHD. Indeed, Shytle, Silver, Wilkinson, and Sanberg (2002) have demonstrated in a double-blind, placebo-controlled randomized pilot trial that transdermal nicotine reduces ADHD symptomatology in children, as measured by the Conners Parent Rating Scale. Unfortunately, the side effects of this treatment reduced the benefit of the intervention. Future investigations of nicotinic ligands may prove beneficial.

Though ADHD is primarily thought of as a childhood disorder, there is increasing evidence that many adults also meet the diagnostic criteria for this syndrome. Nicotinic agonist ABT-418 improves attention in adults with ADHD (Wilens et al., 1999). In a placebo-controlled, double-blind study, smoking and nonsmoking adults were given either placebo or nicotine patches in counterbalanced order roughly one week apart (Conners et al., 1996; Levin et al, 1996). There was significant improvement in attentional symptoms both in smokers and nonsmokers, relative to placebo, as measured by the Global Impressions Scale. Similar improvement in nonsmokers suggests that the effect was not merely due to withdrawal relief. There was reduced variability on the CPT as well and this effect also occurs with chronic 4-week administration (Levin, Conners, Silva, Canu, & March, 2001). Interestingly, nicotine did not reduce errors of omission, as it did with normal adults and patients with Alzheimer's disease. This could be because of greater severity of attentional deficits in ADHD patients, or because of a different mechanism of action.

Parkinson's disease

Several epidemiological studies have noted an inverse relationship between premorbid cigarette smoking and the occurrence of Parkinson's disease, sometimes in a dose-related fashion (Gorell, Rybicki, Johnson, & Peterson, 1999; Hellenbrand et al., 1997; Morens, Grandinetti, Davis, Ross, White, & Reed, 1996), though this may be true only in younger patients (Tzourio et al., 1997). As with Alzheimer's disease, there is a marked reduction in cortical nicotinic receptor binding in Parkinson's disease that corresponds to the degree of dementia and increasing age (Aubert, Araujo, Cecyre, Robitaille,

Gauthier, & Quirion, 1992; Whitehouse et al., 1988). Furthermore, nicotine activates striatal and mesolimbic dopamine-secreting neurons in experimental animals (Pidoplichko, DeBiasi, Williams, & Dani, 1997). Preliminary studies have shown positive effects of nicotine administration on tremor (Fagerstrom, Polerleau, Giordani, & Stelson, 1994; Ishikawa & Miyatake, 1993; Marshall & Schnieden, 1966) and disorganized thinking (Fagerstrom et al., 1994), although well-controlled studies have demonstrated negative findings with regard to motor and affective symptoms in these patients (Clemens, Baron, Coffey, & Reeves, 1995; Lemay et al., 2004; Vieregge, Sieberer, Jacobs, Hagenah, & Vieregge, 2001). In a study more specific to cognitive function, Kelton, Kahn, Conrath, and Newhouse (2000) gave nicotine intravenously at various doses acutely, followed by chronic administration via a patch for 2 weeks to nondemented early to patients with moderate Parkinson's disease, and reported acute facilitative effects on choice reaction time in a U-shaped function with dose-related improvement at the low and mid-doses and slowing at higher doses. Nicotine also improved performance on a critical flicker fusion task which assesses attention and arousal. There was no improvement on measures of semantic fluency or divided attention. Two weeks after patch removal, these patients were re-tested. It was found that performance on several motor measures had improved (e.g., stand–walk–sit test), although practice effects are a consideration.

Summary of nicotine as a treatment

Exciting new research suggests that nicotine effectively remediates the cognitive deficits observed in a wide variety of neuropsychiatric disorders. Indeed, in preliminary research, individuals with Alzheimer's disease, age-associated memory impairment, schizophrenia, ADHD, and Parkinson's disease have demonstrated improvements in cognitive function following nicotine administration. It remains to be seen whether these improvements will translate into improved ability to manage various functional activities (e.g., activities of daily living).

Summary

In summary, nicotine facilitates acute improvements in speed of processing and attention. There is some suggestion that nicotine exerts positive effects on attention via attentional narrowing and increased perceptual processing capacity (Kassel, 1997), though this remains speculative. A priori investigations of nicotine's effects on specific task components will resolve this question (Heishman, 1999). Brain imaging studies suggest the possibility that these facilitative effects are due to brain "activation," though the identification of the mechanism(s) by which nicotine influences cognitive performance requires additional research.

Research has also demonstrated the potential for using nicotine in the treatment of cognitive disorders across a spectrum of neuropsychiatric disorders. Indeed, in preliminary research, individuals with Alzheimer's disease, age-associated memory impairment, schizophrenia, ADHD, and Parkinson's disease have benefited cognitively from nicotine administration. As in studies conducted with normal individuals, most facilitative effects have been demonstrated on tasks of attention and/or processing speed. Studies are needed to study other cognitive domains, as well as the potential mediating effects of mood.

Chronically, nicotine seems to have adverse, albeit small, effects on cognitive functioning. Structural neuroimaging studies suggest the possibility that these adverse effects are the result of increased WMH and atrophy associated with smoking. Bauman, Koch, and Fisher (1989) found that as smoking among household members increased from 0 to >2 packs per day, achievement performance in children declined even when potential mediators were controlled (such as age, sex, parental education, race, and personality variables). This study illustrates the importance of the chronic effects of nicotine even among "passive smokers."

References

Abdulla, F. A., Bradbury, E., Calaminici, M. R., Lippiello, P. M., Wonnacott, S., Gray, J. A., et al. (1996). Relationship between up-regulation of nicotine binding sites in rat brain and delayed cognitive enhancement observed after chronic or acute nicotinic receptor stimulation. *Psychopharmacology*, *124*, 323–331.

Adler, L. E., Hoffer, L. D., Wiser, A., & Freedman, R. (1993). Normalization of auditory physiology by cigarette smoking in schizophrenic patients. *American Journal of Psychiatry*, *150*, 1856–1861.

Andersson, K., & Post, B. (1974). Effects of cigarette smoking on verbal rote learning and physiological arousal. *Scandanavian Journal of Psychology*, *15*, 263–267.

Ashby, F. G., Isen, A. M., & Turken, A. U. (1999). A neuropsychological theory of positive affect and its influence on cognition. *Psychological Review*, *106*, 529–550.

Attaway, C. M., Compton, D. M., & Turner, M. D. (1999). The effects of nicotine on learning and memory: A neuropsychological assessment in young and senescent Fischer 344 rats. *Physiology and Behavior*, *67*, 421–431.

Aubert, I., Araujo, D. M., Cecyre, D., Robitaille, Y., Gauthier, S., & Quirion, R. (1992). Comparative alterations of nicotinic and muscarinic binding sites in Alzheimer's and Parkinson's diseases. *Journal of Neurochemistry*, *58*, 529–541.

Baldinger, B., Hasenfratz, M., & Battig, K. (1995). Comparison of the effects of nicotine on a fixed rate and a subject-paced version of the rapid visual information processing task. *Psychopharmacology*, *121*, 396–400.

Baker, P. J., & Walsh, T. (1996). Smoking a cigarette has no effect on visual temporal order discrimination in regular smokers. *Addiction*, *91*, 879–884.

Bates, T., Mangan, G., Stough, C., & Corballis, P. (1995). Smoking, processing speed and attention in a choice reaction time task. *Psychopharmacology*, *120*, 209–212.

Bauman, K. E., Koch, G. G., & Fisher, L. A. (1989). Family cigarette smoking and test performance by adolescents. *Health Psychology*, *8*, 97–105.

Bell, S. L., Taylor, R. C., Singleton, E. G., Henningfield, J. E., & Heishman, S. J.

(1999). Smoking after nicotine deprivation enhances cognitive performance and decreases tobacco craving in drug abusers. *Nicotine and Tobacco Research, 1,* 45–52.

Benowitz, N. L., Kuyt, F., & Jacob, P. (1982). Circadian blood nicotine concentrations during cigarette smoking. *Clinical Pharmacology and Therapeutics, 32,* 758–764.

Berkman, L. F., Seeman, T. E., Albert, M., Blazer, D., Kahn, R., Mohs, R., et al. (1993). High, usual and impaired functioning in community-dwelling older men and women: Findings from the MacArthur Foundation Research Network on Successful Aging. *Journal of Clinical Epidemiology, 46,* 1129–1140.

Bontempi, B., Whelan, K. T., Risbrough, V. B., Lloyd, G. K., & Menzaghi, F. (2003). Cognitive enhancing properties and tolerability of cholinergic agents in mice: A comparative study of nicotine, donepezil, and SIB-1553A, a subtype-selective ligand for nicotinic acetylcholine receptors. *Neuropsychopharmacology, 28,* 1235–1246.

Breslau, N., Davis, G. C., & Schultz, L. R. (2003). Posttraumatic stress disorder and the incidence of nicotine, alcohol, and other drug disorders in persons who have experienced trauma. *Archives of General Psychiatry, 60,* 289–294.

Breslau, N., Johnson, E. O., Hiripi, E., & Kessler, R. (2001). Nicotine dependence in the United States: Prevalence, trends and smoking persistence. *Archives of General Psychiatry, 58,* 810–816.

Breslau, N., Peterson, E. L., Schultz, L. R., Chilcoat, H. D., & Andreski, P. (1998). Major depression and stages of smoking: A longitudinal investigation. *Archives of General Psychiatry, 55,* 161–166.

Brody, A. L., Mandelkern, M. A., Jarvik, M. E., Lee, G. S., Smith, E. C., Huang, J. C., et al. (2004). Differences between smokers and nonsmokers in regional gray matter volumes and densities. *Biological Psychiatry, 55,* 77–84.

Brown, R. W., Beale K. S., & Jay Frye G. D. (2002). Mecamylamine blocks enhancement of reference memory but not working memory produced by post-training injection of nicotine in rats tested on the radial arm maze. *Behavioral Brain Research, 21,* 259–265.

Brown, R. A., Lewinsohn, P. M., Seeley, J. R., & Wagner, E. F. (1996). Cigarette smoking, major depression, and other psychiatric disorders among adolescents. *Journal of the American Academy of Child and Adolescent Psychiatry, 35,* 1602–1610.

Buccafusco, J. J., & Terry, A. V. (2003). The potential role of cotinine in the cognitive and neuroprotective actions of nicotine. *Life Sciences, 72,* 2931–2942.

Cahill, L., & McGaugh, J. L. (1995). A novel demonstration of enhanced memory associated with emotional arousal. *Consciousness and Cognition, 4,* 410–421.

Carmelli, D., Swan, G. E., LaRue, A., & Eslinger, P. J. (1997). Correlates of change in cognitive function in survivors from the Western Collaborative Group Study. *Neuroepidemiology, 16,* 285–295.

Carmelli, D., Swan, G. E., Reed, T., Schellenberg, G. D., & Christian, J. C. (1999). The effect of apolipoprotein E epsilong4 in the relationships of smoking and drinking to cognitive function. *Neuroepidemiology, 18,* 125–133.

Cerhan, J. R., Folsom, A. R., Mortimer, J. A., Shahar, E., Knopman, D. S., McGovern, P. G., et al. (1998). Correlates of cognitive function in middle-aged adults. Atherosclerosis Risk in Communities (ARIC) Study Investigators. *Gerontology, 44,* 95–105.

Cervilla, J. A., Prince, M., Joels, S., Lovestone, S., & Mann, A. (2000). Long-term predictors of cognitive outcome in a cohort of older people with hypertension. *British Journal of Psychiatry, 177,* 66–71.

Chen, W. T., Wang, P. N., Wang, S. J., Fuh, J. L., Lin, K. N., & Liu, H. C. (2003). Smoking and cognitive performance in the community elderly: A longitudinal study. *Journal of Geriatric Psychiatry and Neurology*, *16*, 18–22.

Clemens, P., Baron, J. A., Coffey, D., & Reeves, A. (1995). The short-term effect of nicotine chewing gum in patients with Parkinson's disease. *Psychopharmacology*, *117*, 253–256.

Colrain, I. M., Mangan, G. L., Pellett, O. L., & Bates, T. C. (1992). Effects of post-learning smoking on memory consolidation. *Psychopharmacology*, *108*, 448–451.

Conners, C. K., Levin, E. D., Sparrow, E., Hinton, S. C., Erhardt, D., Meck, W. H., et al. (1996). Nicotine and attention in adult ADHD. *Psychopharmacology Bulletin*, *32*, 67–73.

Cook, M. R., Gerkovich, M. M., Graham, C., Hoffman, S. J., & Peterson, R. C. (2003). Effects of the nicotine patch on performance during the first week of smoking cessation. *Nicotine and Tobacco Research*, *5*, 169–180.

Court, J. A., Lloyd, S., Thomas, N., Piggott, M. A., Marshall, E. F., Morris, C. M., et al. (1998). Dopamine and nicotinic receptor binding and the levels of dopamine and homovanillic acid in human brain related to tobacco use. *Neuroscience*, *87*, 63–78.

Deary, I. J., Pattie, A., Taylor, M. D., Whiteman, M. C., Starr, J. M., & Whalley, L. J. (2003). Smoking and cognitive change from age 11 to age 80. *Journal of Neurology, Neurosurgery and Psychiatry*, *74*, 1003–1007.

Decker, M. W., Brioni, J. D., Bannon, A. W., and Arneric, S. P. (1995). Diversity of neuronal nicotinic acetylcholine receptors: Lessons from behavior and implications for CNS therapeutics – minireview. *Life Sciences*, *56*, 545–570.

De Leon, J., Becona, E., Gurpegui, M., Gonzalez-Pinto, A., & Diaz, F. J. (2002). The association between high nicotine dependence and severe mental illness may be consistent across countries. *Journal of Clinical Psychiatry*, *63*, 812–816.

Depatie, L., O'Driscoll, G. A., Holahan, A. L., Atkinson, V., Thavundayil, J. X., Kin, N. N., et al. (2002). Nicotine and behavioral markers of risk for schizophrenia: A double-blind, placebo-controlled, cross-over study. *Neuropsychopharmacology*, *27*, 1056–1070.

Dierker, L. C., Avenevoli, S., Stolar, M., & Merikangas, K. R. (2002). Smoking and depression: An examination of mechanisms of comorbidity. *American Journal of Psychiatry*, *159*, 947–953.

Difranza, J. R., & Guerrera, M. P. (1990). Alcoholism and smoking. *Journal of Studies on Alcohol*, *51*, 130–135.

Dinn, W. M., Aycicegi, A., & Harris, C. L. (2004). Cigarette smoking in a student sample: Neurocognitive and clinical correlates. *Addictive Behaviors*, *29*, 107–126.

Domino, E. F., Minoshima, S., Guthrie, S., Ohl, L., Ni, L., Koeppe, R. A., et al. (2000). Nicotine effects on regional cerebral blood flow in awake, resting tobacco smokers. *Synapse*, *38*, 313–321.

Domino, E. F., Ni, L., Xu, Y., Koeppe, R. A., Guthrie, S., & Zubieta, J. K. (2004). Regional cerebral blood flow and plasma nicotine after smoking tobacco cigarettes. *Progress in Neuropsychopharmacology and Biological Psychiatry*, *28*, 319–327.

Donny, E. C., Caggiula, A. R., Rowell, P. P., Gharib, M. A., Maldovan, V., Booth, S., et al. (2000). Nicotine self-administration in rats: Estrous cycle effects, sex differences and nicotinic receptor binding. *Psychopharmacology*, *151*, 392–405.

Due, D. L., Huettel, S. A., Hall, W. G., & Rubin, D. C. (2002). Activation in mesolimbic and visuospatial neural circuits elicited by smoking cues: Evidence from functional magnetic resonance imaging. *American Journal of Psychiatry, 159*, 954–960.

Dunne, M. P., MacDonald, D., & Hartley, L. R. (1986). The effects of nicotine upon memory and problem solving performance. *Physiology and Behavior, 37*, 849–854.

Edelstein, S. L., Kritz-Silverstein, D., & Barrett-Connor, E. (1998). Prospective association of smoking and alcohol use with cognitive function in an elderly cohort. *Journal of Women's Health, 7*, 1271–1281.

Edwards, J. A., Wesnes, K., Warburton, D. M., & Gale, A. (1985). Evidence of more rapid stimulus evaluation following cigarette smoking. *Addictive Behaviors, 10*, 113–126.

Elrod, K., Buccafusco, J. J., & Jackson, W. J. (1988). Nicotine enhances delayed matching-to-sample performance by primates. *Life Sciences, 43*, 277–287.

Elwood, P. C., Gallacher, J. E. J., Hopkinson, C. A., Pickering, J., Rabbitt, P., Stollery, B., et al., (1999). Smoking, drinking, and other life style factors and cognitive function in men in the Caerphilly cohort. *Journal of Epidemiology and Community Health, 53*, 9–14.

Ernst, M., Heishman, S. J., Spurgeon, L., & London, E. D. (2001a). Smoking history and nicotine effects on cognitive performance. *Neuropsychopharmacology, 25*, 313–319.

Ernst, M., Matochik, J. A., Heishman, S. J., Van Horn, J. D., Jons, P. H., Henningfield, J. E., et al. (2001b). Effect of nicotine on brain activation during performance of a working memory task. *Proceedings of the National Academy of Sciences, 98*, 4728–4733.

Fagerstrom, K. O., Pomerleau, O., Giordani, B., & Stelson, F. (1994). Nicotine may relieve symptoms of Parkinson's disease. *Psychopharmacology, 116*, 117–119.

File, S. E., Dinnis, A. K., Heard, J. E., & Irvine, E. E. (2002). Mood differences between male and female light smokers and nonsmokers. *Pharmacology, Biochemistry and Behavior, 72*, 681–689.

Fleming, S. E., & Lombardo, T. W. (1987). Effects of cigarette smoking on phobic anxiety. *Addictive Behaviors, 12*, 195–198.

Foulds, J., Stapleton, J., Swettenham, J., Bell, N., McSorley, K., & Russell, M. A. (1996). Cognitive performance effects of subcutaneous nicotine in smokers and never-smokers. *Psychopharmacology, 127*, 31–38.

Foulds, J., Stapleton, J., Swettenham, J., Jarvis, M. J., & Russell, M. A. H. (1997). Mood and physiological effects of subcutaneous nicotine in smokers and never-smokers. *Drug and Alcohol Dependence, 44*, 105–115.

Freedman, R., Hall, M., Adler, L. E., & Leonard, S. (1995). Evidence in postmortem brain tissue for decreased numbers of hippocampal nicotinic receptors in schizophrenia. *Biological Psychiatry, 38*, 22–33.

Fukuda, H., & Kitani, M. (1996). Cigarette smoking is correlated with the periventricular hyperintensity grade on brain magnetic resonance imaging. *Stroke, 27*, 645–649.

Galanis, D. J., Petrovitch, H., Launer, L. J., Harris, T. B., Foley, D. J., & White, L. R. (1997). Smoking history in middle age and subsequent cognitive performance in elderly Japanese-American men. The Honolulu-Asia Aging Study. *American Journal of Epidemiology, 145*, 507–515.

Ghatan, P. H., Ingvar, M., Eriksson, L., Stone-Elander, S., Serrander, M., Ekberg, K., et al. (1998). Cerebral effects of nicotine during cognition in smokers and non-smokers. *Psychopharmacology, 136*, 179–189.

Gilbert, D. G. (1995). *Smoking: Individual differences, psychopathology and emotion.* Washington, DC: Taylor and Francis.

Gilbert, D. G. (1997). The situation X trait adaptive response (STAR) model of drug use effects and craving. *Human Psychopharmacology, 12*, S89–S102.

Gilbert, D. G., Estes, S. L., & Welser, R. (1997). Does noise stress modulate effects of smoking/nicotine? Mood, vigilance, and EEG responses. *Psychopharmacology, 129*, 382–389.

Gill, T. M., Sarter, M., & Givens, B. (2000). Sustained visual attention performance-associated prefrontal neuronal activity: Evidence for cholinergic modulation. *Journal of Neuroscience, 20*, 4745–4757.

Gorell, J. M., Rybicki, B. A., Johnson, C. C., & Peterson, E. L. (1999). Smoking and Parkinson's disease: A dose-response relationship. *Neurology, 52*, 115–119.

Granon, S., Faure, P., & Changeux, J. P. (2003). Executive and social behaviors under nicotinic receptor regulation. *Proceedings of the National Academy of Sciences of the United States of America, 100*, 9596–9601.

Gray, R., Rajan, A. S., Radcliffe, K. A., Yakehiro, M., & Dani, J. A. (1996). Hippocampal synaptic transmission enhanced by low concentrations of nicotine. *Nature, 38*, 713–716.

Griesar, W. S., Zajdel, D. P., Oken, B. S. (2000). Nicotine effects on alertness and spatial attention in non-smokers. *Nicotine and Tobacco Research, 4*, 185–194.

Grottick, A. J., Wyler, R., & Higgins, G. A. (2000). The alpha4beta2 agonist SIB 1765F, but not the alpha7 agonist AR-R 17779, cross-sensitizes to the psychostimulant effects of nicotine. *Psychopharmacology, 150*, 233–236.

Grunberg, N., Winders, S., & Wewers, M. E. (1991). Gender differences in tobacco use. *Health Psychology, 10*, 143–153.

Haan, M. N., Shemanski, L., Jagust, W. J., Manolio, T. A., & Kuller, L. (1999). The relationship between alcohol consumption, cognitive performance, and daily functioning in an urban sample of older black Americans. *Journal of the American Geriatrics Society, 44*, 1158–1165.

Hale, C. R., Gentry, M. V., & Meliska, C. J. (1999). Effects of cigarette smoking on lexical decision-making. *Psychological Reports, 84*, 117–120.

Hamid, S., Dawe, G. S., Gray, J. A., & Stephenson, J. D. (1997). Nicotine induces long-lasting potentiation in the dentate gyrus of nicotine-primed rats. *Neuroscience Research, 29*, 81–85.

Hasenfratz, M., & Battig, K. (1992). Action profiles of smoking and caffeine: Stroop effect, EEG, and peripheral physiology. *Pharmacology, Biochemistry and Behavior, 42*, 155–161.

Heilman, K. M., & Van Den Abell, T. (1980). Right hemisphere dominance for attention: the mechanism underlying hemispheric asymmetries of inattention (neglect). *Neurology, 30*, 327–330.

Heishman, S. J. (1999). Behavioral and cognitive effects of smoking: Relationship to nicotine addiction. *Nicotine and Tobacco Research, 1*, S143–S147.

Heishman, S. J., & Henningfield, J. E. (2000). Tolerance to repeated nicotine administration on performance, subjective, and physiological responses in nonsmokers. *Psychopharmacology, 152*, 321–333.

Heishman, S. J., Snyder, F. R., & Henningfield, J. E. (1993). Performance, subjective, and physiological effects of nicotine in nonsmokers. *Drug and Alcohol Dependence, 34*, 11–18.

Heishman, S. J., Taylor, R. C., & Henningfield, J. E. (1994). Nicotine and smoking: A review of effects on human performance. *Experimental Clinical Psychopharmacology, 2*, 345–395.

Hellenbrand, W., Seidler, A., Robra, B. P., Vieregge, P., Oertel, W. H., Joerg, J., et al. (1997). Smoking and Parkinson's disease: A case-control study in Germany. *International Journal of Epidemiology, 26*, 328–339.

Heller, W., Etienne, M. A., & Miller, G. A. (1995). Patterns of perceptual asymmetry in depression and anxiety: Implications for neuropsychological models of emotion and psychopathology. *Journal of Abnormal Psychology, 104*, 327–333.

Henningfield, J. E. (1994). Comments on West's editorial "Beneficial effects of nicotine: Fact or fiction?" *Addiction, 89*, 135–146.

Henningfield, J. E., Miyasato, K., & Jasinski, D. R. (1985). Abuse liability and pharmacodynamic characteristics of intravenous and inhaled nicotine. *Journal of Pharmacology and Experimental Therapeutics, 234*, 1–12.

Herbert, M., Foulds, J., & Fife-Schaw, C. (2001). No effect of cigarette smoking on attention or mood in non-deprived smokers. *Addiction, 96*, 1349–1356.

Herbert, L. E., Scherr, P. A., Beckett, L. A., Albert, M. S., Rosner, B., Taylor, J. O., et al. (1993). Relation of smoking and low-to-moderate alcohol consumption to change in cognitive function: a longitudinal study in a defined community of older persons. *American Journal of Epidemiology, 137*, 881–891.

Herning, R. I., & Pickworth, W. B. (1985). Nicotine gum improved stimulus processing during tobacco withdrawal. *Psychophysiology, 22*, 594.

Higa, M., & Davanipour, Z. (1991). Smoking and stroke. *Neuroepidemiology, 10*, 211–222.

Hill, R. D., Nilsson, L., Nyberg, L., & Backman, L. (2003). Cigarette smoking and cognitive performance in healthy Swedish adults. *Age and Ageing, 32*, 548–550.

Hindmarch, I., Kerr, J. S., & Sherwood, N. (1990). Effects of nicotine gum on psychomotor performance in smokers and non-smokers. *Psychopharmacology, 100*, 535–541.

Houlihan, M. E., Pritchard, W. S., & Robinson, J. H. (1996). Faster P300 latency after smoking in visual but not auditory oddball tasks. *Psychopharmacology, 123*, 231–238.

Howe, M. N., & Price, I. R. (2001). Effects of transdermal nicotine on learning, memory, verbal fluency, concentration, and general health in a healthy sample at risk for dementia. *International Psychogeriatrics, 13*, 465–475.

Hughes, J. R. (1986). Genetics of smoking: A brief review. *Behavior Therapy, 17*, 335–345.

Hughes, J. R., Hatsukami, D. K., Mitchell, J. E., & Dahlgren, L. A. (1996). Prevalence of smoking among psychiatric outpatients. *American Journal of Psychiatry, 143*, 993–997.

Ishikawa, A., & Miyatake, T. (1993). Effects of smoking in patients with early-onset Parkinson's disease. *Journal of Neurological Science, 117*, 28–32.

Isensee, B., Wittchen, H. U., Stein, M. B., Hofler, M., & Lieb, R. (2003). Smoking increases the risk of panic: Findings from a prospective community study. *Archives of General Psychiatry, 60*, 692–700.

Jarrard, L. E. (1995). What does the hippocampus really do? *Behavioral Brain Research, 71*, 1–10.

Jensen, M. K., Sorensen, M. T., Andersen, A. T., Thorsen, T., Tolstrup, J. S., Godtfredsen, N. S., & Gronbaek, M. (2003). A prospective study of the association between smoking and later alcohol drinking in the general population. *Addiction, 98*, 355–363.

Jones, G. M., Sahakian, B. J., Levy, R., Warburton, D. M., & Gray, J. A. (1992). Effects of acute subcutaneous nicotine on attention, information processing and short-term memory in Alzheimer's disease. *Psychopharmacology, 108*, 485–494.

Kalmijn, S., van Boxtel, M. P., Verschuren, M. W., Jolles, J., & Launer, L. J. (2002). Cigarette smoking and alcohol consumption in relation to cognitive performance in middle age. *American Journal of Epidemiology, 15*, 936–944.

Kandel, D. B., Johnson, J. G., Bird, H. R., Canino, G., Goodman, S., Lahey, B., Regier, D., & Schwab-Stone, M. (1997). Psychiatric disorders associated with substance use among children and adolescents: Findings from the Methods for the Epidemiology of Child and Adolescent Mental Disorders (MECA) Study. *Journal of Abnormal Child Psychology, 25*, 121–132.

Kassel, J. D. (1997). Smoking and attention: A review and reformulation of the stimulus-filter hypothesis. *Clinical Psychology Review, 17*, 451–478.

Kassel, J. D., & Shiffman, S. (1997). Attentional mediation of cigarette smoking's effect on anxiety. *Health Psychology, 16*, 359–368.

Kelton, M. C., Kahn, H. J., Conrath, C. L., & Newhouse, P. A. (2000). The effects of nicotine on Parkinson's disease. *Brain and Cognition, 43*, 274–282.

Kendler, K. S., Neale, M. C., MacLean, C. J., Heath, A. C., Eaves, L., & Kessler, R. (1993). Smoking and major depression: A causal analysis. *Archives of General Psychiatry, 50*, 36–43.

Kerr, J. S., Sherwood, N., & Hindmarch, I. (1991). Separate and combined effects of the social drugs on psychomotor performance. *Psychopharmacology, 104*, 113–119.

Kilander, L., Nyman, H., Boberg, M., & Lithell, H. (1997). Cognitive function, vascular risk factors and education. A cross-sectional study based on a cohort of 70-year-old men. *Journal of Internal Medicine, 242*, 313–321.

Kilander, L., Nyman, H., & Lithell, M. B. (1997). Cognitive function, vascular risk factors and education. A cross-sectional study based on a cohort of 70-year-old men. *Journal of Internal Medicine, 242*, 313–321.

Knott, V. J. (1986). Tobacco effects on cortical evoked potentials to task stimuli. *Addictive Behaviors, 11*, 219–223.

Knott, V., Bosman, M., Mahoney, C., Ilivitsky, V., & Quirt, K. (1999). Transdermal nicotine: Single dose effects on mood, EEG, performance, and event-related potentials. *Pharmacology, Biochemistry and Behavior, 63*, 253–261.

Kos, J., Hasenfratz, M., & Battig, K. (1997). Effects of a 2-day abstinence from smoking on dietary, cognitive, subjective, and physiologic parameters among younger and older female smokers. *Physiology and Behavior, 61*, 671–678.

Krebs, S. J., Petros, T. V., & Beckwith, B. E. (1994). Effects of smoking on memory for prose passages. *Physiology and Behavior, 56*, 723–727.

Ksir, C., Hakan, R., & Kellar, K. J. (1987). Chronic nicotine and locomotor activity: Influences of exposure dose and test dose. *Psychopharmacology, 92*, 25–29.

Kumari, V., Gray, J. A., Fytche, D. H., Mitterschiffthaler, M. T., Das, M., Zachariah, E., et al. (2003). Cognitive effects of nicotine in humans: An fMRI study. *Neuroimage, 19*, 1002–1013.

Landers, D. M., Crews, D. J., Boutcher, S. H., Skinner, J. S., & Gustafsen, S. (1992). The effects of smokeless tobacco on performance and psychophysiological response. *Medicine and Science in Sports and Exercise, 24*, 895–903.

Launer, L. J., Feskens, E. J. M., Kalmijn, S., & Kromhout, D. (1996). Smoking, drinking, and thinking: The Zutphen Elderly Study. *American Journal of Epidemiology, 143*, 219–227.

Lawrence, N. S., Ross, T. J., & Stein, E. A. (2002). Cognitive mechanisms of nicotine on visual attention. *Neuron, 36*, 539–548.

Leibovici, D., Ritchie, K., Ledesert, B., & Touchon, J. (1999). The effects of wine and tobacco consumption on cognitive performance in the elderly: a longitudinal study of relative risk. *International Journal of Epidemiology, 28*, 77–81.

Le Houezec, J., Halliday, R., Benowitz, N. L., Callaway, E., Naylor, H., & Herzig, K. (1994). A low dose of subcutaneous nicotine improves information processing in non-smokers. *Psychopharmacology, 114*, 628–634.

Lemay, S., Chouinard, S., Blanchet, P., Masson, H., Soland, V., Beuter, A., et al. (2004). Lack of efficacy of a nicotine transdermal treatment on motor and cognitive deficits in Parkinson's disease. *Progress in Neuropsychopharmacology and Biological Psychiatry, 28*, 31–39.

Levin, E. D., Conners, C. K., Silva, D., Canu, W., & March, J. (2001). Effects of chronic nicotine and methylphenidate in adults with attention deficit/hyperactivity disorder. *Experimental and Clinical Psychopharmacology, 9*, 83–90.

Levin, E. D., Conners, C. K., Silva, D., Hinton, S. C., Meck, W., March, J., & Rose, J. E. (1998). Transdermal nicotine effects on attention. *Psychopharmacology, 140*, 135–141.

Levin, E. D., Conners, C. K., Sparrow, E., Hinton, S. C., Erhardt, D., Meck, et al. (1996). Nicotine effects on adults with attention-deficit/hyperactivity disorder. *Psychopharmacology, 123*, 55–63.

Levin, E. D., Kaplan, S., & Boardman, A. (1997). Acute nicotine interactions with nicotinic and muscarinic antagonists: Working and reference memory effects in the 16-arm radial maze. *Behavioral Pharmacology, 8*, 236–242.

Levin, E. D., Kim, P., & Meray, R. (1996). Chronic nicotine effects on working memory and reference memory in the 16-arm radial maze: Interactions with D1 agonist and antagonist drugs. *Psycopharmacology, 127*, 25–30.

Levin, E. D., Lee, C., Rose, J. E., Reyes, A., Ellison, G., Jarvik, M., et al. (1990). Chronic nicotine and withdrawal effects on radial-arm maze performance in rats. *Behavioral and Neural Biology, 53*, 269–276.

Levin, E. D., & Simon, B. B. (1998). Nicotinic acetylcholine involvement in cognitive function in animals. *Psychopharmacology, 138*, 369–373.

Levin, E. D., & Torry, D. (1996). Acute and chronic nicotine effects on working memory in aged rats. *Psychopharmacology, 123*, 88–97.

Levin, E. D., Wilson, W., Rose, J., & McEvoy, J. (1996). Nicotine-haloperidol interactions and cognitive performance in schizophrenics. *Neuropsychopharmacology, 15*, 429–436.

Li, M. D., Cheng, R., Ma, J. Z., & Swan, G. E. (2003). A meta-analysis of estimated genetic and environmental effects on smoking behavior in male and female adult twins. *Addiction, 98*, 23–31.

Liao, D., Cooper, L., Cai, J., Toole, J., Bryan, N., Burke, G., et al. (1997). The prevalence and severity of white matter lesions, their relationship with age, ethnicity, gender, and cardiovascular disease risk factors: the ARIC Study. *Neuroepidemiology, 16*, 149–162.

Longstreth, W. T., Arnold, A. M., Manolio, T. A., Burke, G. L., Bryan, N., Jungreis, C. A., et al. (2000). Clinical correlates of ventricular and sulcal size on cranial magnetic resonance imaging of 3,301 elderly people: The cardiovascular health study. *Neuroepidemiology, 19*, 30–42.

Longstreth, W. T., Diehr, P., Manolio, T. A., Beauchamp, N. J., Jungreis, C. A., & Lefkowitz, D. (2001). Cluster analysis and patterns of findings on cranial magnetic resonance imaging of the elderly: The cardiovascular health study. *Archives of Neurology, 58*, 635–640.

Mancuso, G., Warburton, D. M., Melen, M., Sherwood, N., & Tirelli, E. (1999). Selective effects of nicotine on attentional processes. *Psychopharmacology, 146*, 199–204.

Mangan, G. L. (1983). The effects of cigarette smoking on verbal learning and retention. *Journal of General Psychology, 108*, 203–210.

Marshall, J., & Schnieden, H. (1966). Effect of adrenaline, noradrenaline, atropine, and nicotine on some types of human tremor. *Journal of Neurological and Neurosurgical Psychiatry, 29*, 214–218.

Martin, B. R., & Aceto, M. D. (1981). Nicotine binding sites and their localization in the central nervous system. *Neuroscience and Biobehavioral Reviews, 5*, 473–478.

Mathieu-Kia, A. M., Kellogg, S. H., Butelman, E. R., & Kreek, M. J. (2002). Nicotine addiction: Insights from recent animal studies. *Psychopharmacology, 162*, 102–118.

McClernon, F. J., Gilbert, D. G., & Radtke, R. (2003). Effects of transdermal nicotine on lateralized identification and memory interference. *Human Psychopharmacology, 18*, 339–343.

Meliska, C. J., & Gilbert, D. G. (1991). Hormonal and subjective effects of smoking the first five cigarettes a day: A comparison in males and females. *Pharmacology, Biochemistry and Behavior, 40*, 229–235.

Mirza, N. R., & Stolerman, I. P. (1998). Nicotine enhances sustained attention in the rat under specific task conditions. *Psychopharmacology, 138*, 266–274.

Morens, D. M., Grandinetti, A., Davis, J. W., Ross, G. W., White, L., & Reed, D. (1996). Evidence against the operation of selective mortality in explaining the association between cigarette smoking and reduced occurrence of idiopathic Parkinson disease. *American Journal of Epidemiology, 144*, 400–404.

Murphy, F. C., & Klein, R. M. (1998). The effects of nicotine on spatial and non-spatial expectancies in a covert orienting task. *Neuropsychologia, 36*, 1103–1114.

Museo, E., & Wise, R. A. (1990). Locomotion induced by ventral tegmental injections of a nicotine agonist. *Pharmacology, Bicochemistry and Behavior, 37*, 113–116.

Nakamura, H., Tanaka, A., Nomoto, Y., Ueno, Y., & Nakayama, Y. (2000). Activation of fronto-limbic system in the human brain by cigarette smoking: Evaluated by a CBF measurement. *Keio Journal of Medicine, 49*, A122–A124.

Newhouse, P. A., Potter, A., & Singh, A. (2004). Effects of nicotinic stimulation on cognitive performance. *Current Opinion in Pharmacology, 4*, 36–46.

Newhouse, P. A., Sunderland, T., Narang, P. K., Mellow, A. M., Fertig, J. B., Lawlor, B. A., et al. (1990). Neuroendrocrine, physiologic, and behavioral responses following intravenous nicotine in nonsmoking healthy volunteers and patients with Alzheimer's disease. *Psychoendocrinology, 15*, 471–484.

Newhouse, P. A., Sunderland, T., Tariot, P. N., Blumhardt, C. L., Weingaartner, H., Mellow, A., et al. (1988). Intravenous nicotine in Alzheimer's disease: A pilot study. *Psychopharmacology, 95*, 171–175.

Noteboom, J. T., Fleshner, M., & Enoka, R. M. (2001). Activation of the arousal response can impair performance on a simple motor task. *Journal of Applied Physiology, 91*, 821–831.

Page R. D., & Cleveland M. F. (1987). Cognitive dysfunction and aging among male alcoholics and social drinkers. *Alcoholism, Clinical and Experimental Research, 11*, 376–384.

Park, S., Knopick, C., McGurk, S., & Meltzer, H. Y. (2000). Nicotine impairs spatial working memory while leaving spatial attention intact. *Neuropsychopharmacology, 22*, 200–209.

Parks, R. W., Becker, R. E., Rippey, R. F., Gilbert, D. C., Matthews, J. R., Kabatay, E., et al. (1996). Increased regional cerebral glucose metabolism and semantic memory performance in Alzheimer's disease: A pilot double blind transdermal nicotine positron emission tomography study. *Neuropsychology Review, 6*, 61–79.

Parrott, A. C. (1993). Cigarette smoking: Effects upon self-rated stress and arousal over the day. *Addictive Behaviors, 18*, 389–395.

Parrott, A. C., & Craig, D. (1992). Cigarette smoking and nicotine gum (0, 2 and 4 mg): Effects upon four visual attention tasks. *Neuropsychobiology, 25*, 34–43.

Parrott, A. C., & Kaye, F. J. (1999). Daily uplifts, hassles, stresses and cognitive failures: In cigarette smokers, abstaining smokers, and non-smokers. *Behavioral Pharmacology, 10*, 639–646.

Parrott, A. C., & Roberts, G. (1991). Smoking deprivation and cigarette reinstatement: Effects upon visual attention. *Journal of Psychopharmacology, 5*, 404–409.

Parrott, A. C., & Winder, G. (1989). Nicotine chewing gum (2 mg, 4 mg) and cigarette smoking: Comparative effects upon vigilance and heart rate. *Psychopharmacology, 97*, 257–261.

Paterson, D., & Nordberg, A. (2000). Neuronal nicotinic receptors in the human brain. *Progress in Neurobiology, 61*, 75–111.

Pauly, J. R., Marks, M. J., Gross, S. D., & Collins, A. C. (1991). An autoradiographic analysis of cholinergic receptors in mouse brain after chronic nicotine treatment. *Journal of Pharmacology and Experimental Therapeutics, 258*, 1127–1136.

Pauly, J. R., Marks, M. J., Robinson, S. F., van de Kamp, J. L., & Collins, A. C. (1996). Chronic nicotine and mecamylamine treatment increase brain nicotinic receptor binding without change alpha 4 or beta 2 mRNA levels. *Journal of Pharmacology and Experimental Therapeutics, 278*, 361–369.

Peeke, S. C., & Peeke, H. S. (1984). Attention, memory and cigarette smoking. *Psychopharmacology, 84*, 205–216.

Perez-Stable, E. J., Herrera, B., Jacob, P., & Benowitz, N. L. (1998). Nicotine metabolism and intake in black and white smokers. *Journal of the American Medical Association, 280*, 152–156.

Perkins, K. A., Epstein, L. H., Stiller, R. L., Sexton, J. E., Debski, T. D., & Jacob, R. G. (1990). Behavioral performance effects of nicotine in smokers and non-smokers. *Pharmacology, Biochemistry and Behavior, 37*, 11–15.

Perkins, K. A., Grobe, J. E., Epstein, L. H., Caggiula, A. R., & Stiller, R. L. (1992). Effects of nicotine on subjective arousal may be dependent on baseline subjective state. *Journal of Substance Abuse, 4*, 131–141.

Perkins, K. A., Grobe, J. E., Fonte, C., Goettler, J., Caggiula, A. R., Reynolds, W. A., et al. (1994). Chronic and acute tolerance to subjective, behavioral and cardiovascular effects of nicotine in humans. *Journal of Pharmacology and Experimental Therapeutics, 270*, 628–638.

Perkins, K. A., Grobe, J. E., Mitchell, S. L., Goettler, J., Caggiula, A., Stiller, R. I., et al. (1995). Acute tolerance to nicotine in smokers: Lack of dissipation within 2 hours. *Psychopharmacology, 118*, 164–170.

Peto, R., Lopez, A. D., Boreham, J., Thun, M., & Heath, C. (1992). Mortality from tobacco in developed countries: Indirect estimation from national vital statistics. *Lancet, 339*, 1268–1278.

Pidoplichko, V. I., DeBiasi, M., Williams, J. T., & Dani, J. A. (1997). Nicotine activates and desensitizes midbrain dopamine neurons. *Nature (London), 390*, 401–404.

Pineda, J. A., Herrera, C., Kang, C., & Sandler, A. (1998). Effects of cigarette smoking and 12-h abstention on working memory during a serial-probe recognition task. *Psychopharmacology, 139*, 311–321.

Pomerleau, C. S., & Pomerleau, O. F. (1987). The effects of psychological stressor on cigarette smoking and subsequent behavioural and physiological responses. *Psychophysiology, 24*, 278–285.

Pomerleau, C. S., Teuscher, F., Goeters, S., & Pomerleau, O. F. (1994). Effects of nicotine abstinence and menstrual phase on task performance. *Addictive Behaviors, 19*, 357–362.

Pomerleau, O. F., & Pomerleau, C. S. (1991). Research on stress and smoking: Progress and problems. *British Journal of Addiction, 86*, 599–603.

Pomerleau, O., Turk, D., & Fertig, J. (1984). The effects of cigarette smoking on pain and anxiety. *Addictive Behaviors, 9*, 256–271.

Pritchard, W. S., Robinson, J. H., & Guy, T. D. (1992). Enhancement of continuous performance task reaction time by smoking in non-deprived smokers. *Psychopharmacology, 108*, 437–442.

Provost, S. C., & Woodwad, R. (1991). Effects of nicotine gum on repeated administration of the Stroop test. *Psychopharmacology, 104*, 536–540.

Quinn, D. I., Wodak, A., & Day, R. O. (1997). Pharmacokinetic and pharmacodynamic principles of illicit drug use and treatment of illicit drug users. *Clinical Pharmacokinetics, 33*, 344–400.

Quirion, R., Martel, J. C., Robitaille, Y., Etienne, P., Wood, P., Nair, N. P., et al. (1986). Neurotransmitter and receptor deficits in senile dementia of the Alzheimer's type. *Canadian Journal of Neurological Sciences, 13*, 503–510.

Rezvani, A. H., & Levin, E. D. (2001). Cognitive effects of nicotine. *Biological Psychiatry, 49*, 258–267.

Richards, M., Jarvis, M. J., Thompson, N., & Wadsworth, M. J. (2003). *American Journal of Public Health, 93*, 994–998.

Riggs, P. D., Mikulich, S. A., Whitmore, E. A., & Crowley, T. J. (1999). Relationship of ADHD, depression, and non-tobacco substance use disorders to nicotine dependence in substance-dependent delinquents. *Drug and Alcohol Dependence, 3*, 195–205.

Robbins, T. W. (1997). Aroual systems and attentional processes. *Biological Psychology, 45*, 57–71.

Roman, G. C. (1987). Senile dementia of the Binswanger type: A vascular form of dementia in the elderly. *Journal of the American Medical Association, 257*, 1782–1788.

Romanelli, L., Ohman, B., Adem, A., & Nordberg, A. (1988). Subchronic treatment of rats with nicotine: Interconversion of nicotinic receptor subtypes in brain. *European Journal of Pharmacology, 148*, 289–291.

Rose, J. E., Behm, F. M., Westman, E. C., & Coleman, R. E. (1999). Arterial nicotine kinetics during cigarette smoking and intravenous nicotine administration: Implications for addiction. *Drug and Alcohol Dependence, 56*, 99–107.

Rose, J. E., Behm, F. M., Westman, E. C., Mathew, R. J., London, E. D., Hawk, T. C., et al. (2003). PET studies of the influence of nicotine on neural systems in cigarette smokers. *American Journal of Psychiatry, 160*, 323–333.

Rose, J. E., & Corrigall, W. A. (1997). Nicotine self-administration in animals and humans: Similarities and differences. *Psychopharmacology, 130*, 28–40.

Rowell, P. P., & Li, M. (1997). Dose-response relationship for nicotine-induced up-regulation of rat brain nicotinic receptors. *Journal of Neurochemistry, 68*, 1982–1989.

Rusted, J., & Eaton-Williams, P. (1991). Distinguishing between attentional and amnestic effects in information processing: The separate and combined effects of scoporamine and nicotine on verbal free recall. *Psychopharmacology (Berlin), 104*, 363–366.

Rusted, J. M., Graupner, L., Tennant, A., & Warburton, D. M. (1998). Effortful processing is a requirement for nicotine-induced improvements in memory. *Psychopharmacology, 138*, 362–368.

Rusted, J. M., Graupner, L., & Warburton, D. (1995). Effects of post-trial administration of nicotine on human memory: Evaluating the conditions for improving memory. *Psychopharmacology (Berlin), 119*, 405–413.

Rusted, J. M., & Wharburton, D. M. (1992). Facilitation of memory by post-trial administration of nicotine: Evidence for an attentional explanation. *Psychopharmacology, 108*, 452–455.

Sahakian, B. J., & Jones, G. M. (1991). The effects of nicotine on attention, information processing, and working memory in patients with dementia of the Alzheimer's type. In F. Adlkofer & K. Thruau (Eds.). *Effects of nicotine on biological systems* (pp. 623–630). Basel, Switzerland: Birkhauser Verlag.

Sahakian, B., Jones, G., Levy, R., Gray, J., & Warburton, D. (1989). The effects of nicotine on attention, information processing, and short-term memory in patients with dementia of the Alzheimer type. *British Journal of Psychiatry, 154*, 797–800.

Sakurai, Y., & Kanazawa, I. (2002). Acute effects of cigarettes in non-deprived smokers on memory, calculation and executive functions. *Human Psychopharmacology, 17*, 369–373.

Sastry, B. V., Chance, M. B., Singh, G., Horn, J. L., & Janson, V. E. (1995). Distribution and retention of nicotine and its metabolite, cotinine, in the rat as a function of time. *Pharmacology, 50*, 128–136.

Schinka, J. A., Belanger, H., Mortimer, J. A., & Graves, A. B. (2003). Effects of the use of alcohol and cigarettes on cognition in elderly African American adults. *Journal of the International Neuropsychological Society, 9*, 690–697.

Schinka, J. A., Vanderploeg, R. D., Rogish, M., Graves, A. B., Mortimer, J. A., & Ordorica, P. I. (2002a). Effects of alcohol and cigarettes on cognition in elderly adults. *Journal of the International Neuropsychology Society, 8*, 811–818.

Schinka, J. A., Vanderploeg, R. D., Rogish, M., & Ordorica, P. I. (2002b). Effects of alcohol and cigarette use on cognition in middle-aged adults. *Journal of the International Neuropsychology Society, 8*, 683–690.

Schneider, N. G., Lunell, E., Olmstead, R. E., & Fagerstrom, K. O. (1996). Clinical pharmacokinetics of nasal nicotine delivery. A review and comparison to other nicotine systems. *Clinical Pharmacokinetics, 31*, 65–80.

Sherwood, N. (1993). Effects of nicotine on human psychomotor performance. *Human Psychopharmacology, 8*, 155–184.

Sherwood, N. (1995). Effects of cigarette smoking on performance in a simulated driving task. *Neuropsychobiology, 32,* 161–165.

Sherwood, N., Kerr, J. S., & Hindmarch, I. (1992). Psychomotor performance in smokers following single and repeated doses of nicotine gum. *Psychopharmacology, 108,* 432–436.

Shim, I., Javaid, J. E., Wirtshafter, D., Jang, S. Y., Shin, K. H., Lee, H. J., et al. (2001). Nicotine-induced behavioral sensitization is associated with extracellular dopamine release expression of c-Fos in the striatum and nucleus accumbens of the rat. *Behavioral Brain Research, 121,* 137–147.

Shimohama, S., Taniguchi, T., Fujiwara, M., & Kameyama, M. (1986). Changes in nicotinic and muscarinic receptors in Alzheimer-type dementia. *Journal of Neurochemistry, 46,* 288–293.

Shinton, R., & Beevers, G. (1989). Meta-analysis of the relation between cigarette smoking and stroke. *British Medical Journal, 298,* 789–794.

Shirtcliff, E. A., & Marrocco, R. T. (2003). Salivary cotinine levels in human tobacco smokers predict the attentional validity effect size during smoking abstinence. *Psychopharmacology, 166,* 11–18.

Shytle, R. D., Silver, A. A., Wilkinson, B. J., & Sanberg, P. R. (2002). A pilot controlled trial of transdermal nicotine in the treatment of attention deficit hyperactivity disorder. *World Journal of Biological Psychiatry, 3,* 150–155.

Skinhoj, E., Olesen, J., & Paulson, O. B. (1973). Influence of smoking and nicotine on cerebral blood flow and metabolic rate of oxygen in man. *Journal of Applied Physiology, 35,* 820–822.

Slater, M. D., Basil, M. D., & Maibach, E. W. (1999). A cluster analysis of alcohol-related attitudes and behaviors in the general population. *Journal of Studies on Alcohol, 60,* 667–674.

Smith, R. C., Singh, A., Infante, M., Khandat, A., & Kloos, A. (2002). Effects of cigarette smoking and nicotine nasal spray on psychiatric symptoms and cognition in schizophrenia. *Neuropsychopharmacology, 27,* 479–497.

Snaedal, J., Johannesson, T., Jonsson, J. E., & Gylfadottir, G. (1996). The effects of nicotine in dermal plaster on cognitive functions in patients with Alzheimer's disease. *Dementia, 7,* 47–52.

Snyder, F. R., Davis, F. C., & Henningfield, J. E. (1989). The tobacco withdrawal syndrome: Performance decrements assessed on a computerized test battery. *Drug and Alcohol Dependence, 23,* 259–266.

Snyder, F. R., & Henningfield, J. E. (1989). Effects of nicotine administration following 12 h of tobacco deprivation: assessment on computerized performance tasks. *Psychopharmacology, 97.* 17–22.

Spilich, G. J., June, L., & Renner, J. (1992). Cigarette smoking and cognitive performance. *British Journal of Addiction, 87,* 1313–1326.

Staley, J. K., Krishnan-Sarin, S., Zoghbi, S., Tamagnan, G., Fujita, M., Seibyl, J. P., et al. (2001). Sex differences in [^{123}I]beta-CIT SPECT measures of dopamine and serotonin transporter availability in healthy smokers and nonsmokers. *Synapse, 41,* 275–284.

Stein, E. A., Pankiewicz, J., Harsch, H. H., Cho, J., Fuller, S. A., Hoffmann, R. G., Hawkins, M., Rao, S. M., Bandettini, P. A., & Bloom, A. S. (1998). Nicotine-induced limbic cortical activation in the human brain: A functional MRI study. *American Journal of Psychiatry, 155,* 1009–1015.

Substance Abuse and Mental Health Services Administration (2001). *Summary of*

Findings from the 2000 National Household Survey on Drug Abuse, NHSDA Series H-13, DHHS Publication no. (SMA) 01-3549. Rockville, MD: Office of Applied Studies.

Sullivan, P. F., & Kendler, K. S. (1999). The genetic epidemiology of smoking. *Nicotine and Tobacco Research, 1*, S51–S57.

Sutter, T. W., Buzzi, R., Woodson, P. P., & Battig, K. (1993). Psychophysiological correlates of conflict solving and cigarette smoking. *Activitas Nervosa Superior, 25*, 261–272.

Swan, G. E., Carmelli, D., & Cardon, L. R. (1996). The consumption of tobacco, alcohol, and caffeine in Caucasian male twins: A multivariate genetic analysis. *Journal of Substance Abuse, 8*, 19–31.

Swan, G. E., DeCarli, C., Miller, B. L., Reed, T., Wolf, P. A., & Carmelli, D. (2000). Biobehavioral characteristics of nondemented older adults with subclinical brain atrophy. *Neurology, 54*, 2108–2114.

Tsushima, Y., Tanizaki, Y., Aoki, J., & Endo, K. (2002). MR detection of microhemorrhages in neurologically healthy adults. *Neuroradiology, 44*, 31–36.

Tucker, D. M., & Williamson, P. A. (1984). Asymmetric neural control systems in human self regulation. *Psychological Review, 91*, 185–215.

Turchi, J., & Sarter, M. (1997). Cortical acetylcholine and processing capacity: Effects of cortical cholinergic deafferentation on crossmodal divided attention in rats. *Cognitive Brain Research, 6*, 147–158.

Tzourio, C., Rocca, W. A., Breteler, M. M., Baldereschi, M., Dartigues, J. F., Lopez-Pousa, S., et al. (1997). Smoking and Parkinson's disease. An age-dependent risk effect? *Neurology, 49*, 1267–1272.

Upadhyaya, H. P., Brady, K. T., Wharton, M., & Liao, J. (2003). Psychiatric disorders and cigarette smoking among child and adolescent psychiatry inpatients. *American Journal of Addiction, 12*, 144–152.

US Department of Health and Human Services (1988). *The health consequences of smoking: Nicotine addiction; A report of the Surgeon General* (pp. 377–392). Rockville, MD: Centers for Disease Control, Office for Smoking and Health.

Vanderploeg, R. D., & Schinka, J. A. (1995). Predicting WAIS-R IQ premorbid ability: combining subtest performance and demographic variable predictors. *Archives of Clinical Neuropsychology, 10*, 225–239.

van Gool, C. H., Kempen, G. I., Penninx, B. W., Deeg, D. J., Beekman, A. T., & van Eijk, J. T. (2003). Relationship between changes in depressive symptoms and unhealthy lifestyles in late middle aged and older persons: Results from the Longitudinal Aging Study Amsterdam. *Age and Ageing, 32*, 81–87.

Vieregge, A., Sieberer, M., Jacobs, H., Hagenah, J. M., & Vieregge, P. (2001). Transdermal nicotine in PD: A randomized, double-blind, placebo-controlled study. *Neurology, 57*, 1032–1035.

Wall, A., Gong, Z. H., Johnson, A. E., Meyerson, B., & Zhang, X. (2000). Cross-tolerance in drug response and differential changes in central nicotinic and N-methyl-D-aspartate receptor binding following chronic treatment with either (+)- or (−)-nicotine. *Psychopharmacology, 148*, 186–195.

Warburton, D. M. (1992). Nicotine as cognitive enhancer. *Progress in NeuroPsychopharmacology and Biological Psychiatry, 16*, 181–191.

Warburton, D. M., & Arnall, C. (1994). Improvements in performance without nicotine withdrawal. *Psychopharmacology, 115*, 539–542.

Warburton, D. M., Rusted, J. M., & Fowler, J. (1992). A comparison of the attentional and consolidation hypothesis for the facilitation of memory by nicotine. *Psychopharmacology (Berlin)*, *108*, 443–447.

Warburton, D. M., Rusted, J. M., & Muller, C. (1992). Patterns of facilitation of memory by nicotine. *Behavioural Pharmacology*, *3*, 375–378.

Warburton, D. M., Skinner, A., & Martin, C. D. (2001). Improved incidental memory with nicotine after semantic processing, but not after phonological processing. *Psychopharmacology*, *153*, 258–263.

Warburton, D. M., Wesnes, K., Shergold, K., & James, M. (1986). Facilitation of learning and state dependency with nicotine. *Psychopharmacology*, *89*, 55–59.

Waters, A. J., & Sutton, S. R. (2000). Direct and indirect effects of nicotine/smoking on cognition in humans. *Addictive Behaviors*, *25*, 29–43.

Wesnes, K., & Revell, A. (1984). The separate and combined effects of scopolamine and nicotine on human information processing. *Psychopharmacology*, *84*, 5–11.

Wesnes, K., & Warburton, D. M. (1983). Effects of smoking on rapid information processing performance. *Neuropsychobiology*, *9*, 223–229.

Wesnes, K., & Warburton, D. M. (1984). Effects of scopolamine and nicotine on rapid information processing performance. *Psychopharmacology*, *82*, 147–150.

Wesnes, K., Warburton, D. M., & Matz, B. (1983). Effects of nicotine on stimulus sensitivity and response bias in a visual vigilance task. *Neuropsychobiology*, *9*, 41–44.

West, R., & Hack, S. (1991). Effect of cigarettes on memory search and subjective ratings. *Pharmacology, Biochemistry, and Behavior*, *38*, 281–286.

West, R. J., & Jarvis, M. J. (1986). Effects of nicotine on finger tapping rate in nonsmokers. *Pharmacology, Biochemistry and Behavior*, *25*, 727–731.

White, H. K., & Levin, E. D. (1999). Four week nicotine skin patch treatment effects on cognitive performance in Alzheimer's disease. *Psychopharmacology*, *143*, 158–165.

White, H. K., & Levin, E. D. (2004). Chronic trandermal nicotine patch treatment effects on cognitive performance in age-associated memory impairment. *Psychopharmacology*, *171*, 465–471.

Whitehouse, P. J., Martino, A. M., Wagster, M. V., Price, D. L., Mayeux, R., Atack, J. R., et al. (1988). Reductions in [^{3}H] nicotinic acetylcholine binding in Alzheimer's disease and Parkinson's disease: An autoradiographic study. *Neurology*, *38*, 720–723.

Wilens, T. E., Biederman, J., Spencer, T. J., Bostic, J., Prince, J., Monuteaux, M. C., et al. (1999). A pilot controlled clinical trial of ABT-418, a cholinergic agonist, in the treatment of adults with attention deficit hyperactivity disorder. *American Journal of Psychiatry*, *156*, 1931–1937.

Wilson, A. L., Langley, L. K., Monley, J., Bauer, T., Rottunda, S., Mcfalls, E., et al. (1995). Nicotine patches in Alzheimer's disease: Pilot study on learning, memory, and safety. *Pharmacology, Biochemistry and Behavior*, *51*, 509–514.

Witte, E. A., Davidson, M. C., & Marrocco, R. T. (1997). Effects of altering brain cholinergic activity on covert orienting of attention: Comparison of monkey and human performance. *Psychopharmacology (Berlin)*, *132*, 324–334.

Wittling, W. (1995). Brain asymmetry in the control of autonomic physiologic activity. In R. J. Davidson & K. Hugdahl (Eds.), *Brain asymmetry* (pp. 305–357). Cambridge, MA: MIT Press.

Wonnacott, S. (1990). The paradox of nicotinic acetylcholine receptor upregulation by nicotine. *Trends in Pharmacological Sciences*, *11*, 216–219.

Yamashita, K., Kobayashi, S., Yamaguchi, S., & Koide, H. (1996). Cigarette smoking and silent brain infarction in normal adults. *Internal Medicine*, *35*, 704–706.

Yetkin, F. Z., Fischer, M. E., Papke, R. A., & Haughton, V. M. (1993). Focal hyperintensities in cerebral white matter on MR images of asymptomatic volunteers: Correlation with social and medical histories. *American Journal of Roentgenology*, *161*, 855–858.

Zhou, H., Deng, J., Li, J., Wang, Y., Zhang, M., & He, H. (2003). Study of the relationship between cigarette smoking, alcohol drinking and cognitive impairment among elderly people in China. *Age and Ageing*, *32*, 205–210.

Zubieta, J., Lombardi, U., Minoshima, S., Guthrie, S., Ni, L., Ohl, L. E., et al. (2001). Regional cerebral blood flow effects of nicotine in overnight abstinent smokers. *Biological Psychiatry*, *49*, 906–913.

9 Opioids

Miriam Z. Mintzer and Matthew W. Johnson

Opioid drugs exert activity on the endogenous opioid system, which has multiple receptor types and ligands (Gutstein & Akil, 2001). Opioids are used medically (e.g., morphine, meperidine, fentanyl and its derivatives, dextropropoxyphene, oxycodone, codeine) for surgical anesthesia, postoperative analgesia, and chronic pain. This chapter focuses on the neuropsychological consequences of opioid abuse. Opioid abuse (primarily heroin) is a significant public health problem, with more than nine million people estimated to abuse heroin worldwide (United Nations Office on Drugs and Crime, 2004), and an estimated 119,000 current heroin users in the United States (Substance Abuse and Mental Health Services Administration, 2004). The most widespread single intervention for opioid dependence is pharmacological treatment (primarily opioid substitution pharmacotherapy) (NIH-CDC, 1997). Thus, many of the studies reviewed in this chapter involve opioid abusers being maintained on an opioid pharmacotherapy medication. Methadone, a long-acting mu-opioid agonist that is well absorbed orally, has been used as a pharmacotherapy for opioid dependence since the mid-1960s (Dole & Nyswander, 1965). Buprenorphine, a mu-opioid partial agonist and kappa antagonist, was approved recently by the Federal Drug Administration (FDA) as an opioid pharmacotherapy (October 2002). In the United States, buprenorphine is approved for sublingual administration alone and in combination with the opioid antagonist naloxone (designed to minimize intravenous abuse of buprenorphine by dependent opioid abusers). [Levomethadyl acetate (LAAM), another opioid pharmacotherapy, has been associated with serious cardiovascular complications (cf. Gonzalez et al., 2002) and was recently taken off the market in the United States.]

Laboratory studies

Pathophysiology

Nonhuman animal models

Data from nonhuman animal studies provide evidence that opioids can produce neurological impairment, as reflected in the effects of opioid administration on tasks of learning and memory, and in the morphological and histological alterations resulting from opioid exposure. These findings may represent analogues and underlying mechanisms for the performance deficits in human opioid abusers reviewed in this chapter.

A host of studies have demonstrated the adverse effects of opioids on learning and memory. For example, rats receiving chronic morphine administration followed by cessation were impaired, relative to control rats receiving vehicle administration, in an operant food acquisition task as well as in a conditioned place preference task, in which time spent in a context previously associated with food administration is measured relative to a nonpaired context (Harris & Aston-Jones, 2003). Spatial learning and memory also appear to be impaired by acute opioid administration. For example, exposure to morphine and etonitazene dose-dependently impaired food-maintained spatial memory in a radial arm maze task (Braida, Gori, & Sala, 1994). Similar results were found with methadone in the Morris water maze task of spatial memory (Hepner, Homewood, & Taylor, 2002). It is noteworthy that learning and memory are not always impaired as a result of opioid administration. For example, morphine-exposed rats upon cessation more rapidly learned to fear a tone (as demonstrated by the suppression of operant food responding) compared to control rats (Harris & Aston-Jones, 2003). This finding suggests that chronic opioid administration may be associated with improved learning for aversive stimuli. Another study found that aversive shock conditioning in a passive avoidance preparation was impaired by morphine administration at testing (retrieval), but not immediately after training (encoding) (Saha, Datta, & Sharma, 1991).

Other studies have provided evidence of central nervous system (CNS) alterations in nonhuman animals following opioid exposure. Using light microscopy, Tapia-Arizmendi, Garcia-Estrada, Feria-Velasco, and Aleman (1987) found structural changes in rats that were chronically administered morphine, relative to vehicle control rats, in brain areas unrelated to opioid receptor density. The morphological alterations were most extensive in the hippocampus, with moderate alterations in the sensory motor cortex and the caudate nucleus. Another study found changes to the cells in some of these areas as well (Garcia-Estrada, Tapia-Arizmendi, Feria-Velasco, & Aleman, 1988). Other evidence shows that rats chronically administered morphine and put into abstinence show development of specific proteins in the brainstem relative to control rats (Rönnbäck, Wikkelso, & Blomstrand, 1983). Rats treated chronically with morphine also show a reduction in dopamine cell size in the ventral tegmental area (Sklair-Tavron, Shi, Lane, Harris, Bunney, & Nestler, 1996). Other studies have demonstrated that morphine administration reduces dendritic spine density and complexity in several areas, including the nucleus accumbens shell (Robinson & Kolb, 1999, 2004). Interestingly, these decrements are more pronounced with self-administration relative to passive administration (Robinson, Gorny, Savage, & Kolb, 2002). Histological evidence suggests that opioids such as fentanyl, alfentanyl, and morphine induce seizures that cause damage in the limbic system and other areas (Ikonomidou-Turski, Cavalheiro, Turski, Bortolotto, & Turski, 1987; Kofke, Garman, Garman, & Rose, 1999; Kofke, Garman, Janosky, & Rose, 1996; Kofke, Garman, Stiller, Rose, & Garman, 1996; Kofke, Garman, Tom, Rose, & Hawkins, 1992; Sinz, Kofke, & Garman, 2000; Turski, Czuczwar, Kleinrok, Schwarz, & Turski, 1983).

Postmortem studies

Postmortem studies offer an opportunity to examine the consequences of chronic opioid abuse on the brain by identifying markers that differentiate between deceased opioid abusers and deceased nondrug-abusing controls. Comparing markers of monoamine neurotransmitters in opioid users who died of causes related to acute narcotic ingestion, and controls who died of other causes and tested negative for abused drugs, Kish and colleagues (2001) found a modest reduction of dopamine and serotonin activity in the striatum of opioid users. Although the authors note that the observed reductions are modest relative to those associated with chronic psychomotor stimulant use (cf., Wilson et al., 1996), they could nonetheless impact behavior, particularly motivational regulation (associated with dopamine) and impulsive behavior (associated with serotonin). Using Western blotting, Garcia-Sevilla, Ventayol, Busquets, La Harpe, Walzer, and Guimon (1997) found a decrease in the neurofilament (NF-L) proteins in the frontal cortex in postmortem brains of individuals who had died of a heroin or methadone overdose compared to nondrug-abusing controls (Garcia-Sevilla et al., 1997). These proteins are thought to be involved in axonal transport and neuronal morphology, suggesting that decreases in NF-L may be associated with functional impairment, particularly executive functions and other cognitive functions associated with the frontal cortex. The decrease in NF-L was not correlated with blood concentration of opioids or delay since death, indicating that the decrease is due to chronic abuse and not acute drug administration. Interestingly, the decrease in NF-L was greater in those who had died of a heroin overdose compared to a methadone overdose, suggesting that resulting cognitive impairment may be greater with chronic heroin use than chronic methadone use. In a review of postmortem opioid overdose cases, Pearson and Richter (1975) note that although a variety of abnormalities were found (such as neuronal depletion in the globus pallidus, brain edema, myelin damage, and astrocytic clasmatodendrosis), there was no consistency across individuals in these abnormalities.

Imaging studies

A variety of neuroimaging techniques have been used to examine the consequences of opioid abuse. Studies examining acute opioid administration have generally found decreased brain activation. Using positron emission tomography (PET), London et al. (1990) found that acute morphine administration decreased glucose metabolism in several cortical areas and the brain as a whole, relative to saline administration. Walsh et al. (1994) found that acute buprenorphine administration reduced global cerebral glucose metabolism. Functional magnetic resonance imaging (fMRI) revealed the presence of decreased activation in the visual cortex as a response to visual stimulation following acute heroin administration (Sell, Simmons, Lemmens, Williams, Brammer, & Strang, 1997).

Observational studies comparing opioid abusers (mostly opioid pharmacotherapy patients or current illicit opioid abusers) to controls have found hypoperfusion (i.e., decreased cerebral blood flow) and other brain abnormalities in opioid abusers. Using single photon emission computed tomography (SPECT), Pezawas et al. (2002) found hypoperfusion in several brain areas, particularly in the prefrontal cortex, in current dependent opioid abusers (a mixed group of methadone maintenance patients and active illicit opioid abusers) compared to nondrug-abusing controls. Additionally, the lateral asymmetry previously observed under nondrug conditions was reversed in the opioid abusers for several cortical areas, such that increased blood flow was observed in the right hemisphere relative to the left hemisphere in the controls, and in the left hemisphere relative to the right hemisphere in the opioid abusers. Danos et al. (1998) also employed SPECT and found hypoperfusion in dependent opioid abusers (most of whom had received levomethadone at the time of scanning) in specific areas that varied across participants (predominantly in the temporal and parietal lobes); however, the lack of a control group makes these results difficult to interpret. Using SPECT, Krystal et al. (1995) found that dependent opioid abusers had lower activity (relative to whole-brain activity) in the parietal and frontal lobes and greater activity in the thalamus compared to nondrug-abusing controls. Another study used phosphorus magnetic resonance spectroscopy to demonstrate that methadone maintenance patients had abnormal brain metabolism and phospholipid balance relative to nondrug-abusing controls (Kaufman et al., 1999). Computerized tomography (CT) was used to show that dependent opioid abusers in an outpatient treatment program (some on methadone or morphine pharmacotherapy, and others undergoing detoxification) had ventricular and cortical volume loss compared to nondrug-abusing controls (Pezawas et al., 1998). Interestingly, frontal lobe loss was greater for opioid abusers who were unable to remain abstinent for one year following previous detoxification attempts, compared to those able to remain abstinent for over a year in previous attempts. Strang and Gurling (1989) found signs of brain atrophy in long-term dependent opioid abusers (who were currently abusing heroin, or had recently stopped) using CT; however, there was no consistent pattern of abnormality. Other studies have failed to find volume loss in dependent opioid abusers (e.g., Amass, Nardin, Mendelson, Teoh, & Woods, 1992; Hill & Mikhael, 1979); however, these studies have been criticized on methodological grounds (Pezawas et al., 1998).

Other studies have utilized neuroimaging techniques to show that the brain changes observed in opioid abusers are partially attenuated with methadone maintenance. Using Doppler sonography, Herning, Better, Tate, Umbricht, Preston, and Cadet (2003) found that polydrug abusers (some on methadone maintenance and others not) had greater blood resistance than nondrug-abusing controls; however, the resistance was lower for those polydrug abusers on methadone. Using PET, Galynker et al. (2000) found decreased glucose metabolism in the anterior cingulate gyrus in dependent opioid abusers not on methadone relative to nondrug-abusing controls. The levels of glucose metabolism in dependent opioid abusers on methadone were intermediate between those of the other two groups. These findings suggest that the brain changes associated with methadone maintenance may be of a lower magnitude than those associated with illicit opioid abuse (cf. Postmortem studies).

Imaging studies have also detected abnormalities during opioid antagonist-precipitated withdrawal (Krystal et al., 1995). Other studies have examined the brain changes that are still present after acute withdrawal symptoms have subsided. Rose et al. (1996) found hypoperfusion in frontal, temporal, and parietal lobes in dependent opioid abusers one week after cessation of heroin use. Two weeks later, a subsequent scan revealed increased blood flow, suggesting that the blood flow abnormalities observed in opioid dependence may resolve when abstinence is sustained; however, this interpretation is complicated by the fact that the initially observed abnormalities may have reflected opioid withdrawal rather than long-term opioid abuse. Moreover, using SPECT, Gerra et al. (1998) found hypoperfusion in dependent opioid abusers who had been abstinent for four months, suggesting that brain changes may persist during abstinence. Interestingly, psychiatric comorbidity moderated these findings such that hypoperfusion was observed in the right frontal and left temporal lobes in opioid abusers with comorbid depression, and in the right frontal lobe only in those with antisocial personality disorder.

Intoxication and withdrawal

Effects of intoxication on cognitive and psychomotor performance: Observational studies

This section reviews observational studies that examined performance (using standardized neuropsychological batteries or other measures of cognitive and/or psychomotor performance) in groups of opioid abusers with current active opioid use relative to various control groups. In most of these studies, opioid-abuser participants consisted of individuals being maintained on an opioid [i.e., methadone, levo-alpha-acetylmethadol (LAAM), buprenorphine] as part of a pharmacotherapy treatment program, but in a few studies active illicit opioid abusers were included. Study details and a summary of results are presented in Table 9.1.

Table 9.1 Observational studies of cognitive and psychomotor performance in opioid abusers with current opioid use

Study	Groups (n)[a]	Opioid pharmacotherapy daily dose[b]	Measures	Results[c]
Rothenberg et al., 1977	MMP (12) Nondrug abusers (12)	(20–70 mg)	Sustained attention, simple visual RT	Unimpaired
Darke et al., 2000	MMP (30) Nondrug abusers (30)	78.6 mg (15–200)	Battery	Impaired on all measures except premorbid intelligence
Specka et al., 2000	MMP (54) Nondrug abusers (54)	93 mg (10–240)	Act-React Test System	Impaired
Mintzer & Stitzer, 2002	MMP (18) Nondrug abusers (21)	67.2 mg (12–100)	Battery	Impaired: psychomotor performance, working memory, metamemory, decision-making
Rotheram-Fuller et al., 2004	MMP/smokers (9) MMP/nonsmokers (9) Nondrug/smokers (9) Nondrug/nonsmokers (10)	Smokers: 68.0 mg (SD: 15.4) Nonsmokers: 55.3 mg (SD: 24.0)	Decision-making, WCST	Impaired: decision-making (MMP smokers)
Madden et al., 1997	BMP (18) Nondrug abusers (38)	Not reported	Delay discounting	Impaired: greater impulsivity
Petry, Bickel, & Arnett, 1998	BMP (34) Nondrug abusers (59)	Not reported	Decision-making	Impaired
Kirby et al., 1999	Opioid abusers (56) Nondrug abusers (60)	Not reported	Delay discounting	Impaired: greater impulsivity

Rounsaville et al., 1982	Opioid abusers (72) Nondrug abusers (29) Epileptics (60)	NA	Battery	Unimpaired
Guerra et al., 1987	Opioid abusers (93) Nondrug abusers (31)	NA	Battery	Impaired: attention, verbal fluency, short-term memory
Strang & Gurling, 1989[d]	Opioid abusers (7)	NA	Battery	Impaired on all measures except visual perception, premorbid intelligence
Gritz et al., 1975	MMP (10) Abstinent abusers (10)	Median: 65 mg (quartile range: 35–85)	Battery	Impaired: perception, word memory (hard, but not easy words), story memory (recall, but not recognition)
Moskowitz & Robinson, 1985	MMP (Exp 1: 12; Exp 2: 15) Abstinent abusers (Exp 1: 12; Exp 2: 15)	(60–100 mg)	Tracking	Unimpaired
Robinson & Moskowitz, 1985	MMP (Exp 1: 15; Exp 2: 12) Abstinent abusers (Exp 1: 16; Exp 2: 12)	(60–80 mg)	Divided attention, visual search, tachistoscopic information processing	Impaired: rate of information processing
Gordon, 1970	MMP (27) Abstinent abusers (39) Nondrug abusers (29)	100 mg	Simple and choice RT	Unimpaired
Appel & Gordon, 1976	MMP (48) Abstinent abusers (24) Nondrug abusers (24)	Not reported	DSST	Unimpaired

(Continued Overleaf)

Table 9.1 (Continued)

Study	Groups (n)[a]	Opioid pharmacotherapy daily dose[b]	Measures	Results[c]
Appel, 1982	MMP (48) Abstinent abusers (24) Nondrug abusers (24)	Modal: 100 mg (70–120)	Sustained attention	Unimpaired
Davis et al., 2002	MMP (15) Abstinent abusers (16) Nondrug abusers (14)	32.5 mg (15–60)	Battery	Impaired: verbal fluency (MMP < abstinent abusers)
Mintzer, Copersino, & Stitzer, 2004[e]	MMP (18) Abstinent abusers (21) Nondrug abusers (20)	67.2 mg (12–100)	Battery	Impaired: conceptual flexibility (MMP < abstinent abusers)
Grevert et al., 1977	MMP (30) LAAM patients (31) Nondrug abusers (26)	MMP: 52 mg (20–80) LAAM patients (3×/wk): (15–100 mg)	Verbal memory, spatial memory	Unimpaired
Soyka et al., 2001	MMP (28) BMP (13)	MMP: 68 mg BMP: 6.5 mg (SD: 5.8)	Act-React Test System	MMP < BMP
Schindler et al., 2004[f]	MMP (15) BMP (15) Nondrug abusers	MMP: 45.7 mg (SD: 21.4) BMP: 10.0 mg (SD: 3.9)	Act-React Test System	MMP < BMP
Korin, 1974	Opioid abusers (27) Nonopioid drug abusers (17)	NA	Bender-Gestalt test	Opioid abusers < nonopioid drug abusers

Hill et al., 1979[g]	Opioid abusers (70; 43 current) Alcohol abusers (23) Nondrug abusers (14)	NA	Battery	Alcohol abusers < opioid abusers < nondrug abusers
Rogers et al., 1999	Opioid abusers (13; 10 MMP) Amphetamine abusers (18) Nondrug abusers (26)	39.5 mg (SD: 9.4)	Decision-making	Impaired: see text for details
Ornstein et al., 2000[h]	Opioid abusers (22; 20 MMP) Amphetamine abusers (23) Nondrug abusers (22)	Not reported	CANTAB battery	Impaired: see text for details

Note: MMP, methadone maintenance patients; BMP, buprenorphine maintenance patients; SD, standard deviation; NA, not applicable; Battery, study used a performance testing battery that included four or more measures (see text for details); RT, reaction time; WCST, Wisconsin Card Sorting Test; CANTAB, Cambridge Neuropsychological Test Automated Battery; DSST, Digit Symbol Substitution Test; LAAM, levo-alpha-acetylmethadol.

[a] Number of participants in each group.
[b] Mean (range in parentheses), unless otherwise noted.
[c] Results of statistical comparison of current opioid abuser group vs. control group, unless otherwise noted; < indicates poorer performance.
[d] The performance of each individual opioid abuser was compared to the mean of a normal age-matched general population sample, and impairment was measured in terms of number of standard deviations from the norm.
[e] See Mintzer & Stitzer (2002) above for results of MMP vs. nondrug abuser comparison.
[f] Each maintenance group participant was matched with a group of nondrug-abusing controls; MMP and BMP were not directly compared but results suggested greater impairment relative to controls in MMP than in BMP (see text for details).
[g] Conclusions regarding differences between opioid abusers and nondrug abusers are based on the current opioid abuser subgroup; conclusions regarding differences between opioid abusers and alcohol abusers are based on the entire opioid abuser group (see text for details).
[h] Different groups of nondrug abusers (each $n = 22$) served as controls for different tasks.

OPIOID ABUSERS VERSUS NONDRUG-ABUSING CONTROLS

A number of studies have examined the performance of methadone maintenance patients (MMP) relative to nondrug-abusing controls (i.e., individuals with no known history of drug abuse). Rothenberg, Schottenfeld, Meyer, Krauss, and Gross (1977) compared MMP who reported having had little or no drug use (other than methadone) for at least one month prior to testing (confirmed via urine analysis), to nondrug-abusing controls in a similar age range. Relative to controls, MMP were unimpaired on a continuous performance test (measuring sustained attention) and actually exhibited *shorter* reaction times on a simple visual reaction time task. While these results provide no evidence for impairment in MMP, interpretation is somewhat limited by the absence of information about matching of the two groups on variables that might affect performance (e.g., years of education, IQ) and the limited range of measures.

Using a standardized neuropsychological battery, Darke, Sims, McDonald, and Wickes (2000) examined the performance of MMP relative to nondrug abusers matched with respect to age, gender, and years of education. The battery included measures of premorbid intelligence, psychomotor performance, information processing, attention, short-term memory, long-term memory, and problem-solving. While the groups did not differ with respect to premorbid intelligence, MMP performed significantly worse than controls on all other measures. The wide range of impaired functions is striking. However, conclusions based on this study are limited for the following reasons. First, a urine drug screen was not performed prior to neuropsychological testing. A larger proportion of MMP than controls in the study reported current use of a variety of drugs, including benzodiazepines which have well-documented performance-impairing effects (see Curran, 2000, for a review); thus, it is difficult to differentiate effects of opioid use from other acute drug effects. Second, there was an exceptionally high prevalence of reported head injury in the MMP group (67% compared to only 20% for controls), which may also have contributed to impaired performance in MMP. Third, testing was conducted prior to daily methadone dosing, raising the possibility that some MMP may have been in early withdrawal during testing.

Using a standardized battery developed by the Austrian Road Safety Board to assess driving-related skills (Act & React Test System), Specka, Finkbeiner, Lodemann, Leifert, Kluwig, and Gastpar (2000) examined the performance of MMP relative to nondrug abusers matched with respect to age, gender, and years of education. An important strength of the study is the relatively large sample size. MMP were impaired relative to controls on a tachistoscopic perception task, a 7-min task in which participants are asked to decide whether comparison patterns are identical to or different from target patterns, and a task requiring the capacity to integrate information under high-pressure conditions. On a choice reaction time task, MMP were faster than controls but produced more errors. On two tasks requiring visual tracking, MMP were more accurate but slower. Although a urine drug screen was performed prior to performance testing, MMP with a positive drug screen (38 out of 54 MMP) were not excluded, again making it difficult to differentiate effects of opioid use from other acute drug effects. It is important to note, however, that analyses comparing MMP with positive drug screens versus negative drug screens at the time of performance testing revealed no significant differences in performance.

In a study conducted in our laboratory (Mintzer & Stitzer, 2002), we examined the performance of MMP relative to nondrug abusers matched with respect to gender, race, age, years of education, current employment status, current reading level, and estimated IQ score. Recent drug abstinence was verified by urine analysis. MMP exhibited impairment relative to controls in psychomotor speed [as assessed by the Digit Symbol Substitution test (DSST) and computerized trail-making tests], working memory (as assessed by the 2-back task, which requires participants to temporarily maintain in memory and continuously update the identity and order of the two previous letters in a sequence of letters presented consecutively on the screen), decision-making [as assessed by a computerized version of the gambling task (Bechara, Damasio, Damasio, & Anderson, 1994; Bechara, Damasio, Tranel, & Anderson, 1998; Bechara, Tranel, & Damasio, 2000), which requires the evaluation of long-term consequences of current decisions], and meta-memory (awareness and knowledge of one's own memory). Results also suggested possible impairment in inhibitory mechanisms (Stroop color-word task), although the effect was not statistically significant. MMP did not exhibit impairment in time estimation, conceptual flexibility, or episodic memory. Like the Darke et al. (2000) study, these results provide evidence for impairment in a wide range of functions.

A few recent studies have specifically examined decision-making in opioid pharmacotherapy patients. Rotheram-Fuller, Shoptaw, Berman, and London (2004) examined performance on a version of Bechara's gambling task as well as the Wisconsin Card Sorting Task (WCST: a measure of conceptual thinking and flexibility) for four groups, matched with respect to age, gender, and estimated IQ score: methadone-maintained tobacco smokers and nonsmokers, and control (nondrug-abusing) smokers and nonsmokers. While there were no significant differences among groups in WCST performance, methadone-maintained smokers (but not nonsmokers) were significantly impaired on the gambling task relative to both control groups. An analysis comparing the two MMP groups indicated that the smokers were also significantly impaired relative to the nonsmokers. These results are consistent with Mintzer and Stitzer's (2002) findings with the gambling task, but additionally suggest that tobacco smoking may be a risk factor for decision-making impairment in MMP. Interestingly, the differences among groups disappeared when participants performed the gambling task a second time after being informed of the optimal strategy for performing the task. This pattern suggests that the impairment in smoking MMP is related to deficient strategy learning rather than to continued use of suboptimal decision-making strategies, despite awareness of consequences. Although MMP were encouraged to abstain from other drug use throughout the study, participants who reported drug use were not excluded, again making it difficult to differentiate effects of opioid use from other acute drug effects.

Madden, Petry, Badger, and Bickel (1997) and Petry, Bickel, and Arnett (1998) examined decision-making in dependent opioid abusers being maintained on daily buprenorphine (buprenorphine maintenance patients: BMP) as participants in clinical trials for buprenorphine. Kirby, Petry, and Bickel (1999) examined decision-making in dependent opioid abusers enrolled in a clinic that offered buprenorphine and naltrexone (antagonist) treatment. Using the delay-discounting task, Madden et al. (1997) compared the rate of temporal discounting of monetary rewards in BMP to that of nondrug-abusing controls matched with respect to age, gender, education, and estimated IQ. BMP discounted the subjective value of hypothetical delayed monetary rewards significantly more (reflecting greater impulsivity) than did controls. Kirby et al. (1999) extended this result to show that opioid abusers also discounted the value of *real* delayed monetary rewards significantly more than age-matched nondrug-abusing controls. Petry, Bickel, and Arnett (1998) compared the performance of BMP to that of nondrug-abusing controls matched with respect to age, gender, education, and estimated IQ on a version of Bechara's gambling task and on the Future Perspective Task (FPT) in which participants are asked to make predictions about the timing and ordering of future events. BMP were less likely than controls to predict events far into the future and to systematically organize events in the future on the FPT (suggesting a shortened time horizon) and were impaired relative to controls on the gambling task [consistent with the Mintzer & Stitzer (2002) and Rotheram-Fuller et al. (2004) studies described above]. No information is provided about the current drug use of the opioid-abuser participants and no urine drug screens are reported prior to testing in these studies, again making it difficult to differentiate effects of opioid use from other acute drug effects.

A few studies have included opioid abusers with current active illicit opioid use (not being maintained on an opioid pharmacotherapy medication). Rounsaville, Jones, Novelly, and Kleber (1982) examined performance on a neuropsychological battery (which included measures of grip strength, rapid alternating movement, rapid visual–tactual motor integration, visual–perceptual function, visual search, speech–language function, new associative learning, and intelligence), of dependent opioid abusers early in treatment ($n = 15$ still using opioids; $n = 37$ recently initiated methadone maintenance; $n = 20$ recently detoxified and participating in treatment) relative to two control groups: nondrug abusers of similar socioeconomic status and patients with epilepsy. Both control groups were matched to the opioid-abuser group with respect to gender, age, education, and handedness. The opioid-abuser group exhibited comparable or superior performance relative to the two control groups, providing no evidence for impairment. Although interpretation of the results is complicated by the inclusion of both current and detoxified users in the opioid-abuser group, it should be noted that analyses comparing opioid abusers with positive versus negative opioid urine screens at the time of neuropsychological testing revealed no significant differences in neuropsychological performance.

Guerra, Sole, Cami, and Tobena (1987) examined the performance of dependent opioid abusers prior to their admission to a detoxification unit, relative to a group of nondrug-abusing controls who were reported to have similar demographic, educational, and cultural characteristics, and similar intelligence (although the actual values are not presented in the paper). At the time of testing, some of the opioid abusers reported acute opioid effects and others reported drug abstinence for a few hours; however, no drug urine screens are reported prior to neuropsychological testing. The opioid-abuser group exhibited impairment relative to controls on all measures on an abbreviated neuropsychological battery (attention, verbal fluency, short-term memory) except long-term memory. Analyses comparing opioid abusers reporting acute opioid effects versus those reporting brief drug abstinence, and comparing opioid abusers reporting heavy heroin use during the week before screening for treatment (defined as more than 500 mg) versus lighter heroin use (defined as less than 500 mg), revealed no significant differences in neuropsychological performance. One limitation of the study is that the opioid abusers were reported to have used barbiturates, other sedatives, and alcohol occasionally and yet no drug urine or breath alcohol tests are reported, making it difficult to differentiate effects of opioid use from other acute drug effects.

Strang and Gurling (1989) examined the performance of an older group of long-term dependent opioid abusers (mean age: 54, range: 40–61; mean duration of heroin abuse: 32 years, range: 20–43) using the computerized Bexley/Maudsley Automated Psychological Screening Battery [which includes measures of visual spatial ability, psychomotor speed (symbol digit coding), visual perceptual analysis, verbal recognition memory, and visual spatial recognition memory], the Bexley/Maudsley Category Sorting Test (which measures conceptual thinking and flexibility; similar to the WCST), the Nelson Adult Reading Test (NART: a measure of premorbid verbal intelligence), and a tactual performance test. At the time of testing, three out of the seven opioid abusers had just recently stopped using opioids, while the remaining four were still abusing opioids; however, no drug urine screens are reported prior to neuropsychological testing. The performance of each individual opioid abuser was compared to the mean of a normal age-matched general population sample. Five of the seven opioid abusers showed considerable neuropsychological impairment. The measures exhibiting greatest impairment were the symbol digit coding test and the verbal recognition memory test, with several participants scoring more than two standard deviations below the norm on these measures. The only measures on which no impairment was reported for any participant were the NART and the visual perception test.

OPIOID ABUSERS WITH CURRENT USE VERSUS ABSTINENT OPIOID ABUSERS

In the studies reviewed above, opioid abusers were compared to nondrug-abusing controls only, making it difficult to differentiate the effects of current opioid use from the effects of a history of long-term opioid abuse. This section reviews studies that included abstinent opioid abusers (i.e., individuals with a history of long-term opioid abuse, but with no current use) as controls.

Using a broad range of measures, Gritz et al. (1975) examined the performance of MMP relative to a control group of former opioid abusers residing in an abstinence colony. The groups did not differ significantly with respect to level of education. Recent drug abstinence was verified in both groups via urine analysis. MMP were impaired relative to controls on measures of perception, story memory (assessed via recall), and memory for difficult pairs of words, but unimpaired on immediate digit span, story memory (assessed via recognition), object recognition memory, memory for easy pairs of words, and the DSST. Robinson and Moskowitz found that MMP were unimpaired, relative to abstinent opioid abusers in a similar age range, on tracking (Moskowitz & Robinson, 1985), divided attention, and visual search tasks (Robinson & Moskowitz, 1985), but that the rate of processing of tachistoscopically-presented information was reduced in the MMP (Robinson & Moskowitz, 1985). Recent drug abstinence was verified in both groups via urine analysis. Gordon and Appel found that MMP were unimpaired relative to control groups of abstinent opioid abusers and nondrug-abusing controls on the DSST (Appel & Gordon, 1976) and the continuous performance task (Appel, 1982), and exhibited comparable or shorter reaction times relative to controls on visual reaction time tasks (Gordon, 1970). Recent drug abstinence was verified via urine analysis.

Davis, Liddiard, and McMillan (2002) examined performance on a neuropsychological battery (which included measures of attention, spatial and verbal learning, immediate and delayed spatial and verbal recall, verbal fluency, and conceptual flexibility) of MMP relative to abstinent opioid abusers enrolled in drug-free treatment programs and nondrug-abusing controls (pain management patients). The MMP and abstinent opioid abusers did not differ significantly in terms of age or estimated IQ score, and had similar histories of drug abuse. MMP were significantly impaired relative to abstinent opioid abusers on the verbal fluency task (a measure of semantic memory, left frontal lobe function), and the overall incidence of impaired performance (defined as a score of two or more standard deviations below published norms on two or more neuropsychological measures) in the abstinent opioid abusers (31%) fell between that in the MMP (60%; highest incidence of impairment) and that in the nondrug-abusing controls (7%: lowest incidence of impairment). The incidence of impairment was significantly different in the MMP versus control groups, but no other paired comparisons were significant. Although the incidence of impairment in the abstinent opioid abuser group was not significantly different from that in the MMP group, the pattern of results suggests that current methadone maintenance may be associated with additional impairment over and above that associated with long-term opioid abuse. It should be noted that no information is provided about the current drug use of the MMP and no drug urine screens are reported prior to testing, making it difficult to differentiate effects of opioid use from other acute drug effects.

We recently completed a study in our laboratory (Mintzer, Copersino, & Stitzer, 2005) in which we compared performance of a control group of currently abstinent, formerly dependent opioid abusers retrospectively to our earlier groups (MMP and nondrug-abusing controls; Mintzer & Stitzer, 2002; cf. previous section on opioid abusers vs. nondrug-abusing controls) on the same battery of performance measures. Consistent with the Davis et al. (2002) study, performance of the abstinent opioid abusers fell between that of the MMP and nondrug-abusing controls on most measures, although MMP were only significantly impaired relative to the abstinent opioid abusers on one measure (conceptual flexibility). While conclusions based on retrospective comparisons are inherently limited, it is important to note that the MMP and abstinent opioid abusers did not differ significantly with respect to gender, race, mean age, years of education, current reading level, or estimated IQ, and had similar histories of drug abuse.

COMPARISONS OF OPIOID ABUSERS BEING MAINTAINED ON DIFFERENT OPIOID PHARMACOTHERAPY MEDICATIONS

A few studies have compared the performance of dependent opioid abusers being maintained on different opioid pharmacotherapy medications. Using an elegant mixed design, Grevert, Masover, and Goldstein (1977) tested the memory performance of MMP and patients being maintained on LAAM at three separate timepoints: prior to beginning pharmacotherapy, and following one and three months of pharmacotherapy. A control group of nondrug abusers who were matched to individual MMP participants with respect to age, gender, education, ethnicity, and employment status were tested at similar intervals. There were no significant differences among groups at any of the three timepoints and no differences within either pharmacotherapy group at the later timepoints relative to pretreatment performance.

Two recent studies examined the performance of patients being maintained on methadone versus buprenorphine (Schindler, Ortner, Peternell, Eder, Opgenoorth, & Fischer, 2004; Soyka, Horak, Dittert, & Kagerer, 2001). As a partial agonist, buprenorphine may produce less performance impairment than full agonists such as methadone and LAAM. Soyka et al. (2001) retrospectively compared the performance of BMP to that of MMP who had been previously tested on the same standardized battery developed by the Austrian Road Safety Board to assess driving-related skills (Act & React Test System: ART-90). MMP exhibited significant impairment relative to BMP on a 7-minute task in which participants are asked to decide whether comparison patterns are identical to or different from target patterns, a task requiring the capacity to integrate information under high-pressure conditions, and a choice reaction time task. Although these results support the hypothesis of less performance impairment with buprenorphine than methadone, conclusions are limited due to the absence of controlled procedures and matching of patients in the two groups.

Schindler et al. (2004) also used a version of the Act & React Test System (ART 2020) to examine the performance of MMP and BMP. Each maintenance group participant was matched with a group of nondrug-abusing controls ($n = 3–56$; the median performance score for the control group was then compared to that of the matched maintenance group participant) with respect to age, gender, and score on a measure of intelligence. The controls were selected from a sample of people who had previously completed the ART 2020 battery. The combined MMP and BMP group exhibited significantly longer mean reaction and decision times relative to controls on a task in which participants are required to respond as quickly as possible to specific stimuli appearing in a video sequence of a city drive from the driver's perspective. In addition, the percentage of incorrect responses was significantly higher in the combined MMP and BMP group relative to controls on a 7-minute task in which participants are asked to decide whether comparison patterns are identical to or different from target patterns. However, the overall number of responses and the number of correct responses were also significantly higher in the combined groups, making this result somewhat difficult to interpret. There were no significant differences between the combined group and the controls on the other four tasks of the ART 2020 battery.

Analyses comparing each pharmacotherapy group separately to controls revealed that the MMP group exhibited the same pattern of impairment relative to controls as described above in the combined group, whereas the BMP group exhibited significant differences relative to controls only on the 7-minute pattern-comparison task (increases in percentage of incorrect responses only). The authors suggest that MMP (and BMP to a lesser degree) may sacrifice accuracy for speed. Although these results support the hypothesis of less performance impairment with buprenorphine than methadone, conclusions are limited for the following reasons. First, the MMP and BMP groups were not directly compared because they were not matched. Second, conclusions regarding differences between MMP and BMP are complicated by the fact that testing began 22 hours after last medication dosing; given the half-life differences between methadone and buprenorphine, it is more likely that MMP than BMP may have started to experience opioid withdrawal symptoms during the test battery, making it difficult to differentiate drug effects from early drug withdrawal effects. Third, although a urine drug screen was performed prior to performance testing, participants with positive drug screens for other drugs were not excluded, making it difficult to differentiate effects of opioid use from other acute drug effects. In fact, MMP/BMP with positive drug screens at the time of neuropsychological testing exhibited greater impairment relative to controls than those with negative drug screens.

OPIOID ABUSERS VERSUS NONOPIOID DRUG ABUSERS

As discussed earlier, some of the studies reviewed above included opioid abusers who also used other (nonopioid) drugs, making it difficult to differentiate effects of opioid abuse from other acute drug effects, particularly when drug urine screens were not reported prior to performance testing. The specificity of the effects of opioid abuse on performance is examined in this section by reviewing studies that examined the performance of opioid abusers relative to abusers of nonopioid drugs.

Using the Bender-Gestalt test (in which participants are asked to reproduce designs presented on cards), Korin (1974) compared inpatient male veterans who had used opioids primarily, but also other drugs, to a group of hospitalized male veterans in the same Veterans Administration hospital who had used nonopioid drugs only and who were reported to be in a similar age range with comparable education levels. The opioid-abuser group exhibited greater impairment than the nonopioid-abuser group. Analyses within the opioid group revealed no performance differences between patients who had been drug free for 1–3 months ($n = 14$) and those who had been using opioids ($n = 13$) when they were admitted to the hospital. Interpretation of the results is complicated by the absence of a nondrug-abusing control group and the inclusion of patients with psychiatric disorders (e.g., schizophrenia).

Using Raven's Progressive Matrices and selected subtests from the Halstead-Reitan Battery, Hill, Reyes, Mikhael, and Ayre (1979) examined the neuropsychological performance of male opioid abusers (without alcohol abuse or extensive abuse of other drugs), alcohol abusers (without opioid abuse or extensive abuse of other drugs), and nondrug-abusing controls who were matched to the opioid and heroin abusers with respect to age, education, race, and socioeconomic status. For purposes of comparison with the nondrug-abusing controls, the opioid and alcohol groups were further subdivided into current users (for the opioid group, defined as those who had abused opioids within the last two months, including those in methadone maintenance) and those in remission (for the opioid group, defined as those who had not abused opioids for at least two months). On Raven's Progressive Matrices (designed to measure abstract cognitive functioning) and the Category subtest (designed to measure abstracting ability and conceptual shifting), the current opioid abusers were impaired relative to controls. On the Tactual Performance subtest, the current opioid abusers were slower than controls in completing the initial task (in which blindfolded participants are required to fit wooden blocks of various shapes into a board) but were unimpaired relative to controls on the subsequent memory test for the identity and location of each shape on the wooden board. The current opioid abusers did not exhibit impairment on the Finger Oscillation subtest, a simple psychomotor task. Results from the group of opioid abusers in remission will be presented in a later section (Residual effects). Comparison of the opioid and alcohol groups as a whole (i.e., including both current users and those in remission) indicated that the opioid group performed significantly better than the alcohol group.

Two recent studies examined performance of opioid abusers (mostly MMP in both studies) relative to amphetamine abusers (Ornstein et al., 2000; Rogers et al. 1999). Using a novel computerized decision-making task, Rogers et al (1999) examined the performance of opioid abusers relative to amphetamine abusers and nondrug-abusing controls. The groups were matched with respect to age and estimated IQ. Both the opioid and amphetamine abusers took significantly longer to deliberate about their decisions than controls. However, a difference between the drug groups also emerged such that the amphetamine abusers made optimal decisions less often than the opioid abusers. In addition, the percentage of optimal decisions was negatively correlated with years of drug abuse for the amphetamine abusers but not the opioid abusers. Using a neuropsychological battery that included some tasks from the Cambridge neuropsychological test automated battery (CANTAB), Ornstein et al. (2000) examined the performance of opioid abusers relative to amphetamine abusers and nondrug-abusing controls. The groups were matched with respect to age and estimated IQ. The drug-abuser groups combined performed significantly worse relative to controls on a pattern recognition memory test (both accuracy and speed measures), were significantly slower on the Tower of London task (a measure of planning), and showed overall impaired performance relative to controls on an attentional set-shifting task (similar to the WCST) and on a visuospatial strategy task. On the attentional set-shifting task, differences between the drug groups also emerged such that the opioid abusers were impaired relative to the amphetamine abusers in the initial intradimensional shift stage (which involves abstraction and learning of a set), whereas the amphetamine abusers were impaired relative to the opioid abusers in the extradimensional shift stage (which involves shifting set; comparable to the category shift in the WCST). In addition, the opioid abusers were impaired relative to the amphetamine abusers in efficient strategy use on a spatial working memory task, and showed less improvement following training on a visuospatial strategy task. The suggestion that abuse of different drugs results in different patterns of impairment is intriguing. However, it should be noted that although care was taken in both studies to ensure that drug abusers were not acutely intoxicated or in withdrawal at the time of testing, drug urine screens were not conducted prior to performance testing.

SUMMARY

The results of observational studies comparing opioid abusers with current active opioid drug use (mostly opioid pharmacotherapy patients) to nondrug abusers or abstinent opioid abusers are inconsistent, with some studies showing impairment in a wide range of functions and some providing no evidence for impairment. However, two conclusions that are supported by several different studies may be drawn. First, opioid abusers appear to exhibit impairment in processing information when performing at high speeds. Given Schindler et al. (2004)'s suggestion that MMP (and BMP to a lesser degree) may sacrifice accuracy for speed, this conclusion is not inconsistent with reports of shorter reaction times for opioid abusers in some reaction time tasks (Gordon, 1970; Rothenberg et al., 1977). Second, opioid abusers appear to exhibit impairment in decision-making tasks. The results of the two studies that compared opioid abusers being maintained on methadone versus buprenorphine provide some support for the hypothesis of less impairment with buprenorphine than methadone, although conclusions are limited due to methodological issues and further research is needed. The results of the few studies comparing opioid abusers to nonopioid drug abusers suggest that opioid abusers are less impaired than alcohol abusers and exhibit a different pattern of impairment relative to amphetamine abusers.

It is important to note that although observational studies can provide valuable, clinically relevant information about performance impairment, the conclusions that can be drawn are limited due to difficulties in differentiating impairments attributable to acute opioid dosing, chronic opioid dosing, polydrug abuse, and other confounding factors (e.g., differences in personality, brain dysfunction, environment). Furthermore, observational studies do not enable differentiation of impairments that are a consequence of opioid abuse versus impairments that predated the opioid abuse. In the case of the observed decision-making deficits, it is possible that the impairment may have predated the opioid abuse and in fact even played a role in its development, rather than being a consequence of the abuse. The next section reviews experimental studies involving performance testing following administration of opioids to opioid abusers.

Effects of intoxication on cognitive and psychomotor performance: Drug administration studies

ACUTE EFFECTS (DEPENDENT OPIOID ABUSERS)

This section reviews studies in which participants were physically dependent on opioids at the time of testing. Given the risk of withdrawal in this population, studies in dependent opioid abusers of the acute effects of opioids typically maintain participants daily on an opioid (e.g., morphine, hydromorphone, methadone, buprenorphine) and examine the acute effects of the test opioid(s) relative to acute placebo administration, during stable opioid maintenance. Study details and a summary of results are presented in Table 9.2.

Table 9.2 Studies of acute effects of opioid drug administration on cognitive and psychomotor performance

Study	Participants (n)	Maintenance drug (dose/day)	Acute test drug	Measures	Results[a]
Lamas et al., 1994	Dependent (6)	Methadone 30 mg PO	Morphine 20–60 mg IM	Maddox Wing	Unimpaired
Preston, Bigelow, Bickel, & Liebson, 1987	Dependent (4)	Methadone 40 or 50 mg PO	Hydromorphone 2.5–14 mg IM	DSST	Unimpaired
Preston et al., 1988a	Dependent (6)	Methadone 30 mg PO	Hydromorphone 6 mg SC	DSST, digit recall	Unimpaired
Preston et al., 1988b	Dependent (5)	Methadone 30 mg PO	Hydromorphone 4, 8 mg IM	DSST, digit recall	Unimpaired
Preston, Bigelow, & Liebson, 1989	Dependent (5)	Methadone 30 mg PO	Hydromorphone 4, 8 mg IM	DSST, digit recall	Unimpaired
Preston et al., 1990	Dependent (5)	Methadone 30 mg PO	Hydromorphone 2.5–10 mg/70 kg IM	DSST	Impaired
Strain et al., 1992	Dependent (6)	Methadone 30 mg PO	Hydromorphone 5, 10 mg IM	DSST, digit recall	Unimpaired
Strain et al., 1993	Dependent (5)	Methadone 30 mg PO	Hydromorphone 5, 10 mg IM	DSST, digit recall	Unimpaired
Strain et al., 1996	Dependent (6)	Methadone 30 mg PO	Hydromorphone 5, 10 mg IM	DSST, digit recall	Unimpaired
Strain et al., 1997	Dependent (8)	Buprenorphine 8 mg SL	Hydromorphone 9, 18 mg IM	DSST, digit recall	Unimpaired
Stoller et al., 2001	Dependent (8)	Hydromorphone 40 mg PO	Hydromorphone 10 mg	DSST, trail-making, circular lights	Impaired: circular lights
Comer et al., 1997	Dependent (5)	Morphine 20–40 mg q.i.d. PO	Heroin 12.5–100 mg IN	Battery	Impaired (100 mg): DSST, divided attention

Study	Population (N)	Drug 1	Drug 2	Test	Result
Walsh et al., 1995	Dependent (13)	Methadone 30 or 60 mg PO	Methadone 15–60 mg PO	DSST, digit recall	Unimpaired
Rothenberg et al., 1977	MMP (12)	Methadone 20–70 mg PO	Methadone 5, 10 mg PO	Sustained attention, simple visual RT	Unimpaired
Curran et al., 1999	MMP (18)	Methadone 20–80 mg PO	Methadone 33% increase in daily dose PO	Battery	Unimpaired
Curran et al., 2001	MMP (20)	Methadone 10–50 mg b.i.d. PO	Methadone dose increase (total daily dose given at one time instead of b.i.d.) PO	Battery	Impaired: delayed prose recall
Preston et al., 1988a	Dependent (6)	Methadone 30 mg PO	Buprenorphine 0.2, 0.3 mg SC	DSST, digit recall	Unimpaired
Strain et al., 1992	Dependent (6)	Methadone 30 mg PO	Buprenorphine 0.5–8 mg IM	DSST, digit recall	Unimpaired
Walsh et al., 1995	Dependent (13)	Methadone 30 or 60 mg PO	Buprenorphine 2–8 mg SL	DSST, digit recall	Unimpaired
Strain et al., 1997	Dependent (8)	Buprenorphine 8 mg SL	Buprenorphine 4–16 mg IM	DSST, digit recall	Unimpaired
Stoller et al., 2001	Dependent (8)	Hydromorphone 40 mg PO	Buprenorphine 8 mg IM, SL	DSST, trail-making, circular lights	Unimpaired
Stoller et al., 2001	Dependent (8)	Hydromorphone 40 mg PO	Buprenorphine/naloxone 1/0.25–16/4 mg IM, SL	DSST, trail-making, circular lights	Impaired: trail-making (8/2, 16/4 mg IM), circular lights (16/4 mg IM)
Strain et al., 1996	Dependent (6)	Methadone 30 mg PO	Dezocine 7.5–60 mg IM	DSST, digit recall	Unimpaired
Preston et al., 1988b	Dependent (5)	Methadone 30 mg PO	Butorphanol 0.375–6 mg IM	DSST, digit recall	Unimpaired
Preston et al., 1990	Dependent (5)	Methadone 30 mg PO	Butorphanol 0.375–1.5 mg/70 kg IM	DSST	Unimpaired

(*Continued Overleaf*)

Table 9.2 (Continued)

Study	Participants (n)	Maintenance drug (dose/day)	Acute test drug	Measures	Results[a]
Preston, Bigelow, & Liebson, 1989	Dependent (5)	Methadone 30 mg PO	Nalbuphine 0.375–3 mg IM	DSST, digit recall	Unimpaired
Preston et al., 1990	Dependent (5)	Methadone 30 mg PO	Nalbuphine 1.05–3 mg/70 kg IM	DSST	Unimpaired
Strain et al., 1993	Dependent (5)	Methadone 30 mg PO	Pentazocine 7.5–120 mg IM	DSST, digit recall	Unimpaired
Lamas et al., 1994	Dependent (6)	Methadone 30 mg PO	Pentazocine 45, 60 mg IM	Maddox Wing	Unimpaired
Hill et al., 1952[b]	Nondependent (22)	NA	Morphine 15 mg SC	Simple visual RT	Impaired
Hill et al., 1955[c,d]	Nondependent (24)	NA	Morphine 15 mg IM	Simple visual RT	Impaired
Hill et al., 1956[c]	Nondependent (117)	NA	Morphine 15 mg IM	Simple visual RT	Results varied by incentive condition
Wikler et al., 1965	Nondependent (10)	NA	Morphine 15, 30 mg IM	Auditory RT	Impaired
Martin et al., 1974	Nondependent (12)	NA	Morphine 8–32 mg IM	Nystagmus	Impaired (32 mg)
Preston, Bigelow, & Liebson, 1987	Nondependent (5)	NA	Morphine 7.5–30 mg IM	Battery	Impaired: digit recall
Foltin & Fishman, 1992	Nondependent (9)	NA	Morphine 5, 10 mg/70 kg IV	Sequence learning	Unimpaired
Higgins et al., 1992	Nondependent (5)	NA	Morphine 4–16 mg/70 kg	DSST	Unimpaired
Petry, Bickel, Huddleston, et al., 1998	Nondependent (9)	NA	Morphine 10–100 mg PO	DSST	Impaired
Preston, Bigelow, Bickel, & Liebson, 1989	Nondependent (6)	NA	Hydromorphone 0.5–3 mg/70 kg IM	DSST	Unimpaired

Reference	Subject type (n)		Drug and dose	Task	Result
Preston et al., 1992	Nondependent (5)	NA	Hydromorphone 0.125–3 mg/70 kg IM	DSST	Unimpaired
Pickworth et al., 1997	Nondependent (8)	NA	Hydromorphone 1, 3 mg PO	Battery	Impaired: visual search accuracy
Strain et al., 2000	Nondependent (7)	NA	Hydromorphone 2, 4 mg IM	DSST, trail-making, circular lights	Unimpaired
Fraser et al., 1963	Nondependent (5)	NA	Heroin 8 mg IV	Pursuit rotor tracking	Unimpaired
Fraser et al., 1964	Nondependent (5)	NA	Heroin 8 mg IV	Sustained attention	Unimpaired
Cone et al., 1993	Nondependent (6)	NA	Heroin 6, 12 mg IN, 6 mg IM	Circular lights	Unimpaired
Walsh et al., 1994	Nondependent (5)	NA	Methadone 15–60 mg PO	DSST	Unimpaired
Preston, Bigelow, Bickel, & Liebson, 1989	Nondependent (4)	NA	Buprenorphine 0.11–0.9 mg/70 kg IM	DSST	Unimpaired
Preston et al., 1992	Nondependent (4)	NA	Buprenorphine 0.05–0.45 mg/70 kg IM	DSST	Unimpaired
Pickworth et al., 1993[d]	Nondependent (6)	NA	Buprenorphine 0.3–1.2 mg IV	Circular lights	Impaired
Walsh et al., 1994	Nondependent (4)	NA	Buprenorphine 1–32 mg SL	DSST	Unimpaired
Strain et al., 2000	Nondependent (7)	NA	Buprenorphine 4–16 mg SL	DSST, trail-making, circular lights	Impaired: circular lights (16 mg)
Strain et al., 2000	Nondependent (7)	NA	Buprenorphine/naloxone 1/0.25–16/4 mg SL	DSST, trail-making, circular lights	Impaired: circular lights (8/2, 16/4 mg), trail-making (16/4 mg)

(*Continued Overleaf*)

Table 9.2 (Continued)

Study	Participants (n)	Maintenance drug (dose/day)	Acute test drug	Measures	Results[a]
Preston, Bigelow, Bickel, & Liebson, 1989	Nondependent (5)	NA	Butorphanol 0.75–6 mg/70 kg IM	DSST	Unimpaired
Preston et al., 1992	Nondependent (5)	NA	Butorphanol 0.375–6 mg/70 kg IM	DSST	Unimpaired
Preston, Bigelow, Bickel, & Liebson, 1989	Nondependent (5)	NA	Nalbuphine 3–24 mg/70 kg IM	DSST	Unimpaired
Preston et al., 1992	Nondependent (5)	NA	Nalbuphine 1.5–24 mg/70 kg IM	DSST	Unimpaired
Preston, Bigelow, & Liebson, 1987	Nondependent (5)	NA	Pentazocine 22.5–90 mg IM	Battery	Impaired: DSST
Preston, Bigelow, Bickel, & Liebson, 1989	Nondependent (6)	NA	Pentazocine 8–45 mg/70 kg IM	DSST	Unimpaired
Preston et al., 1992	Nondependent (5)	NA	Pentazocine 4–45 mg/70 kg IM	DSST	Unimpaired

Note: Dependent, dependent opioid abusers (i.e., physically dependent on opioids at the time of testing); Nondependent, nondependent opioid abusers (i.e., with a history of opioid abuse, but not physically dependent on opioids at the time of testing); MMP, methadone maintenance patients; NA, not applicable; IM, intramuscular; SC, subcutaneous; IN, intranasal; PO, per oral; SL, sublingual; IV, intravenous; b.i.d., two times per day; q.i.d., four times per day; Battery, study used a performance testing battery that included four or more measures (see text for details); DSST, Digit Symbol Substitution Test; RT, reaction time.

[a] Results of within-subject statistical comparison of drug vs. placebo condition, unless otherwise noted.
[b] Drug vs. no-drug condition (instead of placebo) comparison.
[c] Between-subject design (drug vs. no-drug group comparison).
[d] No statistics reported.

Acute morphine administration did not affect the extraocular muscle balance of the eyes (as measured by the Maddox Wing test: exophoria or eye divergence is considered an index of psychomotor impairment; Lamas, Farre, & Cami, 1994). Hydromorphone did not impair DSST (Preston, Bigelow, Bickel, & Liebson, 1987; Preston, Bigelow, & Liebson, 1988a, 1988b, 1989, 1990; Stoller, Bigelow, Walsh, & Strain, 2001; Strain, Preston, Liebson, & Bigelow, 1992, 1993, 1996; Strain, Walsh, Preston, Liebson, & Bigelow, 1997), short-term memory (as measured by an immediate digit recall task; Preston, Bigelow, & Liebson, 1988a, 1988b, 1989; Strain et al., 1992, 1993, 1996, 1997), or trail-making performance (Stoller et al., 2001), but did impair performance on a measure of psychomotor tracking/speed (circular lights; Stoller et al., 2001). Acute administration of a high heroin dose (100 mg) impaired DSST and divided attention performance but did not impair performance on a rapid information processing task (measuring sustained attention and working memory) or a repeated acquisition task involving learning of a 10-response sequence of button presses (Comer, Collins, & Fischman, 1997).

Acute methadone did not impair DSST or short-term memory performance (Walsh, June, Schuh, Preston, Bigelow, & Stitzer, 1995). Three studies examined acute effects of an additional methadone dose on performance in dependent opioid abusers being maintained clinically on methadone. Rothenberg et al. (1977) found that an additional dose of up to 10 mg had no effect on simple visual reaction time or sustained attention in MMP being maintained on 20–70 mg methadone/day. Using a battery of tasks that included finger tapping, simple visual reaction time, the DSST, digit cancellation (measuring sustained attention), and immediate and delayed prose recall, Curran and colleagues examined the effects of increasing the MMP daily dose. They found that increasing patients' usual dose by 33% did not affect performance in MMP being maintained on 20–80 mg methadone/day (mean daily dose: 44 mg; Curran, Bolton, Wanigaratne, & Smyth, 1999). However, administering the full daily dose on a single occasion to MMP accustomed to receiving 50% of their dose at each of two occasions during the day significantly impaired delayed recall of prose in a task that has been shown to be a good predictor of everyday memory performance (mean daily dose: 33 mg, range: 10–50 mg; Curran, Kleckham, Bearn, Strang, & Wanigaratne, 2001). Acute buprenorphine did not impair DSST (Preston et al., 1988a; Stoller et al., 2001; Strain et al., 1992, 1997; Walsh et al., 1995), short-term memory (Preston et al., 1988a; Strain et al., 1992, 1997; Walsh et al., 1995), trail-making, or circular lights performance (Stoller et al., 2001). Acute administration of the buprenorphine/naloxone combination also did not impair DSST or short-term memory performance (Stoller et al., 2001). Interestingly, buprenorphine/naloxone impaired trail-making and circular lights performance when administered intramuscularly but not when administered sublingually (Stoller et al., 2001). In other studies, acute administration of dezocine, butorphanal, nalbuphine, or pentazocine did not impair performance (Lamas et al., 1994; Preston, Bigelow, & Liebson, 1989; Preston et al., 1988b, 1990; Strain et al., 1993, 1996).

ACUTE EFFECTS (NONDEPENDENT OPIOID ABUSERS)

This section reviews studies in which participants had a history of opioid abuse but were not physically dependent on opioids at the time of testing. Studies in nondependent opioid abusers typically administer somewhat lower doses than those in dependent opioid abusers due to concerns of toxicity in this less-tolerant population. Study details and a summary of results are presented in Table 9.2.

Three early studies (Hill, Belleville, & Wikler, 1955, 1957; Hill, Kornetsky, Flanary, & Wikler, 1952) examined the effects of acute morphine administration on simple visual reaction time. In the first two studies (Hill et al., 1952, 1955) reaction time was increased following morphine. In the third study (Hill et al., 1957) the authors tested the role of motivation in morphine's effects by examining the effects under different incentive conditions, and demonstrated that reaction time was increased, unchanged, or decreased following morphine depending on the incentive condition. Acute administration of morphine impaired auditory reaction time (Wikler, Haertzen, Chessick, Hill, & Pescor, 1965), nystagmus (Martin, Thompson, & Fraser, 1974), and short-term memory (Preston, Bigelow, & Liebson, 1987), but did not impair performance on sequence learning (Foltin & Fischman, 1992), circular lights, or choice reaction time tasks (Preston, Bigelow, & Liebson, 1987). Morphine did not impair performance on the DSST in two studies (Higgins, Preston, Cone, Henningfield, & Jaffe, 1992; Preston, Bigelow, & Liebson, 1987; up to 30 mg), but did impair DSST performance in another study that tested higher doses (Petry, Bickel, Huddleston, Tzanis, & Badger, 1998; up to 100 mg).

Hydromorphone did not impair performance on circular lights (Pickworth et al., 1997; Strain et al., 2000), a card sorting task requiring conceptual thinking (Pickworth, Rohrer, & Fant, 1997), an arithmetic task (Pickworth et al., 1997), trail-making (Strain, Stoller, Walsh, & Bigelow, 2000), or the DSST (Pickworth et al., 1997; Preston, Bigelow, Bickel, & Liebson, 1989; Preston, Liebson, & Bigelow, 1992; Strain et al., 2000). On a visual search task, hydromorphone impaired accuracy but not reaction time (Pickworth et al., 1997). Heroin administration did not impair performance on a pursuit rotor tracking task (Fraser, Jones, Rosenberg, & Thompson, 1963), a 12-minute number cancellation task measuring sustained attention (Fraser, Jones, Rosenberg, & Thompson, 1964), or circular lights (Cone, Holicky, Grant, Darwin, & Goldberger, 1993). Methadone did not impair DSST performance (Walsh et al., 1994). Acute administration of buprenorphine impaired performance on circular lights (Pickworth, Johnson, Holicky, & Cone, 1993; Strain et al., 2000) but not the DSST (Preston, Bigelow, Bickel, & Liebson, 1989; Preston et al., 1992; Strain et al., 2000; Walsh et al., 1994) or trail-making (Strain et al., 2000). Buprenorphine/naloxone impaired performance on circular lights and trail-making but not the DSST (Strain et al., 2000). Butorphanal and nalbuphine did not impair DSST performance (Preston, Bigelow, Bickel, & Liebson, 1989; Preston et al., 1992). Pentazocine impaired DSST (Preston, Bigelow, & Liebson, 1987; but not at lower doses: Preston, Bigelow, Bickel, & Liebson, 1989; Preston et al., 1992) but not short-term memory, circular lights, or visual choice reaction time performance (Preston, Bigelow, & Liebson, 1987).

CHRONIC EFFECTS

In two early studies, Fraser and colleagues examined the effects of chronic heroin administration on performance in nondependent opioid abusers (Fraser et al., 1963, 1964). Following 30 days of placebo (saline injections four times a day), the opioid abusers were administered heroin intravenously four times a day for 60 days (beginning with an average total daily dose of 10 mg, increasing to an average total daily dose of 95 mg by the 18th day, and maintained at that level for the remaining 42 days). Performance on a 12-minute number cancellation task measuring sustained attention was not impaired during the chronic heroin administration phase relative to the initial placebo phase (Fraser et al., 1964). Performance on a pursuit rotor tracking task was reduced nonsignificantly during the first 12 days of the heroin phase relative to placebo, but then returned to preheroin phase levels and was not impaired during the rest of the heroin phase (Fraser et al., 1963).

Results of an early study in which 15 nondependent opioid abusers were given doses of up to 400 mg methadone/day for a period ranging from 28 to 186 days show that following chronic methadone administration participants performed arithmetic and coordination tests at similar rates of speed as at baseline, but with substantially more errors, and that participants' mean IQ (measured by the Otis intelligence test) decreased by 7 points relative to baseline (Isbell, Wilker, Eisenman, Daingerfield, & Frank, 1948). Although this is the only published experimental study to provide information about chronic dosing effects of methadone at such high doses, results must be interpreted cautiously due to lack of statistical analysis and controlled procedures (e.g., daily dose and duration of treatment were not consistent across participants).

More recently, Lenne, Dietze, Rumbold, Redman, and Triggs (2003) used an independent group design to test dependent opioid abusers randomly assigned to three months of daily dosing of methadone ($n = 10$; mean daily dose: 48 mg) or buprenorphine ($n = 11$; mean daily dose: 14.4 mg) on simulated driving, and found no performance differences between the methadone and buprenorphine groups. In addition, neither pharmacotherapy group performed significantly worse than a group of nondrug-abusing age-matched controls. While these results support the hypothesis of limited impairment with buprenorphine, conclusions are limited by the lack of impairment in the methadone group (possibly due to the low methadone doses). We recently completed a study in our laboratory (Mintzer, Correia, & Strain, 2004) that evaluated the chronic dose-effects of buprenorphine/naloxone (8/2, 16/4, 32/8 mg, sublingual tablets) in dependent opioid abusers on performance of a broad range of psychomotor and cognitive tasks, following a period of 7–10 days of repeated dosing at each dose, in a double-blind, within-subject, crossover design. Results indicated only one significant effect: impairment in episodic memory performance for 32/8 relative to 8/2 and 16/4 mg buprenorphine/naloxone. The absence of impairment on most measures, and the finding of impairment in episodic memory only at the highest dose (32/8 mg; doses of 4–24 mg buprenorphine are recommended for opioid pharmacotherapy) support the hypothesis of limited impairment with buprenorphine. However, these null effects should be interpreted cautiously due to the absence of a placebo condition or control group.

SUMMARY

Results of studies in dependent opioid abusers (tested during daily stable opioid maintenance) indicate that acute opioid dosing produces little or no performance impairment in this population, suggesting that tolerance develops to the performance-impairing effects of opioids. Likewise, results of the few studies that have examined effects of chronic dosing in opioid abusers suggest that performance effects are minimal. Although a review of the effects of opioids in pain patients who are maintained chronically on opioids is beyond the scope of this chapter (and interpretation of the results of studies in chronic pain patients is complicated by the possible role of pain), results in that population also provide evidence for little or no performance impairment, supporting the notion of tolerance development (cf. Zacny, 1995). Results of studies in nondependent abusers provide more evidence for impairment in this less-tolerant population. A review of the effects of opioids in nondrug-abusing volunteers is also beyond the scope of this chapter. However, results of studies in nondrug abusers generally reveal greater performance impairment following acute opioid administration in this non-tolerant population than that observed in abusers (cf. Zacny, 1995). To our knowledge, only one study has directly compared acute effects of opioids in opioid abusers versus nondrug abusers (Rothenberg et al., 1977). As mentioned above, acute doses of up to 10 mg methadone did not impair performance in MMP in that study. However, when the same acute doses were administered to nondrug-abusing volunteers, impaired performance was observed.

It is important to note that conclusions based on the drug administration literature are limited due to the narrow range of performance tasks used in these studies (cf. Zacny, 1995, for a similar critique). In addition, results may not generalize to illicit use where opioid doses may be considerably higher than those safely administered in the laboratory.

Effects of withdrawal on cognitive and psychomotor performance

Three studies have examined the performance of dependent opioid abusers following short-term abstinence (Folli et al., 1992; Kelly, Welch, & McKnelley, 1978; Lyvers & Yakimoff, 2003). Based on the timing of performance testing, participants may have been in early withdrawal during testing, although it should be noted that no withdrawal symptom values are reported by the authors to enable confirmation of withdrawal status. Using a 30-minute sustained-attention reaction time task, Folli et al. (1992) examined the performance of eight male dependent opioid abusers who reportedly had used 1.5–2 g of street heroin daily (2–3 times a day) for more than three years until the day before testing, relative to eight male age-matched nondrug-abusing controls. The opioid abusers were required to abstain from heroin use for 12 hours prior to testing. The opioid abusers showed no impairment relative to controls.

Using a within-subject design, Kelly et al. (1978) examined the performance of 30 MMP (mean daily methadone dose: 63 mg, range: 20–120; mean duration of methadone maintenance treatment: 240 days, range: 28–874) tested 1 hour versus 25 hours (short-term abstinence) after daily methadone dosing. The battery included measures of auditory threshold, distance perception, reaction time, time perception, digit span, and attention span. The only measure that showed an effect of time of testing was distance perception, and interpretation of the direction of the effect is ambiguous. Using an independent group design, Lyvers and Yakimoff (2003) compared performance on the WCST of a group of MMP tested 90 minutes after daily methadone dosing ($n = 21$; peak methadone effect) and a group tested 24 hours after daily methadone dosing ($n = 18$; short-term abstinence). For both groups, participants had to be stabilized on at least 25 mg daily methadone (mean = 66.9) for at least one month prior to testing. MMP with excessive alcohol consumption, recent use of drugs other than methadone, or a history of treatment for alcohol or nonopioid drug-related problems were excluded from participation. MMP tested 24 hours after methadone dosing exhibited significantly higher rates of perseverative responses and errors (considered measures of impaired frontal lobe functioning) relative to MMP tested 90 minutes after methadone dosing. There were no differences in rates of nonperseverative errors.

Withdrawal effects on performance have also been examined using opioid antagonists to precipitate withdrawal in dependent opioid abusers. The opioid antagonist naloxone administered 20 hours or more after methadone dosing in opioid abusers maintained on daily methadone has been shown to precipitate symptoms of withdrawal as assessed by standard objective and subjective scales, but not to impair performance as assessed by the DSST (Preston, Bigelow, & Liebson, 1989; Preston et al., 1988a, 1988b; Strain et al., 1992, 1993, 1996), immediate digit recall (Preston, Bigelow, & Liebson, 1989; Preston et al., 1988a, 1988b; Strain et al., 1992, 1993, 1996), the Maddox

Wing test (Lamas et al., 1994), the Stroop test, or the digit span test (Kanof, Handelsman, Aronson, Ness, Cochrane, & Rubinstein, 1992).

To summarize, of the three studies that tested performance following short-term opioid abstinence, only one provides evidence of impairment (Lyvers & Yakimoff, 2003). Studies of opioid-precipitated withdrawal provide no evidence of performance impairment. The suggestion that withdrawal may be associated with selective impairment in measures of frontal lobe functioning (Lyvers & Yakimoff, 2003) is intriguing and warrants further research.

Effects of intoxication on mood

Effects of opioid intoxication on mood were first systematically characterized in the 1950s and 1960s. These early studies were typically conducted in individuals with a history of opioid abuse, and showed that acute administration of opioid agonists such as morphine, heroin, and methadone caused euphoric mood changes [e.g., increases in the Addiction Research Center Inventory (ARCI) morphine-benzedrine group: MBG], and to a lesser degree relaxation and sedation (e.g., increases in the ARCI pentobarbital-chlorpromazine-alcohol group: PCAG) (Haertzen, Meketon, & Hooks, 1963; Lasagna, von Felsinger, & Beecher, 1955). The acute mood-elevating effects of opioids in opioid abusers appear robust and have been demonstrated with a variety of standardized subjective measures, such as the ARCI, the Profile of Mood States (POMS), and various visual analogue scales (e.g., Cone et al., 1993; Heishman, Schuh, Schuster, Henningfield, & Goldberg, 2000; Jasinski & Preston, 1986; Martin & Fraser, 1961; Martin et al., 1973; McCaul, Bigelow, Stitzer, & Liebson, 1982; Walsh et al., 1995). A review of the mood effects of opioids in nondrug-abusing volunteers is beyond the scope of this chapter. However, it is interesting to note that although acute administration of opioids has been shown to increase ratings of positive mood and "high" in nondrug-abusing volunteers, such increases are often inconsistent, moderate, transient, and accompanied by concurrent increases in ratings of dysphoric mood, sedation, mental clouding, and impairment (e.g., Gravenstein, Smith, Sphire, Isaacs, & Beecher, 1956; Lasagna et al., 1955; Smith & Beecher, 1959, 1962; von Felsinger, Lasagna, & Beecher, 1955; Walker & Zacny, 1998; Zacny, Lichtor, Flemming, Coalson, & Thompson, 1994; Zacny, Lichtor, Zaragoza, & de Wit, 1992).

There is evidence that opioids differ in their acute effects on mood and that these differences may be at least partially accounted for by receptor affinity and action. The mu agonists (e.g., morphine, heroin, methadone, fentanyl, hydromorphone) are associated primarily with euphoria and appear qualitatively similar in their mood effects (Jasinski & Preston, 1986; Martin & Fraser, 1961). However, differences have been found between agonists and mixed agonist/antagonists (e.g., buprenorphine, pentazocine), and among the mixed agonist/antagonists (e.g., Greenwald & Stitzer, 1998; Jasinski, Martin,

& Hoeldtke, 1970; Jasinski & Mansky, 1972; Lamas et al., 1994; Preston, Bigelow, Bickel, & Liebson, 1989; Preston, Bigelow, & Liebson, 1987, 1989, 1990, 1992; Strain et al., 1992, 1996; Walsh et al., 1994, 1995). Interestingly, dysphoric and psychotomimetic effects [e.g. increases in the ARCI lysergic acid diethylamide (LSD) scale] are found with opioids with kappa agonist activity (e.g., Jasinski et al., 1970; Preston, Bigelow, & Liebson, 1989). Consistent with reports of psychotomimetic effects with kappa agonists is the recent identification of a kappa opioid agonist, salvinorin A, in the herb salvia divinorum. This highly selective kappa agonist induces a hallucinogenic state characterized by distortions of space and time perception. Native religious users of the herb in the Oaxaca region of Mexico consider these profound changes in consciousness a mystical, divinatory state (Siebert, 1994; Yan & Roth, 2004).

Effects of chronic administration of opioids on mood may differ from the acute effects. Fraser et al. (1963) administered placebo for 30 days and then heroin for 60 days to opioid abusers. Compared to placebo, heroin administration caused measures of physical activity to increase during the first four days of administration. However, after four days, heroin caused reduced activity, increased social isolation, and irritability with social interaction. Haertzen and Hooks (1969) found that acute morphine administration increased euphoria in nondependent opioid abusers; however, during chronic morphine administration (for an average duration of 3.5 months), euphoria was attenuated, somatic concern increased, and motivation for activity and social interaction decreased. A series of studies allowed detoxified opioid abusers to self-administer heroin (within constraints) with escalating doses during a 10-day period while mood was assessed (Mirin, Meyer, & McNamee, 1976; Mirin, Meyer, McNamee, & McDougle, 1976; McNamee, Mirin, Kuehnle, & Meyer, 1976). During the early part of the 10-day period, mood was elevated, while anxiety and somatic concerns decreased relative to the preheroin baseline. Toward the end of the 10-day period, although mood remained elevated, dysphoric symptoms such as somatic concerns, anxiety, depression, negativism, lack of emotion, and social isolation increased. Interestingly, other research suggests that chronic opioid abuse may be associated with impaired social interaction, including impaired facial recognition in MMP and detoxified opioid abusers (Kornreich et al., 2003), and increased interrogative suggestibility in dependent opioid abusers compared to formerly dependent opioid abusers (Murakami, Edelmann, & Davis, 1996). These various results suggest that although acute opioid administration in opioid abusers increases euphoria, chronic administration may increase dysphoria and social isolation.

Effects of withdrawal on mood

In addition to a wide array of physical symptoms (e.g., sweating, vomiting, diarrhea, goose bumps, muscle aches), a body of work provides evidence that withdrawal from opioids, whether from illicit use or opioid pharmacotherapy, is characterized by an array of subjective mood changes. Although affective states prior to abstinence (e.g., anxiety concerning future withdrawal) may be related to the severity of subsequent withdrawal (e.g., Phillips, Gossop, & Bradley, 1986), the focus here will be affective states as withdrawal symptoms themselves. An early study by Haertzen and Hooks (1969) noted the presence of affective withdrawal symptoms. Opioid abusers were injected with heroin or morphine daily for an average of 3.5 months, and were then measured on the ARCI and other self-report measures before, and after, a 10-day dose reduction period. Symptoms such as depression, anxiety, and irritability were present following detoxification, in addition to classic physical withdrawal symptoms. Results of subsequent studies suggest that negative subjective mood symptoms are associated both with spontaneous opioid withdrawal (e.g., Cushman & Dole, 1973; Gold, Sorensen, McCanlies, Trier, & Dlugosch, 1988; Handelsman, Aronson, Ness, Cochrane, & Kanof, 1992; Kleber, 1997; Price, Moran, Crunican, Rothenberg, & Cutter, 1975) and with opioid antagonist-precipitated withdrawal (e.g., Gerra et al, 2003; Handelsman, et al., 1992; Heishman, Stitzer, Bigelow, & Liebson, 1990; Kanof et al., 1992).

Results of two studies suggest that patients may experience the mood symptoms associated with opioid withdrawal as more severe than the physical symptoms. Cohen, Klett, and Ling (1983) had 15 clinicians experienced with opioid-dependence treatment rank the severity of a list of commonly reported opioid withdrawal symptoms, based on previous experience. One-hundred and fifty MMP rated the same symptoms, using retrospective evaluations of previous methadone dose reductions or periods of opioid abstinence. Clinicians rated physical symptoms such as diarrhea, abdominal cramps, and nausea/vomiting as more severe than the patients. The patients, however, rated subjective symptoms, including mood symptoms such as irritability and anxiety, as more severe than the clinicians. Eklund, Hiltunen, Melin, & Borg (1997) examined ten MMP with the objective to cease methadone maintenance. Patient-rated symptoms were assessed via visual analogue scales including 12 psychological symptoms (including mood symptoms such as depression, aggression, stress sensitivity, and irritability) and 12 physiological symptoms. Questionnaires were completed three days before and seven days after each dose reduction, with the number and frequency of dose reductions determined individually for each patient (average of one reduction per two months for 11 months). Overall, psychological symptoms were rated as more severe than classic physiological symptoms during methadone dose reduction.

Much of the information on the timecourse of opioid withdrawal focuses on methadone due to its use in opioid pharmacotherapy. Although the onset of withdrawal symptoms following methadone discontinuation is later relative to withdrawal onset following morphine discontinuation (Martin et al., 1973), there is evidence that methadone is associated with affective withdrawal symptoms even within a 24-hour period. Dyer, White, Foster, Bochner, Menelaou, and Somogyi (2001) administered the POMS to MMP and nondrug-abusing controls on several occasions throughout a 24-hour period following daily methadone dosing. The MMP also gave blood samples for the analysis of plasma methadone concentrations. MMP provided higher ratings of anger, depression, tension, confusion, and fatigue, and decreased ratings of vigor relative to controls. Consistent with previous demonstrations of an association between mood and plasma methadone concentration (Hiltunen et al., 1995), the greatest differences were found at the times of lowest methadone concentrations.

Latowsky (1996) reviewed the evidence that a protracted opioid withdrawal syndrome may be associated with affective symptoms. Specifically, withdrawal may consist of two phases: a primary abstinence phase and a secondary, prolonged abstinence phase (Martin, 1968; Martin & Jasinski, 1969; Martin & Sloan, 1968; Price et al., 1975). The primary phase starts within two days of drug cessation and lasts up to four weeks, consisting of physical symptoms such as vomiting, restlessness, poor appetite, gooseflesh, dilated pupils, tremor, perspiration, rhinorrhea, lacrimation, yawning, increased body temperature, respiration, and systolic blood pressure, and a decrease in body weight. The secondary, prolonged phase starts at 6–9 weeks and lasts up to 30 months, consisting of relatively low-magnitude physiological symptoms such as low blood pressure, pulse rate, and body temperature. Affective disturbances may be one aspect of this protracted syndrome (Latowsky, 1996; Price et al., 1975). Although the classification of such a protracted mood syndrome as a distinct diagnostic entity has not achieved consensus, such affective disturbances are considered clinically relevant (Latowsky, 1996). Support for the concept of a protracted opioid withdrawal syndrome associated with affective disturbances is also found in a study by Kanof, Aronson, and Ness (1993). That study examined MMP who underwent gradual dose reduction from an average of 39 mg/day by 5 mg/week until a level of 15 mg/day was achieved, at which point reduction proceeded at 3 mg/week until complete detoxification. The study attempted to maintain participation for an additional 12 weeks upon complete detoxification. Detoxification was associated with impairment in mood as measured by all six POMS subscales: tension–anxiety, depression–dejection, anger–hostility, vigor, fatigue, and confusion. Data presented from one representative participant showed that these dysphoric symptoms peaked 10–11 weeks after complete detoxification. Other scales utilized included two scales measuring subjective symptoms, including mood symptoms – the lengthened version of the Subjective Opiate Withdrawal Scale (Handelsman, Cochrane, Aronson, Ness, Rubinstein, & Kanof, 1987) and the Weak Opiate Withdrawal Scale (Haertzen et al., 1970) – and a scale measuring physical opioid withdrawal symptoms: Objective Opiate Withdrawal Scale (Handelsman et al., 1987). Both the Subjective Opiate Withdrawal Scale and the Weak Opiate Withdrawal Scale revealed increasing withdrawal during detoxification, while the Objective Opiate Withdrawal Scale showed little change in physical withdrawal symptoms. The authors argued that this pattern of results reflects an organic mood syndrome resulting from methadone maintenance detoxification. Other work suggests that anger may play a part in this possible protracted mood syndrome. Powell and Taylor (1992) examined speech samples, made immediately after detoxification and 4–5 weeks after detoxification, from 60 patients in an inpatient drug detoxification unit. Analysis with the methods of Gottschalk and Gleser (1969) indicated that although ratings of depression, anxiety, and anger increased immediately upon detoxification, depression and anxiety eventually subsided whereas anger remained. Price et al. (1975) found that the pretreatment Anger subscale of the POMS was positively correlated with treatment program retention and detoxification completion. Although Price et al. state that the relationship may have resulted from group treatment sessions that encouraged acceptance of feelings, the results may also indicate that anger plays a complicated role in the withdrawal process.

Residual effects

To assess the neuropsychological effects that are still present after opioid use has been discontinued (and after acute withdrawal symptoms have subsided), this section reviews observational studies that examined performance in abstinent opioid abusers relative to control participants. Study details and a summary of results are presented in Table 9.3.

In an early study, Brown and Partington (1942) used a battery of tasks assessing abstract thinking, set shifting, attention, memory, spatial orientation, and psychomotor coordination and speed to compare former opioid abusers who had been drug abstinent for at least six months to nondrug-abusing controls matched with respect to age, education, and IQ. No performance differences were found between the groups. In another early study, Pfeffer and Ruble (1946) used the Shipley-Hartford Scale to compare hospitalized dependent opioid abusers to nondrug-abusing controls (hospital attendants at the same institution) matched with respect to age and education. No performance differences were found between the groups. Although the specific duration of drug abstinence is not provided, information in the Discussion suggests that the opioid abusers had been abstinent for at least six weeks. Using the Halstead-Reitan Neuropsychological Battery, Fields and Fullerton (1975) compared inpatient opioid-dependent male veterans to a control group of hospitalized male veterans in the same Veterans Administration hospital. No performance differences were reported. No information is provided about the opioid abusers' current opioid use or abstinence status; however, given that they were hospitalized, it may be assumed that they were detoxified prior to testing.

Table 9.3 Observational studies of cognitive and psychomotor performance in abstinent opioid abusers

Study	Groups (n)[a]	Duration of opioid abuse (years)[b]	Duration of drug abstinence[b]	Measures	Results[c]
Brown & Partington, 1942	Abstinent abusers (42) Nondrug abusers (42)	Not reported	≥ 6 months	Battery	Unimpaired
Pfeffer & Ruble, 1946	Abstinent abusers (25) Nondrug abusers (25)	12.7 (3–20)	Not reported	Shipley-Hartford Scale	Unimpaired
Fields & Fullerton, 1975	Abstinent abusers (25) Nondrug abusers (25)	4.9	Not reported	Battery	Unimpaired
Gerra et al., 1998	Abstinent abusers (27) Nondrug abusers (9)	4.7 (4–6)	4 months	Vocabulary, digit symbol, category	Unimpaired
Pau et al., 2002	Abstinent abusers (30) Nondrug abusers (25)	4.7	13.7 months	Battery	Impaired: impulse control
Hill et al., 1979[d]	Abstinent abusers (27) Nondrug abusers (14)	6.3 (2–22)	1.7 years (2 months–5 years)	Battery	Impaired: tactual performance
Davis et al., 2002	Abstinent abusers (16) Nondrug abusers (14)	11.5 (3–30)	26 weeks (6–56)	Battery	Unimpaired
Mintzer, Stitzer, & Copersino, 2004	Abstinent abusers (21) Nondrug abusers (20)	16.9 (2–37)	36 weeks (3.3–144)	Battery	Impaired: psychomotor speed

Note: Battery, study used a performance testing battery that included four or more measures (see text for details).
[a] Number of participants in each group.
[b] Mean (range in parentheses), unless otherwise noted.
[c] Results of statistical comparison of abstinent opioid abusers vs. nondrug abusers.
[d] Information about duration of opioid abuse is reported by Hill et al., 1979 only for the entire opioid abuser group (n = 70; which consisted of both current and abstinent opioid abusers; cf. Intoxication section above).

Using the Vocabulary and Digit Symbol subtests from the Wechsler Adult Intelligence Scale and the Category test, Gerra et al. (1998) examined the performance of dependent opioid abusers who had been abstinent for four months, relative to nondrug-abusing controls matched with respect to age. Prior to neuropsychological testing, the opioid abusers were detoxified and then admitted to a long-term residential program where their urine was tested for drugs of abuse three times weekly to ensure their abstinence throughout the four months. Opioid abusers with a history of use of drugs of abuse other than heroin, or excessive alcohol use, were excluded. The neuropsychological performance of the abstinent opioid abusers was worse than that of the controls, but the difference was not statistically significant. Interestingly, the performance of a subgroup of abstinent opioid abusers who were diagnosed with antisocial personality disorder was significantly worse relative to the control group, suggesting that antisocial personality disorder may be a risk factor for impairment in this population. Using a battery of tasks designed to measure frontal executive functions (sustained attention, divided attention, impulse control, mental flexibility/abstract reasoning), Pau, Lee, and Chan (2002) compared the performance of abstinent opioid abusers to nondrug-abusing controls, matched with respect to gender. There were significant differences between the groups in age and education, so these variables were controlled statistically. The opioid abusers were significantly impaired relative to controls on a measure of impulse control but not on measures of attention or mental flexibility/abstract reasoning.

Results of the Hill et al. (1979) study described earlier in which a group of opioid abusers was subdivided into current users and users in remission (defined as those who had not abused opioids for at least two months) indicated that in contrast to current opioid abusers, who were impaired on a number of different neuropsychological measures, opioid abusers in remission were impaired relative to controls only on the Tactual Performance subtest, suggesting that recovery of functioning occurs during abstinence. In contrast, a comparison within the group of alcohol abusers of current users versus users in remission revealed no differences in the pattern of impairment relative to controls. As described earlier, results of two recent studies that included MMP, abstinent opioid abusers, and nondrug-abusing controls indicated that the performance of the abstinent opioid abusers generally fell between that of the MMP and controls, suggesting that some recovery of functioning may occur during abstinence (Davis et al., 2002: abstinent opioid abusers were unimpaired relative to nondrug-abusing controls; Mintzer, Copersino, & Stitzer, 2004: the only significant impairment for abstinent abusers relative to nondrug-abusing controls was in psychomotor speed; cf. Table 9.3).

Also relevant to the issue of residual effects is a large, multisite study that was conducted in polydrug abusers (Collaborative Neuropsychological Study of Polydrug Users). In that study, Grant, Adams, Carlin, Rennick, Judd, and Schooff (1978) used the Halstead-Reitan Neuropsychological Battery to examine the performance of polydrug abusers, psychiatric patients, and demographically similar nondrug-abusing, psychiatrically healthy controls. Participants were re-tested three months after the initial testing. For the polydrug abusers, the initial testing was conducted 21–30 days after they enrolled in a detoxification program. Neuropsychological impairment at initial testing was found in 37% of polydrug abusers, 26% of psychiatric patients, and 8% of controls. Most relevant for the present purpose is that heavy use of opioids was significantly related to neuropsychological impairment both at initial testing and at a three-month follow-up. Little change was observed in the polydrug abusers at the three-month follow-up, suggesting that the effects persist during drug abstinence (at least during the first three months).

To summarize, most of the studies reviewed in this section suggest that recovery of functioning occurs during opioid drug abstinence and that residual performance impairment is minimal. One notable exception is the Grant et al. (1978) study that suggests that performance impairment is present following three months of abstinence. An important strength of the Grant et al. (1978) study is its use of a controlled longitudinal design. However, results are difficult to interpret in the present context given that the study was conducted in polydrug abusers, rather than in opioid abusers. To our knowledge, no longitudinal studies have been conducted in opioid abusers to examine the timecourse of recovery following detoxification. As discussed in the section on intoxication, it is important to note that conclusions based on observational studies are limited due to difficulties in differentiating between impairments that are a consequence of opioid abuse versus impairments that predated the abuse. For example, it is possible that the impairment in impulse control reported by Pau et al. (2002) may have predated the opioid abuse and in fact even played a role in its development, rather than being a residual effect of the abuse.

Risk factors for impairment

In this section, we summarize potential risk factors for neuropsychological impairment in opioid abusers that are suggested by results of subgroup and correlational analyses conducted in studies that have examined performance in this population. It should be noted that such analyses may underestimate the contribution of some factors due to small sample sizes and restricted ranges. Of the demographic variables that have been examined, level of education appears to be most consistently related to performance impairment (i.e., performance is more impaired in opioid abusers with lower levels of education) (Grant et al., 1978; Guerra et al., 1987; Rounsaville et al., 1981, 1982). Increasing age was positively related to performance impairment in one study (Grant et al., 1978). The failure to observe a relationship between age and performance impairment in other studies may be due to the exclusion of elderly adults from participation.

Drug use/history variables have also been examined. Duration of opioid abuse was positively related to performance impairment in one study (Hill et al., 1979), and severity of opioid dependence was positively related to perseverative responses and errors on the WCST in another study (Lyvers & Yakimoff, 2003). The daily dose of methadone in MMP appears to have only a weak positive relationship to performance impairment (Darke et al., 2000; Specka et al., 2000), although it is possible that a stronger relationship would be observed if MMP maintained on a wider range of doses were tested. Current use of other drugs (Grevert et al., 1977; Schindler et al., 2004), particularly alcohol (Darke et al., 2000; Rounsaville et al., 1982), tobacco smoking (Rotheram-Fuller et al., 2004), a history of heroin overdoses (Darke et al., 2000), and heavy abuse of alcohol (Darke et al., 2000; Rounsaville et al., 1981) or cocaine (Rounsaville et al., 1981), also appear to be risk factors for cognitive impairment. Other variables that have emerged as risk factors for cognitive impairment in opioid abusers include a history of childhood hyperactivity (Rounsaville et al., 1981), antisocial personality disorder (Gerra et al., 1998), HIV infection (Boccellari et al., 1994; Margolin, Avants, Warburton, & Hawkins, 2002; Woods et al., 1991), and premorbid medical factors (Grant et al., 1978).

Association between neuropsychological profile and imaging

Findings of hypoperfusion and other brain changes in opioid abusers with current active use relative to nondrug-abusing controls (cf. Pathophysiology: Imaging studies) are consistent with findings of impaired performance in current opioid abusers (cf. Effects of intoxication on cognitive and psychomotor performance: Observational studies). Furthermore, the finding that brain changes are particularly pronounced in frontal and temporal areas is consistent with observed deficits in decision-making and memory in some studies in current opioid abusers. The suggestion of improvement in brain functioning with abstinence (Rose et al., 1996) is consistent with the recovery of functioning observed during abstinence (cf. Residual effects). The lateralization pattern observed in opioid abusers relative to nondrug abusers (Pezawas et al., 2002) may be related to the mood effects of opioids (cf. Mood) given that greater activation in the left than the right hemisphere is hypothesized to be associated with positive moods (cf. Pezewas et al., 2002).

A few studies have specifically examined the association between performance impairment and abnormalities detected via brain imaging techniques. Strang and Gurling (1989) did not observe an association between neuropsychological performance impairment and CT scan changes. Likewise, in the Gerra et al. (1998) study, no relationship was found between neuropsychological performance impairment and cerebral blood flow changes using SPECT. In the Hill et al. (1979) study in which a subset of the participants (a mixed group of opioid and alcohol abusers) were given CT scans, a significant correlation was observed between CT scan changes and the number of errors on the category test. Using event-related functional magnetic resonance imaging (fMRI), Forman et al. (2004) examined performance on a Go/No-Go task and the associated brain activity of dependent opioid abusers shortly after intake at a methadone maintenance program ($n = 13$; mean duration of methadone maintenance treatment: 15.5 days, range: 0–21; mean duration of opioid use: 16.3 years, SD: 11.0) relative to nondrug-abusing controls ($n = 13$), matched with respect to age, gender, ethnicity, and parental education, but not socioeconomic status. The opioid abusers all had opioid dependence as their primary current substance abuse diagnosis but seven also had a secondary current substance use disorder (4 out of 7 cocaine). In the Go/No-Go task, participants are presented with a continuous stream of stimuli (letters in this study) sequentially and are instructed to respond to specified target stimuli and to suppress responding to nontarget stimuli. The opioid abusers exhibited impairment relative to controls in discriminating between target and nontarget stimuli, and exhibited a decrease relative to controls in the anterior cingulate cortex activation that is normally associated with false alarm responses to nontarget stimuli (considered an error "signal"). Furthermore, there was a relationship between anterior cingulate cortex activity and between-group differences in task performance. Given that response suppression in this task is considered a measure of behavioral control, these results support the notion that impaired behavioral control is associated with impaired anterior cingulate activity as assessed by fMRI.

To summarize, there is evidence both from neuroimaging studies and from studies specifically examining the association between performance impairment and brain changes that there is a relationship between the neuropsychological profile and brain changes associated with opioid abuse.

Epidemiological studies

Thus far, we have examined the neuropsychological consequences of opioid abuse by reviewing studies that tested performance in the laboratory environment. Although some of these studies provide evidence for impairment on laboratory tasks of performance (particularly observational studies in current opioid users and drug administration studies in nondependent opioid abusers), a critical issue is the extent to which opioid abuse may be associated with functional impairment in a patient's natural environment. Given that an important benefit of opioid pharmacotherapy is that it provides the stability necessary to initiate lifestyle changes, obtain steady employment, and function in society, the question of functional impairment is particularly important with respect to opioid pharmacotherapy patients.

A useful source of information regarding functional performance impairment is the body of epidemiological data on the incidence of accidents (traffic accidents, falls). Results of studies that have analyzed biological fluid samples (i.e., blood, urine) from drivers injured or killed in traffic accidents typically indicate that the rate of samples positive for opioids is low relative to that for other drugs (e.g., Budd, Muto, & Wong, 1989; Christensen, Nielsen, & Nielsen, 1990; Cimbura, Lucas, Bennett, Warren, & Simpson, 1982; Garriott, DiMaio, Zumwalt, & Petty, 1977; Gjerde, Beylich, & Morland, 1993; Honkanen et al., 1980; Mason & McBay, 1984). However, results of a study in Switzerland in drivers suspected of driving under drug-impaired conditions found that the rate of samples positive for opioids (36%) was comparable to that for alcohol (Augsburger & Rivier, 1997). Although the rate of methadone-positive samples in that study was relatively low (10%), it is interesting to note that all methadone-positive samples were also positive for an additional drug, raising concerns about possible potentiation of performance impairment (cf. next section). Results of studies that have examined the rate of traffic accidents or serious motor vehicle violations in opioid users typically indicate that opioid users do not have higher rates of traffic accidents or serious motor vehicle violations relative to nonusers (Babst, Newman, Gordon, & Warner, 1973; Blomberg & Preusser, 1974; Maddux, Williams, & Ziegler, 1977; Ray, Fought, & Decker, 1992). Although the results of one study suggest that opioid use does not increase the risk of traffic accidents in older adults (Ray et al., 1992), the results of two other studies suggest that opioid use increases the risk of traffic accidents (Leveille, Buchner, Koepsell, McCloskey, Wolf, & Wagner, 1994) and falls (Shorr, Griffin, Daugherty, & Ray, 1992) in older adults. Interestingly, in the Shorr et al. (1992) study, the risk of falls (in older adults) was much higher following initial doses than subsequent doses, again supporting the notion that tolerance develops to the performance-impairing effects of opioids.

From these epidemiological data, one can infer that opioid pharmacotherapy patients would likely be at minimal risk for impairment (as measured by accident rates) during the stable maintenance phase, but might be at increased risk during the initial medication induction phase or following dose escalation, and that the risk of impairment may be higher in older adults. Unfortunately, there are limited data concerning the effects of specific methadone dose increases on performance in MMP. Results of the few studies that have been conducted in MMP suggest that acute increases of up to 33% of the daily maintenance dose do not impair performance, whereas increases of 100% of the daily dose may impair performance (Curran, Bolton, Wanigaratne, & Smyth, 1999; Curran, Kleckham, Bearn, Strang, & Wanigaratne, 2001; see Effects of intoxication on cognitive and psychomotor or performance: Drug administration studies). To our knowledge, no studies have examined the performance effects of acute buprenorphine dose increases in BMP.

Recommendations for further study

Use of more sophisticated performance testing techniques

As mentioned earlier, one limitation of the laboratory-study literature on cognitive and psychomotor consequences of opioid abuse is the narrow range of performance tasks used in many studies, particularly in studies examining effects of opioid drug administration. In fact, many of the drug administration studies were not specifically designed to address the issue of performance effects but rather were primarily focused on other issues (e.g., drug discrimination, abuse liability) and simply included a few performance tasks secondarily as part of a larger battery of measures. To provide a better understanding of the specificity of the performance effects of opioid abuse, there is a need for additional studies that are specifically designed to address this issue, that use a wide range of sophisticated performance tasks tapping specific functions (including standard neuropsychological batteries), and that are informed by methodological and theoretical advances in the cognitive, neuropsychological, and neuroimaging fields.

Use of controlled longitudinal designs

Studies that employ controlled longitudinal designs would be useful in a number of different areas. First, to better understand the effects of opioid pharmacotherapies on performance, there is a need for studies that test performance in dependent opioid abusers prior to beginning opioid pharmacotherapy and at multiple timepoints during the course of opioid pharmacotherapy treatment. To our knowledge, the only study that used a longitudinal design in opioid pharmacotherapy patients was an early study that only tested memory performance (Grevert et al., 1977). Second, to provide a better understanding of the timecourse of recovery of functioning following detoxification and of the residual effects of long-term opioid abuse, there is a need for studies that test performance at multiple timepoints for at least one year following detoxification. To our knowledge, the only study that used a controlled longitudinal design to test performance at multiple timepoints following opioid detoxification was conducted in polydrug abusers rather than in opioid abusers and only followed participants for three months after detoxification (Grant et al., 1978). Large-scale prospective studies in which performance testing is initiated in adolescents prior to onset of drug use would be ideal (although complicated logistically), as they may also enable differentiation of impairments that are a consequence of opioid abuse versus impairments that predated the abuse. Third, longitudinal designs are needed to better understand the timecourse of mood effects following detoxification and to shed light on a possible protracted affective withdrawal syndrome (cf. Mood).

Studies of high-dose methadone

The original methadone dose recommendation made by Dole and colleagues (Dole & Nyswander, 1966) was 80–120 mg/day (with some patients requiring higher doses), and the superior efficacy of doses ≥ 80 mg relative to lower doses was supported by subsequent clinical research (Ling, Wesson, Charuvastra, & Klett, 1996; Strain, Bigelow, Liebson, & Stitzer, 1999; cf. Payte & Khuri, 1993). In the 1980s, there were attempts to reduce methadone doses in many clinics, such that a survey conducted in 1988 found that the average maintenance dose was 50 mg/day or less at 68% of US methadone maintenance treatment clinics (D'Aunno & Vaughn, 1992). Although the issue of optimal methadone dosing is still controversial (Blaney & Craig, 1999; Cooper, 1992; D'Aunno & Pollack, 2002; Joseph, Stancliff, & Langrod, 2000; Leavitt, Shinderman, Maxwell, Eap, & Paris, 2000), recently there has been a trend toward using increasingly higher maintenance doses. An informal national survey found that the average daily methadone dose in US clinics increased from 45 mg in 1988 to 56.6 mg in 1993 to 69.4 mg in 1998 (Leavitt, 1998). This trend is supported by recent clinical data suggesting that some patients require doses considerably higher than the 100 mg "glass ceiling" common in the 1980s (higher than 200 mg/day, and as high as 1100 mg/day in some cases; Maxwell & Shinderman, 1999, 2002; Robles, Miller, Gilmore-Thomas, & McMillan, 2001). Increasingly higher doses may also be needed due to higher dependence levels resulting from increased purity of street heroin (Bach & Lantos, 1999). Given that patients being maintained on high methadone doses would be expected to be most vulnerable to performance impairment, information about the effects of methadone at high doses is now needed. Yet, with the exception of the Isbell et al. (1948) study that examined effects of doses as high as 400 mg, most studies of methadone have examined low to moderate doses (cf. Table 9.1), and none has examined multiple doses to provide information about performance dose–effect functions.

Dose-transition studies with opioid pharmacotherapies

Data from both laboratory and epidemiological studies suggest that opioid pharmacotherapy patients would likely be at increased risk for performance impairment following dose escalation. Yet, to our knowledge, there are little or no data on the effects of specific methadone or buprenorphine dose increases on performance in MMP or BMP (cf. Effects of intoxication on cognitive and psychomotor performance: Drug administration studies). There is a need for studies in which the effects of specific opioid pharmacotherapy dose increases and decreases on performance are examined. Data from such studies may aid clinicians in making decisions about opioid pharmacotherapy dosing schedules, particularly in patients with additional risk factors for impairment (cf. Risk factors for impairment).

Interaction studies of opioid pharmacotherapies with alcohol and benzodiazepines

Polydrug abuse is common in dependent opioid abusers. Clinical surveys indicate that rates of alcohol and benzodiazepine abuse are particularly high in MMP (Bleich, Gelkopf, Schmidt, Hayward, Bodner, & Adelson, 1999; Hillebrand, Marsden, Finch, & Strang, 2001; Iguchi, Handelsman, Bickel, & Griffiths, 1993; Stastny & Potter, 1991). Relative to other MMP, patients who abuse benzodiazepines and/or alcohol exhibit a more severe profile of symptoms, including greater psychopathology, more HIV risk-taking behavior, poorer health and social functioning, and a greater mortality risk (Best, Gossop, Lehmann, Harris, & Strang, 1999; Bleich et al., 1999; Chatham, Rowan-Szal, Joe, Brown, & Simpson, 1995; Chutuape, Brooner, & Stitzer, 1997; Darke, Swift, & Hall, 1994; El-Bassel, Schilling, Turnbull, & Su, 1993). For both alcohol and benzodiazepines, patients commonly report using the drugs to "boost" the effects of their daily methadone (Iguchi et al., 1993; Kreek, 1984; Stitzer, Griffiths, McLellan, Grabowski, & Hawthorne, 1981). These clinical observations are supported by evidence that experimental administration of the benzodiazepine diazepam potentiates the subjective and physiological (e.g., pupil constriction) effects of methadone and decreases methadone self-administration in MMP (Preston, Griffiths, Stitzer, Bigelow, & Liebson, 1984; Spiga, Huang, Meisch, & Grabowski, 2001).

Given that alcohol and benzodiazepines are both known to profoundly impair performance after acute administration (cf. Curran, 2000; Finnigan & Hammersley, 1992), potentiation of performance-impairing effects of opioid pharmacotherapies could have serious consequences. To our knowledge, only one study (Lenne et al., 2003) has examined interactive effects of alcohol on performance in MMP and BMP, and none has examined interactive effects of a benzodiazepine. As noted earlier, Lenne et al. reported that opioid abusers receiving daily chronic dosing of methadone or buprenorphine were unimpaired on simulated driving relative to controls. Although acute alcohol dosing impaired simulated driving in all three groups, it did not differentially affect performance of the pharmacotherapy groups relative to controls. While these results do not provide support for the hypothesis of additive interactions between methadone/buprenorphine and alcohol, conclusions are limited by the lack of impairment in the pharmacotherapy groups in the absence of alcohol and the relatively low alcohol dose (at or below 0.05% blood alcohol). Linnoila and colleagues (Linnoila & Hakkinen, 1974; Linnoila & Mattila, 1973) demonstrated that another opioid, codeine, potentiated the performance-impairing effects of alcohol on simulated driving, supporting the hypothesis of additive interactions between opioids and alcohol. In addition, the finding in an epidemiological study of suspected drug-impaired drivers that all methadone-positive samples were also positive for an additional drug raises concerns about possible functional performance impairment associated with methadone/drug combinations (Augsburger & Rivier, 1997).

Comparison of opioid pharmacotherapies with alcohol and other drugs

A critical issue is the extent to which opioid abuse may be associated with functional impairment in a patient's natural environment, particularly for opioid pharmacotherapy patients. As discussed above, one useful source of information regarding functional performance impairment is the body of epidemiological data on incidence of accidents. Another way to address the issue of functional impairment is to estimate the degree of expected impairment in the environment by directly comparing the performance deficits to those produced by other drugs that have already been established as producing clinically significant impairment. The World Health Organization has recommended that alcohol (which has a well-established association with traffic accidents and driving impairment) be used as a reference drug against which to compare other drugs with respect to performance impairment (Willette & Walsh, 1983). Likewise, the International Council on Alcohol, Drugs and Traffic Safety has proposed that categories of drug-induced driving-related impairment be defined in reference to specific blood alcohol levels, and researchers have recommended that alcohol be included as an active drug control when evaluating effects of drugs on driving (Alvarez & del Rio, 2002). This approach of using alcohol as a reference drug for assessing performance impairment has been employed by researchers to estimate the impairment associated with opioid analgesics and other drugs used as anesthetics during ambulatory surgical procedures (Thapar, Zacny, Choi, & Apfelbaum, 1995a; Thapar, Zacny, Thompson, & Apfelbaum, 1995b). However, to our knowledge, it has not been applied to pharmacotherapies for opioid dependence. Some investigators have also argued for the usefulness of establishing a hierarchy of performance impairment in which drugs are ranked relative to each other with respect to their performance-impairing effects (Hindmarch, Kerr, & Sherwood, 1991; Zacny, 1995). Such a hierarchy was attempted with alcohol, benzodiazepines, antihistamines, caffeine, and nicotine, but opioids were not included (Hindmarch et al., 1991).

References

Alvarez, J. F., & del Rio, M. C. (2002). Medicinal drugs and driving: From research to clinical practice. *Trends in Pharmacological Sciences, 23*, 441–443.

Amass, L., Nardin, R., Mendelson, J. H., Teoh, S. K., & Woods, B. T. (1992). Quantitative magnetic resonance imaging in heroin- and cocaine-dependent men: a preliminary study. *Psychiatry Research, 45*, 15–23.

Appel, P. W. (1982). Sustained attention in methadone patients. *International Journal of Addiction, 17*, 1313–1327.

Appel, P. W., & Gordon, N. B. (1976). Digit-symbol performance in methadone-treated ex-heroin addicts. *American Journal of Psychiatry, 133*, 1337–1340.

Augsburger, M., & Rivier, L. (1997). Drugs and alcohol among suspected impaired drivers in Canton de Vaud (Switzerland). *Forensic Science International, 85*, 95–104.

Babst, D. V., Newman, S., Gordon, N., & Warner, A. (1973). Driving records of methadone maintenance patients in New York State. *Journal of Drug Issues, 3,* 285–292.

Bach, P. B., & Lantos, J. (1999). Methadone dosing, heroin affordability, and the severity of addiction. *American Journal of Public Health, 89,* 662–665.

Bechara, A., Damasio, A. R., Damasio, H., & Anderson, S. W. (1994). Insensitivity to future consequences following damage to human prefrontal cortex. *Cognition 50,* 7–15.

Bechara, A., Damasio, H., Tranel, D., & Anderson, S. W. (1998). Dissociation of working memory from decision making within the human prefrontal cortex. *Journal of Neuroscience, 18,* 428–437.

Bechara, A., Tranel, D., & Damasio, H. (2000). Characterization of the decision-making deficit of patients with ventromedial prefrontal cortex lesions. *Brain 123,* 2189–2202.

Best, D., Gossop, M., Lehmann, P., Harris, J., & Strang, J. (1999). The relationship between overdose and alcohol consumption among methadone maintenance patients. *Journal of Substance Use, 4,* 41–44.

Blaney, T., & Craig, R. J. (1999). Methadone maintenance. Does dose determine differences in outcome? *Journal of Substance Abuse Treatment, 16,* 221–228.

Bleich, A., Gelkopf, M., Schmidt, V., Hayward, R., Bodner, G., & Adelson, M. (1999). Correlates of benzodiazepine abuse in methadone maintenance treatment. A 1 year prospective study in an Israeli clinic. *Addiction, 94,* 1533–1540.

Blomberg, R. D., & Preusser, D. F. (1974). Narcotic use and driving behavior. *Accident Analysis and Prevention, 6,* 23–32.

Boccellari, A. A., Chambers, D. B., Dilley, J. W., Shore, M. D., Tauber, M. A., Moss, A. R., et al. (1994). Relationship of B_2 microglobulin and CD4 counts to neuropsychological performance in HIV-1-infected intravenous drug users. *Journal of Acquired Immune Deficiency Syndrome, 7,* 1040–1049.

Braida, D., Gori, E., & Sala, M. (1994). Relationship between morphine and etonitazene-induced working memory impairment and analgesia. *European Journal of Pharmacology, 271,* 497–504.

Brown, R. R., & Partington, J. E. (1942). A psychometric comparison of narcotic addicts with hospital attendants. *Journal of General Psychology, 27,* 71–79.

Budd, R. D., Muto, J. J., & Wong, J. K. (1989). Drugs of abuse found in fatally injured drivers in Los Angeles County. *Drug and Alcohol Dependance, 23,* 153–158.

Chatham, L. R., Rowan-Szal, G. A., Joe, G. W., Brown, B. S., & Simpson, D. D. (1995). Heavy drinking in a population of methadone-maintained clients. *Journal of Studies on Alcohol, 56,* 417–422.

Christensen, L. Q., Nielsen, L. M., & Nielsen, S. L. (1990). Traffic accidents and drivers suspected for drug influence. *Forensic Science International, 45,* 273–280.

Chutuape, M. A., Brooner, R. K., & Stitzer, M. (1997). Sedative use disorders in opiate-dependent patients: association with psychiatric and other substance use disorders. *Journal of Nervous and Mental Disorders, 185,* 289–297.

Cimbura, G., Lucas, D. M., Bennett, R. C., Warren, R. A., & Simpson, H. M. (1982). Incidence and toxicological aspects of drugs detected in 484 fatally injured drivers and pedestrians in Ontario. *Journal of Forensic Science, 27,* 855–867.

Cohen, A. J., Klett, C. J., & Ling, W. (1983). Patient perspectives of opiate withdrawal. *Drug and Alcohol Dependence, 12,* 167–172.

Comer, S. D., Collins, E. D., & Fischman, M. W. (1997). Choice between money and intranasal heroin in morphine-maintained humans. *Behavioral Pharmacology*, *8*, 677–690.

Cone, E. J., Holicky, B. A., Grant, T. M., Darwin, W. D., & Goldberger, B. A. (1993). Pharmacokinetics and pharmacodynamics of intranasal "snorted" heroin. *Journal of Analytical Toxicology*, *17*, 327–337.

Cooper, J. R. (1992). Ineffective use of psychoactive drugs. Methadone treatment is no exception. *Journal of the American Medical Association*, *267*, 281–282.

Curran, H. V. (2000). Psychopharmacological approaches to human memory. In M. S. Gazzaniga (Ed.) *The new cognitive neurosciences* (2nd edn, pp. 797–804). Boston: MIT Press.

Curran, H. V., Bolton, J., Wanigaratne, S., & Smyth, C. (1999). Additional methadone increases craving for heroin: a double-blind, placebo-controlled study of chronic opiate users receiving methadone substitution treatment. *Addiction*, *94*, 665–674.

Curran, H. V., Kleckham, J., Bearn, J., Strang, J., & Wanigaratne, S. (2001). Effects of methadone on cognition, mood and craving in detoxifying opiate addicts: a dose–response study. *Psychopharmacology (Berlin)*, *154*, 153–160.

Cushman, P., & Dole, V. P. (1973). Detoxification of rehabilitated methadone-maintained patients. *Journal of the American Medical Association*, *226*, 747–752.

Danos, P., Kasper, S., Grunwald, F., Klemm, E., Krappel, C., Broich, K., et al. (1998). Pathological regional cerebral blood flow in opiate-dependent patients during withdrawal: a HMPAO-SPECT study. *Neuropsychobiology*, *37*, 194–199.

Darke, S., Sims, J., McDonald, S., & Wickes, W. (2000). Cognitive impairment among methadone maintenance patients. *Addiction*, *95*, 687–695.

Darke, S., Swift, W., & Hall, W. (1994). Prevalence, severity and correlates of psychological morbidity among methadone maintenance clients. *Addiction*, *89*, 211–217.

D'Aunno, T., & Pollack, H. A. (2002). Changes in methadone treatment practices: results from a national panel study, 1988–2000. *Journal of the American Medical Association*, *288*, 850–856.

D'Aunno, T., & Vaughn, T. E. (1992). Variations in methadone treatment practices. Results from a national study. *Journal of the American Medical Association*, *267*, 253–258.

Davis, P. E., Liddiard, H., & McMillan, T. M. (2002). Neuropsychological deficits and opiate abuse. *Drug and Alcohol Dependence*, *67*, 105–108.

Dole, V. P., & Nyswander, M. E. (1965). A medical treatment for diacetylmorphine (heroin) addiction: A clinical trial with methadone hydrochloride. *Journal of the American Medical Association*, *193*, 80–84.

Dole, V. P., & Nyswander, M. E. (1966). Rehabilitation of heroin addicts after blockade with methadone. *New York State Journal of Medicine*, *66*, 2011–2017.

Dyer, K. R., White, J. M., Foster, D. J., Bochner, F., Menelaou, A., & Somogyi, A. A. (2001). The relationship between mood state and plasma methadone concentration in maintenance patients. *Journal of Clinical Psychopharmacology*, *21*, 78–84.

Eklund, C., Hiltunen, A. J., Melin, L., & Borg, S. (1997). Patient perceptions of psychological and physiological withdrawal symptoms and positive factors associated with gradual withdrawal from methadone maintenance treatment: a prospective study. *Substance Use and Misuse*, *32*, 1599–1618.

El-Bassel, N., Schilling, R. F., Turnbull, J. E., & Su, K. H. (1993). Correlates of alcohol use among methadone patients. *Alcohol Clinical Experimental Research*, *17*, 681–686.

Fields, F. R., & Fullerton, J. R. (1975). Influence of heroin addiction on neuropsychological functioning. *Journal of Consulting Clinical Psychology, 43*, 114.

Finnigan, F., & Hammersley, R. (1992). The effect of alcohol on performance. In A. P. Smith & D. M. Jones (Eds.), *Handbook of human performance, health and performance 2* (pp. 73–126). London: Academic Press.

Folli, D., Mutti, A., Van der Venne, M. T., Berlin, A., Gerra, G., Cavazzini, S., et al. (1992). Neuroendocrine response to psychological performance testing. *Psychoneuroendocrinology, 17*, 467–474.

Foltin, R. W., & Fischman, M. W. (1992). The cardiovascular and subjective effects of intravenous cocaine and morphine combinations in humans. *Journal of Pharmacology and Experimental Therapeutics, 261*, 623–632.

Forman, S. D., Dougherty, G. G., Casey, B. J., Siegle, G. J., Braver, T. S., Barch, D. M., et al. (2004). Opiate addicts lack error-dependent activation of rostral anterior cingulate. *Biological Psychiatry, 55*, 531–537.

Fraser, H. F., Jones, B. E., Rosenberg, D. E., & Thompson, A. K. (1963). Effects of addiction to intravenous heroin on patterns of physical activity in man. *Clinical Pharmacology and Therapeutics, 4*, 188–196.

Fraser, H. F., Jones, B. E., Rosenberg, D. E., & Thompson, A. K. (1964). Effect of a cycle of addiction to intravenous heroin on certain physiological measurements. *Bulletin of Narcotics, 16*, 17–23.

Galynker, I. I., Watras-Ganz, S., Miner, C., Rosenthal, R. N., Des Jarlais, D. C., Richman, B. L., et al. (2000). Cerebral metabolism in opiate-dependent subjects: effects of methadone maintenance. *Mount Sinai Journal of Medicine, 67*, 381–387.

Garcia-Estrada, J., Tapia-Arizmendi, G., Feria-Velasco, A., & Aleman, V. (1988). Ultrastructural alterations in caudate nucleus, cerebral cortex and hippocampus produced by morphine. *General Pharmacology, 19*, 841–848.

Garcia-Sevilla, J. A., Ventayol, P., Busquets, X., La Harpe, R., Walzer, C., & Guimon, J. (1997). Marked decrease of immunolabelled 68 kDa neurofilament (NF-L) proteins in brains of opiate addicts. *Neuroreport, 8*, 1561–1565.

Garriott, J. C., DiMaio, V. J., Zumwalt, R. E., & Petty, C. S. (1977). Incidence of drugs and alcohol in fatally injured motor vehicle drivers. *Journal of Forensic Science, 22*, 383–389.

Gerra, G., Calbiani, B., Zaimovic, A., Sartori, R., Ugolotti, G., Ippolito, L., et al. (1998). Regional cerebral blood flow and comorbid diagnosis in abstinent opioid addicts. *Psychiatry Research, 83*, 117–126.

Gerra, G., Ceresini, S., Esposito, A., Zaimovic, A., Moi, G., Bussandri, M., et al. (2003). Neuroendocrine and behavioural responses to opioid receptor-antagonist during heroin detoxification: Relationship with personality traits. *International Clinical Psychopharmacology, 18*, 261–269.

Gjerde, H., Beylich, K.-M., & Morland, J. (1993). Incidence of alcohol and drugs in fatally injured car drivers in Norway. *Accident Analysis and Prevention, 25*, 479–483.

Gold, M. L., Sorensen, J. L., McCanlies, N., Trier, M., & Dlugosch, G. (1988). Tapering from methadone maintenance: attitudes of clients and staff. *Journal of Substance Abuse Treatment, 5*, 37–44.

Gonzalez, G., Oliveto, A., & Kosten, T. R. (2002). Treatment of heroin (diamorphine) addiction. Current approaches and future prospects. *Drugs, 62*, 1331–1343.

Gordon, N. B. (1970). Reaction-times of methadone treated ex-heroin addicts. *Psychopharmacologia, 16*, 337–344.

Gottschalk, L. A., & Gleser, G. C. (1969). *The measurement of psychological states through the content analysis of verbal behavior*, Berkeley, CA: University of California Press.

Grant, I., Adams, K. M., Carlin, A. S., Rennick, P. M., Judd. L. L., & Schooff, K. (1978). The collaborative neuropsychological study of polydrug users. *Archives of General Psychiatry, 35*, 1063–1074.

Gravenstein, J. S., Smith, G. M., Sphire, R. D., Isaacs, J. P., & Beecher, H. K. (1956). Dihydrocodeine; further development in measurement of analgesic power and appraisal of psychologic side effects of analgesic agents. *New England Journal of Medicine, 254*, 877–885.

Greenwald, M. K., & Stitzer, M. L. (1998). Butorphanol agonist effects and acute physical dependence in opioid abusers: comparison with morphine. *Drug and Alcohol Dependence, 53*, 17–30.

Grevert, P., Masover, B., & Goldstein, A. (1977). Failure of methadone and levomethadyl acetate (levo-alpha-acetylmethadol, LAAM) maintenance to affect memory. *Archives of General Psychiatry, 34*, 849–853.

Gritz, E. R., Shiffman, S. M., Jarvik, M. E., Haber, J., Dymond, A. M., Coger, R., et al. (1975). Physiological and psychological effects of methadone in man. *Archives of General Psychiatry, 32*, 237–242.

Guerra, D., Sole, A., Cami, J., & Tobena, A. (1987). Neuropsychological performance in opiate addicts after rapid detoxification. *Drug and Alcohol Dependence, 20*, 261–270.

Gutstein, H. B., & Akil, H. (2001). Opioid analgesics. In *Goodman & Gilman's, The pharmacological basis of therapeutics* (10th edn, pp. 569–619). New York: McGraw-Hill.

Haertzen, C. A., Hill, H. E., & Belleville, R. E. (1963). Development of the addiction research center inventory (ARCI): Selection of items that are sensitive to the effects of various drugs. *Psychopharmacologia, 4*, 155–166.

Haertzen, C. A., & Hooks, N. T., Jr. (1969). Changes in personality and subjective experience associated with the chronic administration and withdrawal of opiates. *Journal of Nervous and Mental Disorders, 148*, 606–614.

Haertzen, C. A., Meketon, M. J., & Hooks, N. T., Jr. (1970). Subjective experiences produced by the withdrawal of opiates. *British Journal of Addiction to Alcohol and Other Drugs, 65*, 245–255.

Handelsman, L., Aronson, M. J., Ness, R., Cochrane, K. J., & Kanof, P. D. (1992). The dysphoria of heroin addiction. *American Journal of Drug and Alcohol Abuse, 18*, 275–287.

Handelsman, L., Cochrane, K. J., Aronson, M. J., Ness, R., Rubinstein, K. J., & Kanof, P. D. (1987). Two new rating scales for opiate withdrawal. *American Journal of Drug and Alcohol Abuse, 13*, 293–308.

Harris, G. C., & Aston-Jones, G. (2003). Altered motivation and learning following opiate withdrawal: evidence for prolonged dysregulation of reward processing. *Neuropsychopharmacology, 28*, 865–871.

Heishman, S. J., Schuh, K. J., Schuster, C. R., Henningfield, J. E., & Goldberg, S. R. (2000). Reinforcing and subjective effects of morphine in human opioid abusers: effect of dose and alternative reinforcer. *Psychopharmacology (Berlin), 148*, 272–280.

Heishman, S. J., Stitzer, M. L., Bigelow, G. E., & Liebson, I. A. (1990). Acute opioid physical dependence in humans: Effect of naloxone at 6 and 24 hours postmorphine. *Pharmacology, Biochemistry and Behavior, 36*, 393–399.

Hepner, I. J., Homewood, J., & Taylor, A. J. (2002). Methadone disrupts performance

on the working memory version of the Morris water task. *Physiology and Behavior*, *76*, 41–49.
Herning, R. I., Better, W. E., Tate, K., Umbricht, A., Preston, K. L., & Cadet, J. L. (2003). Methadone treatment induces attenuation of cerebrovascular deficits associated with the prolonged abuse of cocaine and heroin. *Neuropsychopharmacology*, *28*, 562–568.
Higgins, S. T., Preston, K. L., Cone, E. J., Henningfield, J. E., & Jaffe, J. H. (1992). Supersensitivity to naloxone following acute morphine pretreatment in humans: behavioral, hormonal and physiological effects. *Drug and Alcohol Dependence*, *30*, 13–26.
Hill, H. E., Belleville, R. E., & Wikler, A. (1955). Studies on anxiety associated with anticipation of pain. II. Comparative effects of pentobarbital and morphine. *AMA Archives of Neurology and Psychiatry*, *73*, 602–608.
Hill, H. E., Belleville, R. E., & Wikler, A. (1957). Motivational determinants in modification of behavior by morphine and pentobarbital. *AMA Archives of Neurology and Psychiatry*, *77*, 28–35.
Hill, H. E., Kornetsky, C. H., Flanary, H. G., & Wikler, A. (1952). Studies on anxiety associated with anticipation of pain. I. Effects of morphine. *AMA Archives of Neurology and Psychiatry*, *67*, 612–619.
Hill, S. Y., & Mikhael, M. A. (1979). Computerized transaxial tomographic and neuropsychol evaluations in chronic alcoholics and heroin abusers. *American Journal of Psychiatry*, *136*, 598–602.
Hill, S. Y., Reyes, R. B., Mikhael, M., & Ayre, F. (1979). A comparison of alcoholics and heroin abusers: computerized transaxial tomography and neuropsychological functioning. *Currents in Alcohol*, *5*, 187–205.
Hillebrand, J., Marsden, J., Finch, E., & Strang, J. (2001). Excessive alcohol consumption and drinking expectations among clients in methadone maintenance. *Journal of Substance Abuse Treatment*, *21*, 155–160.
Hiltunen, A. J., Lafolie, P., Martel, J., Ottosson, E. C., Boreus, L. O., Beck, O., et al. (1995). Subjective and objective symptoms in relation to plasma methadone concentration in methadone patients. *Psychopharmacology*, *118*, 122–126.
Hindmarch, I., Kerr, J. S., & Sherwood, N. (1991). The effects of alcohol and other drugs on psychomotor performance and cognitive function. *Alcohol and Alcoholism*, *26*, 71–79.
Honkanen, R., Ertama, L., Linnoila, M., Alha, A., Lukkari, I., Karlsson, M., et al. (1980). Role of drugs in traffic accidents. *British Medical Journal*, *281*, 1309–1312.
Iguchi, M. Y., Handelsman, L., Bickel, W. K., & Griffiths, R. R. (1993). Benzodiazepine and sedative use/abuse by methadone maintenance clients. *Drug and Alcohol Dependence*, *32*, 257–266.
Ikonomidou-Turski, C., Cavalheiro, E. A., Turski, W. A., Bortolotto, Z. A., & Turski, L. (1987). Convulsant action of morphine, [D-ALA, D-LEU]-enkephalin and naloxone in the rat amygdala: Electroencephalographic, morphological and behavioural sequelae. *Neuroscience*, *20*, 671–686.
Isbell, H., Wilker, A., Eisenman, A. J., Daingerfield, M., & Frank, K. (1948). Liability of addiction to 6-dimethylamino-4-4-diphenyl-3-heptanone (methadon, "amidone" or "10820") in man. *Archives of Internal Medicine*, *82*, 362–392.
Jasinski, D. R., & Mansky, P. A. (1972). Evaluation of nalbuphine for abuse potential. *Clinical Pharmacology and Therapeutics*, *13*, 78–90.
Jasinski, D. R., Martin, W. R., & Hoeldtke, R. D. (1970). Effects of short- and

long-term administration of pentazocine in man. *Clinical Pharmacology and Therapeutics, 11*, 385–403.

Jasinski, D. R., & Preston, K. L. (1986). Comparison of intravenously administered methadone, morphine and heroin. *Drug and Alcohol Dependence, 17*, 301–310.

Joseph, H., Stancliff, S., & Langrod, J. (2000). Methadone maintenance treatment (MMT): a review of historical and clinical issues. *Mount Sinai Journal of Medicine, 67*, 347–364.

Kanof, P. D., Aronson, M. J., & Ness, R. (1993). Organic mood syndrome associated with detoxification from methadone maintenance. *American Journal of Psychiatry, 150*, 423–428.

Kanof, P. D., Handelsman, L., Aronson, M. J., Ness, R., Cochrane, K. J., & Rubinstein, K. J. (1992). Clinical characteristics of naloxone-precipitated withdrawal in human opioid-dependent subjects. *Journal of Pharmacology and Experimental Therapeutics, 260*, 355–363.

Kaufman, M. J., Pollack, M. H., Villafuerte, R. A., Kukes, T. J., Rose, S. L., Mendelson, J. H., et al. (1999). Cerebral phosphorus metabolite abnormalities in opiate-dependent polydrug abusers in methadone maintenance. *Psychiatry Research, 90*, 143–152.

Kelly, D., Welch, R., & McKnelley, W. (1978). Methadone maintenance: an assessment of potential fluctuations in behavior between doses. *International Journal of Addiction, 13*, 1061–1068.

Kirby, K. N., Petry, N. M., & Bickel, W. K. (1999). Heroin addicts have higher discount rates for delayed rewards than non-drug-using controls. *Journal of Experimental Psychology: General, 128*, 78–87.

Kish, S. J., Kalasinsky, K. S., Derkach, P., Schmunk, G. A., Guttman, M., Ang, L., et al. (2001). Striatal dopaminergic and serotonergic markers in human heroin users. *Neuropsychopharmacology, 24*, 561–567.

Kleber, H. D. (1977). Detoxification from methadone maintenance: the state of the art. *International Journal of Addiction, 12*, 807–820.

Kofke, W. A., Garman, R. H., Garman, R., & Rose, M. E. (1999). Opioid neurotoxicity: fentanyl-induced exacerbation of cerebral ischemia in rats. *Brain Research, 818*, 326–334.

Kofke, W. A., Garman, R. H., Janosky, J., & Rose, M. E. (1996). Opioid neurotoxicity: Neuropathologic effects in rats of different fentanyl congeners and the effects of hexamethonium-induced normotension. *Anesthesia and Analgesia, 83*, 141–146.

Kofke, W. A., Garman, R. H., Stiller, R. L., Rose, M. E., & Garman, R. (1996). Opioid neurotoxicity: fentanyl dose-response effects in rats. *Anesthesia and Analgesia, 83*, 1298–1306.

Kofke, W. A., Garman, R. H., Tom, W. C., Rose, M. E., & Hawkins, R. A. (1992). Alfentanil-induced hypermetabolism, seizure, and histopathology in rat brain. *Anesthesia and Analgesia, 75*, 953–964.

Korin, H. (1974). Comparison of psychometric measures in psychiatric patients using heroin and other drugs. *Journal of Abnormal Psychology, 83*, 208–212.

Kornreich, C., Foisy, M. L., Philippot, P., Dan, B., Tecco, J., Noel, X. et al. (2003). Impaired emotional facial expression recognition in alcoholics, opiate dependence subjects, methadone maintained subjects and mixed alcohol-opiate antecedents subjects compared with normal controls. *Psychiatry Research, 119*, 251–260.

Kreek, M. J. (1984). Opioid interactions with alcohol. *Advances in Alcohol and Substance Abuse, 3*, 35–46.

Krystal, J. H., Woods, S. W., Kosten, T. R., Rosen, M. I., Seibyl, J. P., van Dyck, C. C., et al. (1995). Opiate dependence and withdrawal: preliminary assessment using single photon emission computerized tomography (SPECT). *American Journal of Drug and Alcohol Abuse, 21*, 47–63.

Lamas, X., Farre, M., & Cami, J. (1994). Acute effects of pentazocine, naloxone and morphine in opioid-dependent volunteers. *Journal of Pharmacology and Experimental Therapeutics, 268*, 1485–1492.

Lasagna, L., von Felsinger, J. M., & Beecher, H. K. (1955). Drug-induced mood changes in man. I. Observations on healthy subjects, chronically ill patients, and postaddicts. *Journal of the American Medical Association, 157*, 1006–1020.

Latowsky, M. (1996). Improving detoxification outcomes from methadone maintenance treatment: the interrelationship of affective states and protracted withdrawal. *Journal of Psychoactive Drugs, 28*, 251–257.

Leavitt, S. B. (1998). Dosage survey '98: Changes for the better. *Addiction Treatment Forum, 7*, 1. Retrieved May 29, 2003, from *http://www.atforum.com*

Leavitt, S. B., Shinderman, M., Maxwell, S., Eap, C. B., & Paris, P. (2000). When "enough" is not enough: new perspectives on optimal methadone maintenance dose. *Mount Sinai Journal of Medicine, 67*, 404–411.

Lenne, M. G., Dietze, P., Rumbold, G. R., Redman, J. R., & Triggs, T. J. (2003). The effects of the opioid pharmacotherapies methadone, LAAM and buprenorphine, alone and in combination with alcohol, on simulated driving. *Drug and Alcohol Dependence, 72*, 271–278.

Leveille, S. G., Buchner, D. M., Koepsell, T. D., McCloskey, L. W., Wolf, M. E., & Wagner, E. H. (1994). Psychoactive medications and injurious motor vehicle collisions involving older drivers. *Epidemiology, 5*, 591–598.

Ling, W., Wesson, D. R., Charuvastra, C., & Klett, C. J. (1996). A controlled trial comparing buprenorphine and methadone maintenance in opioid dependence. *Archives of General Psychiatry, 53*, 401–407.

Linnoila, M., & Hakkinen, S. (1974). Effects of diazepam and codeine, alone and in combination with alcohol, on simulated driving. *Clinical Pharmacology and Therapeutics, 15*, 368–373.

Linnoila, M., & Mattila, M. J. (1973). Interaction of alcohol and drugs on psychomotor skills as demonstrated by a driving simulator. *British Journal of Pharmacology, 47*, 671P–672P.

London, E. D., Broussolle, E. P. M., Links, J. M., Wong, D. F., Cascella, N. G., Dannals, R. F., et al. (1990). Morphine-induced metabolic changes in human brain. *Archives of General Psychiatry, 47*, 73–81.

Lyvers, M., & Yakimoff, M. (2003). Neuropsychological correlates of opioid dependence and withdrawal. *Addiction and Behavior, 28*, 605–611.

Madden, G. J., Petry, N. M., Badger, G. J., & Bickel, W. K. (1997). Impulsive and self-control choices in opioid-dependent patients and non-drug-using control participants: drug and monetary rewards. *Experiments in Clinical Psychopharmacology, 5*, 256–262.

Maddux, J. F., Williams, T. R., & Ziegler, J. A. (1977). Driving records before and during methadone maintenance. *American Journal of Drug and Alcohol Abuse, 4*, 91–100.

Margolin, A., Avants, S. K., Warburton, L. A., & Hawkins, K. A. (2002). Factors affecting cognitive functioning in a sample of human immunodeficiency virus-positive injection drug users. *AIDS Patient Care and STDs, 16*, 255–267.

Martin, W. R. (1968). A homeostatic and redundancy theory of tolerance to and dependence on narcotic analgesics. In A. Wikler (Ed.) *The addictive states: Proceedings of the association for research in nervous and mental disease, December 2 and 3, 1966, New York, NY* (pp. 206–223). Baltimore: Williams and Wilkins.

Martin, W. R., & Fraser, H. F. (1961). A comparative study of physiological and subjective effects of heroin and morphine administered intravenously in postaddicts. *Journal of Pharmacology and Experimental Therapeutics, 133*, 388–399.

Martin, W. R., & Jasinski, D. R. (1969). Physiological parameters of morphine dependence in man – tolerance, early abstinence, protracted abstinence. *Journal of Psychiatric Research, 7*, 9–17.

Martin, W. R., Jasinski, D. R., Haertzen, C. A., Kay, D. C., Jones, B. E., Mansky, P. A., et al. (1973). Methadone – a reevaluation. *Archives of General Psychiatry, 28*, 286–295.

Martin, W. R., & Sloan, J. W. (1968). The pathophysiology of morphine dependence and its treatment with opioid antagonists. *Pharmakopsychiatrie/Neuropsychopharmakologie, 1*, 260–270.

Martin, W. R., Thompson, W. O., & Fraser, H. F. (1974). Comparison of graded single intramuscular doses of morphine and pentobarbital in man. *Clinical Pharmacology and Therapeutics, 15*, 623–630.

Mason, A. P., & McBay, A. J. (1984). Ethanol, marijuana, and other drug use in 600 drivers killed in single-vehicle crashes in North Carolina, 1978–1981. *Journal of Forensic Science, 29*, 987–1026.

Maxwell, S., & Shinderman, M. (1999). Optimizing response to methadone maintenance treatment: use of higher-dose methadone. *Journal of Psychoactive Drugs, 31*, 95–102.

Maxwell, S., & Shinderman, M. S. (2002). Optimizing long-term response to methadone maintenance treatment: a 152-week follow-up using higher-dose methadone. *Journal of Addictive Diseases, 21*, 1–12.

McCaul, M. E., Bigelow, G. E., Stitzer, M. L., & Liebson, I. (1982). Short-term effects of oral methadone in methadone maintenance subjects. *Clinical Pharmacology and Therapeutics, 31*, 753–761.

McNamee, H. B., Mirin, S. M., Kuehnle, J. C., & Meyer, R. E. (1976). Affective changes in chronic opiate use. *British Journal of Addiction to Alcohol and Other Drugs, 71*, 275–280.

Mintzer, M. Z., Copersino, M. L., & Stitzer, M. L. (2005). Opioid abuse and cognitive performance. *Drug and Alcohol Dependence, 78*, 225–230.

Mintzer, M. Z., Correia, C. J., & Strain, E. C. (2004). A dose-effect study of repeated administration of buprenorphine/naloxone on performance in opioid-dependent volunteers. *Drug and Alcohol Dependence, 74*, 205–209.

Mintzer, M. Z., & Stitzer, M. L. (2002). Cognitive impairment in methadone maintenance patients. *Drug and Alcohol Dependence, 67*, 41–51.

Mirin, S. M., Meyer, R. E., & McNamee, H. B. (1976). Psychopathology and mood during heroin use: acute vs chronic effects. *Archives of General Psychiatry, 33*, 1503–1508.

Mirin, S. M., Meyer, R. E., McNamee, H. B., & McDougle, M. (1976). Psychopathology, craving, and mood during heroin acquisition: an experimental study. *International Journal of Addiction, 11*, 525–544.

Moskowitz, H., & Robinson, C. D. (1985). Methadone maintenance and tracking

performance. In S. Kaye & G. W. Meier (Eds.), *Alcohol, drugs and traffic safety* (pp. 995–1004). Washington, DC: US Department of Transportation.
Murakami, A., Edelmann, R. J., & Davis, P. E. (1996). Interrogative suggestibility in opiate users. *Addiction, 91*, 1365–1373.
NIH-CDC (1997). Effective medical treatment of heroin addiction. *NIH consensus statement*. Bethesda, MD: National Institutes of Health.
Ornstein, T. J., Iddon, J. L., Baldacchino, A. M., Sahakian, B. J., London, M., Everitt, B. J., et al. (2000). Profiles of cognitive dysfunction in chronic amphetamine and heroin abusers. *Neuropsychopharmacology, 23*, 113–126.
Pau, C. W., Lee, T. M., & Chan, S. F. (2002). The impact of heroin on frontal executive functions. *Archives of Clinical Neuropsychology, 17*, 663–670.
Payte, J. E., & Khuri, E. T. (1993). Principles of methadone dose determination. In M. W. Parrino (Ed.), *CSAT State methadone treatment guidelines*, Treatment Improvement Protocol (TIP) Series 1, US Department of Health and Human Services 1993:47–58, USPHS Publication (SMA) 93–1991. Rockville, MD: Center for Substance Abuse Treatment.
Pearson, J., & Richter, R. W. (1975) Neuropathological effects of opiate addiction, In R. W. Richter (Ed.), *Medical aspects of drug abuse* (pp. 308–319). Hagerstown: Harper & Row.
Petry, N. M., Bickel, W. K., & Arnett, M. (1998). Shortened time horizons and insensitivity to future consequences in heroin addicts. *Addiction, 93*, 729–738.
Petry, N. M., Bickel, W. K., Huddleston, J., Tzanis, E., & Badger, G. J. (1998). A comparison of subjective, psychomotor and physiological effects of a novel muscarinic analgesic, LY297802 tartrate, and oral morphine in occasional drug users. *Drug and Alcohol Dependence, 50*, 129–136.
Pezawas, L. M., Fischer, G., Diamant, K., Schneider, C., Schindler, S. D., Thurnher, M., et al. (1998). Cerebral CT findings in male opioid-dependent patients: stereological, planimetric and linear measurements. *Psychiatry Research, 83*, 139–147.
Pezawas, L., Fischer, G., Podreka, I., Schindler, S., Brucke, T., Jagsch, R., et al. (2002). Opioid addiction changes cerebral blood flow symmetry. *Neuropsychobiology, 45*, 67–73.
Pfeffer, A. Z., & Ruble, D. C. (1946). Chronic psychoses and addiction to morphine. *Archives of Neurology and Psychiatry, 56*, 665–672.
Phillips, G. T., Gossop, M., & Bradley, B. (1986). The influence of psychological factors on the opiate withdrawal syndrome. *British Journal of Psychiatry, 149*, 235–238.
Pickworth, W. B., Johnson, R. E., Holicky, B. A., & Cone, E. J. (1993). Subjective and physiologic effects of intravenous buprenorphine in humans. *Clinical Pharmacology and Therapeutics, 53*, 570–576.
Pickworth, W. B., Rohrer, M. S., & Fant, R. V. (1997). Effects of abused drugs on psychomotor performance. *Experimental and Clinical Psychopharmacology, 5*, 235–241.
Powell, J. E., & Taylor, D. (1992). Anger, depression, and anxiety following heroin withdrawal. *International Journal of Addiction, 27*, 25–35.
Preston, K. L., Bigelow, G. E., Bickel, W., & Liebson, I. A. (1987). Three-choice drug discrimination in opioid-dependent humans: hydromorphone, naloxone and saline. *Journal of Pharmacology and Experimental Therapeutics, 243*, 1002–1009.
Preston, K. L., Bigelow, G. E., Bickel, W. K., & Liebson, I. A. (1989). Drug

discrimination in human postaddicts: agonist-antagonist opioids. *Journal of Pharmacology and Experimental Therapeutics, 250,* 184–196.

Preston, K. L., Bigelow, G. E., & Liebson, I. A. (1987). Comparative evaluation of morphine, pentazocine and ciramadol in postaddicts. *Journal of Pharmacology and Experimental Therapeutics, 240,* 900–910.

Preston, K. L., Bigelow, G. E., & Liebson, I. A. (1988a). Buprenorphine and naloxone alone and in combination in opioid-dependent humans. *Psychopharmacology (Berlin), 94,* 484–490.

Preston, K. L., Bigelow, G. E., & Liebson, I. A. (1988b). Butorphanol-precipitated withdrawal in opioid-dependent human volunteers. *Journal of Pharmacology and Experimental Therapeutics, 246,* 441–448.

Preston, K. L., Bigelow, G. E., & Liebson, I. A. (1989). Antagonist effects of nalbuphine in opioid-dependent human volunteers. *Journal of Pharmacology and Experimental Therapeutics, 248,* 929–937.

Preston, K. L., Bigelow, G. E., & Liebson, I. A. (1990). Discrimination of butorphanol and nalbuphine in opioid-dependent humans. *Pharmacology, Biochemistry and Behavior, 37,* 511–522.

Preston, K. L., Griffiths, R. R., Stitzer, M. L., Bigelow, G. E., & Liebson, I. A. (1984). Diazepam and methadone interactions in methadone maintenance. *Clinical Pharmacology and Therapeutics, 36,* 534–541.

Preston, K. L., Liebson, I. A., & Bigelow, G. E. (1992). Discrimination of agonist-antagonist opioids in humans trained on a two-choice saline-hydromorphone discrimination. *Journal of Pharmacology and Experimental Therapeutics, 261,* 62–71.

Price, B. B., Moran, S., Crunican, M. A., Rothenberg, S., & Cutter, H. S. (1975). Mood, primary heroin withdrawal, and acute methadone administration. *International Journal of Addiction, 10,* 613–631.

Ray, W. A., Fought, R. L., & Decker, M. D. (1992). Psychoactive drugs and the risk of injurious motor vehicle crashes in elderly drivers. *American Journal of Epidemiology, 136,* 873–883.

Robinson, C. D., & Moskowitz, H. (1985). Methadone maintenance treatment and aspects of skilled performance. In S. Kaye & G. W. Meier (Eds.), *Alcohol, drugs and traffic safety* (pp. 1145–1157). Washington, DC: US Department of Transportation.

Robinson, T. E., Gorny, G., Savage, V. R., & Kolb, B. (2002). Widespread but regionally specific effects of experimenter- versus self-administered morphine on dendritic spines in the nucleus accumbens, hippocampus, and neocortex of adult rats. *Synapse, 46,* 271–279.

Robinson, T. E., & Kolb, B. (1999). Morphine alters the structure of neurons in the nucleus accumbens and neocortex of rats. *Synapse, 33,* 160–162.

Robinson, T. E., &, Kolb, B. (2004). Structural plasticity associated with exposure to drugs of abuse. *Neuropharmacology, 47,* 33–46.

Robles, E., Miller, F. B., Gilmore-Thomas, K. K., & McMillan, D. E. (2001). Implementation of a clinic policy of client-regulated methadone dosing. *Journal of Substance Abuse and Treatment, 20,* 225–231.

Rogers, R. D., Everitt, B. J., Baldacchino, A., Blackshaw, A. J., Swainson, R., Wynne, K., et al. (1999). Dissociable deficits in the decision-making cognition of chronic amphetamine abusers, opiate abusers, patients with focal damage to prefrontal cortex, and tryptophan-depleted normal volunteers: evidence for monoaminergic mechanisms. *Neuropsychopharmacology, 20,* 322–339.

Rönnbäck, L., Wikkelso, C., & Blomstrand, C. (1983). Macromolecular changes in brain stem of morphinized rats. *Neurochemistry Research, 8,* 1487–1495.

Rose, J. S., Branchey, M., Buydens-Branchey, L., Stapleton, J. M., Chasten, K., Werrell, A., et al. (1996). Cerebral perfusion in early and late opiate withdrawal: a technetium-99m-HMPAO SPECT study. *Psychiatry Research, 67,* 39–47.

Rothenberg, S., Schottenfeld, S., Meyer, R. E., Krauss, B., & Gross, K. (1977). Performance differences between addicts and non-addicts. *Psychopharmacology (Berlin), 52,* 299–306.

Rotheram-Fuller, E., Shoptaw, S., Berman, S. M., & London, E. D. (2004). Impaired performance in a test of decision-making by opiate-dependent tobacco smokers. *Drug and Alcohol Dependence, 73,* 79–86.

Rounsaville, B. J., Jones, C., Novelly, R. A., & Kleber, H. (1982). Neuropsychological functioning in opiate addicts. *Journal of Nervous and Mental Disorders, 170,* 209–216.

Rounsaville, B. J., Novelly, R. A., Kleber, H. D., & Jones, C. (1981). Neuropsychological impairment in opiate addicts: risk factors. *Annals of the New York Academy of Sciences, 362,* 79–80.

Saha, N., Datta, H., & Sharma, P. L. (1991). Effects of morphine on memory: interactions with naloxone, propranolol and haloperidol. *Pharmacology, 42,* 10–14.

Schindler, S. D., Ortner, R., Peternell, A., Eder, H., Opgenoorth, E., & Fischer, G. (2004). Maintenance therapy with synthetic opioids and driving aptitude. *European Addiction Research, 10,* 80–87.

Sell, L. A., Simmons, A., Lemmens, G. M., Williams, S. C., Brammer, M., & Strang, J. (1997). Functional magnetic resonance imaging of the acute effect of intravenous heroin administration on visual activation in long-term heroin addicts: results from a feasibility study. *Drug and Alcohol Dependence, 49,* 55–60.

Shorr, R. I., Griffin, M. R., Daugherty, J. R., & Ray, W. A. (1992). Opioid analgesics and the risk of hip fracture in the elderly: codeine and propoxyphene. *Journal of Gerontology, 47,* M111–115.

Siebert, D. J. (1994). Salvia divinorum and salvinorin A: new pharmacologic findings. *Journal of Ethnopharmacology, 43,* 53–56.

Sinz, E. H., Kofke, W. A., & Garman, R. H. (2000). Phenytoin, midazolam, and naloxone protect against fentanyl-induced brain damage in rats. *Anesthesia and Analgesia, 91,* 1443–1449.

Sklair-Tavron, L., Shi, W. X., Lane, S. B., Harris, H. W., Bunney, B. S., & Nestler, E. J. (1996). Chronic morphine induces visible changes in the morphology of mesolimbic dopamine neurons. *Proceedings of the National Academy of Sciences of the USA, 93,* 11202–11207.

Smith, G. M., & Beecher, H. K. (1959). Measurement of mental clouding and other subjective effects of morphine. *Journal of Pharmacology and Experimental Therapeutics, 126,* 50–62.

Smith, G. M., & Beecher, H. K. (1962). Subjective effects of heroin and morphine in normal subjects. *Journal of Pharmacology and Experimental Therapeutics, 136,* 47–52.

Soyka, M., Horak, M., Dittert, S., & Kagerer, S. (2001). Less driving impairment on buprenorphine than methadone in drug-dependent patients? *Journal of Neuropsychiatry and Clinical Neuroscience, 13,* 527–528.

Specka, M., Finkbeiner, T., Lodemann, E., Leifert, K., Kluwig, J., & Gastpar, M. (2000). Cognitive-motor performance of methadone-maintained patients. *European Addiction Research, 6,* 8–19.

Spiga, R., Huang, D. B., Meisch, R. A., & Grabowski, J. (2001). Human methadone self-administration: effects of diazepam pretreatment. *Experimental and Clinical Psychopharmacology, 9*, 40–46.

Stastny, D., & Potter, M. (1991). Alcohol abuse by patients undergoing methadone treatment programmes. *British Journal of Addiction, 86*, 307–310.

Stitzer, M. L., Griffiths, R. R., McLellan, A. T., Grabowski, J., & Hawthorne, J. W. (1981). Diazepam use among methadone maintenance patients: patterns and dosages. *Drug and Alcohol Dependence, 8*, 189–199.

Stoller, K. B., Bigelow, G. E., Walsh, S. L., & Strain, E. C. (2001). Effects of buprenorphine/naloxone in opioid-dependent humans. *Psychopharmacology (Berlin), 154*, 230–242.

Strain, E. C., Bigelow, G. E., Liebson, I. A., & Stitzer, M. L. (1999). Moderate- vs high-dose methadone in the treatment of opioid dependence: a randomized trial. *Journal of the American Medical Association, 281*, 1000–1005.

Strain, E. C., Preston, K. L., Liebson, I. A., & Bigelow, G. E. (1992). Acute effects of buprenorphine, hydromorphone and naloxone in methadone-maintained volunteers. *Journal of Pharmacology and Experimental Therapeutics, 261*, 985–993.

Strain, E. C., Preston, K. L., Liebson, I. A., & Bigelow, G. E. (1993). Precipitated withdrawal by pentazocine in methadone-maintained volunteers. *Journal of Pharmacology and Experimental Therapeutics, 267*, 624–634.

Strain, E. C., Preston, K. L., Liebson, I. A., & Bigelow, G. E. (1996). Opioid antagonist effects of dezocine in opioid-dependent humans. *Clinical Pharmacology and Therapeutics, 60*, 206–217.

Strain, E. C., Stoller, K., Walsh, S. L., & Bigelow, G. E. (2000). Effects of buprenorphine versus buprenorphine/naloxone tablets in non-dependent opioid abusers. *Psychopharmacology (Berlin), 148*, 374–383.

Strain, E. C., Walsh, S. L., Preston, K. L., Liebson, I. A., & Bigelow, G. E. (1997). The effects of buprenorphine in buprenorphine-maintained volunteers. *Psychopharmacology (Berlin), 129*, 329–338.

Strang, J., & Gurling, H. (1989). Computerized tomography and neuropsychological assessment in long-term high-dose heroin addicts. *British Journal of Addiction, 84*, 1011–1019.

Substance Abuse and Mental Health Services Administration (2004). *Results from the 2003 National Survey on Drug Use and Health: national findings*, Office of Applied Studies, NSDUH Series H-25, DHHS Publication No. SMA 04-3964. Rockville, MD: SAMHSA.

Tapia-Arizmendi, G., Garcia-Estrada, J., Feria-Velasco, A., & Aleman, V. (1987). Structural changes in caudate nucleus, cerebral cortex and hippocampus induced by morphine. Light microscopy study. *General Pharmacology, 18*, 321–325.

Thapar, P., Zacny, J. P., Choi, M., & Apfelbaum, J. L. (1995a). Objective and subjective impairment from often-used sedative/analgesic combinations in ambulatory surgery, using alcohol as a benchmark. *Ambulatory Anesthesia, 80*, 1092–1098.

Thapar, P., Zacny, J. P., Thompson, W., & Apfelbaum, J. L. (1995b). Using alcohol as a standard to assess the degree of impairment induced by sedative and analgesic drugs used in ambulatory surgery. *Anesthesiology, 82*, 53–59.

Turski, W. A., Czuczwar, S. J., Kleinrok, Z., Schwarz, M., & Turski, L. (1983). Intraamygdaloid morphine produces seizures and brain damage in rats. *Life Sciences, 33*(Suppl. 1), 615–618.

United Nations Office on Drugs and Crime (2004). *United Nations Office on Drugs and Crime World Drug Report 2004, Volume 1*, United Nations Publication No. E.04.XI.16. Vienna, Austria: UNODC.

Von Felsinger, J. M., Lasagna, L., & Beecher, H. K. (1955). Drug-induced mood changes in man. II. Personality and reactions to drugs. *Journal of the American Medical Association, 157*, 1113–1119.

Walker, D. J., & Zacny, J. P. (1998). Subjective, psychomotor, and analgesic effects of oral codeine and morphine in healthy volunteers. *Psychopharmacology (Berlin), 140*, 191–201.

Walsh, S. L., Gilson, S. F., Jasinski, D. R., Stapleton, J. M., Phillips, R. L., Dannals, R. F., et al. (1994). Buprenorphine reduces cerebral glucose metabolism in polydrug abusers. *Neuropsychopharmacology, 10*, 157–170.

Walsh, S. L., June, H. L., Schuh, K. J., Preston, K. L., Bigelow, G. E., & Stitzer, M. L. (1995). Effects of buprenorphine and methadone in methadone-maintained subjects. *Psychopharmacology (Berlin), 119*, 268–276.

Wikler, A., Haertzen, C. A., Chessick, R. D., Hill, H. E., & Pescor, F. T. (1965). Reaction time ("mental set") in control and chronic schizophrenic subjects and in postaddicts under placebo, LSD-25, morphine, pentobarbital and amphetamine. *Psychopharmacologia, 7*, 423–443.

Willette, R. E., & Walsh, J. M. (1983). *Drugs, driving and traffic safety*, Publication No. 78. Geneva, Switzerland: World Health Organization.

Wilson, J. M., Kalasinsky, K. S., Levey, A. I., Bergeron, C., Reiber, G., Anthony, R. M., et al. (1996). Striatal dopamine nerve terminal markers in human, chronic methamphetamine users. *Nature Medicine, 2*, 699–703.

Woods, S. W., O'Malley, S. S., Martini, B. L., McDougle, C. J., Price, L. H., Krystal, J. H. et al., (1991). Spect regional cerebral blood flow and neuropsychological testing in non-demented HIV-positive drug abusers: Preliminary results. *Progress in Neuropsychopharmacology and Biological Psychiatry, 15*, 649–662.

Yan, F., & Roth, B. L. (2004). Salvinorin A: a novel and highly selective kappa-opioid receptor agonist. *Life Sciences, 75*, 2615–2619.

Zacny, J. P. (1995). A review of the effects of opioids on psychomotor and cognitive functioning in humans. *Experimental and Clinical Psychopharmacology, 3*, 432–466.

Zacny, J. P., Lichtor, J. L., Flemming, D., Coalson, D. W., & Thompson, W. K. (1994). A dose–response analysis of the subjective, psychomotor and physiological effects of intravenous morphine in healthy volunteers. *Journal of Pharmacology and Experimental Therapeutics, 268*, 1–9.

Zacny, J. P., Lichtor, J. L., Zaragoza, J. G., & de Wit, H. (1992). Subjective and behavioral responses to intravenous fentanyl in healthy volunteers. *Psychopharmacology (Berlin), 107*, 319–326.

Part II

Populations of Interest

10 Substance use and neuropsychological disorders in aging

Dylan G. Harwood, Ari Kalechstein, and David L. Sultzer

The United States is currently witnessing the "graying of America," with the elderly population expected to increase dramatically during the coming decades. This may be attributed to a host of factors, including the aging of the baby boomers, advances in medicine and health care, increased awareness in exercise, and improved diet. Census estimates indicate that there are currently over 30 million elderly in this country and the number is projected to increase to nearly 80 million by the year 2050, with the greatest growth between 2010 and 2030 (US Department of Health and Human Services, 1993; US Census Bureau, 2000).

The aging trend in this country suggests that issues related to mental health in the elderly are of increasing importance from both a clinical and research standpoint. A review of the extant literature indicates a wealth of studies addressing issues such as mood disorders and cognitive dysfunction in older adults; however, there is a dearth of research focusing specifically on substance use disorders in late-life. Indeed, an expert panel recently identified that substance abuse in aging "remains underestimated, underidentified, underdiagnosed, and undertreated" (US Department of Health and Human Services, 2001). In light of the demonstrated link between substance use and increased medical and psychological morbidity and mortality, a careful delineation of this body of research is warranted.

The present review will focus primarily on alcohol and tobacco, two of the most frequently abused substances in the elderly in this country. Importantly, research has documented a high comorbidity in relation to these two substances, as older adults that abuse alcohol are far more likely to use nicotine than their age-matched peers (Colsher & Wallace, 1990; Finlayson, Hurt, Davis, & Morse, 1988). The use of benzodiazepine medications in older adults will also be discussed, given the putative link between benzodiazepine use and cognitive decline (Paterniti, Dufoil, & Alpérovitch, 2002) and possibly the development of dementia (Lagnaoui et al., 2002). Issues related to epidemiology, diagnosis, and association with subacute, acute, and chronic neurobehavioral syndromes will be addressed. This review will also describe recent advances in treatment, the relationship with functional outcomes, and areas warranting future research. The primary purpose of this review is to provide an overview of three specific substances in relation to neuropsychological disorders in aging rather than a comprehensive review of substance abuse in the elderly. Moreover, while it is recognized that the issue of polypharmacy is important in terms of neurocognitive functioning in older adults (Meader, 1998; Starr, McGurn, Whiteman, Pattie, Whalley, & Deary, 2004), a comprehensive discussion of this topic is beyond the scope of the present review. Lastly, acute conditions such as substance intoxication, withdrawal syndromes, and acute confusional states (i.e., delirium) also will not be reviewed.

Epidemiology of alcohol use in older adults

The prevalence of daily alcohol consumption in older adults is estimated to be between 10% and 20% (Beresford & Gomberg, 1995). The 2003 National Survey on Drug Use and Health (NSDUH) reported prevalence rates of 34.3% for current alcohol use (one or more drinks in the past 30 days), 9.4% for binge alcohol use (five or more drinks on the same occasion at least once in the past 30 days), and 2.5% for heavy alcohol use (five or more drinks on the same occasion on at least five different days in the past 30 days) in individuals 60–64 years old (Substance Abuse and Mental Health Services Administration, 2004). These rates were 27.2%, 5.4%, and 1.8% in individuals aged 65 or older (Substance Abuse and Mental Health Services Administration, 2004). Overall, total consumption of alcohol in the US population has been shown to decline with advancing age (Rigler, 2000).

Risk factors for alcohol abuse in older adults include male gender, loss of a spouse, low income, poor education, and psychiatric comorbidity, such as depression and anxiety (US Department of Health and Human Services, 2001). Research indicates that the comorbidity of alcohol problems and other psychiatric disorders in late life is between 10% and 15% (Finlayson et al., 1988). Of particular importance, alcohol use has been associated with a number of subacute, acute, and chronic neurobehavioral syndromes, including Alzheimer's disease (AD) and vascular dementia (VaD), which are the two most common forms of dementia in older adults in this country (Hendrie, 1998). Thus, exploring the impact of alcohol in the development of late-life neurocognitive disorders is particularly relevant.

Epidemiology of smoking in older adults

Tobacco dependence represents the most prevalent substance-use disorder in older adults. The 2003 NSDUH reported prevalence rates of 4.5% for cigarette use over the past month and 12.0% had nicotine (cigarette) dependence over the past month among 60–64-year-olds (Substance Abuse and Mental Health Services Administration, 2004). The corresponding prevalence rates were 3.6% and 6.4% among persons aged 65 or older (Substance

Abuse and Mental Health Services Administration, 2004). Although tobacco use continues to be a major public health concern, overall rates of smoking have decreased over the past 30 years (Smith & Fiore, 1999).

Smoking in older adults has been linked with heightened morbidity and mortality. For instance, smoking has been identified as a major risk factor for at least six of the fourteen leading causes of death in older adults over 60 years of age (Cox, 1993). Tobacco consumption has particular relevance in terms of cognitive functioning in older adults. Similar to alcohol use, this substance has been implicated in the development of both VaD and AD (e.g., Gorelick et al., 1993; Launer et al., 1999). The available data suggest that clarifying the role of smoking in the pathogenesis of VaD and AD as well as identifying the impact of smoking cessation on risk are particularly relevant issues at this time.

Epidemiology of benzodiazepine use in older adults

Benzodiazepines (e.g., Valium [diazepam], Xanax [alprazolam], Ativan [lorazepam], Librium [chlordiazepoxide], and Serax [oxazepam]) are generally prescribed for anxiety or insomnia. They also may be prescribed as a principal pharmacological treatment for alcohol withdrawal. While the Food and Drug Administration (FDA) recommends that benzodiazepine use be limited to less than four months (Food and Drug Administration, 1980), research suggests that many elderly patients are prescribed these medications for longer periods of time (Kirby, Denihan, Bruce, Radic, Coakley, & Lawlor, 1999). In older adults, short-acting benzodiazepines have been recommended relative to longer-acting benzodiazepines to reduce the potential for excessive sedation (Dufour & Fuller, 1995). Prevalence studies from the United States and Canada indicate that over 20% of community-dwelling older adults have used a benzodiazepine over the past year (Hogan et al., 2003; Mayer-Oakes et al., 1993). This class of medication has been associated with heightened morbidity in older adults. Cross-sectional and longitudinal studies have suggested a link between benzodiazepine use and poorer neurocognitive functioning. Benzodiazepine use may also impact the risk for developing dementia.

Alcohol use and neurocognitive disorders in aging

Diagnosis of alcoholism

A chronic and maladaptive pattern of alcohol use may represent alcoholism, or alcohol dependence as cited in the DSM-IV TR (American Psychiatric Association, 2000). The diagnosis of alcohol abuse shares several common symptoms with alcohol dependence, although dependence is considered to be relatively more severe and marked by tolerance, withdrawal, and a pattern of compulsive use (American Psychiatric Association, 2000). It has been proposed that 10% of patients diagnosed with alcohol dependence are likely to evidence a severe cognitive disorder (Rourke & Løberg, 1996), including Wernicke-Korsakoff's syndrome (alcohol-induced persisting amnestic disorder) and alcohol-related dementia (alcohol-induced persisting dementia) (American Psychiatric Association, 2000).

Alcohol-related neuropsychiatric conditions

Chronic heavy use of alcohol has been linked with a host of cognitive disorders secondary to toxic-metabolic effects. A number of acute, subacute, and chronic alcohol-related neurobehavioral syndromes have been identified, including pellagra, alcohol hallucinosis, acquired hepatocerebral degeneration, alcoholic cardiomyopathy, pancreatic encephalopathy, central pontine myelinolysis, delirium tremens, hepatic encephalopathy, alcohol-related dementia (ARD), Wernicke-Korsakoff's syndrome (WKS), and Marchiafava-Bignami disease (MBD) (Mendez & Cummings, 2003). Several alcohol-related conditions will be discussed in this chapter due to their prevalence and/or specific impact on neurocognition in older adults. A growing body of literature has implicated chronic alcohol use with heightened risk of developing the two most common causes of dementia in late-life, AD and VaD. Thus, the specific role of ethanol in AD and VaD will also be addressed.

General cognitive functioning

Research indicates that moderate amounts of current alcohol (2–4 drinks per day) use may improve cognitive functioning on measures of basic neurocognition (Mini-Mental State Exam; Cognitive Abilities Screening Instrument), attention/information processing, executive skills, and memory (Bond et al., 2003; Dufouil, Decimetiere, & Alperovitch, 1997; Elias, Elias, D'Agostino, Silberhatz, & Wolf, 1999). A U-shaped dose–response effect between earlier alcohol consumption and neuropsychological functioning has also been reported in the literature among older adults, with greatest risk observed among abstainers and heavy drinkers (Edelstein, Kritz-Silverstein, & Barrett-Connor, 1998; Launer, Feskens, Kalmijn, & Kromhout, 1996). A recent population-based prospective study further documented the U-shaped association between alcohol use in middle age and neuropsychological functioning over two decades later. Anttila and colleagues (2004) observed that frequent (defined as several times per month) alcohol use in middle age increased the risk for developing mild cognitive impairment (MCI) in older age, utilizing the criteria for MCI established by the Mayo Clinic (Peterson et al., 2001). Participants who abstained from drinking or drank alcohol frequently in middle age were noted to be twice as likely to develop incident MCI later in life relative to individuals who drank infrequently (defined as less than once per month) earlier in life. As the conversion rate to dementia for patients with MCI is much greater than that observed for cognitively intact older adults (Peterson et al., 2001), it is likely that the mechanisms underlying the risk for MCI conferred by alcohol use are the same as those identified for dementia. These putative mechanisms are delineated later in the section addressing AD.

Hepatic encephalopathy

A significant proportion of individuals who chronically abuse alcohol will eventually develop cirrhosis of the liver. Liver dysfunction has been linked with hepatic encephalopathy, which represents a chronic and fluctuating neuropsychiatric disorder. Hepatic encephalopathy is marked by changes in consciousness ranging from mild disorientation in subclinical encephalopathy (grades 0 and I) to coma (grade IV) (Watanabe, 1998). The neurocognitive changes associated with hepatic encephalopathy are believed to be secondary to increases in nitrogenous compounds (e.g., gamma-aminobutyric acid) and decreases in the synthesis of protein (Moss, Tarter, Yao, & Van Thiel, 1992). Characteristic neuropsychological deficits in this condition include changes in memory, psychomotor speed, and executive skills (Catafau et al., 2000; O'Carroll, 1993).

Specific biochemical measures of hepatic function have implications in terms of the unique patterns of neuropsychological dysfunction in patients with chronic liver disease and subclinical hepatic encephalopathy (Moss et al., 1992). For instance, impaired hepatic protein synthesis has been correlated with poor performance on measures of language efficiency, perceptual speed, and psychomotor efficiency, and impaired processing of nitrogenous compounds has been linked with poor performance on measures of visuospatial functioning. In hepatic encephalopathy, liver transplantation may result in an amelioration of some of the neuropsychological deficits; however, residual memory difficulties have been observed (Arria, Tarter, Starzl, & Van Thiel, 1991).

Among patients with chronic liver disease, hepatic dysfunction has been linked with characteristic deficits in cerebral functioning. Studies using single photon emission computed tomography (SPECT) have demonstrated decreased cerebral blood flow in the basal ganglia and frontal, temporal, and parietal lobe regions (Nakagawa, Matsumura, Iwasa, Kaito, Adachi, & Takeda, 2004; Trzepacz, Tarter, Shah, Tringali, Faett, & Van Thiel, 1994). Positron emission tomography (PET) techniques have revealed decreased metabolism in the frontal and temporal cortices, as well as the basal ganglia (Kato, Suzuki, Kaneta, Obara, Fujishima, & Sato, 2000). Research also indicates that among patients with cirrhosis, liver transplantation may normalize cortical regional blood flow deficits one year following successful surgery (Dam et al., 1998). However, patients with alcoholic cirrhosis evidence greater impairment in frontal lobe functioning at follow-up relative to individuals with nonalcoholic cirrhosis, which may represent the possible irreversible neurotoxic action of ethanol on cerebral functioning.

Wernicke-Korsakoff's syndrome

Older adults with a history of heavy alcohol use are at risk for WKS (alcohol-induced persisting amnestic disorder in the DSM-IV TR; American Psychiatric Association, 2000). This disorder is marked by a pure amnestic state secondary to severe thiamine (vitamin B_1) depletion (Victor, Adams, & Collins, 1989). Patients with WKS evidence a host of neuropathological changes in structures relevant to learning and memory, including the mammillary bodies, dorsomedial nucleus of the thalamus, periaqueductal gray matter, locus coeruleus, dorsal raphe nucleus, and basal nucleus of Meynert (Sahin, Gurvit, Bilgic, Hanagasi, & Emre, 2002). Cerebral changes evidenced on magnetic resonance imaging (MRI) include atrophy of the anterior diencephalon and mammillary bodies, and enlargement of the third ventricle with hypodense areas in its walls and surrounding the aqueduct of Sylvius (Mendez & Cummings, 2003).

Clinically, patients with WKS evidence an abrupt onset of ophthalmoplegia, ataxia, and delirium (Wernicke's encephalopathy) that is often followed by an enduring amnestic disorder (Korsakoff's disorder) (Mendez & Cummings, 2003). Among patients with acute Wernicke's encephalopathy that survive, approximately three-quarters of them will eventually develop Korsakoff's disorder (Phillips, Ingram, & Grammer, 1994). Individuals diagnosed with WKS demonstrate a characteristic pattern of memory impairment, marked by severe anterograde amnesia and a temporally graded retrograde amnesia (Butters, 1981). Visuospatial deficits (Jacobson, Acker, & Lishman, 1990; Krabbendam et al., 2000) and poorer visual working memory abilities (van Asselen, Kessels, Wester, & Postma, 2005) have also been documented in WKS. Executive deficits are commonly documented among these patients and likely stem from putative frontal lobe dysfunction (Brand, Fujiwara, Borsutzky, Kessler, & Markowitsch, 2005; Brokate, Hildebrandt, Eling, Fichtner, Runge, & Timm, 2003; Krabbendam et al., 2000). This executive dysfunction has been shown to be more severe among Korsakoff versus non-Korsakoff alcoholics (Oscar-Berman, Kirkley, Gansler, & Couture, 2004).

Alcohol-related dementia

Heavy use of alcohol may also give rise to a mild and minimally progressive dementia syndrome. The diagnosis of ARD remains controversial and it has been questioned whether a persistent dementia syndrome can develop from the direct toxic effects of alcohol on the brain, due to the lack of a distinctive, well-defined pathology (Victor, 1994). Moreover, there are no specific autopsy studies of ARD at this time. The specific impact of heavy alcohol use as a risk factor for the development of dementia has not been determined. For instance, a large retrospective analysis of patients referred to a neuropsychology unit secondary to suspected alcohol brain dysfunction found that while frontal lobe dysfunction (34%) and short-term memory deficits (32%)

were common, the presence of dementia was rare (4%) (Tuck & Jackson, 1991). In contrast, Finlayson and colleagues (1988) reported that approximately 25% of older adults with alcoholism evidence ARD. Moreover, it has been noted that heavy alcohol use is a contributing factor in over 20% of cases of dementia (Smith & Atkinson, 1995).

The most commonly utilized definition for ARD is found in the DSM-IV TR (American Psychiatric Association, 2000). Provisional diagnostic criteria have been developed more recently to guide clinicians and researchers in distinguishing ARD from other causes of dementia (Oslin, Atkinson, Smith, & Hendrie, 1998). The Oslin criteria for ARD are based on the DSM-IV TR criteria and the relationship between alcohol use and dementia is defined using four categories: Definite, Probable, Possible, and Contributing. The diagnostic criteria also include a category for mixed dementia for cases in which several factors appear to be underlying the current dementia syndrome. A recent longitudinal study of long-term care patients offered support for the validation of the criteria for ARD (e.g., stabilization of cognitive and functional symptoms in ARD versus decline in both domains in AD and VaD) (Oslin & Cary, 2003).

The rate of dementia secondary to alcoholism is not well characterized. One large longitudinal study of community-dwelling older adults (n=1070) reported that the overall incidence of dementia, clinically confirmed by six-year follow-up, was 9.2/1000 per year (AD=6.3; VaD=1.9; ARD=1.0) (Copeland et al., 1992). Clinical case series have reported that ARD represents between 4% (Larson, Kukull, & Katzman, 1984; Renvoize, Gaskell, & Klar, 1985) and 10% (Wells, 1979) of all documented dementia cases. More recent studies in long-term-care residents have confirmed the high prevalence of ARD among older adults. For instance, Oslin and Cary (2003) reported a prevalence rate of 10.1% among demented nursing home residents. Moreover, a study of cognitively impaired long-term-care residents documented a prevalence rate of 24% for ARD (Carlen et al., 1994). Given that much of the prevalence data for ARD is several decades old, additional studies addressing the current rates of this disorder are warranted.

Patients with ARD demonstrate characteristic neuropsychiatric changes, such as symptoms of circumstantiality and perseveration (Mendez & Cummings, 2003). The pattern of neuropsychological deficits associated with ARD reportedly is consistent with both cortical (e.g., Alzheimer's disease) and subcortical (e.g., Parkinson's disease) dementia processes, including difficulties in the areas of verbal memory, visual memory, visuoconstruction, and psychomotor speed (Munro, Saxton, & Butters, 2001). Patients with ARD do not generally differ from normal controls on measures of confrontation naming, category fluency, verbal recognition, and procedural memory (Munro et al., 2001). A number of investigations have documented the distinct neuropsychological profiles between older adults diagnosed with ARD versus AD. For instance, AD patients show greater decrements on tasks of recognition memory versus verbal learning and recall (Munro et al., 2001;

Saxton, Munro, Butters, Schramke, & McNeal, 2000) and anomia (Atkinson & Ganzini, 1994). Prospectively, older adults with ARD also demonstrate less overall cognitive impairment and reduced decline over time of both cognitive and functional symptoms in comparison to patients with other forms of dementia, including AD and VaD (Oslin & Cary, 2003). Further support for differences in the clinical course of ARD and AD is offered by a retrospective study of 120 cases from a dementia registry, which found no decline on the Mini-Mental State Exam on serial testing among patients with ARD over a 20-month period (Atkinson & Ganzini, 1994). In contrast, AD patients with no history of prior alcohol use and AD patients with a history of alcohol consumption of more than 3–4 drinks per day during some previous period showed a progressive decline in basic cognition. This finding is limited by the lack of more sensitive and comprehensive neuropsychological measures in measuring change in this study. The lack of neuropsychological decline in patients with ARD is likely to be secondary to decreased risk for ethanol-related neurotoxicity and cerebrovascular changes following cessation.

Alzheimer's disease

One of the consequences of an aging society is an increase in the prevalence of dementing illness such as AD. It is the most frequently occurring dementing illness and the most common cause of disability in persons over age 85 (Larson, Kukull, & Katzman, 1992). Alzheimer's disease currently affects an estimated 4.5 million Americans and the number of people suffering from this disease is expected to grow to over 13 million by the middle of next century (Hebert, Scherr, Bienias, Bennett, & Evans, 2003).

Several sets of criteria have been developed for the diagnosis of AD. The two most often utilized are those formulated by the National Institute of Neurological and Communicative Disorders and Stroke and the Alzheimer's Disease and Related Disorders Association Joint Task Force (NINCDS-ADRDA; McKhann, Drachman, Folstein, Katzman, Price, & Stadian, 1984), and, most recently, the criteria included in the DSM-IV TR (American Psychiatric Association, 2000). The DSM-IV TR criteria identify AD as a dementing disorder characterized primarily by the development of multiple cognitive deficits. These include memory impairment (impaired ability to learn new information or to recall previously learned information) and other cognitive disturbances such as aphasia (language disturbance), apraxia (impaired ability to carry out motor activities despite intact motor function), agnosia (failure to recognize or identify objects despite intact sensory function), or disturbance in executive functioning such as planning, sequencing, organizing, and abstracting (American Psychiatric Association, 2000). The criteria also identify the course of the disease as being characterized by an insidious onset with continued cognitive decline.

The NINCDS-ADRDA criteria are more detailed than those formulated by the DSM-IV TR. The diagnosis is designated as "definite", "probable", or "possible" AD. Criteria for the diagnosis of "definite" AD include autopsy or biopsy confirmation, whereas the criteria for "probable" AD do not include pathological confirmation; however, it does include an insidious onset of decline in memory as well as impairment in at least one other area of cognition, a preserved level of consciousness, a progressive course, and the exclusion of other conditions that may cause symptoms of dementia. The diagnosis of "possible" AD is reserved for clinical circumstances marked by an atypical onset, presentation, or course, by focal neurological findings, or by evidence of a gradually progressive cognitive deficit in the absence of other identifiable causes (McKhann et al., 1984).

The findings of studies addressing the association between alcohol use and AD have been inconsistent. The inconsistency is probably underlined by methodological differences across studies. For instance, cross-sectional investigations addressing the relationship between AD and alcohol use have been negative. The EURODEM meta-analysis of five case–control studies failed to show a significant link between alcohol consumption and risk for AD (Graves et al., 1991). In contrast, the findings from prospective studies indicate that alcohol use in the elderly may decrease the risk for developing AD. Several studies have reported a relationship between overall alcohol use, rather than focusing on the type of beverage consumed, and the development of AD. One study found reduced risk for AD among light to moderate drinkers compared to nondrinkers (Huang, Qiu, Winblad, & Fratiglioni, 2002). The prospective, population-based Cardiovascular Health Study also reported a relation between lower levels of alcohol consumption and decreased risk of incident AD compared with abstention (Mukamal, Kuller, Fitzpatrick, Longstreth, Mittleman, & Siscovick, 2003). Other investigations have suggested that the putative risk for AD conferred by alcohol may be specific to the type of beverage consumed. For example, mild to moderate intake of wine has been shown to lower the risk of incident AD, specifically in older adults without the ε_4 allele of the apolipoprotein gene (Luchsinger, Tang, Siddiqui, Shea, & Mayeux, 2004). Intake of liquor, beer, and total alcohol reportedly was not linked with a lower risk of developing AD in follow-up analyses. The association between mild to moderate consumption of wine and lower risk for developing AD has received further support (Orgozo et al., 1997) and remained significant in follow-up analyses that controlled for additional potential confounding factors (Lemeshow, Letenneur, Dartigues, Orgogozu, & Commenges, 1998).

Research suggests that alcohol consumption may alter the expression of AD. For instance, a large clinic-based study of AD patients found that alcoholism was associated with a significantly lower age of onset for the disease (~5 years; Cantillon, Barker, Harwood, Espinosa, Kumar, & Duara, 1996). This finding was also reported in the multi-site Mirage Study (Rao et al., 1995). Thus, while alcohol consumption may decrease the likelihood of developing AD, heavy drinking may also impact the clinical phenotype among patients in the early stages of the disease by altering the age at which the clinical symptoms are expressed.

Several mechanisms have been offered to explain the association between alcohol use and decreased risk for AD or dementia (nonspecific classification). For instance, alcohol may affect cognition by decreasing cardiovascular risk factors (e.g., reducing platelet adhesion or by lowering serum cholesterol and triglycerides) implicated in AD and VaD (e.g., Luchsinger & Mayeux, 2004). Alcohol may also impact cognition directly by affecting the release of acetylcholine in certain areas of the brain such as the hippocampus (Letenneur, Larrieu, & Barberger-Gateau, 2004; Ruitenberg et al., 2003). Finally, the presence of flavenoids contained in wine may lower the risk for dementia secondary to antioxidant properties (Letenneur et al., 2004; Ruitenberg et al., 2003).

Vascular dementia

Dementia secondary to cerebrovascular disease, or vascular dementia (VaD), has been identified as the second most common cause of late-life cognitive impairment in this country (Skoog, 1998). Several sets of criteria have been developed to establish the diagnosis of VaD. The three most often employed in research include those formulated by the National Institute of Neurological Disorders and Stroke and the Association Internationale pour la Recherche et l'Enseignement en Neurosciences (NINDS-AIREN; Roman et al., 1993), the State of California Alzheimer's Disease Diagnostic Treatment Centers (ADDTC; Chui et al., 1992), and the DSM-IV TR (American Psychiatric Association, 2000). Criteria for VaD are also included in the ICD-10, which was developed by the World Health Organization (Wetterling, Kanitz, & Borgis, 1994). The DSM-IV TR applies the clinical criteria for AD to patients who have experienced some degree of cerebrovascular disease. However, the criteria specify that the clinical presentation is characterized by a stepwise deterioration, "patchy" distribution of deficits in intellectual functioning associated with focal neurological signs and symptoms, and evidence of cerebrovascular disease (American Psychiatric Association, 1994). While VaD may represent a distinct neuropsychological entity, there can be significant overlap between the clinical manifestations of VaD, AD, and mixed dementia (i.e., AD with co-occurring cerebrovascular disease) (Zekry, Hauw, & Gold, 2002). Moreover, cerebrovascular disease likely contributes to the expression of AD (Snowden, Greiner, Mortimer, Riley, Greiner, & Markesbery, 1997).

Researchers have focused on further refining the diagnostic criteria employed to characterize the cognitive and functional deficits among patients with cerebrovascular disease. This has included developing criteria to address more homogenous groups, such as those patients with subcortical small-vessel ischemic lesions (i.e., Binswanger's disease, lacunar state) (Erkinjuntti et al., 2000). Additionally, vascular cognitive impairment (VCI) has been proposed as a diagnostic term to classify individuals experiencing a range of neurocognitive deficits secondary to cerebrovascular disease, ranging from mild cognitive deficits to frank dementia (Roman et al., 2004).

Patients with VaD may evidence a host of neuropsychological difficulties over the course of their dementia syndrome, including deficits in the areas of memory, attention and information processing, language, visuospatial skills, and executive skills. The neurocognitive deficits witnessed in VaD may be very similar to those seen in AD depending on the underlying severity and location of cerebrovascular disease. For instance, pronounced clinical differences can be seen between AD patients and patients diagnosed with the subcortical variant of VaD. The latter group often has greater difficulties on measures associated with disruption of frontal-subcortical pathways in the brain, such as information processing, sustained attention, motor programming, perseveration, and executive functioning (Cummings, 1994). Neuropsychological tests may have clinical utility in differentiating patients with VaD from those with AD. For instance, a review indicated that after matching for age, education, and severity of dementia, VaD patients performed better on measures of long-term memory and had more pronounced difficulties with executive or frontal lobe skills (Looi & Sachdev, 1999). Of additional importance, neurological symptoms and signs, such as focal motor or sensory deficits, dysarthria, gait disturbance, or tremor, have shown diagnostic utility in differentiating VaD from AD (Cummings, 1994; Verghese, Lipton, Hall, Kuslansky, Katz, & Buschke, 2002).

In recent years, an emerging literature has focused on identifying risk factors for VaD, including alcohol use. This area of study is based on the strong association between alcohol consumption and cerebrovascular disease. Heavy alcohol use has been linked with hemorrhagic (Klatsky, Armstrong, Friedman, & Sidney, 2002) and nonhemorrhagic stroke (Gill et al., 1991). In contrast, a lower risk of ischemic stroke has been witnessed in mild to moderate drinkers in comparison to nondrinkers or heavy drinkers (Lee et al., 2000; Stampfer, Colditz, Willett, Speizer, & Hennekens, 1988). Beverage-specific analyses indicate that the decreased risk for ischemic stroke associated with alcohol use may only occur with wine rather than beer or spirits (Djousse, Ellison, Beiser, Scaramucci, D'Agostino, & Wolf, 2002; Truelsen, Gronbaek, Schnohr, & Boysen, 1998).

The putative link between alcohol and cerebral ischemia (Gill et al., 1991; Klatsky et al., 2002; Lee et al., 2000; Stampfer et al., 1988) suggests that a history of heavy ethanol use in older adults likely represents a factor in the etiology of vascular dementia. The direct relationship between high alcohol consumption and VaD has been established in several investigations (Lindsay, Hebert, & Rockwood, 1997; Meyer, Judd, Tawakina, Rogers, & Mortel, 1986; Yoshitake et al., 1995). Moreover, light to moderate drinking has been associated with a lower risk of any dementia and VaD specifically regardless of type of alcoholic beverage (Ruitenberg et al., 2003).

Treatment

Research has addressed the efficacy of pharmacotherapy in targeting the cognitive and functional symptoms associated with several alcohol-related neuropsychiatric conditions. Patients diagnosed with WKS often receive supplemental thiamine to address the prominent nutritional deficiency (Cook & Thomson, 1997; Thomson et al., 2002). The administration of thiamine generally results in an amelioration of the acute symptoms of Wernicke's encephalopathy over the course of several days. Once the acute symptoms of encephalopathy have improved, the pervasive memory symptoms of Korsakoff's amnesia generally manifest.

Research has clearly documented that the three commonly used acetylcholinesterase inhibitors (donepezil, galantamine, and rivastigmine) and one NMDA antagonist (memantine) exert a positive effect on global cognition in patients with AD (Ritchie, Ames, Clayton, & Lai, 2004). The efficacy of acetylcholinesterase inhibitors and memantine among patients with cognitive decline secondary to VaD has also been documented (Malouf & Birks, 2004; Wilcock et al., 2002), although these medications are not FDA-approved for this use. Because patients with WKS may show neurochemical deficits in the cholinergic system secondary to lesions in the basal nucleus of Meynert (Sahin, Gurvit, Bilgic, Hanagasi, & Emre, 2002), studies have investigated the therapeutic effects of cholinergic agents on the neurocognitive deficits seen in WKS. Some have shown a lack of benefit with respect to acetylcholinesterase inhibitors and neuropsychological functioning in patients with alcohol-related WKS (O'Donnell, Pitts, & Fann, 1986) and nonalcoholic WKS (Sahin et al., 2002). However, several recent case reports have identified improved functioning in WKS patients treated with donepezil, galantamine, and rivastigmine (Angunawela & Baker, 2001; Iga, Araki, Ishimoto, & Ohmori, 2001; Phillips, Ingram, & Grammer, 2004). Because the data have been equivocal, additional controlled studies are warranted. Memantine may also ameliorate overall neurocognitive functioning in patients with WKS (Rustembegovic, Kundurovic, Sapcanin, & Sofic, 2003). In terms of ARD, a recent case report documented improved cognitive performance after treatment with donepezil (Kim, Ke, & Adkins, 2004). There are no data at this time addressing memantine and ARD.

The issue of abstinence should always be addressed when considering treatment for putative alcohol-related neuropsychiatric conditions. Overall, research suggests that heavy alcohol consumption results in cerebral atrophic effects involving the gray and white matter, particularly in the frontal lobes, cerebellum, and limbic structures (Mukamal, 2004). However, cessation has been linked with significant volumetric increases in both the white and gray matter structures in abstinent alcoholics as well as a reduction in cerebrospinal fluid volume (Agartz et al., 2003; Pfefferbaum, Sullivan, Mathalon, Shear, Rosenbloom, & Lim, 1995; Schroth, Naegle, Klose, Mann, & Peterson, 1988; Shear, Jernigan, & Butters, 1994). These data indicate that some of the neuropsychological deficits witnessed in chronic alcoholics may be partially ameliorated through abstinence due to the effects of cerebral recovery. The specific clinical response to abstinence among older adults with alcohol-related deficits of sufficient severity to warrant a diagnosis of ARD has not been reported. However, the neuropsychological deficits in patients with ARD that are no longer abusing alcohol have been shown to plateau or stabilize over a several-year period (Atkinson & Ganzini, 1994).

Smoking and neurocognitive disorders in aging

Vascular dementia

Smoking has been linked with increased risk for stroke (Wolf, D'Agostino, Kannel, Bonita, & Belanger, 1988), myocardial infarction (Jajich, Ostfeld, & Freeman, 1984), and diabetes mellitus (Sairenchi et al., 2004). These medical conditions, in turn, have all been implicated in the development of VaD (Skoog, 1998). In addition to conferring risk for VaD indirectly through the aforementioned medical conditions, cross-sectional and prospective research has documented a direct link between tobacco use and the development of VaD. For instance, a case–control study of hospital-based patients with multiple cerebral infarcts found that recent smoking was associated with heightened risk for dementia secondary to ischemic lesions (Gorelick et al., 1993). Moreover, a longitudinal study of cognitive functioning in older adults reported that compared with never smokers, current smokers evidenced an increased risk for incident VaD over a two-year period (Juan, Zhou, Li, Wang, Goa, & Chen, 2004). Cigarette smoking may affect cognition by reducing cerebral circulation; research indicates that elderly smokers evidence lower regional cerebral blood flow relative to elderly nonsmokers (Yamashita, Kobayashi, Yamaguchi, Kitani, & Tsunematsu, 1988). Also, among older adults who have smoked for three to four decades, abstaining from cigarette smoking can result in significant improvements in cerebral circulation within one year following cessation (Rogers, Meyer, Judd, & Mortel, 1985). Other research indicates that while improved cerebral circulation occurs following smoking cessation, this effect may require several years (Yamashita, Kobayashi, & Yamaguchi, 2000).

Specific brain regions are particularly susceptible to hypoperfusion and ischemia, including the periventricular white matter, basal ganglia, and hippocampus (Roman, 2004). Moreover, ischemic lesions may result in the development of vascular cognitive impairment (e.g., ranging from VCI-ND to VaD) secondary to disruption of prefrontal-basal ganglia circuits. Patients with the subcortical form of VaD secondary to frontal-subcortical dysfunction generally present with a distinct clinical profile, which may include executive slowing, forgetfulness, dysarthria, mood changes, urinary symptoms, and short-stepped gait (Roman, Erkinjuntti, Wallin, Pantoni, & Chui, 2002). Taken together, the extant empirical literature indicates that cigarette dependence represents an important and potentially modifiable risk factor for the second most common cause of late-life dementia in this country.

Alzheimer's disease

Studies have investigated whether a history of smoking may alter the risk for AD. The large EURODEM meta-analysis, which incorporated data from eight case–control studies of AD, showed that smoking was linked with a decreased risk for AD (Graves et al., 1991). However, the effect size was small and none of the eight studies individually showed significant findings. This risk was also observed to be limited to patients with no first-degree relatives with dementia (van Duijn et al., 1994). The association between smoking and decreased risk for AD has been attributed to several factors. For instance, the protective effect conferred by tobacco use vis-à-vis AD has been hypothesized to be secondary to differential mortality (Wang, Fratiglioni, Frisoni, Viitanen, & Winblad, 1999). Moreover, there is evidence that the negative risk related to smoking disappears after controlling for potential confounding factors, such as educational level and occupational category (Letenneur et al., 1994). Alternatively, nicotine exposure in smokers may delay the onset of AD or confer protection by altering the cholinergic deficit seen in this disease (Letenneur et al., 2004). Similarly, both retrospective and prospective epidemiological studies indicate that cigarette smoking may reduce the risk for developing Parkinson's disease and a neuroprotective role for nicotine has been suggested (Ross & Petrovitch, 2001).

Prospective studies have also reported that smoking may increase rather than decrease the risk for developing AD (Juan et al., 2004). Results from the EURODEM group that pooled analysis of four European population-based prospective studies indicated that current smoking increased the risk of incident AD (Launer et al., 1999). The empirical literature showed that smoking may also interact with genotype to impact clinical phenotype. For instance, Ott et al. (1998) documented a link between current smoking and heightened risk for incident AD only among noncarriers of the APOE ε_4 allele (Ott et al., 1998). Past smoking patterns may also impact later cognition, as mid-life smoking has been linked with late-life AD as well as the number of neuritic plaques on neuropathological evaluation (Tyas et al., 2003). Taken together, the available research suggests that while smoking may confer greater risk for developing AD in later life, protective effects have also been observed and additional investigations are warranted.

Treatment

Older adults diagnosed with VaD may receive pharmacotherapy with the three commonly prescribed acetylcholinesterase inhibitors and/or memantine, although these medications have not been FDA-approved for this patient population. Although acetylcholinesterase inhibitors were developed initially to target patients with AD secondary to the profound loss of cholinergic neurons in this disease (Ritchie et al., 2004), acetylcholinesterase inhibitors treatment has been shown to improve cognitive and functional symptoms in patients with VaD (Malouf & Birks, 2004). The efficacy of ChIs in patients with VaD is believed to be secondary to an amelioration of cholinergic deficits associated with ischemia of basal forebrain nuclei and cholinergic pathways (Erkinjuntti, Roman, & Gauthier, 2004).

In terms of smoking and VaD, prevention represents the most promising option. For instance, the regional cerebral blood flow deficits that are observed in elderly smokers (Yamashita et al., 1988) and appear to place them at increased risk for the subcortical variant of this disorder (Roman, 2004; Roman et al., 2002) may be ameliorated through smoking cessation. Indeed, as mentioned previously, abstaining from cigarette smoking can result in significant improvements in cerebral circulation within one year following cessation among older adults who have smoked for three to four decades (Rogers et al., 1985). Other research indicates that while improved cerebral circulation occurs following smoking cessation, this effect may require several years to manifest (Yamashita et al., 2000). Regarding prevention, smoking cessation has also been shown to reduce the risk of stroke among men (Wannamethee, Shaper, Whincup, & Walker, 1995) and women (Kawachi et al., 1993). Abstinence may also decrease the likelihood of heart disease in older adults (Jajich et al., 1984). Thus, modification of smoking habits can impact the development or course of VaD through decreased risk for chronic cerebral hypoperfusion, myocardial infarction, and stroke.

Benzodiazepine use and neurocognitive disorders in aging

Research has addressed the impact of benzodiazepine use on functioning in older adults. In terms of morbidity, benzodiazepine use has been linked with a host of deleterious outcomes in the elderly, including postoperative confusion (Kudoh, Takase, Takahira, & Yakazawa, 2004), urinary incontinence (Landi et al., 2002), motor vehicle accidents (Hemmelgarn, Suissa, Huang, Boivin, & Pinard, 1997), hip fractures (Wagner et al., 2004), and heightened risk for decline in physical performance (Gray et al., 2003). Benzodiazepine use was shown to be common (43%) among elderly patients presenting to an emergency room for treatment (Verhaeghe, Mets, & Corne, 1996). There is also evidence that approximately 15% of older alcoholics misuse other drugs, such as benzodiazepines (Finlayson et al., 1988).

Significant neurocognitive sequelae have been associated with benzodiazepine use in older adults, although the results have been equivocal. The acute cognitive effects of benzodiazepines in humans are well documented, and include decreased attention and memory (Buffett-Jerrott & Stewart, 2002). With regard to longer term use, a recent meta-analysis that did not focus specifically on older adults evaluated cognitive performance associated with long-term use of benzodiazepine medications in 13 studies utilizing neuropsychological testing (Barker, Greenwood, Jackson, & Crowe, 2004a). The authors found that long-term benzodiazepine users, relative to controls, performed consistently worse across all cognitive domains, including sensory processing, psychomotor speed, nonverbal memory, visuospatial functioning, speed of processing, problem-solving, attention/concentration, verbal memory, general intelligence, motor control/performance, working memory, and verbal reasoning. A follow-up meta-analysis by Barker and colleagues (2004b) revealed that cognitive functioning in long-term benzodiazepine users improved following withdrawal, particularly for the domains of visuospatial skills, attention/concentration, general intelligence, psychomotor speed, and nonverbal memory; however, a significant degree of impairment remained in most areas of cognition vis-à-vis controls or normative data sets.

Several studies have addressed whether long-term benzodiazepine use in older adults represents a significant risk factor for cognitive decline and dementia. In a study of 1176 noninstitutionalized older adults in Connecticut, Paterniti et al. (2002) found that cognitive decline was twice as likely among chronic users versus nonusers over a four-year period. In contrast, a large population-based study from France did not report a significant association between benzodiazepine use and neuropsychological decline over a six-year period (Dealberto, Mcavay, Seeman, & Berkman, 1997). Moreover, in a community-based study of 2765 elders from North Carolina, Hanlon et al. (1998) documented that previous and current use of benzodiazepines was not associated with cognitive decline over a three-year period. Allard, Artero, and Ritchie (2003) also reported a negligible relationship between chronic use of benzodiazepines and cognitive decline over a two-year period in a cohort of 372 older adults recruited from a regional network of general practitioners in France. Taken together, the available data remain equivocal with respect to the relationship between long-term use of this class of medication and neurocognition in older adults; however, the majority of studies have not documented a clear association.

There is also evidence that benzodiazepine use may impact the risk for late-life dementia syndromes. For instance, a recent case–control study of 3777 older adults in France followed over an eight-year period found that former and ever usage of benzodiazepines, but not current usage, was a risk factor for developing dementia (Lagnaoui et al., 2002). This finding contrasted with an earlier study of 242 community-dwelling elders in Sweden, which suggested a protective effect of benzodiazepines against dementia, with the incidence of dementia significantly lower in users compared to nonusers (Fastbom, & Forsell, Winblad, 1998). In terms of their findings, Fastbom et al. (1998) hypothesized that this class of medications may decrease the risk for developing dementia by protecting against glutamate toxicity associated with increased GABA transmission. Overall, the discrepant findings in relation to benzodiazepine use and cognitive decline in older adults may be secondary to methodological differences (e.g., definition of drug exposure and cognitive outcome employed) (Verdoux, Lagnaoui, &

Begaud, 2005). Given the high frequency of benzodiazepine use among the elderly (Hogan et al., 2003; Mayer-Oakes et al., 1993; Verhaeghe et al., 1996), additional prospective studies are warranted in order to further clarify the relationship between usage and cognitive decline and incident dementia.

The relationship between benzodiazepine use and neurocognition is likely to be confounded by the issue of polypharmacy. For instance, a large cross-sectional study of community-dwelling older adults in southern California found that elderly benzodiazepine users were more than twice as likely to take ten or more drugs (Mayer-Oakes et al. 1993). Clearly, the use of multiple substances in older adults has clinical import and places them at particular risk for neurocognitive deficits (Meader, 1998; Starr et al., 2004). This is especially true with respect to the use of anticholinergic drugs, which have been shown to be widely used in community-dwelling older adults (Ness, Hoth, Barnett, Shorr, & Kabuli, 2006). Anticholinergic toxicity is not uncommon in this population and has been associated with several adverse effects, including urinary retention, constipation, visual impairments, dry mouth, and confusion/delirium (Tune, 2001). Moreover, in older adults with established dementia, anticholinergic activity has been linked with poorer cognitive functioning (Chew, Mulsant, & Pollack, 2005).

Summary

This review described the prevalence of alcohol, tobacco, and benzodiazepine use among older adults as well as some of the neurocognitive disorders associated with these substances, such as hepatic encephalopathy, WKS, ARD, AD, and VaD. Ethanol and tobacco both appear to modify the risk for developing AD and VaD, the two most common causes of late-life dementia in this country. Moreover, the observed relationships are likely related to the pattern of use. For instance, mild to moderate drinking has been shown to decrease the risk of developing AD and VaD. Conversely, high alcohol consumption may increase the risk of VaD. There is also evidence that cigarette smoking may increase the risk for incident AD and VaD. While the relationship between benzodiazepine use and poorer cognitive functioning is suggested, the association between usage of this class of medication and the development of dementia is inconclusive. Overall, substance use is relevant to neuropsychological functioning in older adults who are at risk for cognitive disorders and have reduced homeostatic mechanisms to preserve brain function in the face of substance use or abuse.

There is a need for additional research addressing substance abuse and neuropsychological functioning in older adults. For instance, the clinical entity of ARD remains controversial and additional empirical information is required to identify the etiological factors, neuropathological/neuroradiological characteristics, clinical course, and behavioral and psychological manifestations of this disorder. Additional research should also address the interaction of ethnicity, substance use, and cognition. This is particularly important because the United States is becoming increasingly ethnoracially diverse and there is evidence that substance use patterns may differ across various groups (Dawson, 1998). It remains to be determined whether differential rates of substance usage in distinct ethnic groups may impact the prevalence or expression of dementia. Lastly, the association between benzodiazepine use, cognitive dysfunction, and dementia warrants clarification in light of the inconsistent findings reported in this area.

References

Agartz, I., Brag, S, Franck, J., Hammarberg, A., Okugawa, G., Svinhufvud, K., et al. (2003). MR volumetry during acute alcohol withdrawal and abstinence: a descriptive study. *Alcohol and Alcoholism, 38*, 71–78.

Allard, J., Artero, S., & Ritchie, K. (2003). Consumption of psychotropic medication in the elderly: a re-evaluation of its effect on cognitive performance. *International Journal of Geriatric Psychiatry, 18*, 874–878.

American Psychiatric Association (2000). *Diagnostic and statistical manual of mental disorders* (DSM-IV TR). Washington, DC: APA.

Angunawela, I., & Barker, A. (2001). Anticholinesterase drugs for alcoholic Korsakoff syndrome. *International Journal of Geriatric Psychiatry, 16*, 338–339.

Antilla, T., Helkala, E-L., Viitanen, M., Kåreholt, I., Fratiglioni, L., Winblad, B., et al. (2004). Alcohol drinking in middle age and subsequent risk of mild cognitive impairment and dementia in old age: a prospective population based study. *British Medical Journal, 329*, 539–545.

Arria, A. M., Tarter, R. E., Starzl, T. E., & Van Thiel, D. H. (1991). Improvement in cognitive functioning of alcoholics following orthotopic liver transplantation. *Alcoholism, Clinical and Experimental Research, 15*, 956–962.

Atkinson, R. M., & Ganzini, L. (1994). Substance abuse. In C. E. Coffey, & J. L. Cummings (Eds.), *Textbook of geriatric neuropsychiatry* (pp. 297–321). Washington, DC: American Psychiatric Press.

Barker, M. J., Greenwood, K. M., Jackson, M., & Crowe, S. F. (2004a). The cognitive effects of long-term benzodiazepine use: A meta-analysis. *CNS Drugs, 18*, 37–48.

Barker, M. J., Greenwood, K. M., Jackson, M., & Crowe, S. F. (2004b). Persistence of cognitive effects after withdrawal from long-term benzodiazepine use: A meta-analysis. *Archives of Clinical Neuropsychology, 19*, 437–454.

Beresford, T., & Gomberg, E. (1995). *Alcohol and aging*. New York: Oxford University Press.

Bond, G. E., Burr, R., Rice, M. M., McCurry, S., Graves, A. B., Teri, L., et al. (2003). Alcohol, aging, and cognitive performance: a cross-cultural comparison. *Journal of Aging and Health, 15*, 371–390.

Brand, M., Fujiwara, E., Borsutzky, S., Kalbe, E., Kessler, J., & Markowitsch, H. J. (2005). Decision-making deficits of Korsakoff patients in a new gambling task with explicit rules: association with executive functions. *Neuropsychology, 19*, 267–277.

Brokate, B., Hildebrandt, H., Eling, P., Fichtner, H. Runge, K., & Timm, C. (2003). Frontal lobe dysfunctions in Korsakoff's syndrome and chronic alcoholism: continuity or discontinuity? *Neuropsychology, 17*, 420–428.

Buffet-Jerrott, S. E., & Stewart, S. H. (2002). Cognitive and sedative effects of benzodiazepine use. *Currents in Pharmacy Design, 8*, 45–58.

Butters, N. (1981). The Wernicke-Korsakoff syndrome: a review of psychological, neuropathological and etiological factors. *Currents in Alcoholism, 8*, 205–232.

Cantillon, M., Barker, W., Harwood, D., Espinosa, J., Kumar, V., & Duara, R. (1996). Earlier onset AD in alcoholics. Poster session presented at the American Association for Geriatric Psychiatry, Tucson, AZ.

Carlen, P. L., McAndrews, M. P., Weiss, R. T., Dongier, M., Hill, J. M., Menzano, E., et al. (1994). Alcohol-related dementia in the institutionalized elderly. *Alcoholism, Clinical and Experimental Research, 18*, 1330–1334.

Catafau, A. M., Kulisevsky, J., Berna, L., Pujol, J, Martin, J. C., Otermin, P., et al. (2000). Relationship between cerebral perfusion in frontal-limbic-basal ganglia circuits to neuropsychologic impairment in patients with subclinical hepatic encephalopathy. *Journal of Nuclear Medicine, 41*, 405–410.

Chew, M. L., Mulsant, B. H., & Pollack, B. G. (2005). Serum anticholinergic activity and cognition in patients with moderate-to-severe dementia. *American Journal of Geriatric Psychiatry, 13*, 535–538.

Chui, H. C., Victoroff, J. I., Margolin, D., Jagust, W., Shankle, R., & Katzman, R. (1992). Criteria for the diagnosis of ischemic vascular dementia proposed by the State of California Alzheimer's Disease Diagnostic Treatment Centers. *Neurology, 42*, 473–480.

Colsher, P. L., & Wallace, R. B. (1990). Elderly men with histories of heavy drinking: correlates and consequences. *Journal of Studies on Alcohol, 51*, 528–535.

Cook, C. C., & Thomson, A. D. (1997). B-complex vitamins in the prophylaxis and treatment of Wernicke-Korsakoff syndrome. *British Journal of Hospital Medicine, 57*, 461–465.

Copeland, J. R., Davidson, J. A., Dewey, M. E., Gilmore, C., Larkin, B. A., McWilliam, C., et al. (1992). Alzheimer's disease, other dementias, depression and pseudodementia: prevalence, incidence, and three-year outcome in Liverpool. *British Journal of Psychiatry, 161*, 230–239.

Cox, J. L. (1993). Smoking cessation in the elderly patient. *Clinics in Chest Medicine, 14*, 423–428.

Cummings, J. L. (1994). Vascular subcortical dementias: clinical aspects. *Dementia, 5*, 177–180.

Dam, M., Burra, P., Tedeschi, U., Cagnin, A., Chierichetti, F., Ermani, M., et al. (1998). Regional cerebral blood flow changes in patients with cirrhosis assessed with 99m Tc-HM-PAO single-photon emission computed tomography: effect of liver transplantation. *Journal of Hepatology, 29*, 78–84.

Dawson, D. A. (1998). Beyond black, white, and Hispanic: race, ethnic origin and drinking patterns in the United States. *Journal of Substance Abuse, 10*, 321–339.

Dealberto, M. J., Mcavay, G. J., Seeman, T., & Berkman, L. (1997). Psychotropic drug use and cognitive decline among older men and women. *International Journal of Geriatric Psychiatry, 12*, 567–574.

Djousse, L., Ellison, R. C., Beiser, A., Scaramucci, A., D'Agostino, R. B., & Wolf, P. A. (2002). Alcohol consumption and risk of ischemic stroke: The Framingham Study. *Stroke, 33*, 907–912.

Dufouil, C., Ducimetiere, P., & Alperovitch, A. (1997). Sex differences in the association between alcohol consumption and cognitive performance. *American Journal of Epidemiology, 146*, 405–412.

Dufour, M., & Fuller, R. K. (1995). Alcohol in the elderly. *Annual Review of Medicine, 46*, 123–132.

Edelstein, S. L., Kritz-Silverstein, D., & Barrett-Connor, C. (1998). Prospective association of smoking and alcohol use with cognitive function in an elderly cohort. *Journal of Women's Health, 7*, 1271–1281.

Elias, P. K., Elias, M. F., D'Agostino, R. B., Silbershatz, H., & Wolf, P. A. (1999). Alcohol consumption and cognitive performance in the Framingham Heart Study. *American Journal of Epidemiology, 150*, 580–589.

Erkinjuntti, T., Inzitari, D., Pantoni, L., Wallin, A., Scheltens, P., Rockwood, K., et al. (2000). Research criteria for subcortical vascular dementia in clinical trials. *Journal of Neural Transmission Supplement, 59*, 23–30.

Erkinjuntti, T., Roman, G. C., & Gauthier, S. (2004). Treatment of vascular dementia – evidence from clinical trials with cholinesterase inhibitors. *Journal of Neurological Science, 226*, 63–66.

Fastbom, J., Forsell, Y., & Winblad, B. (1998). Benzodiazepines may have protective effects against Alzheimer disease. *Alzheimer Disease and Associated Disorders, 12*, 14–17

Finlayson, R. E., Hurt, R. D., Davis, L. J., & Morse, R. M. (1988). Alcoholism in elderly persons: a study of the psychiatric and psychosocial features of 216 inpatients. *Mayo Clinic Proceedings, 63*, 761–768.

Food and Drug Administration (1980). Prescribing of minor tranquilizers. *FDA Drug Bulletin, 10*, 2–3.

Gill, J. S., Shipley, M. J., Tsementzis, S. A., Hornby, R. S., Gill, S. K., Hitchcock, E. R., et al. (1991). Alcohol consumption – a risk factor for hemorrhagic and non-hemorrhagic stroke. *American Journal of Medicine, 90*, 489–497.

Gorelick, P. B., Brody, J., Cohen, D., Freels, S., Levy, P., Dollear, W., et al. (1993). Risk factors for dementia associated with multiple cerebral infarcts. A case control study in predominantly African-American hospital-based patients. *Archives of Neurology, 50*, 714–720.

Graves, A. B., van Duijn, C. M., Chandra, V., Fratiglioni, L., Heyman, A., Jorm, A. F., et al. (1991). Alcohol and tobacco consumption as risk factors for Alzheimer's disease: a collaborative re-analysis of case control studies. *International Journal of Epidemiology, 20*, S48–S57.

Gray, S. L., Penninx, B. W., Blough, D. K., Artz, M. B., Guralnik, J. M., Wallace, R. B., et al. (2003). Benzodiazepine use and physical performance in community-dwelling older women. *Journal of the American Geriatrics Society, 51*, 1563–1570.

Hanlon, J., Horner, R., Schmader, K., Fillenbaum, G. G., Lewis, I. K., Wall, W. E., et al. (1998). Benzodiazepine use and cognitive function among community-dwelling elderly. *Clinical Pharmacology and Therapeutics, 64*, 684–692.

Hebert, L. E., Scherr, P. A., Bienias, J. L., Bennett, D. A., & Evans, D. (2003). Alzheimer's disease in the US population: prevalence estimates using the 2000 Census. *Archives of Neurology, 60*, 1119–1122.

Hemmelgarn, B., Suissa, S., Huang, A., Boivin, J. F., & Pinard, G. (1997). Benzodiazepine use and the risk of motor vehicle crash in the elderly. *Journal of the American Medical Association, 278*, 27–31.

Hendrie, H. C. (1998). Epidemiology of dementia and Alzheimer's disease. *American Journal of Geriatric Psychiatry, 6*, S3–S18.

Hogan, D. B., Maxwell, C. J., Fung, T. S., Ebly, E. M., & the Canadian Study on Health and Aging. (2003). Prevalence and potential consequences of benzodiazepine use in senior citizens: results from the Canadian Study of Health and Aging. *Canadian Journal of Clinical Pharmacology, 10*, 72–77.

Huang, W., Qiu, C., Winblad, B., & Fratiglioni, L. (2002). Alcohol consumption and incidence of dementia in a community sample aged 75 years and older. *Journal of Clinical Epidemiology, 55,* 959–964.

Iga, J., Araki, M., Ishimoto, Y., & Ohmori, T. (2001). A case of Korsakoff's syndrome improved by high doses of donepezil. *Alcohol and Alcoholism, 36,* 553–555.

Jacobson, R. R., Acker, C. F., & Lishman, W. W. (1990). Patterns of neuropsychological deficit in alcoholic Korsakoff's syndrome. *Psychological Medicine, 20,* 321–334.

Jajich, C. L., Ostfeld, A. M., & Freeman, D. H. (1984). Smoking and coronary artery disease mortality in the elderly. *Journal of the American Medical Association, 252,* 2831–2834.

Juan, D., Zhou, D. H., Li, J., Wang, J. Y., Goa, C., & Chen, M. (2004). A 2-year follow-up study of cigarette smoking and risk of dementia. *European Journal of Neurology, 11,* 277–282.

Kato, A., Suzuki, K., Kaneta, H., Obara, H., Fujishima, Y., & Sato, S. (2000). Regional differences in cerebral glucose metabolism in cirrhotic patients with subclinical hepatic encephalopathy using positron emission tomography. *Hepatology Research, 17,* 237–245.

Kawachi, I., Colditz, G. A., Sampfer, M. J., Willett, W. C., Manson, J. E., Rosner, D., et al. (1993). Smoking cessation and decreased risk of stroke in women. *Journal of the American Medical Association, 269,* 232–236.

Kim, K. Y., Ke, V., & Adkins, L. M. (2004). Donepezil for alcohol-related dementia: a case report. *Pharmacotherapy, 24,* 419–421.

Kirby, M., Denihan, A., Bruce, I., Radic, A., Coakley, D., & Lawlor, B. (1999). Benzodiazepine use among the elderly in the community. *International Journal of Geriatric Psychiatry, 14,* 280–284.

Klatsky, A. L., Armstrong, M. A., Friedman, G. D., & Sidney, S. (2002). Alcohol drinking and risk of hemorrhagic stroke. *Neuroepidemiology, 21,* 115–122.

Krabbendam, L., Visser, P. J., Derix, M. M., Verhey, F., Hofman, P., Verhoeven Tuinier, S., et al. (2000). Normal cognitive performance in patients with chronic alcoholism in contrast to patients with Korsakoff's syndrome. *Journal of Neuropsychiatry and Clinical Neurosciences, 12,* 44–50.

Kudoh, A., Takase, H., Takahira, Y., & Yakazawa, T. (2004). Postoperative confusion increases in elderly long-term benzodiazepine users. *Anesthesia and Analgesia, 99,* 1674–1678.

Lagnaoui, R., Bégaud, B., Moore, N., Chaslerie, A., Fourrier, A., Letenneur, L., et al. (2002). Benzodiazepine use and risk of dementia: a nested case-control study. *Journal of Clinical Epidemiology, 55,* 314–318.

Landi, F., Cesari, M., Russo, A., Onder, G., Sgadari, A., Bernabei, R., et al. (2002). Benzodiazepines and the risk of urinary incontinence in frail older persons living in the community. *Clinical Pharmacology and Therapeutics, 72,* 729–734.

Larson, E. B., Kukull, W. A., & Katzman, R. L. (1992). Cognitive impairment: Dementia and Alzheimer's disease. *Annual Review of Public Health, 13,* 431–449.

Larson, E. B., Reifler, B. V., Featherstone, H. J., & English, D. R. (1984). Dementia in elderly outpatients: a prospective study. *Annals of Internal Medicine, 100,* 417–423.

Launer, L. J., Andersen, K., Dewey, M. E., Letenneur, L., Ott, A., Amaducci, L. A., et al. (1999). Rates and risk factors for dementia and Alzheimer's disease: results from EURODEM pooled analyses. EURODEM Incidence Research Group and Work Groups. European Studies of Dementia. *Neurology, 52,* 78–84.

Launer, L. J., Feskens, E. J. M., Kalmijn, S., & Kromhout, D. (1996). Smoking, drinking, and thinking: The Zutphen Elderly Study. *American Journal of Epidemiology, 143*, 219–227.

Lee, S. C., Park, S-J., Ki, H-K., Gwon, H-C., Chung, C-S., Byun, J. S., et al. (2000). Prevalence and risk factors of silent cerebral infarction in apparently normal adults. *Hypertension, 36*, 73–77.

Lemeshow, S., Letenneur, L., Dartigues, J. F., Orgogozu, J. M., & Commenges, D. (1998). An illustration of analysis taking into account complex survey considerations: the association between wine consumption and dementia in the Paquid study. *American Journal of Epidemiology, 148*, 298–306.

Letenneur, L., Dartigues, J. F., Commenges, D., Gagnon, M., Barberger-Gateau, P., Tessier, J. F., et al. (1994). Tobacco consumption and cognitive impairment in elderly people. A population-based study. *Annals of Epidemiology, 4*, 449–454.

Letenneur, L., Larrieu, S., & Barberger-Gateau, P. (2004). Alcohol and tobacco consumption as risk factors of dementia: a review of epidemiological studies. *Biomedicine and Pharmacotherapy, 58*, 95–99.

Lindsay, J., Hebert, R., & Rockwood, K. (1997). The Canadian Study on Health and Aging: risk factors for vascular dementia. *Stroke, 28*, 526–530.

Looi, J. C., & Sachdev, P. S. (1999). Differentiation of vascular dementia from AD on neuropsychological tests. *Neurology, 53*, 670–678.

Luchsinger, J. A., & Mayeux, R. (2004). Cardiovascular risk factors and Alzheimer's disease. *Current Atherosclerosis Reports, 6*, 261–266.

Luchsinger, J. A., Tang, M. X., Siddiqui, M., Shea, S., & Mayeux, R. (2004). Alcohol intake and risk of dementia. *Journal of the American Geriatric Society, 52*, 540–546.

Malouf, R., & Birks, J. (2004). Donepezil for vascular cognitive impairment. *Cochrane Database Systematic Reviews*, CD004395.

Mayer-Oakes, S. A., Kelman, G., Beers, M. H., De Jong, F., Matthias, R., Atchiso, K. A., et al. (1993). Benzodiazepine use in older, community-dwelling southern Californians: prevalence and clinical correlates. *Annals of Pharmacotherapy, 27*, 416–421.

McKhann, G., Drachman, D., Folstein, M. F., Katzman, R., Price, D., & Stadian, E. (1984). Clinical diagnosis of Alzheimer's disease: Report of the NINCDS-ADRDA Work Group under the auspices of Department of Health and Human Services Task Force on Alzheimer's disease. *Neurology, 34*, 939–944.

Meader, K. J. (1998). Cognitive side effects of medications. *Neurology Clinics, 16*, 141–155.

Mendez, M. F., & Cummings, J. L. (2003). *Dementia: a clinical approach* (3rd ed.). Philadelphia, PA: Butterworth Heinemann.

Meyer, J. S., Judd, B. W., Tawakina, T., Rogers, R. L., & Mortel, K. F. (1986). Improved cognition after control of risk factors for multi-infarct dementia. *Journal of the American Medical Association, 256*, 2203–2209.

Moss, H. B., Tarter, R. E., Yao, J. K., & Van Thiel D. H. (1992). Subclinical hepatic encephalopathy: relationship between neuropsychological deficits and standard laboratory tests assessing hepatic status. *Archives of Clinical Neuropsychology, 7*, 419–429.

Mukamal, K. J. (2004). Alcohol consumption and abnormalities of brain structure and vasculature. *American Journal of Geriatric Cardiology, 13*, 22–28.

Mukamal, K. J., Kuller, L. H., Fitzpatrick, A. L., Longstreth, W. T., Mittleman, M. A., & Siscovick, D. S. (2003). Prospective study of alcohol consumption and risk of dementia in older adults. *Journal of the American Medical Association, 289*, 1405–1413.

Munro, C. A., Saxton, J., & Butters, M. A. (2001). Alcohol dementia: "cortical" or "subcortical" dementia? *Archives of Clinical Neuropsychology, 16*, 523–533.

Nakagawa, Y., Matsumura, K., Iwasa, M., Kaito, M., Adachi, Y., & Takeda, K. (2004). Single photon emission computed tomography and statistical parametric mapping analysis in cirrhotic patients with and without minimal hepatic encephalopathy. *Annals of Nuclear Medicine, 18*, 123–129.

Ness, J., Hoth, A., Barnett, M. J., Shorr, R. I., & Kaboli, P. J. (2006). Anticholinergic medication in community-dwelling veterans: prevalence of anticholinergic symptoms, symptom burden, and adverse drug events. *American Journal of Geriatric Pharmacotherapy, 4*, 42–51.

O'Carroll, R. (1993). Neuropsychological and neuroimaging aspects of latent hepatic encephalopathy. *Alcohol and Alcoholism Supplement, 2*, 191–195.

O'Donnell, V. M., Pitts, W. M., & Fann, W. E. (1986). Noradrenergic and cholinergic agents in Korsakoff's syndrome. *Clinical Neuropharmacology, 9*, 65–70.

Orgogozo, J. M., Dartigues, J. F., Lafont, S., Letenneur, L., Commenges, D., Salamon, R., et al. (1997). Wine consumption and dementia in the elderly: a prospective community study in the Bordeaux area. *Review of Neurology, 153*, 185–192.

Oscar-Berman, M., Kirkley, S. M., Gansler, D. A., & Couture, A. (2004). Comparisons of Korsakoff and non-Korsakoff alcoholics on neuropsychological tests of prefrontal brain functioning. *Alcoholism, Clinical and Experimental Research, 28*, 667–675.

Oslin, D., Atkinson, R. M., Smith, D. M., & Hendrie, H. (1998). Alcohol Related Dementia: proposed clinical criteria. *International Journal of Geriatric Psychiatry, 13*, 203–212.

Oslin, D., & Cary, M. S. (2003). Alcohol-Related Dementia: validation of diagnostic criteria. *American Journal of Geriatric Psychiatry, 11*, 441–447.

Ott, A., Slooter, A. J., Hofman, V., van Harskamp, F., Witteman, J. C., Van Broeckhoven, C., et al. (1998). Smoking and risk of dementia and Alzheimer's disease in a population-based cohort study: the Rotterdam Study. *Lancet, 351*, 1840–1843.

Paterniti, S., Dufouil, C., & Alpérovitch, A. (2002). Long-term benzodiazepine use and cognitive decline in the elderly: the Epidemiology of Vascular Aging Study. *Journal of Clinical Psychopharmacology, 22*, 285–293.

Peterson, R. C., Doody, R., Kurz, A., Mohs, R. C., Morris, J. C., Rabins, P. V., et al. (2001). Current concepts in mild cognitive impairment. *Archives of Neurology, 58*, 1985–1992.

Pfefferbaum, A., Sullivan, E. V., Mathalon, D. H., Shear, P. K., Rosenbloom, M. J., & Lim, K. O. (1995). Longitudinal changes in magnetic resonance imaging brain volumes in abstinent and relapsed alcoholics. *Alcoholism, Clinical and Experimental Research, 19*, 1177–1191.

Phillips, B. K., Ingram, M. V., & Grammer, G. G. (2004). Wernicke-Korsakoff syndrome and galantamine. *Psychosomatics, 45*, 366–368.

Rao, V. S., Cupples, L. A., Auerbach, S. A., Becker, R., Burke, J., Chui, H., et al (1995). Age at onset of Alzheimer's disease is influenced by multiple genetic and non-genetic factors: The Mirage Study. *Alzheimer's Research, 1*, 159–168.

Renvoize, E. B., Gaskell, R. K., & Klar, H. M. (1985). Results of investigations in 150 demented patients consecutively admitted to a psychiatric hospital. *British Journal of Psychiatry, 147*, 204–205.

Rigler, S. K. (2000). Alcoholism in the elderly. *American Family Physician, 61*, 1710–1716.

Ritchie, C. W., Ames, D., Clayton, T., & Lai, R. (2004). Meta-analysis of randomized trials of the efficacy and safety of donepezil, galantamine, and rivastigmine for the treatment of Alzheimer disease. *American Journal of Geriatric Psychiatry, 12*, 358–369.

Rogers, R. L., Meyer, J. S., Judd, B. W., & Mortel, K. F. (1985). Abstention from cigarette smoking improves cerebral perfusion among elderly chronic smokers. *Journal of the American Medical Association, 253*, 2970–2974.

Roman, G. C. (2004). Brain hypoperfusion: a critical factor in vascular dementia. *Neurological Research, 26*, 454–458.

Roman, G. C., Erkinjuntti, T., Wallin, A., Pantoni, L., & Chui, H. C. (2002). Subcortical ischaemic vascular dementia. *Lancet Neurology, 1*, 426–436.

Roman, G. C., Sachdev, P., Royall, D. R., Bullock, R. A., Orogozo, J. M., Lopez-Pousa, S., et al. (2004). Vascular cognitive disorder: a new diagnostic category updating vascular cognitive impairment and vascular dementia. *Journal of Neurological Science, 226*, 81–87.

Roman, G. C., Tatemichi, T. K., Erkinjuntti, T., Cummings, J. L., Masdeu, J. C., Garcia, J. H., et al. (1993). Vascular dementia: diagnostic criteria for research studies. Report of the NINDS-AIREN International Workshop. *Neurology, 43*, 250–260.

Ross, G. W., & Petrovitch, H. (2001). Current evidence for a neuroprotective effect of nicotine and caffeine against Parkinson's disease. *Drugs and Aging, 18*, 797–806.

Rourke, S. B., & Løberg, T. (1996). The neurobehavioral correlates of alcoholism. In I. Grant & K. M. Adams (Eds.), *Neuropsychological assessment of neuropsychiatric disorders* (pp. 423–485). New York, NY: Oxford University Press.

Ruitenberg, A., van Swieten, J. C., Witteman, J. C., Mehta, K. M., van Duijn, C. M., Hofman, A., et al. (2003). Alcohol consumption and the risk of dementia: the Rotterdam Study. *Journal of the American Medical Association, 289*, 1405–1413.

Rustembegovic, A., Kundurovic, Z., Sapcanin, A., & Sofic, E. (2003). A placebo-controlled study of memantine (Ebixa) in dementia of Wernicke-Korsakoff syndrome. *Medicinski Arhiv, 57*, 149–150.

Sahin, H. A., Gurvit, H., Bilgic, B., Hanagasi, H. A., & Emre, M. (2002). Therapeutic effects of an acetylcholinesterase inhibitor (Donepezil) on memory in Wernicke-Korsakoff's disease. *Clinical Neuropharmacology, 25*, 16–20.

Sairenchi, T., Iso, H., Nishimura, A., Hosoda, T., Irie, F., Saito, Y., et al. (2004). Cigarette smoking and risk of type 2 diabetes mellitus among middle-aged and elderly Japanese men and women. *American Journal of Epidemiology, 160*, 158–162.

Saxton, J., Munro, C. A., Butters, M. A., Schramke, C., & McNeal, M. A. (2000). *Journal of Geriatric Psychiatry and Neurology, 13*, 141–149.

Schroth, G., Naegele, T., Klose, U., Mann, K., & Peterson, D. (1988). Reversible brain shrinkage in abstinent alcoholics, measured by MRI. *Neuroradiology, 30*, 385–389.

Shear, P. K., Jernigan, T. L., & Butters, N. (1995). Volumetric magnetic resonance imaging quantification of longitudinal brain changes in abstinent alcoholics. *Alcoholism, Clinical and Experimental Research, 18*, 172–176.

Skoog, I. (1998). Status of risk factors for vascular dementia. *Neuroepidemiology, 17*, 2–9.

Smith, D. M., & Atkinson, R. M. (1995). Alcoholism and dementia. *International Journal of Addiction, 30*, 1843–1869.

Smith, S. S., & Fiore, M. C. (1999). The epidemiology of tobacco use, dependence, and cessation in the United States. *Primary Care, 26*, 433–461.

Snowden, D. A., Greiner, L. H., Mortimer, J. A., Riley, K. P., Greiner, P. A., & Markesbery, W. R. (1997). Brain infarction and the clinical expression of Alzheimer disease. The Nun Study. *Journal of the American Medical Association, 278*, 813–817.

Stampfer, M. J., Colditz, G. A., Willett, W. C., Speizer, F. E., & Hennekens, C. H. (1988). A prospective study of moderate alcohol consumption and the risk of coronary disease and stroke in women. *New England Journal of Medicine, 319*, 267–273.

Starr, J. M., McGurn, B., Whiteman, M., Pattie, A., Whalley, L. J., & Deary, I. J. (2004). Life long changes in cognitive ability are associated with prescribed medications in old age. *International Journal of Geriatric Psychiatry, 19*, 327–332.

Substance Abuse and Mental Health Services Administration (2004). *Results from the 2003 National Survey on Drug Use and Health: national findings* (Office of Applied Studies NSDUH Series H–25, DHHS Publication No. SMA 04–3964). Rockville, MD: SAMHSA.

Thomson, A. D., Cook, C. C., Touquet, R., Henry, J. A., & the Royal College of Physicians, London (2002). The Royal College of Physicians report on alcohol: guidelines for managing Wernicke's encephalopathy in the Accident and Emergency Department. *Alcohol and Alcoholism, 37*, 513–521.

Trzepacz, P. T., Tarter, R. E., Shah, A., Tringali, R., Faett, D. G., & Van Thiel, D. H. (1994). SPECT scan and cognitive findings in subclinical hepatic encephalopathy. *Journal of Neuropsychiatry and Clinical Neurosciences, 6*, 170–175.

Truelsen, T., Gronbaek, M., Schnohr, P., & Boysen, G. (1998). Intake of beer, wine, and spirits and risk of stroke: the Copenhagen City Heart Study. *Stroke, 29*, 2467–2472.

Tuck, R. R., & Jackson, M. (1991). Social, neurological and cognitive disorders in alcoholics. *Medical Journal of Australia, 19*, 225–229.

Tune, L. E. (2001). Anticholinergic effects of medication in elderly patients. *Journal of Clinical Psychiatry, 62* (Suppl. 21), 11–14.

Tyas, S. L., White, L. R., Petrovitch, H., Webster, R. G., Foley, D. J., Heimovitz, H. K., et al. (2003). Mid-life smoking and late-life dementia: the Honolulu-Asia Aging Study. *Neurobiology and Aging, 24*, 589–596.

US Department of Health and Human Services (1993). *Special report on aging* (NIH Publication No. 92-3409). Washington, DC: US Government Printing Office.

US Department of Health and Human Services (2001). *Substance abuse among older adults* (Treatment Improvement Protocol Series). Washington, DC: US Government Printing Office.

US Census Bureau (2000). *United States Census 2000*. Retrieved January 1, 2006, from http://www.census.gov/main/www/cen2000.html.

Van Asselen, M., Kessels, R. P., Wester, A. J., & Postma, A. (2005). Spatial working memory and contextual cueing in patients with Korsakoff amnesia. *Journal of Clinical and Experimental Neuropsychology, 27*, 645–655.

Van Diujn, C. M., Clayton, D. G., Chandra, V., Fratiglioni, L., Graves, A. B., Heyman, A., et al. (1994). Interaction between genetic and environmental risk factors for Alzheimer's disease: a reanalysis of case-control studies. EURODEM Risk Factors Research Group. *Genetic Epidemiology, 11*, 539–551

Verdoux, H., Lagnaoui, R., & Begaud, B. (2005). Is benzodiazepine use a risk factor for cognitive decline and dementia: a literature review of epidemiological studies. *Psychological Medicine, 35,* 307–315.

Verghese, J., Lipton, R. B., Hall, C. B., Kuslansky, G., Katz, M. J., & Buschke, H. (2002). Abnormality of gait as a predictor of non-Alzheimer's dementia. *New England Journal of Medicine, 347,* 1761–1768.

Verhaeghe, W., Mets, T., & Corne, L. (1996). Benzodiazepine use among elderly patients presenting at an emergency room. *Archives of Gerontology and Geriatrics, 22,* 55–62.

Victor, M. (1994). Alcoholic dementia. *Canadian Journal of Neurological Science, 21,* 88–99.

Victor, M., Adams, R. D., & Collins, G. H. (1989). *The Wernicke-Korsakoff Syndrome. A clinical and pathological study of 245 patients, 82 with postmortem examinations* (2nd ed.). Philadelphia, PA: F. A. Davis.

Wagner, A. K., Zhang, F., Soumerai, S. B., Walker, A. M., Gurwitz, J. H., Glynn, R., et al. (2004). Benzodiazepine use and hip fractures in the elderly: who is at greatest risk. *Archives of Internal Medicine, 164,* 1567–1572.

Wang, H. X., Fratiglioni, L., Frisoni, G. B., Viitanen, M., & Winblad, B. (1999). Smoking and the occurrence of Alzheimer's disease: cross-sectional and longitudinal data in a population-based study. *American Journal of Epidemiology, 149,* 640–644.

Wannamethee, S. G., Shaper, A. G., Whincup, P. H., & Walker, M. (1995). Smoking cessation and the risk of stroke in middle-aged men. *Journal of the American Medical Association, 274,* 155–160.

Watanabe, A. (1998). Cerebral changes in hepatic encephalopathy. *Journal of Gastroenterology and Hepatology, 13,* 752–760.

Wells, C. E. (1979). Diagnosis of dementia. *Psychosomatics, 20,* 517–522.

Wetterling, T., Kanitz, R. D., & Borgis, K. J. (1994). The ICD-10 criteria for vascular dementia. *Dementia, 5,* 185–188.

Wilcock, G., Mobius, H. J., Stoffler, A., & MMM 500 Group (2002). A double-blind, placebo-controlled multicentre study of memantine in mild to moderate vascular dementia (MMM500). *International Clinical Psychopharmacology, 17,* 297–305.

Wolf, P. A., D'Agostino, R. B., Kannel, W. B., Bonita, R., & Belanger, A. J. (1988). Cigarette smoking as a risk factor for stroke. The Framingham Study. *Journal of the American Medical Association, 259,* 1025–1029.

Yamashita, K., Kobayashi, S., Yamaguchi, S., Kitani, M., & Tsunematsu, T. (1988). Effect of smoking on regional cerebral blood flow in the normal aged volunteers. *Gerontologist, 34,* 199–204.

Yamashita, K., Kobayashi, S., & Yamaguchi, S. (2000). Cerebral blood flow and cessation of cigarette smoking in healthy volunteers. *Internal Medicine, 39,* 891–893.

Yoshitake, T., Kiyohara, Y., Kato, I., Ohmura, T., Iwamoto, H., Nakayama, K., et al. (1995). Incidence and risk factors of vascular dementia and Alzheimer's disease in a defined elderly Japanese population: The Hisayama Study. *Neurology, 45,* 1161–1168.

Zekry, D., Hauw, J-J., & Gold, G. (2002). Mixed dementia: epidemiology, diagnosis, and treatment. *Journal of the American Geriatrics Society, 50,* 1431–1438.

11 Neurobehavioral consequences of substance abuse and HIV infection

Michael R. Basso, Robert A. Bornstein, and Taeh Ward

It is widely recognized that neurobehavioral deficits are associated with human immunodeficiency virus (HIV) infection (e.g., Grant & Heaton, 1990; Heaton et al., 1995; Reger, Welsh, Razani, Martin, & Boone, 2002). Given that this point is well established, more recent studies have sought to determine if there are factors that exacerbate the impairments that occur as a result of HIV. One factor that has only recently received attention is substance abuse. This is somewhat surprising, because drug abuse is highly prevalent among cohorts of individuals with HIV (cf. Rosenberger et al., 1993). Notably, many abused substances are associated with diminished neuropsychological functioning. In the present review, we will summarize literature concerning the effects of both HIV and substance abuse on neuropsychological function, and we will suggest potential mechanisms by which substance abuse may exacerbate neurobehavioral deficits in individuals infected with HIV.

Neurobehavioral effects of HIV

Among individuals with HIV, the cognitive domains that are most likely to be affected include attention, speed of information processing, psychomotor speed, memory, concept formation, and abstract reasoning (cf. Heaton et al., 1995). Generally, the prevalence and severity of these deficits increase as the disease progresses (cf. Levin et al., 1990). For example, neurobehavioral abnormalities tend to be mild or nonexistent in asymptomatic individuals (e.g., Bornstein, Nasrallah, Para, Whitacre, Rosenberger, & Fass, 1993; Collier et al., 1992; Martin, Robertson, Sorensen, Jagust, Mallon, & Chirurgi, 1993; Reger et al., 2002; van Gorp et al., 1991), whereas symptomatic individuals tend to demonstrate more pronounced cognitive and sensorimotor (e.g., sensorineuropathy, motor slowing) impairments. Among people who have progressed to AIDS, a severe and pervasive pattern of neuropsychological dysfunction is often observed (Grant et al., 1987; Heaton et al., 1995), with marked deficits manifest in motor function (Reger et al., 2002).

At present, the precise cause of HIV-related neurobehavioral abnormalities is unknown, though a number of potential etiological factors have been identified. Based upon observations that HIV is present in brain tissue soon after seroconversion, it was initially hypothesized that the neurobehavioral abnormalities occurred as a result of direct viral interaction with brain tissue (Kure, Lyman, Weidenheim, & Dickson, 1990; Lyman, Kress, Kure, Rashbaum, Rubinstein, & Soeiro, 1990; Wiley, Belman, Dickson, Rubinstein, & Nelson, 1990). More recent studies have implied that the neuropathogenesis of HIV occurs via indirect mechanisms (e.g., McArthur, 1994). In particular, the virus is tropic for glial cells, macrophages, and endothelial cells within the brain rather than neurons, and the amount of neurological damage is disproportionate to the presence of HIV in the brain (Navia Jordan, & Price, 1986). Viral proteins or other cellular mediated substances are shown to exert pathological changes upon cerebral structure and function. For instance, HIV mediates the release of cytokines, tumor necrosis factor, and granulocyte–monocyte colony-stimulating factors, which in turn may be toxic to neuronal activity, modify neurotransmitter function, increase the likelihood of secondary inflammation (e.g., encephalitis), or cause leukoencephalopathy (McArthur, 1994). At the structural level, these pathological changes tend to correlate with several abnormalities, most occurring during later and more severe stages of the disease course (cf. McArthur, 1994). For instance, cerebral atrophy is relatively common among individuals with AIDS, as is the presence of multinucleated giant cells. Additionally, leukoencephalopathy (myelin pallor), gliosis, and microglial nodules also are apt to be present. These structural abnormalities tend to coincide with abnormalities in cerebrospinal fluid, on structural and functional imaging studies, and on electroencephalogram (EEG) recordings (McArthur, 1994).

Although cerebral abnormalities associated with HIV have been demonstrated in a large number of studies, not all infected individuals display neuropsychological impairment. Perhaps reflecting the inconsistent presence of compromised cerebral integrity, only some infected individuals display neuropsychological abnormalities. As many as 10–20% of patients who are in relatively early stages of HIV infection may show subtle cognitive impairment (Heaton et al., 1995). Among those who have progressed to AIDS, some studies estimate that approximately 55–86% have pronounced cognitive deficits (Grant et al., 1987; Heaton et al., 1995; Reger et al., 2002).

These findings have prompted attempts to identify risk factors for developing neurobehavioral dysfunction in HIV infection, with most studies having focused on disease-related markers. For instance, increasingly rapid rates of decline in immunity indicators are associated with greater frequency of cognitive deficits (Bornstein, Nasrallah, Para, Fass, Whitacre, & Rice, 1991). Moreover, increased viral load is associated with greater levels of neurobehavioral dysfunction (Chang, Ernst, Witt, Ames, Gaiefsky & Miller, 2002; McArthur et al., 1997). The combination of diminished immunity function and secondary infection also increases the risk of neuropsychological dysfunction (Basso & Bornstein, 2000a). Furthermore, as more time elapses since seroconversion, neurobehavioral abnormalities tend to occur more frequently (Bornstein, Nasrallah, Para, Whitacre, & Fass, 1994). Additionally, a premorbid level of intelligence seems to moderate the risk of developing neurobehavioral deficits. Specifically, as the disease progresses, individuals with lower levels of premorbid intelligence are more vulnerable to having neuropsychological deficits than are those with higher levels of premorbid intellect (Basso & Bornstein, 2000b).

Substance abuse

As previously stated, substance misuse is a factor that may exacerbate the neuropsychological abnormalities that occur as a result of HIV. A developing literature reveals that dependence on particular drugs is associated with diminished neuropsychological functioning. Additionally, there are suggestions that substance abuse may diminish immune response, which, in turn, may increase the likelihood of further neurobehavioral dysfunction through secondary infection (e.g., toxoplasmosis, cytomegalovirus, etc.).

Notably, a large proportion of individuals infected with HIV are past or current abusers of drugs. For instance, Rosenberger et al. (1993) found that approximately 75% of 250 HIV seropositive individuals had lifetime diagnoses of drug and/or alcohol abuse. Because so many infected people have significant histories of substance abuse, they may consequently show an increased propensity for neuropsychological impairment compared to their nondrug-abusing counterparts; yet, there is relatively little research concerning the neuropsychological consequences of comorbid substance abuse and HIV infection. Indeed, much of the initial research concerning neuropsychological impairment in HIV concerned injection drug users exclusively (e.g., Marder et al., 1995; Selnes et al., 1997). Although these investigations demonstrated meaningful impairment in users infected with HIV, the unique effects of drug use could not be examined. In particular, nondrug-using comparison groups were not used.

In this review, we survey the literature concerning the neurobehavioral and immunological effects of drugs that are popularly abused by individuals infected with HIV. These include cocaine, opiates, alcohol, marijuana, and amphetamines. In doing so, we hope to suggest mechanisms by which abuse of these substances may exacerbate or contribute to neurobehavioral dysfunction in HIV infection. Because the pathophysiology of these drugs will be discussed in other chapters, this topic will be reviewed only briefly in this chapter.

Cocaine

Cerebral morphology and function

Cocaine has its most salient influence upon the dopaminergic system. Indeed, cocaine addicts tend to show elevated dopamine metabolite levels, thereby suggesting dopamine dysfunction (Roy, Berman, Williams, Kuhn, &

Gonzalez, 2002). With chronic use, resulting changes in dopaminergic response are thought to be most prominent in the basal ganglia, orbitofrontal cortex, and cingulate gyrus (Hartman, 1995). Perhaps corresponding with these effects, acute intoxication decreases brain activation in the frontal lobes and basal ganglia (Pearlson, Jeffery, Harris, Ross, Fischman, & Camargo, 1993), and such hypometabolism may persist long after cocaine intoxication (cf. Browndyke et al., 2004; Strickland et al., 1993; Volkow, Mullani, Gould, Adler, & Krajewski, 1988). Apart from functional changes, chronic cocaine use may also alter brain structure, with anomalies occurring in white matter as well as in cortical and subcortical gray matter, especially in the frontal lobes (Bartzokis et al., 1999; Bolla, Cadet, & London, 1998; Franklin et al., 2002; Jacobsen, Giedd, Kreek, Gottschalk, & Kosten, 2001; O'Neill, Cardenas, & Meyerhoff, 2001).

Neuropsychological effects

To our knowledge, only one study has specifically examined the effects of cocaine use and HIV infection on neuropsychological function. Durvasula et al. (2000) administered a relatively broad battery of neuropsychological tests to nearly 240 African-American men, 172 of which were HIV seropositive. Approximately 71% of the sample were either current or past cocaine users. Regardless of HIV status, moderate to heavy users of cocaine demonstrated psychomotor slowing. Regardless of recency or pattern of cocaine use, symptomatic individuals also demonstrated psychomotor slowing. There was no interaction of HIV status and cocaine use, however, which raises questions as to whether cocaine and HIV infection may exert synergistic effects upon neurobehavioral status. It is important to note that the authors did not distinguish patients with AIDS from those in earlier disease stages. Stratification of the sample according to HIV disease status might have yielded different results. Additionally, the sample may possess limited generalizability, as it was comprised entirely of young, moderately educated, African-American gay or bisexual men.

Immune function

In HIV-seronegative individuals, cocaine abuse affects immune response, initially via an acute suppression of T-cell response (Karlix et al., 1998). Overall, immune system integrity is diminished, as a variety of immune cell interactions are affected by cocaine use (Baldwin, Roth, & Tashkin, 1998). The degree of immunosuppression may also be related to the amount of cocaine used (Delafuente & DeVane, 1991). Even after cocaine use is terminated, there is a residual suppression of immune function for at least a few days afterwards (Avila, Alonzo, & Bayer, 2004; Avila, Morgan, & Bayer, 2003).

Such cocaine-related immunosuppression is also observed among individuals with HIV. For example, cocaine use is linked to higher rates of HIV seropositivity and more rapid progression to AIDS (cf. Friedman, Newton, & Klein, 2003; Webber, Schoenbaum, Gourevitch, Buono, & Klein, 1999). Furthermore, in at least one study, cocaine abuse has been shown to intensify replication of HIV throughout the body (Peterson, Gekker, Chao, Schut, Molitor, & Balfour, 1991), although it is unclear whether it similarly increases replication in the central nervous system.

In addition to systemic immune response, cocaine seems to increase the susceptibility of the brain to infection. For example, cocaine increases the permeability of the blood–brain barrier to various viruses, including HIV (Nottet et al., 1996; Zhang et al., 1998). Some researchers have hypothesized that cocaine abuse may contribute to the development of HIV-related neurobehavioral abnormalities by facilitating entrance of the virus into the brain (Zhang et al., 1998).

Collectively, these findings suggest that cocaine abuse may adversely and synergistically influence brain function among HIV-infected individuals in at least two ways. In a direct manner, cocaine is toxic to brain tissue through a negative influence on neurotransmitter function, brain metabolism, and cerebral structure. In an indirect fashion, cocaine abuse may adversely influence neurobehavioral function by its effect upon the immune system. Specifically, it compromises the integrity of the blood–brain barrier, and it decreases systemic immune response. Because neurobehavioral deficits are more common during symptomatic than asymptomatic stages of HIV infection, cocaine abuse may consequently result in diminished neuropsychological function, though this hypothesis was not supported in the single study that focused on this issue (cf. Durvasula et al., 2000).

Opiates

Cerebral morphology and function

Studies of opiate abuse on brain structure have produced inconsistent results. Indeed, a number of researchers acknowledge that relatively little is known concerning the long-term effects of opiate use on the brain (cf. Franken, Stam, Hendriks, & van den Brink, 2004), and existing studies reveal often conflicting findings (cf. Pezawas et al., 1998; Rose et al., 1996). Apart from structural abnormalities, there are suggestions that chronic opiate use corresponds with functional anomalies. In particular, hypometabolism seems to occur in a diffuse pattern, but especially in the frontal, parietal, and temporal lobes (cf. Danos et al., 1998; Pezawas et al., 2002; Rose et al., 1996). Thus, opiates appear to have a potentially diffuse effect upon brain function.

Neuropsychological function

A number of studies have examined neuropsychological function among HIV-infected opiate abusers. The findings from these studies were inconsistent.

For instance, a subset of these studies compared seropositive and seronegative opiate abusers on measures of neuropsychological function and generally found that opiate misuse was not a risk factor for increased neuropsychological impairment (e.g., Concha et al., 1992; Del Pesce et al., 1993; Kovner et al., 1992; Wellman, 1992). Although these findings suggest that opiate abuse does not contribute to neuropsychological deficits in HIV, this is likely due to limitations related to the methodologies employed in these studies. Specifically, the investigators did not examine whether opiate abuse may interact with HIV status to exacerbate neurobehavioral deficits. Rather, only the main effects of substance abuse and infection status were examined. The investigators did not compare seropositive opiate abusers to seropositive individuals who did not abuse opiates. Additionally, sensitivity of neuropsychological measures may have been wanting. For example, screening instruments were employed in some of these studies (e.g., Del Pesce et al., 1993). Such measures are sometimes criticized as possessing insufficient sensitivity and breadth to detect subtle neuropsychological deficits associated with HIV or drug abuse (cf. Bornstein et al., 1993).

Immune function

Although the existing literature is somewhat limited (cf. Friedman et al., 2003), experimental and clinical data indicate that opiate abuse is immunosuppressive. In general, two of the most misused opiates, morphine and heroin, yield similar reductions in CD4 T lymphocyte counts and other indices of immune system integrity (for reviews, see Arora, Fride, Petitto, Waggie, & Skolnick, 1990; Rouveix, 1992). For instance, Freier and Fuchs (1994) reported that natural killer cell activity decreased in a dose–response relationship to morphine administration in mice. However, immunosuppression was blocked when opiate antagonists naloxone and naltrexone were administered simultaneously with the morphine. Heroin addiction in people can create a persistent reduction in CD4 T-lympohcyte cell count despite abstinence for several months (Govitrapong, Suttitum, Kotchabhakdi, & Uneklabh, 1998). The synergistic and immunosuppressive effects of opiates may be particularly significant in HIV infection. Morphine stimulates the replication of the HIV virus (Schweitzer et al., 1991). Moreover, continued opiate abuse after seroconversion may increase the likelihood that an infected individual will progress to AIDS (Di Franco, Marlink, Hunter, Tosteson, Mayer, & Essex, 1993). Additionally, initiating the use of opiates and other drugs seems to contribute to increasing rates of medical illness besides AIDS in HIV-seropositive individuals (Lucas, Gebo, Chaisson, & Moore, 2002).

In this context, opiate agonist treatment, namely methadone, has been used to decrease symptoms of withdrawal as well as behaviors that increase risk of HIV transmission. There are some indications that antiretroviral treatment may reduce serum levels of methadone in seropositive individuals, but this occurs without subsequent withdrawal symptoms (Francis, 2003).

Furthermore, despite methadone maintenance, antiretroviral therapies continue to decrease HIV burden (Lucas, Weidle, Hader, & Moore, 2004). As such, it seems reasonable to maintain seropositive patients on methadone and antiretroviral treatments simultaneously. In doing so, positive health outcomes may be increased for seropositive opiate misusers, and rates of HIV transmission in the population may be reduced (De Castro & Sabate, 2003).

Taken together, these findings fail to provide a consensus regarding the effects of opiate abuse on neuropsychological function. At present, it is unclear as to whether the lack of consistency across studies reflects weaknesses or differences in research methodology or if opiate use actually yields no neuropsychological impairment in people infected with HIV. Notably, there is growing evidence that neuropsychological deficits occur in seronegative individuals who abuse opiates (cf. Mintzer & Stitzer, 2002). Such studies have employed highly sensitive measures, and deficits in memory, speed, and decision-making were observed (cf. Mintzer & Stitzer, 2002). Studies of opiate-related deficits in seropositive individuals have used measures that are arguably less sensitive, and this may explain the different outcomes between studies (Concha et al., 1992; Del Pesce et al., 1993; Kovner et al., 1992; Wellman, 1992). Furthermore, the interactive effects of HIV status and drug use history have not been addressed.

At present, it is uncertain whether the interaction of serostatus and opiate abuse influences neuropsychological function. Regardless, there is a growing consensus that opiate abuse diminishes immune response, and may partially underlie the deterioration to a more severe disease stage. Insofar as individuals with AIDS have worse neurobehavioral impairment than other seropositive individuals, opiate abuse may indirectly contribute to worsening neuropsychological function. Future studies using rigorous study designs can test this assertion.

Alcohol

Rates of alcohol abuse or dependence are substantially higher among people with HIV than among the general population (Rosenberger et al., 1993). Indeed, lifetime prevalence of such disorders ranges from 29% to 60% of people with HIV, whereas prevalence in the general population approaches 15% (Petry, 1999). As such, alcohol abuse and dependence are among the most common comorbid disorders among people infected with HIV.

Cerebral morphology and function

A compelling body of evidence suggests that alcohol misuse corresponds with meaningful cerebral pathology (cf. Jernigan et al., 1991; Sullivan, 2003; Wilkinson, 1987). Structural imaging studies indicate that tissue loss occurs in cortex and white matter, and this seems to occur most commonly in the frontal and parietal lobes. Other structures appear diminished, including the mammillary bodies, basal ganglia, thalamus, pons, and cerebellum, and some assert that alcohol tends to disrupt frontal–brainstem–cerebellum circuits with great saliency (Sullivan, 2003). In addition to structural effects, alcohol misuse seems to diminish brain function. It seems to influence a broad array of neurotransmitter systems, including acetylcholine, norepinephrine, glutamate, and GABA, with chronic abuse resulting in sustained alterations and damage to these systems (Hartman, 1995). Studies employing functional imaging methods (e.g., fMRI, PET, SPECT) have similarly found abnormalities in alcoholics. For instance, a number of investigations indicate that alcoholism is associated with hypometabolism in the frontal and parietal lobes (Adams et al., 1993; Mathew & Wilson, 1991; Volkow et al., 1994).

Neuropsychological function

An extensive literature has shown that alcohol misuse is associated with deleterious effects upon neurobiological and neuropsychological function; yet, whether alcohol misuse increases the risk of neuropsychological deficit in individuals with HIV is largely untested. Among the few studies in this area, Green, Saveanu, and Bornstein (2004) compared four groups of homosexual men on a battery of neuropsychological tests. The men were either HIV positive or negative, and they had either a positive or negative history of past alcohol abuse. A main effect of past alcohol abuse was observed on measures reflecting verbal intelligence, concept formation, auditory working memory, and reaction time, whereas a main effect of HIV status was found on measures of verbal learning and motor speed. Notably, a significant interaction between HIV status and history of alcohol abuse was observed such that HIV-seropositive participants with a history of alcohol abuse demonstrated poorer performance on measures of verbal intelligence, concept formation, and visual reaction time relative to the comparison groups. Additionally, in the HIV negative group, history of alcohol abuse had no significant effect. In a more recent study, Rothlind et al. (2005) administered an extensive neuropsychological battery to four groups of mostly male homosexuals. Similar to Green et al.'s study, participants were either HIV positive or negative, and they were either heavy alcohol consumers or light/nondrinkers. Notably, heavy alcohol use was defined as the consumption of more than 100 alcoholic beverages monthly for the past three years. After controlling for age, education, and estimated premorbid IQ, Rothlind et al. found significant main effects of alcohol use on measures of working memory, motor control, and executive function, with heavy alcohol use corresponding with worse neuropsychological performance. Additionally, seropositive individuals had poorer performance on measures of working memory and speed of information processing. Notably, Rothlind et al. performed supplementary analyses to examine the effects of recent heavy drinking. In particular, they identified individuals who reported an average of more than six alcoholic beverages per occasion during the week preceding participation. Compared to the other groups, current heavy drinkers who were seropositive performed significantly worse on measures of information processing speed and motor speed. Thus, these data imply that heavy sustained alcohol use may act synergistically with HIV status to exacerbate some aspects of neurobehavioral function.

Such findings notwithstanding, several large-scale and well-controlled investigations have concluded that neurobehavioral abnormalities in HIV are not attributable to alcohol abuse (Bornstein et al., 1993; Concha et al., 1997; Heaton et al., 1995). Similarly, imaging studies of cerebral structure and function in HIV have shown either no effect of alcohol abuse (McArthur et al., 1990) or main effects of alcohol abuse and HIV status (Meyerhoff et al., 1995). These studies generally compared seronegative and seropositive subjects on neuropsychological measures, and examined whether alcohol use accounted for deficits shown by the HIV-seropositive individuals. These studies did not determine whether alcohol abuse exacerbated neuropsychological dysfunction within a sample of HIV-infected individuals (e.g., comparing alcoholic and nonalcoholic seropositives). Consequently, there is presently at least one study showing that alcohol abuse exacerbates neuropsychological function in seropositive individuals (Green et al., 2004). Although intriguing, this finding awaits replication.

Immune function

Recent data show that chronic alcohol misuse is associated with increased immunosuppression, both through direct and indirect effects. The durability of this immunosuppression is unknown, though research suggests that the condition reverses after several months of abstinence (Tonnesen, Kaiser, Nielsen, & Pedersen, 1992). Alcoholics are increasingly susceptible to bacterial infections such as pneumonia and tuberculosis as well as viral diseases. Regulation and function of a number of immune responses are also altered (Cook, 1998; Jerrells, Slukvin, Sibley, & Fuseler, 1994; Kronfol, Nair, Hill, Kroll, Brower, & Grenden, 1993; Szabo, 1999; Watson et al., 1994). For instance, chronic moderate use of alcohol suppresses monocytes, macrophages, and lymphocytes, including T-cell responses, and these declines in immune response are not entirely due to malnutrition or other medical comorbidities of alcoholism (Szabo, 1999; Thiele, Szabo, Kovacs, Bautista, Sosa, & Jerrells, 2002). Moreover, Spies et al. (2004) compared postoperative infection rates in chronic alcoholics and a control group who underwent resection of aerodigestive tract tumor. Not only were cellular immune response indicators suppressed in the alcoholics, but they had a higher rate of postoperative infection than the nonalcoholic group.

In the last decade, investigators have begun characterizing the manner in which alcohol further compromises immune function in individuals with HIV. Taking into consideration the suppressive effect of alcohol upon immune response, Wang, Liang, and Watson (1997) suggest that alcohol abuse in seropositive individuals may promote a more rapid progression from asymptomatic to symptomatic illness, and eventually to AIDS. Alcohol abuse induces a synergistic effect with HIV by increasing the rate of HIV replication in the face of progressive immunodeficiency, thereby hastening declines in health status (Bagasra, Kajdacsy-Balla, Lischner, & Pomerantz, 1993). Moreover, alcohol abuse seems to compromise the endothelial cells of the vasculature, consequently increasing the permeability of the blood–brain barrier to infectious agents that potentially cause cerebral dysfunction (Witte, Borgs, Way, Ramirez, Witte, & Bernas, 1994). Bagby et al. (2003) studied the effects of sustained alcohol intoxication on rhesus macaques which were infected with simian immunodeficiency virus (SIV), a model of HIV in non-human primates. The authors administered moderate daily doses of alcohol to macaques for three months, after which the macaques were infected with SIV. Compared to a control group, alcohol-consuming macaques sustained a 60-times higher viral load, and immune response was diminished within two weeks of seroconversion. Two months later, the between-group differences presenting immune function had resolved and the groups were comparable in terms of viral load and immune response.

In a compelling review of the literature, Dingle and Oei (1997) examined whether disease progression in HIV may be moderated by alcohol use. They found that alcohol use may hasten seroconversion and disease progression to AIDS in animals. Surprisingly, similar findings have not been observed in humans. For example, Kaslow et al. (1989) and Penkower et al. (1995) found no evidence that HIV disease progression is accelerated as a result of alcohol misuse. Dingle and Oei recognize that there are reasons to expect a synergistic relationship between HIV and alcohol misuse; however, because few studies have been published on the topic, future investigation will be required to clarify this issue.

Overall, a compelling body of evidence indicates that neuropsychological function is compromised secondary to heavy alcohol misuse. There are at least initial indications (e.g. Dingle & Oei, 1997; Green et al., 2004; Rothlind et al., 2005) that such abuse may interact in a manner that increases the risk for demonstrating neuropsychological impairment. At present, this literature provides only tentative implications and few conclusive assertions, and additional research will be necessary to clarify matters.

Marijuana

Cerebral morphology and function

Similar to opiates, the principal psychoactive ingredient of marijuana (delta-9 tetrahydrocannabinol: THC) has receptors throughout the brain (Iversen, 2003). Marijuana abuse also seems to act as an antagonist for acetylcholine (Hartman, 1995), with some research showing acute inhibition of hippocampal acetylcholine release in response to THC administration. THC is also an antagonist for dopamine, with this effect being most apparent in the medial prefrontal cortex (Jentsch, Dazzi, Chatwal, Verrico, & Roth, 1998).

Functional imaging methods have also been used to study brain function among marijuana users. Effects of marijuana vary as a function of use. During intoxication, brain activation increases diffusely (Mathew, Wilson, Turkington, & Coleman, 1998; Mathew et al., 2002; O'Leary et al., 2000, 2002, 2003), especially in the frontal lobes and right hemisphere (Mathew & Wilson, 1993; Mathew et al., 1992, 1997). In contrast to intoxication, marijuana users show hypoactivation during periods of abstinence (Amen & Waugh, 1998; Lundqvist, Jonsson, & Warkentin, 2001; Tunving, Thulin, Risberg, & Warkentin, 1986). Regarding structural imaging, to our knowledge, there is only one study that has found any abnormalities. Specifically, cortical atrophy was demonstrated in a sample of chronic abusers who were selected for inclusion in the study in part because they demonstrated neurological symptoms (Campbell, Evans, Thomson, & Williams, 1971). However, this finding has apparently not been replicated (cf. Hannerz & Hindmarsh, 1983). Indeed, a recent study by Block et al. (2000) used magnetic resonance imaging to assess brain volumes in 18 chronic marijuana users and 13 control subjects. Across a wide variety of regions, no differences between groups were detected.

Neuropsychological function

To our knowledge, there is at least one investigation which has investigated whether marijuana abuse interacts with HIV serostatus to exacerbate neurobehavioral abnormalities. In a study by Cristiani, Pukay-Martin, and Bornstein (2004), 282 homosexual men were administered a broad battery of neuropsychological tests. Individuals who used marijuana less than once per month over the year preceding study participation comprised a no/minimal marijuana use group, and those who used at least once weekly comprised the frequent marijuana use group. Groups were also classified according to HIV status, with participants being categorized as seronegative, seropositive-asymptomatic, and seropositive-symptomatic. After controlling for depression, anxiety, and alcohol use in the groups, effects of HIV status and marijuana use upon neuropsychological performance were examined. Main effects of HIV status were observed on nearly all measures, including those assessing intellect, executive function, working memory, new learning, speed of information processing, and motor speed. Specifically seropositive-symptomatic participants performed worse than the control group. Additionally, main effects of marijuana use were observed, with participants who frequently used marijuana performing worse than nonusers on measures of new learning and auditory working memory. Notably, HIV status interacted with marijuana use on a global index of impaired neuropsychological test scores. Essentially, marijuana use corresponded with increasing impairment across the three HIV groups, with the seropositive-symptomatic group performing significantly worse than the asymptomatic or seronegative groups.

Among those who did not use marijuana, worsening disease status did not yield a meaningful increase in neuropsychological impairment. Thus, marijuana use appeared to increase the likelihood that HIV infection would exert a negative effect upon mental status.

Immune function

An emerging literature suggests that marijuana use is associated with diminished immune function. Klein and colleagues have demonstrated that marijuana abuse modulates T and B lymphocytes and cytokine response, and it decreases natural killer cell activity (Klein, Friedman, & Specter, 1998; Klein, Newton, & Friedman, 1987). Other researchers have found similar outcomes, and have hypothesized that marijuana may diminish immunity to infection (Pacifici et al., 2003; Pillai, Nair, & Watson, 1991; Srivastava, Srivastava, & Brouhard, 1998). Inasmuch as this is true, the risk of becoming symptomatic or converting to AIDS will increase in an HIV-seropositive individual who uses marijuana.

Overall, there is little research examining the effects of marijuana misuse and HIV on neuropsychological function. Studies reviewed elsewhere in this volume have shown that marijuana abuse corresponds with abnormalities on functional imaging studies and measures of neuropsychological ability. In at least one study (Cristiani et al., 2004), marijuana use exacerbated the presence of neuropsychological impairment among seropositive individuals. Additionally, immune function deteriorates as a function of marijuana misuse, though most evidence suggests that these abnormalities are associated primarily with chronic heavy abuse, and there are few indications that they remain after sustained abstinence. Nonetheless, because marijuana dependence is associated with neuropsychological impairment and immunosuppression, marijuana may increase the likelihood that HIV-infected individuals will show neuropsychological impairment. Further studies are needed to address this interaction.

Amphetamine

Cerebral morphology and function

Amphetamine and methamphetamine act upon dopamine and norepinephrine, causing leakage of these neurotransmitters from presynaptic terminals, enhancing their release during action potentials, and blocking their reuptake from the synaptic cleft (Feldman & Quenzer, 1984; Nordahl, Salo, & Leamon, 2003). These drugs can also deplete the amount of norepinephrine and dopamine in the brain via direct toxicity to cell bodies (cf. Sekine et al., 2003; Villemagne et al., 1998). Perhaps associated with dopamine depletion, investigations using functional imaging methods demonstrate that amphetamine and methamphetamine abusers display abnormal patterns of activation

(Iyo, Namba, Yanagisawa, Hirai, Yui, & Fukui, 1997; Kao, Wang, & Yeh, 1994). However, the precise nature of these changes in brain function appears to vary across studies. Among drug-naïve humans who are acutely intoxicated with amphetamine, generalized cerebral hypoactivation has been reported (Kahn, Prohovnik, Lucas, & Sackeim, 1989). In contrast, other research has demonstrated selective decreases in temporal lobe activation and increased activation in the frontal lobes, cerebellum, cingulate, caudate, and thalamus (Ernst et al., 1997; Vollenweider, Maguire, Leenders, Mathys & Angst, 1998). These anomalies also occur in abstinent users (Iyo et al., 1997; Wang et al., 2004). These functional abnormalities notwithstanding, there is little evidence that chronic amphetamine or methamphetamine abuse yields structural abnormalities.

Neuropsychological function

HIV status may interact with methamphetamine use to influence neuropsychological function. Rippeth et al. (2004) administered a battery of neuropsychological tests to individuals who varied according to HIV serostatus and history of methamphetamine use. Nearly 60% of the patients who were HIV seropositive and methamphetamine dependent were impaired, whereas only 20% of the control group (HIV seronegative and nonmethamphetamine dependent) displayed impairment. Among individuals who were HIV seropositive/nonmethamphetamine dependent and those who were HIV seronegative/methamphetamine dependent, approximately 40% were impaired. As such, there seems to be a synergistic influence of HIV seropositivity and methamphetamine use on neuropsychological function. More recently, Cherner et al. (2005) examined the effects of HIV, methamphetamine dependence, and hepatitis C infection in a sample of 430 participants, 222 of whom were seropositive. Due to the distribution of these three factors among the participants, interaction effects of these characteristics could not be assessed directly. However, their individual and combined effects upon neuropsychological function were examined. Similar to prior research, each of these risk factors independently predicted cognitive impairment. However, as participants had greater numbers of these risk factors, neurobehavioral impairment worsened. Together, these studies imply that methamphetamine use and HIV infection yield a synergistic effect upon neuropsychological function, but additional studies are required to confirm this suggestion.

Immune function

In the last decade, several studies have been published that examined the interactive effects of methamphetamine use and HIV on immune function. Generally, these investigations indicate that amphetamine use results in immunosuppression. For instance, in studies of rodents, acute amphetamine administration decreased T-lymphocyte response and increased flu virus replication (Basso, Gioino, Molina, & Cancela, 1999; Nunez et al., 1993). In humans, methamphetamine use diminished natural-killer cell activity (Nunez-Iglesias et al., 1996). Chronic amphetamine abuse is linked to changes in hormonal and lymphocytic activity that reflects immunosuppression (Freire-Garabal et al., 1991; Swerdlow, Hauger, Irwin, Koob, Britton, & Pulvirenti, 1991). *In vitro* application of HIV and methamphetamine resulted in neuronal cell death, with combined effects of HIV and methamphetamine yielding greater cell death than either effect alone (Turchan et al., 2001).

Overall, these findings imply that amphetamines act as an immunosuppressive agent. In the context of HIV infection, a single study revealed that methamphetamine acts synergistically with the virus to yield significant neuropsychological impairment (Rippeth et al., 2004). These initial findings are not conclusive, but they provide preliminary support for the assertion that amphetamine abuse adversely influences neurobehavioral and immune function.

Conclusions

Based on the findings of our review, we offer the following conclusions. First, the extant literature regarding the neuropsychology of HIV reveals that the disease is a risk factor for neuropsychological impairment. Additionally, the risk for impairment increases commensurately with disease progression. Moreover, the available epidemiological research revealed marked levels of drug use among individuals with HIV. As reviewed elsewhere in this volume, many of the more popular drugs of abuse exert significant neuropsychological and concomitant cerebral dysfunction. Yet, to our knowledge, no studies have examined the interactive effects of HIV and commonly abused drugs such as marijuana, MDMA, or amphetamine. Furthermore, few studies have examined the interactive effects of HIV and other drugs such as cocaine, methamphetamine, opiates, or alcohol. Among these studies, there are at least tentative indications that abuse of some drugs (e.g., alcohol, methamphetamine) exacerbates neurocognitive impairment in HIV.

Regarding immune function, a growing consensus suggests that immune status is compromised as a function of the chronicity of substance misuse. Whether substance use results in durable immunocompromise following cessation of use is less clear, though a number of studies suggest that resumption of substance use may precipitate deterioration in immune function. Such immunocompromise may contribute to diminished neurobehavioral status in HIV through direct effects of infection upon brain function or through co-factors (i.e., opportunistic infections with central nervous system involvement); however, to our knowledge, this topic has not been studied systematically.

In considering this literature, a salient limitation should be acknowledged. In particular, despite the best efforts of researchers, it is difficult to identify individuals who have misused a single substance. Although many studies have attempted to equate groups of drug abusers according to number of other substances abused, this bias is difficult to eradicate. This shortcoming notwithstanding, the findings summarized herein may provide a sufficient basis for future inference.

Consistent with the existing literature, we hypothesize that symptomatic HIV-seropositive individuals will have worse cognitive deficits than seropositive asymptomatics and seronegatives. Moreover, current drug abusers are inclined to display worse neurobehavioral dysfunction than drug-naïve individuals. Considering the combined effects of HIV and substance abuse, neurobehavioral dysfunction is expected to be most prominent in symptomatic individuals who are current substance abusers. In contrast, cognitive deficits may be least apparent in people who are seronegative and drug naïve. Neuropsychological dysfunction associated with HIV and drug use will likely be most pronounced on measures of motor speed, speed of information processing, attention, memory, working memory, and executive function.

As we have acknowledged, few studies have fully addressed this hypothesis. Some research has examined only the main effects of serostatus in substance misusers (Concha et al., 1992; Del Pesce et al., 1993; Kovner et al., 1992; Wellman, 1992), but they have not examined the combined effects of opiates and HIV status. Thus, these investigations provide neither confirmatory nor disconfirmatory evidence. Some studies have examined the interactive effects of HIV status and drug misuse (e.g., Durvasula et al., 2000; Green et al., 2004; Rippeth et al., 2004), and their results have varied. Nevertheless, these studies have failed to elaborate the full range of HIV disease progression or recency of substance misuse. Specifically, they did not examine the effects of progression to AIDS or current substance misuse. Some research (Basso & Bornstein 2000a) indicates that people with AIDS-defining illness are likely to manifest neuropsychological impairment, even more so than seropositive-symptomatic individuals. As a result, it may be that this particular subgroup of individuals will be most likely to be affected by the interaction of substance misuse and HIV infection. Moreover, individuals who are current substance misusers may be more likely to show neuropsychological impairment. It may be that salient vulnerabilities associated with current substance misuse and HIV infection may only be manifest in people who have progressed to AIDS, yet there is little research which addresses this issue.

Basso and Bornstein (2003) attempted to determine whether HIV stage interacted with drug use history to affect neurobehavioral status. We examined performance of symptomatic, asymptomatic, and seronegative individuals who were either past drug abusers or drug naïve on a broad battery of neuropsychological tests. The nature of abuse was varied, with most participants abusing marijuana, cocaine, and/or alcohol. Consistent with expectations, symptomatic individuals were impaired relative to asymptomatic and seronegative groups, and these effects were most pronounced on measures of working memory and executive function. Yet, there were no effects of drug abuse history on performance. This may not be entirely surprising, as past research concerning these drugs suggests that impairment, albeit present, tends to improve with abstinence. Participants with a history of drug abuse had not consumed them for at least six months prior to neuropsychological assessment, and it may be that the effects of substance abuse had largely remitted. Consistent with this assertion, we conducted follow-up analyses, and included a sample of individuals who had recently abused drugs. The sample size was relatively small, and recency of drug use varied. Essentially, we examined individuals who had used drugs within six months of testing, and their drugs of abuse were similar to the original sample. With the inclusion of recent drug users, we found an interaction of HIV and drug use history. In particular, the seropositive-symptomatic subjects who were recent drug abusers tended to have the worst performance of all. Although these findings are consistent with expectations, they are preliminary and await replication with larger samples and better classification of recent drug use.

In addition to the above predictions, it seems likely that the moderating effects of substance abuse will vary according to drug type and chronicity of use. For instance, there is moderate support for the assertion that cocaine, alcohol, and methamphetamine misuse results in cognitive difficulties and changes in cerebral function and morphology, whereas there is less conclusive evidence concerning opiates and marijuana. Furthermore, based upon prior findings, polysubstance abusers tend to have worse impairment than those who abuse a single substance (e.g., Bondi, Drake, & Grant, 1998). As such, seropositive individuals who abuse multiple substances may be at increased risk of cognitive impairment than their drug-naïve counterparts. Moreover, longer chronicity of substance abuse and greater drug consumption are also associated with cognitive impairment. Hence, with longer histories of more severe abuse (cf. Ardila, Rosselli, & Strumwasser, 1991), seropositive individuals will be at increasing risk of neuropsychological deficits.

Elaborating upon these predictions, it seems likely that substances with dopaminergic effects may be potent mediators of neurobehavioral deficit in HIV infection (see Nath et al., 2000). Nath and colleagues (Berger & Nath, 1997; Mirsattari, Power, & Nath, 1998; Nath, Jankovic, & Pettigrew, 1987) have documented that HIV has a particular affinity for dopaminergic neurons in the basal ganglia. As these cells are damaged, symptoms of motor impairment tend to appear. Insofar as cocaine and amphetamine damage these neurons (cf. Hartman, 1995), their abuse may potentiate the severity of psychomotor symptoms associated with HIV. Other substances which have a less deleterious effect upon dopaminergic neurons (e.g., heroin, marijuana) may have a lower likelihood of exacerbating these symptoms.

Besides mediating the severity of impairment, substance abuse may also hasten the onset of neurobehavioral deficits in HIV infection. Most of the substances summarized in this review tend to either decrease immune response or increase HIV replication. Furthermore, there are indications that drug use in seropositive individuals diminishes adherence to antiretroviral therapies (cf. Hinkin et al., 2004; Levine et al., 2005). Notably, some data imply that strict adherence to treatment is required to suppress HIV replication (Paterson et al., 2000). As a consequence, substance abuse may yield an earlier onset of symptomatic illness in infected individuals. As infected individuals become symptomatic, their risk of developing neuropsychological deficit increases (cf. Heaton et al., 1995). Thus, seropositive individuals who abuse drugs may sustain an earlier onset of neurobehavioral impairment than those who abstain from such abuse.

Owing to the high prevalence of substance abuse among HIV-infected individuals, it is notable that so little research has examined the neurobehavioral consequences of substance abuse and HIV. This is especially so when considering the potentially great implications that comorbid substance abuse and HIV infection may have for treatment management, adaptive function, and ultimate morbidity. It is hoped that the inferences provided in this review will serve as an impetus for future research.

References

Adams, K. M., Gilman, S., Koeppe, R. A., Kluin, K. J., Brunberg, J. A., Dede, D., et al. (1993). Neuropsychological deficits are correlated with frontal hypometabolism in positron emission tomography studies of older alcoholic patients. *Alcoholism, Clinical and Experimental Research, 17,* 205–210.

Amen, D. G., & Waugh, M. (1998). High resolution brain SPECT imaging of marijuana smokers with AD/HD. *Journal of Psychoactive Drugs, 30,* 209–214.

Ardila, A., Rosselli, M., & Strumwasser, S. (1991). Neuropsychological deficits in chronic cocaine abusers. *International Journal of Neuroscience, 57,* 73–79.

Arora, P. K., Fride, E., Petitto, J., Waggie, K., & Skolnick, P. (1990). Morphine-induced immune alterations in vivo. *Cell Immunology, 126,* 343–353.

Avila, A. H., Alonzo, N. C., & Bayer, B. M. (2004). Immune cell activity during the initial stages of withdrawal from chronic exposure to cocaine or morphine. *Journal of Neuroimmunology, 147,* 109–113.

Avila, A. H., Morgan, C. A., & Bayer, B. M. (2003). Stress-induced suppression of the immune system after withdrawal from chronic cocaine. *Journal of Pharmacology and Experimental Therapeutics, 305,* 290–297.

Bagasra, O., Kajdacsy-Balla, A., Lischner, H. W., & Pomerantz, R. J. (1993). Alcohol intake increases human immunodeficiency virus type 1 replication in human peripheral blood mononuclear cells. *Journal of Infections Diseases, 167,* 789–797.

Bagby, G. J., Stoltz, D. A., Zhang, P., Kolls, J. K., Brown, J., Bohm, R. P., et al. (2003). The effect of chronic binge ethanol consumption on the primary stage of SIV infection in rhesus macaques. *Alcoholism, Clinical and Experimental Research, 27,* 495–502.

Baldwin, G. C., Roth, M. D., & Tashkin, D. P. (1998). Acute and chronic effects of cocaine on the immune system and the possible link to AIDS. *Journal of Neuroimmunology, 83,* 133–138.

Bartzokis, G., Goldstein, I. B., Hance, D. B., Beckson, M., Shapiro, D., Lu, P. H., et al. (1999). The incidence of T2-weighted MR imaging signal abnormalities in the brain of cocaine-dependent patients is age-related and region-specific. *American Journal of Neuroradiology, 20,* 1628–1635.

Basso, A. M., Gioino, G., Molina, V. A., & Cancela, L. M. (1999). Chronic amphetamine facilitates immunosuppression in response to a novel aversive stimulus: reversal by haloperidol pretreatment. *Pharmacology, Biochemistry and Behavior, 62,* 307–314.

Basso, M. R., & Bornstein, R. A. (2000a). Effects of immunosuppression and disease severity upon neuropsychological function in HIV infection. *Journal of Clinical and Experimental Neuropsychology, 22,* 104–114.

Basso, M. R., & Bornstein, R. A. (2000b). Estimated premorbid intelligence mediates neurobehavioral change in individuals infected with HIV across 12-months. *Journal of Clinical and Experimental Neuropsychology, 22,* 208–218.

Basso, M. R., & Bornstein, R. A. (2003). Effects of past noninjection drug abuse upon executive function and working memory in HIV infection. *Journal of Clinical and Experimental Neuropsychology, 25,* 893–903.

Berger, J. R., & Nath, A. (1997). HIV dementia and the basal ganglia. *Intervirology, 40,* 122–131.

Block, R. I., O'Leary, D. S., Ehrhardt, J. C., Augustinack, J. C., Ghoneim, M. M., Arndt, S., et al. (2000). Effects of frequent marijuana use on brain tissue volume and composition. *Neuroreport, 11,* 491–496.

Bolla, K. I., Cadet, J. L., & London, E. D. (1998). The neuropsychiatry of chronic cocaine abuse. *Journal of Neuropsychiatry and Clinical Neurosciences, 10,* 280–289.

Bondi, M. W., Drake, A. I., & Grant, I. (1998). Verbal learning and memory in alcohol abusers and polysubstance abusers with concurrent alcohol abuse. *Journal of the International Neuropsychological Society, 4,* 319–328.

Bornstein, R. A., Nasrallah, H. A., Para, M. F., Fass, R. J., Whitacre, C. C., & Rice, R. R. (1991). Rate of CD4 decline and neuropsychological performance in HIV infection. *Archives of Neurology, 48,* 704–707.

Bornstein, R. A., Nasrallah, H. A., Para, M. F., Whitacre, C. C., & Fass, R. J. (1994). Duration of illness and neuropsychological performance in asymptomatic HIV infection. *Journal of Neuropsychology and Clinical Neurosciences, 6,* 160–164.

Bornstein, R. A., Nasrallah, H. A., Para, M. F., Whitacre, C. C., Rosenberger, P., & Fass, R. J. (1993). Neuropsychological performance in symptomatic and asymptomatic HIV infection. *AIDS, 7,* 519–524.

Browndyke, J. N., Tucker, K. A., Woods, S. P., Beauvals, J., Cohen, R. A., Gottschalk, P. C., et al. (2004). Examining the effect of cerebral perfusion abnormality magnitude on cognitive performance in recently abstinent chronic cocaine abusers. *Journal of Neuroimaging, 14,* 162–169.

Campbell, A. M., Evans, M., Thomson, J. L., & Williams, M. J. (1971). Cerebral atrophy in young cannabis smokers. *Lancet, 2,* 1219–1224.

Chang, L., Ernst, T., Witt, M. D., Ames, N., Gaiefsky, M., & Miller, E. (2002). Relationships among brain metabolites, cognitive function, and viral loads in antiretroviral-naive HIV patients. *Neuroimage, 17,* 1638–1648.

Cherner, M., Letendre, S., Heaton, R. K., Durelle, J., Marquie-Beck, J., Gragg, B., et al. (2005). Hepatitis C augments cognitive deficits associated with HIV infection and methamphetamine. *Neurology, 64,* 1343–1347.

Collier, A. C., Marra, C., Coombs, R. W., Claypoole, K., Cohen, W., Longstreth, W. T., et al. (1992). Central nervous system manifestations in human immunodeficiency virus infection without AIDS. *Journal of Acquired Immune Deficiency Syndrome, 5,* 229–241.

Concha, M., Graham, N. M., Munoz, A., Vlahov, D., Royal, W. III, Updike, M., et al.

(1992). Effect of chronic substance abuse on the neuropsychological performance of intravenous drug users with a high prevalence of HIV-1 seropositivity. *American Journal of Epidemiology, 136,* 1338–1348.

Concha, M., Selnes, O. A., Vlahov, D., Nance-Sproson, T., Updike, M., Royal, W., et al. (1997). Comparison of neuropsychological performance between AIDS-free injecting drug users and homosexual men. *Neuroepidemiology, 16,* 78–85.

Cook, R. T. (1998). Alcohol abuse, alcoholism, and damage to the immune system – a review. *Alcoholism, Clinical and Experimental Research, 22,* 1927–1942.

Cristiani, S. A., Pukay-Martin, N. D., & Bornstein, R. A. (2004). Marijuana use and cognitive function in HIV-infected people. *Journal of Neuropsychiatry and Clinical Neurosciences, 16,* 330–335.

Danos, P., Kasper, S., Grunwald, F., Klemm, E., Krappel, C., Broich, K., et al. (1998). Pathological regional cerebral blood flow in opiate-dependent patients during withdrawal: a HMPAO-SPECT study. *Neuropsychobiology, 37,* 194–199.

De Castro, S., & Sabate, E. (2003). Adherence to heroin dependence therapies and human immunodeficiency virus/acquired immunodeficiency syndrome infection rates among drug abusers. *Clinical and Infectious Disease, 37,* S464–S467.

Del Pesce, M., Franciolini, B., Censori, B., Bartolini, M., Ancarani, F., Petrelli, E., et al. (1993). Cognitive behavior in asymptomatic (CDC stage II and III) HIV–seropositive intravenous drug users (IVDUs). *Italian Journal of Neurological Science, 14,* 619–625.

Delafuente, J. C., & DeVane, C. L. (1991). Immunologic effects of cocaine and related alkaloids. *Immunopharmacology and Immunotoxicology, 13,* 11–23.

Di Franco, M. J., Marlink, R., Hunter, D. J., Tosteson, T., Mayer, K., & Essex, M. (1993). Association of immune activation with intravenous heroin use and methadone treatment in HIV-1 seropositive and seronegative subjects. *Journal of Acquired Immune Deficiency Syndrome, 6,* 1297–1300.

Dingle, G. A., & Oei, T. P. (1997). Is alcohol a cofactor of HIV and AIDS?: Evidence from immunological and behavioral studies. *Psychological Bulletin, 122,* 56–71.

Durvasula, R. S., Myers, H. F., Satz, P., Miller, E. N., Morgenstern, H., Richardson, M. A., et al. (2000). HIV-1, cocaine, and neuropsychological performance in African American men. *Journal of the International Neuropsychological Society, 6,* 322–335.

Ernst, M., Zametkin, A. J., Matochik, J., Schmidt, M., Jons, P. H., Liebenauer, L. L., et al. (1997). Intravenous dextroamphetamine and brain glucose metabolism. *Neuropsychopharmacology, 17,* 391–401.

Feldman, R. S., & Quenzer, L. F. (1984). *Fundamentals of neuropsychopharmacology.* Sunderland, MA: Sinauer Associates.

Francis, H. (2003). Substance abuse and HIV infection. *Topics in HIV Medicine, 11,* 20–24.

Franken, I. H., Stam, C. J., Hendriks, V. M., & van den Brink, W. (2004). Electroencephalographic power and coherence analyses suggest altered brain function in abstinent male heroin-dependent patients. *Neuropsychobiology, 49,* 105–110.

Franklin, T. R., Acton, P. D., Maldjian, J. A., Gray, J. D., Croft, J. R., Dackis, C. A., et al. (2002). Decreased gray matter concentration in the insular, orbitofrontal, cingulate, and temporal cortices of cocaine patients. *Biological Psychiatry, 51,* 134–142.

Freier, D. O., & Fuchs, B. A. (1994). A mechanism of action for morphine-induced immunosuppression: corticosterone mediates morphine-induced suppression of natural killer cell activity. *Journal of Pharmacology and Experimental Therapeutics, 270,* 1127–1133.

Freire-Garabal, M., Balboa, J. L., Nunez, M. J., Castano, M. T., Llovo, J. B., Fernandez-Rial, J. C., et al. (1991). Effects of amphetamine on T-cell immune response in mice. *Life Sciences, 49,* 107–112.

Friedman, H., Newton, C., & Klein, T. W. (2003). Microbial infections, immunomodulation, and drugs of abuse. *Clinical Microbiology Review, 16,* 209–219.

Govitrapong, P., Suttitum, T., Kotchabhakdi, N., & Uneklabh, T. (1998). Alterations of immune functions in heroin addicts and heroin withdrawal subjects. *Journal of Pharmacology and Experimental Therapeutics, 286,* 883–889.

Grant, I., Atkinson, J. H., Hesselink, J. R., Kennedy, C. J., Richman, D. D., Spector, S. A., et al. (1987). Evidence for early central nervous system involvement in the acquired immunodeficiency syndrome (AIDS) and other human immunodeficiency virus (HIV) infections. *Annals of Internal Medicine, 107,* 828–836.

Grant, I., & Heaton, R. K. (1990). Human immunodeficiency virus-type 1 (HIV-1) and the brain. *Journal of Consulting and Clinical Psychology, 58,* 22–30.

Green, J. E., Saveanu, R. V., & Bornstein, R. A. (2004). The effect of previous alcohol abuse on cognitive function in HIV Infection. *American Journal of Psychiatry, 161,* 249–254.

Hannerz, J., & Hindmarsh, T. (1983). Neurological and neuroradiological examination of chronic cannabis smokers. *Annals of Neurology, 13,* 207–210.

Hartman, D. E. (1995). *Neuropsychological toxicology* (2nd ed.). New York: Plenum.

Heaton, R. K., Grant, I., Butters, N., White, D. A., Kirson, D., Atkinson, J. H., et al. (1995). The HNRC 500 – neuropsychology of HIV infection at different disease stages. *Journal of the International Neuropsychological Society, 1,* 231–251.

Hinkin, C. H., Hardy, D. J., Mason, K. I., Castellon, S. A., Durvasula, R. S., Lan, M. N. et al. (2004). Medication adherence in HIV-infected adults: effect of patient age, cognitive status, and substance abuse. *AIDS, 18,* S19–S25.

Iversen, L. (2003). Cannabis and the brain. *Brain, 126,* 1252–1270.

Iyo, M., Namba, H., Yanagisawa, M., Hirai, S., Yui, N., & Fukui, S. (1997). *Progress in Neuropsychopharmacology and Biological Psychiatry, 21,* 789–796.

Jacobsen, L. K., Giedd, J. N., Kreek, M. J., Gottschalk, C., & Kosten, T. R. (2001). Quantitative medial temporal lobe brain morphology and hypothalamic-pituitary-adrenal axis function in cocaine dependence: a preliminary report. *Drug and Alcohol Dependence, 62,* 49–56.

Jentsch, J. D., Dazzi, L., Chatwal, J. P., Verrico, C. D., & Roth, R. H. (1998). Reduced prefrontal cortical dopamine, but not acetylcholine, release in vivo after repeated, intermittent phencyclidine administration to rats. *Neuroscience Letters, 258,* 175–178.

Jernigan, T. L., Butters, N., DiTraglia, G., Schafer, K., Smith, T., Irwin, M., et al. (1991). Reduced cerebral grey matter observed in alcoholics using magnetic resonance imaging. *Alcoholism, Clinical and Experimental Research, 15,* 418–427.

Jerrells, T. R., Slukvin, I., Sibley, D., & Fuseler, J. (1994). Increased susceptibility of experimental animals to infectious organisms as a consequence of ethanol consumption. *Alcohol and Alcoholism Supplement, 2,* 425–430.

Kahn, D. A., Prohovnik, I., Lucas, L. R., & Sackeim, H. A. (1989). Dissociated effects of amphetamine on arousal and cortical blood flow in humans. *Biological Psychiatry, 25,* 755–767.

Kao, C. H., Wang, S. J., & Yeh, S. H. (1994). Presentation of regional cerebral blood flow in amphetamine abusers by 99Tcm-HMPAO brain SPECT. *Nuclear Medicine Communication, 15*, 94–98.

Karlix, J. L., Behnke, M., Davis-Eyler, F., Wobie, K., Adams, V., Freiburger, B., et al. (1998). Cocaine suppresses fetal immune system. *Pediatric Research, 44*, 43–46.

Kaslow, R. A., Blackwelder, W. C., Ostrow, D. G., Yerg, D., Palenicek, J., Coulson, A. H., et al. (1989). No Evidence for a Role of Alcohol or Other Psychoactive Drugs in Accelerating Immunodeficiency in HIV-1-Positive Individuals. *Journal of the American Medical Association, 261*, 3424–3430.

Klein, T. W., Friedman, H., & Specter, S. (1998). Marijuana, immunity and infection. *Journal of Neuroimmunology, 83*, 102–115.

Klein, T. W., Newton, C., & Friedman, H. (1987). Inhibition of natural killer cell function by marijuana components. *Journal of Toxicology and Environmental Health, 20*, 321–332.

Kovner, R., Lazar, J. W., Lesser, M., Perecman, E., Kaplan, M. H., Hainline, B., et al. (1992). Use of the Dementia Rating Scale as a test for neuropsychological dysfunction in HIV-positive i.v. drug abusers. *Journal of Substance Abuse and Treatment, 9*, 133–137.

Kronfol, Z., Nair, M., Hill, E., Kroll, P., Brower, K., & Grenden, J. (1993). Immune function in alcoholism: a controlled study. *Alcoholism, Clinical and Experimental Research, 17*, 279–283.

Krystal, J. H., Woods, S. W., Kosten, T. R., Rosen, M. I., Seibyl, J. P., van Dyck, C. C., et al. (1995). Opiate dependence and withdrawal: preliminary assessment using single photon emission computerized tomography (SPECT). *American Journal of Drug and Alcohol Abuse, 21*, 47–63.

Kure, K., Lyman, W. D., Weidenheim, W. M., & Dickson, D. W. (1990). Cellular localization of an HIV-1 antigen in subacute AIDS encephalitis using an improved double labeling immunohistochemical method. *American Journal of Pathology, 136*, 1085–1092.

Levin, H. S., Williams, D. H., Borucki, M. J., Hillman, G. K., Williams, J. B., Guinto, F. C., Jr, et al. (1990). Magnetic resonance imaging and neuropsychological findings in human immunodeficiency virus infection. *Journal of Acquired Immune Deficiency Syndrome, 3*, 757–762.

Levine, A. J., Hinkin, C. H., Castellon, S. A., Mason, K. I., Lam, M. N., Perkins, A., et al. (2005). Variations in patterns of highly active antiretroviral therapy (HAART) adherence. *AIDS and Behavior, 9*, 355–362.

Lucas, G. M., Gebo, K. A., Chaisson, R. E., & Moore, R. D. (2002). Longitudinal assessment of the effects of drug and alcohol abuse on HIV-1 treatment outcomes in an urban clinic. *AIDS, 16*, 767–774.

Lucas, G. M., Weidle, P. J., Hader, S., & Moore, R. D. (2004). Directly administered antiretroviral therapy in an urban methadone maintenance clinic: A nonrandomized comparative study. *Clinical and Infectious Disease, 38*, S409–S413.

Lundqvist, T., Jonsson, S., & Warkentin, S. (2001). Frontal lobe dysfunction in long-term cannabis users. *Neurotoxicology and Teratology, 23*, 437–443.

Lyman, W. D., Kress, Y., Kure, K., Rashbaum, W. K., Rubinstein, A., & Soeiro, R. (1990). Detection of HIV in fetal central nervous system tissue. *AIDS, 4*, 917–920.

Marder, K., Liu, X., Stern, Y., Malouf, R., Dooneief, G., Bell, K., et al. (1995). Risk of human immunodeficiency virus type 1-related neurologic disease in a cohort of intravenous drug users. *Archives of Neurology, 52*, 1174–1182.

Martin, E. M., Robertson, L. C., Sorensen, D. J., Jagust, W. J., Mallon, K. F., & Chirurgi, V. A. (1993). Speed of memory scanning is not affected in early HIV-1 infection. *Journal of Clinical and Experimental Neuropsychology, 15*, 311–320.

Mathew, R. J., & Wilson, W. H. (1991). Substance abuse and cerebral blood flow. *American Journal of Psychiatry, 148*, 292–305.

Mathew, R. J., & Wilson, W. H. (1993). Acute changes in cerebral blood flow after smoking marijuana. *Life Sciences, 52*, 757–767.

Mathew, R. J., Wilson, W. H., Coleman, R. E., Turkington, T. G., & DeGrado, T. R. (1997). Marijuana intoxication and brain activation in marijuana smokers. *Life Sciences, 60*, 2075–2089.

Mathew, R. J., Wilson, W. H., Humphreys, D. F., Lowe, J. V., & Wiethe, K. E. (1992). Regional cerebral blood flow after marijuana smoking. *Journal of Cerebral Blood Flow and Metabolism, 12*, 750–758.

Mathew, R. J., Wilson, W. H., Turkington, T. G., & Coleman, R. E. (1998). Cerebellar activity and disturbed time sense after THC. *Brain Research, 797*, 183–189.

Mathew, R. J., Wilson, W. H., Turkington, T. G., Hawk, T. C., Coleman, R. E., DeGrando, T. R., et al. (2002). Time course of tetrahydrocannabinol-induced changes in regional cerebral blood flow measured with positron emission tomography. *Psychiatry Research, 116*, 173–185.

McArthur, J. C. (1994). Neurological and neuropathological manifestations of HIV infection. In I. Grant and A. Martin (Eds.) *Neuropsychology of HIV infection* (pp. 56–107). New York: Oxford.

McArthur, J. C., Kumar, A. J., Johnson, D. W., Selnes, O. A., Becker, J. T., Herman, C., et al. (1990). Incidental white matter hyperintensities on magnetic resonance imaging in HIV-1 infection. Multicenter AIDS Cohort Study. *Journal of Acquired Immune Deficiency Syndrome, 3*, 252–259.

McArthur, J. C., McClernon, D. R., Cronin, M. F., Nance-Sproson, T. E., Saah, A. J., St. Clair, M., et al. (1997). Relationship between human immunodeficiency virus-associated dementia and viral load in cerebrospinal fluid and brain. *Annals of Neurology, 42*, 689–698.

Meyerhoff, D. J., MacKay, S., Sappey-Marinier, D., Deicken, R., Calabrese, G., Dillon, W. P., et al. (1995). Effects of chronic alcohol abuse and HIV infection on brain phosphorus metabolites. *Alcoholism, Clinical and Experimental Research, 19*, 685–692.

Mintzer, M. Z., & Stitzer, M. L. (2002). Cognitive impairment in methadone maintenance patients. *Drug and Alcohol Dependence, 67*, 41–51.

Mirsattari, S. M., Power, C., & Nath, A. (1998). Parkinsonism with HIV infection. *Movement Disorders, 13*, 684–689.

Nath, A., Anderson, C., Jones, M., Maragos, W., Booze, R., Mactutus, C., et al. (2000). Neurotoxicity and dysfunction of dopaminergic systems associated with AIDS dementia. *Journal of Psychopharmacology, 14*, 222–227.

Nath, A., Jankovic, J., & Pettigrew, L. C. (1987). Movement disorders and AIDS. *Neurology, 37*, 37–41.

Navia, B., Jordan, B., & Price, R. (1986). The AIDS dementia complex: I. Clinical Features. *Annals of Neurology, 19*, 517–524.

Nordahl, T. E., Salo, R., & Leamon, M. (2003). Neuropsychological effects of chronic methamphetamine use on neurotransmitters and cognition: a review. *Journal of Neuropsychiatry and Clinical Neurosciences, 15*, 317–325.

Nottet, H. S., Persidsky, Y., Sasseville, V. G., Nukuna, A. N., Bock, P., Zhai, Q. H., et al. (1996). Mechanisms for the transendothelial migration of HIV-1-infected monocytes into brain. *Journal of Immunology, 156,* 1284–1295.

Nunez, M. J., Fernandez-Rial, J. C., Couceiro, J., Suarez, J. A., Gomez-Fernandez, D. E., Rey-Mendez, M., et al. (1993). Effects of amphetamine on influenza virus infection in mice. *Life Sciences, 52,* 73–78.

Nunez-Iglesias, M. J., Castro-Bolano, C., Losada, C., Pereiro-Raposo, M. D., Riveiro, P., Sanchez-Sebio, P., et al. (1996). Effects of amphetamine on cell mediated immune response in mice. *Life Sciences, 58,* 29–33.

O'Leary, D. S., Block, R. I., Flam, M., Schultz, S. K., Boles Ponto, L. L. Watkins, G. L., et al. (2000). Acute marijuana effects on rCBF and cognition: a PET study. *Neuroreport, 11,* 3835–3841.

O'Leary, D. S., Block, R. I., Koeppel, J. A., Flam, M., Schultz, S. K., Andreasen, N. C., et al. (2002). Effects of smoking marijuana on brain perfusion and cognition. *Neuropsychopharmacology, 26,* 802–816.

O'Leary, D. S., Block, R. I., Turner, B. M., Koeppel, J., Magnotta, V. A., Ponto, L. B., et al. (2003). Marijuiana alters the human cerebellar clock. *Neuroreport, 14,* 1145–1151.

O'Neill, J., Cardenas, V. A., & Meyerhoff, D. J. (2001). Separate and interactive effects of cocaine and alcohol dependence on brain structures and metabolites: quantitative MRI and proton MR spectroscopic imaging. *Addiction Biology, 6,* 347–361.

Pacifici, R., Zuccaro, P., Pichini, S., Roset, P. N., Poudevida, S., Farré, M., et al. (2003). Modulation of the immune system in cannabis users. *Journal of the American Medical Association, 289,* 1929–1931.

Paterson, D. L., Swindells, S., Mohr, J., Brester, M., Vergis, R., Squier, C., et al. (2000). Adherence to protease inhibitors, HIV-1 viral load, and development of drug resistance in an indigent population. *AIDS, 14,* 357–366.

Pearlson, G. D., Jeffery, P. J., Harris, G. J., Ross, C. A., Fischman, M. W., & Camargo, E. E. (1993). Correlation of acute cocaine-induced changes in local cerebral blood flow with subjective effects. *American Journal of Psychiatry, 150,* 495–497.

Penkower, L., Dew, M. A., Kingsley, L., Zhou, S. Y., Lyketsos, C. G., Wesch, J., et al. (1995). Alcohol consumption as a cofactor in the progression of HIV infection and AIDS. *Alcohol, 12,* 547–552.

Peterson, P. K., Gekker, G., Chao, C. C., Schut, R., Molitor, T. W., & Balfour, H. H. Jr (1991). Cocaine potentiates HIV-1 replication in human peripheral blood mononuclear cell cocultures. Involvement of transforming growth factor-beta. *Journal of Immunology, 146,* 81–84.

Petry, N. M. (1999). Alcohol use in HIV patients: what we don't know may hurt us. *International Journal of STD AIDS, 10,* 561–570.

Pezawas, L. M., Fischer, G., Diamant, K., Schneider, C., Schindler, S. D., Thurnher, M., et al. (1998). Cerebral CT findings in male opioid-dependent patients: stereological, planimetric and linear measurements. *Psychiatry Research, 83,* 139–147.

Pezawas, L. M., Fischer, G., Podreka, I., Schindler, S., Brucke, T., Jagsch, R., et al. (2002). Opioid addiction changes cerebral blood flow symmetry. *Neuropsychobiology, 45,* 67–73.

Pillai, R., Nair, B. S., & Watson, R. R. (1991). AIDS, drugs of abuse and the immune system: a complex immunotoxicological network. *Archives of Toxicology, 65,* 609–617.

Reger, M., Welsh, R., Razani, J., Martin, D. J., & Boone, K. B. (2002). A meta-analysis of the neuropsychological sequelae of HIV infection. *Journal of the International Neuropsychological Society, 8,* 410–424.

Rippeth, J. D., Heaton, R. K., Carey, C. L., Marcotte, T. D., Moore, D. J., Gonzalez, R., et al. (2004). *Journal of the International Neuropsychological Society, 10,* 1–14.

Rose, J. S., Branchey, M., Buydens-Branchey, L., Stapleton, J. M., Chasten, K., Werrell, A., et al. (1996). Cerebral perfusion in early and late opiate withdrawal: a technetium-99m-HMPAO SPECT study. *Psychiatry Research, 67,* 39–47.

Rosenberger, P. H., Bornstein, R. A., Nasrallah, H. A., Para, M. F., Whitaker, C. C., Fass, R. J., et al. (1993). Psychopathology in human immunodeficiency virus infection: lifetime and current assessment. *Comparative Psychiatry, 34,* 150–158.

Rothlind, J. C., Greenfield, T. M., Bruce, A. V., Meyerhoff, D. J., Flenniken, D. L., Lindgren, J. A., et al. (2005). Heavy alcohol consumption in individuals with HIV infection: Effects on neuropsychological performance. *Journal of the International Neuropsychological Society, 11,* 70–83.

Rouveix, B. (1992). Opiates and immune function. Consequences on infectious diseases with special reference to AIDS. *Therapie, 47,* 503–512.

Roy, A., Berman, J., Williams, R., Kuhn, C., & Gonzalez, B. (2002). Higher levels of CSF homovanillic acid in recently abstinent cocaine-dependent patients. *American Journal of Psychiatry, 159,* 1053–1055.

Schweitzer, C., Keller, F., Schmitt, M. P., Jaeck, D., Adloff, M., Schmitt, C., et al. (1991). Morphine stimulates HIV replication in primary cultures of human Kupffer cells. *Research in Virology, 142,* 189–195.

Sekine, Y., Minabe, Y., Ouchi, Y., Takei, N., Iyo, M., Nakamura, K., et al. (2003). Association of Dopamine Transporter Loss in the Orbitofrontal and Dorsolateral Prefrontal Cortices With Methamphetamine-Related Psychiatric Symptoms. *American Journal of Psychiatry, 160,* 1699–1703.

Selnes, O. A., Galai, N., McArthur, J. C., Cohn, S., Royal, W., Esposito, D., et al. (1997). HIV infection and cognition in intravenous drug users: Long-term follow-up. *Neurology, 48,* 223–230.

Spies, C. D., von Dossow, V., Eggers, V., Jetschmann, G., El-Hilali, R., Egert, J., et al. (2004). Altered cell-mediated immunity and increased postoperative infection rate in long-term alcoholic patients. *Anesthesiology, 100,* 1088–1100.

Srivastava, M. D., Srivastava, B. I., & Brouhard, B. (1998). Delta-9 tetrahydrocannabinol and cannabidiol alter cytokine production by human immune cells. *Immunopharmacology, 40,* 179–185.

Strickland, T. L., Mena, I., Villanueva-Meyer, J., Miller, B., Cummings, J., Mehringer, C. M., et al. (1993). Cerebral perfusion and neuropsychological consequences of chronic cocaine use. *Journal of Neuropsychology and Clinical Neurosciences, 5,* 419–427.

Sullivan, E. V. (2003). Compromised pontocerebellar and cerebellothalamocortical systems: speculations on their contributions to cognitive and motor impairment in nonamnesic alcoholism. *Alcoholism, Clinical and Experimental Research, 27,* 1409–1419.

Swerdlow, N. R., Hauger, R., Irwin, M., Koob, G. F., Britton, K. T., & Pulvirenti, L. (1991). Endocrine, immune, and neurochemical changes in rats during withdrawal from chronic amphetamine intoxication. *Neuropsychopharmacology, 5,* 23–31.

Szabo, G. (1999). Consequences of alcohol consumption on host defense. *Alcohol and Alcoholism, 34,* 830–841.

Thiele, G. M., Szabo, G., Kovacs, E. J., Bautista, A. P., Sosa, L., & Jerrells, T. R. (2002). Modulation of immunity and viral-host interactions by alcohol. *Alcoholism, Clinical and Experimental Research, 26*, 1897–1908.

Tonnesen, H., Kaiser, A. H., Nielsen, B. B., & Pedersen, A. E. (1992). Reversibility of alcohol-induced immune depression. *British Journal of Addiction, 87*, 1025–1028.

Tunving, K., Thulin, S. O., Risberg, J., & Warkentin, S. (1986). Regional cerebral blood flow in long-term heavy cannabis use. *Psychiatry Research, 17*, 15–21.

Turchan, J., Anderson, C., Hauser, K. F., Sun, Q., Zhang, J., Liu, Y., et al. (2001). Estrogen protects against the synergistic toxicity by HIV proteins, methamphetamine and cocaine. *BMC Neuroscience, 2*, 3.

Van Gorp, W. G., Satz, P., Hinkin, C., Selnes, O., Miller, E. N., McArthur, J., et al. (1991). Metacognition in HIV-1 seropositive asymptomatic individuals: Self-ratings versus objective neuropsychological performance. *Journal of Clinical and Experimental Neuropsychology, 13*, 812–819.

Villemagne, V., Yuan, J., Wong, D. F., Dannals, R. F., Hatzidimitriou, G., Mathews, W. B., et al. (1998). Brain dopamine neurotoxicity in baboons treated with doses of methamphetamine comparable to those recreationally abused by humans: evidence from [11C]WIN-35,428 positron emission tomography studies and direct in vitro determinations. *Journal of Neuroscience, 18*, 419–427.

Volkow, N. D., Mullani, N., Gould, K. L., Adler, S., & Krajewski, K. (1988). Cerebral blood flow in chronic cocaine users: A study with positron emission tomography. *British Journal of Psychiatry, 152*, 641–648.

Volkow, N. D., Wang, G. J., Hitzemann, R., Fowler, J. S., Overall, J. E., Burr, G., et al. (1994). Recovery of brain glucose metabolism in detoxified alcoholics. *American Journal of Psychiatry, 151*, 178–183.

Vollenweider, F. X., Maguire, R. P., Leenders, K. L., Mathys, K., & Angst, J. (1998). Effects of high amphetamine dose on mood and cerebral glucose metabolism in normal volunteers using positron emission tomography (PET). *Psychiatry Research, 83*, 149–162.

Wang, G. Y., Liang, B., & Watson, R. R. (1997). Alcohol consumption alters cytokine release during murine AIDS. *Alcohol, 14*, 155–159.

Wang, G. Y., Volkow, N. D., Chang, L., Miller, E., Sedler, M., Hitzemann, R., et al. (2004). Partial recovery of brain metabolism in methamphetamine abusers after protracted abstinence. *American Journal of Psychiatry, 161*, 242–248.

Watson, R. R., Borgs, P., Witte, M., McCuskey, R. S., Lantz, C., Johnson, M. I., et al. (1994). Alcohol, immunomodulation, and disease. *Alcohol and Alcoholism, 29*, 131–139.

Webber, M. P., Schoenbaum, E. E., Gourevitch, M. N., Buono, D., & Klein, R. S. (1999). A prospective study of HIV disease progression in female and male drug users. *AIDS, 13*, 257–262.

Wellman, M. C. (1992). Neuropsychological impairment among intravenous drug users in pre-AIDS stages of HIV infection. *International Journal of Neuroscience, 64*, 183–194.

Wiley, C. A., Belman, A. L., Dickson, D. W., Rubinstein, A., & Nelson, J. A. (1990). Human immunodeficiency virus within the brains of children with AIDS. *Clinical Immunopathology, 9*, 1–6.

Wilkinson, D. A. (1987). Discussion: CT scan and neuropsychological assessments of alcoholism. In O. A. Parsons, N. Butters, & P. E. Nathan (Eds.) *Neuropsychology of alcoholism: Implications for diagnosis and treatment* (pp. 76–102). New York: Guilford Press.

Witte, M. H., Borgs, P., Way, D. L., Ramirez, G. Jr, Witte, C. L., & Bernas, M. J. (1994). AIDS, alcohol, endothelium, and immunity. *Alcohol, 11*, 91–97.

Zhang, L., Looney, D., Taub, D., Chang, S. L., Way, D., Witte, M. H., et al. (1998). Cocaine opens the blood-brain barrier to HIV-1 invasion. *Journal of Neurovirology, 4*, 619–626.

12 The neurocognitive consequences of substance use in schizophrenia: Are there additive effects?

Kari Tervo

The substantial co-occurrence of substance use disorders and schizophrenia is a source of great concern amongst researchers of psychopathology. Epidemiological studies reveal a high prevalence rate regarding the co-occurrence of the two disorders. One investigation found that approximately 65% of individuals with schizophrenia have a co-occurring substance use disorder (Mueser, Yarnold, Levinson, & Singh, 1990), and the Epidemiological Catchment Area study (Regier et al., 1990) concluded that alcohol and drug use disorders are three and six times more likely, respectively, to occur in individuals with schizophrenia than in the general population.

The findings from these epidemiological studies justify concern about the possible consequences of substance use disorders in individuals with schizophrenia. For example, studies have shown that the combination of these disorders is associated with higher rates of homelessness (Drake, Osher, & Wallach, 1991) and unemployment (Soyka, Albus, Kathmann, & Finelli, 1993). Moreover, a review of the literature (Negrete, 2003) concluded that co-occurrence is associated with more severe symptoms and poorer treatment response. In addition, it appears that the combination of substance use and cognitive impairment may have an additive effect; substance use disorders and impairments in nonverbal concept formation are both associated with longer hospitalizations (Jackson, Fein, Essock, & Mueser, 2001).

It is noteworthy, however, that among individuals with schizophrenia, a co-occurring substance use disorder does not uniformly translate into a poorer outcome. Other studies have shown that substance abuse in schizophrenia is unrelated to symptom presentation and level of functioning (Kovasznay, Bromet, Schwartz, & Ram, 1993). That is, substance abuse was not a predictor of age of onset of psychotic symptoms, severity of positive symptoms, or social and occupational functioning. In addition, males with a history of substance abuse in that study had fewer negative symptoms than those who had never abused substances. However, substance-abusing patients in this study had more symptoms of depression and anxiety. Thus, while substance abuse in patients with co-occuring schizophrenia did not have a worse outcome with regard to psychotic symptoms, they did have a higher incidence of other clinical symptoms. Adding to this diversity in outcome is evidence that substance abuse in remission in those with psychiatric disorders is associated with better instrumental role functioning (i.e., effectiveness in performance as a worker, student, etc.) than in those with psychiatric disorders who never abused substances (Carey, Carey, & Simons, 2003). Furthermore, it is unclear that estimates of prevalence are veridical representations of the true state of nature; for example, Blanchard, Brown, Horan, and Sherwood (2000) note that methodological issues such as ascertaining samples from places which are more likely to house the most severely pathological individuals (e.g. treatment facilities, prisons) can result in overestimates of co-occurrence. Moreover, studies may have varying definitions of what constitutes the syndrome of schizophrenia. Hambrecht and Häfner (2000) contend that many studies define the onset of schizophrenia as the onset of psychotic symptoms, whereas the onset of the disorder may actually be more insidious and could be indicated by other symptoms, such as flat affect or anhedonia. Operationally defining the onset of schizophrenia by the appearance of psychotic symptoms could capture a group that had already progressed into a more severe form of the disorder.

Given that a co-occurring substance use disorder is not a definitive risk factor for poorer outcomes among individuals with schizophrenia, it is important to explore which characteristics might account for this variability in outcome. This chapter provides an evaluation of the extant research to determine whether substance abuse is a risk factor for increased neurocognitive impairment for individuals diagnosed with schizophrenia. Because each disorder has been identified as a risk factor for neurocognitive deficits (as was detailed in earlier chapters regarding substance use disorders, and will be discussed below with regard to schizophrenia), it is plausible that a neurocognitive profile of the combination of the two might emerge. An understanding of this profile can be used as a guidepost for further investigation and treatment efforts.

First, however, in order to understand the scope of the problem, it is necessary to discuss theoretical models that attempt to answer the question of why these disorders co-occur. Then, a background on the neurocognitive profiles associated with schizophrenia will be given (refer to earlier chapters for discussion of neurocognitive impairments and substance use). After this, comparative investigations on the neurocognitive testing results of individuals with schizophrenia and those with both disorders will be reviewed. Finally, treatment will be given to scientific and treatment considerations elicited by these data and others.

Why do substance use and schizophrenia co-occur?

Various research groups have generated models in order to explain the vexing problem of why substance use disorders are over-represented in the population of individuals with schizophrenia. The most thorough compendia of these models have been presented by Tracy, Josiassen, and Bellack (1995) and

Blanchard and colleagues (2000). Although several of these models will be touched upon here, the reader is referred to these papers for a more extensive treatment. To date, these models remain largely theoretical and have not been empirically validated; however, they provide a springboard for future research, and are compelling in their consideration of a variety of factors that may contribute to the co-occurrence of schizophrenia and substance use disorders.

First, there is a possibility that the two disorders have a shared neurobiological substrate (Tracy et al., 1995). This model proposes that substance use and schizophrenia arise from a single biological anomaly (or a cluster of anomalies) that potentiates the appearance of both disorders. Perhaps genetic factors, playing a role both in schizophrenia (Gottesman & Shields, 1972) and substance abuse (Kendler, 1995), could lead to the appearance of the disorders. It could be, however, that certain individuals share separate genetic risk factors for both disorders (Kendler, 1985).

Another model proposes that substance abuse leads to schizophrenia. Certain drugs of abuse, such as cocaine and methamphetamine, can produce a transient psychosis; is it possible that the use of such substances can potentiate schizophrenia and all its attendant psychotic symptoms? Administration of Δ-9-tetrahydrocannabinol, one of the active components of cannabis, has been shown to induce psychotomimetic effects in individuals without a psychiatric diagnosis (D'Souza et al., 2004). It is hypothesized that the binding of this substance to cannabinoid receptors increases dopamine production in the mesolimbic system and hippocampus. This may serve as the primary mechanism of substance-induced psychosis in otherwise healthy individuals (D'Souza et al., 2004), as hyper-dopaminergic activity is often presented as one of the causes of psychotic symptoms in schizophrenia patients.

Despite accounts of tolerance to marijuana with frequent use, prolonged exposure to the drug in animals has been shown to have a sensitizing effect (e.g., Rubino, Vigano, Massi, & Parolaro, 2001). Given that positive symptom presentation in schizophrenia may have a neurotoxic effect (e.g., Smythies, 1997), preexisting neurological vulnerabilities to psychosis could be exacerbated by the potential psychosis-kindling effects of chronic marijuana use. Stimulants such as cocaine (Izenwasser, 2004) and methamphetamine (Shi, Pun, & Zhu, 2004) also increase dopamine activity. Thus, the same mechanisms may also be responsible for the potential schizophrenia-inducing effects of those drugs. The same mechanisms of psychosis-induction in healthy individuals, coupled with the neurotoxic effects of schizophrenia-related psychosis, could serve as support for the contention that substances of abuse can cause schizophrenia.

This theory is compelling; however, most empirical investigations of the hypothesis that drug use leads to schizophrenia have failed to show a temporal connection between substance use and the onset of schizophrenia (Blanchard et al., 2000). As an example, Hambrecht and Häfner (2000) found that while chronic marijuana use is correlated with the onset of schizophrenia, the temporal relationship between substance abuse and schizophrenia can take different forms, depending on the characteristics of the individual (i.e., substance use can occur either before or after schizophrenia onset). Furthermore, calcyon, a protein with a possible role in the dopamine-mediated reward-producing effects in the ventral tegmental area, does not have a gene-related association with either schizophrenia or substance abuse (Luo et al., 2004). This points to the possibility that enduring hyper-dopaminergic activity is a consequence, not a cause, of drug-induced and schizophrenia-related psychosis.

Recently, one study (Bühler, Hambrecht, Löffler, van der Heiden, & Häfner, 2002) found that substance abuse onset and schizophrenia onset occurred within the same month; however, there was no temporal association between abuse onset and the first psychotic episode. At five-year follow-up, substance-abusing patients demonstrated more positive symptoms than did patients who did not abuse drugs; however, based on this finding, it is not reasonable to assert that substance abuse leads to psychosis. For example, a third variable could contribute to both, or the premorbid characteristics of schizophrenia, such as anhedonia, could contribute to substance use (Blanchard et al., 2000). Simply demonstrating that substance use precedes schizophrenia onset is not sufficient to prove that the substance use was causal; a variety of factors could contribute to both disorders' appearance.

A third theory is that schizophrenia leads to substance abuse; this is called the self-medication hypothesis (Blanchard et al., 2000) and the theory proposes that schizophrenia patients use substances to counteract symptoms such as anhedonia, poor social functioning, and the side effects produced by neuroleptics. In particular, it has been proposed that these side effects potentiate response to drugs such as cocaine; however, this theory has not been empirically validated (Blanchard et al., 2000). Although Serper, Alpert, Richardson, and Dickson (1995) found that abstinent cocaine users had showed a decrease in negative symptoms compared to current cocaine users at a one-month follow-up, with no group differences in symptoms at that time, their contention that users intentionally used the substance to ameliorate symptoms cannot be supported by the data, according to Blanchard et al. (2000). That is, it is possible that the cocaine-abusing patients simply had fewer negative symptoms to begin with, independent of use (Blanchard et al., 2000).

Furthermore, the self-medication hypothesis is not consistent with the fact that drugs of abuse can induce dopaminergic activity consistent with the presentation of psychotic symptoms. Given that symptoms such as paranoia can lead to social withdrawal, drug use could potentiate the same effects that the self-medication hypothesis proposes that drugs reduce (e.g., Potvin, Stip, & Roy, 2003). In addition, although the self-medication theory is partially informed by patients' reports that they use drugs to increase pleasure and reduce depression, they also report that drug use can increase depression, as well as exacerbate positive symptoms (Addington & Duchak, 1997). This paradoxical finding indicates that patient report of reasons for drug use may not be reliable.

Instead, Blanchard and colleagues (2000) propose that dispositional individual difference factors interact with a diminished capacity to respond to disorder-related and environmental stressors, which results in the use of substances. For example, trait negative affectivity and disinhibition/impulsivity are theorized to contribute to the response to internal (mood-related) and external (e.g., social) stressors pursuant to and exacerbated by deficits in social and problem-solving skills. This model has yet to be empirically supported, although it is certainly testable. In addition, it does not take into account neuropsychological factors that may interact with personality and skills deficits. Later, after neuropsychological findings related to substance abuse and schizophrenia are covered, this theory will be extended to include neurocognitive variables.

A final theory of the co-occurrence of substance abuse and schizophrenia integrates the vulnerability–stress–coping model of the onset of mental illness (Zubin & Spring, 1977) with data from substance-abusing schizophrenia patients. The vulnerability–stress–coping model posits that those who possess the diathesis for mental illness have varying capacities for dealing with stress. Once an individual's stress threshold is reached, he or she may develop a mental illness. The latency to threshold and the propensity to develop an illness, however, are moderated by an individual's personal coping mechanisms (Zubin & Spring, 1977). In terms of the association between schizophrenia and substance use, Hambrecht and Häfner (2000) found that in some individuals schizophrenia onset may be precipitated by years of drug use that may reduce a vulnerability threshold. Other individuals experience the onset of substance abuse and schizophrenia concurrently; in this case, acute substance use poses a dopaminergic stress factor which invites psychosis. As predicted by earlier theories, some patients begin substance abuse after the appearance of psychosis; in this case, the individuals may be trying to cope with their symptoms.

In sum, competing theories of schizophrenia and substance use co-occurrence propose different directions of causality – that schizophrenia causes substance abuse, and vice versa. Elaborations of these theories posit that individual difference factors, such as negative affect, may account for co-occurrence (Blanchard et al., 2000), while others hold that different factors can be held accountable for the variance in temporal relationships between substance use onset and schizophrenia onset (e.g., lowering of vulnerability threshold, acute stressors; Hambrecht & Häfner, 2000).

The neurocognitive profile of schizophrenia

Schizophrenia is associated with a wide range of neurological abnormalities. These abnormalities and deficits are pervasive, appearing in multiple brain regions and influencing performance on neurocognitive tasks. Postmortem studies of schizophrenia patients have revealed subtle cellular anomalies, an imbalance in afferent neuron connections, cortical degeneration, and neuronal loss (Goldman-Rakic, 1996). Positron emission tomography studies revealed diminished blood flow in the frontal (e.g., Andreasen, Rezai, & Alliger, 1992, Tamminga, Thaker, & Buchanan, 1992) and left temporal regions (e.g., Cannon, 1996).

These structural and metabolic abnormalities have been linked to symptom presentation. For example, working memory dysfunction has been shown to be a mediator of psychotic thinking subsequent to negative family interactions (Rosenfarb, Neuchterlein, Goldstein, & Subotnik, 2000). Although some investigators have attempted to localize neurocognitive dysfunction in schizophrenia, the pattern of deficits appears to be generalized, encompassing domains as distinct as motor, sensory, and perceptual functioning, memory (Blanchard & Neale, 1994), and executive functioning (Randolph, Gold, Carpenter, Goldberg, & Weinberger, 1993). Certain specific areas of executive functioning in which investigators have found deficits are verbal fluency (Gruzelier, Seymour, Wilson, Jolley, & Hirsch, 1988; Hoff, Riordan, O'Donnell, Morris, & Delisi, 1992) and strategic planning (Andreasen et al., 1992).

Given the heterogeneity of the syndrome of schizophrenia (i.e., variability in symptom presentation), it follows that individuals with different types of symptoms may have different neurocognitive profiles. Basso, Nasrallah, Olson, and Bornstein (1998) found that those with a negative cluster of symptoms (anhedonia, alogia, and affective flattening) tend to show deficits on measures of executive functioning, sustained attention, and sensory motor functioning. In contrast, the thought disorder and bizarre behaviors of the disorganized subtype are associated with attention span and sensory motor functioning. Surprisingly, hallucinations and delusions do not appear to be associated with a particular neurocognitive deficit.

In general, although neurocognitive deficits in schizophrenia appear to be pervasive and generalized, there is particularly strong evidence for the involvement of prefrontal deficits in schizophrenia. Similarities in the performance and characteristics of schizophrenia patients and frontal lobe-damaged patients abound (Goldman-Rakic & Selemon, 1997), and many studies point to a pathological change in the dorsolateral prefrontal region in schizophrenia (Goldman-Rakic, 1991). In fact, there is diminished metabolic activity in the dorsolateral prefrontal cortex (DLPC) in schizophrenia patients, as evidenced by functional magnetic resonance imaging (fMRI; Goldman-Rakic, 1996; Perlstein, Carter, Noll, & Cohen, 2001).

Studies of eye-tracking and executive functioning provide additional evidence suggesting the presence of hypofrontality in schizophrenia. Abnormalities in smooth pursuit eye movement (SPEM) and other measures of eye tracking, including saccadic suppression, have been found in individuals with schizophrenia, schizophrenia spectrum personality disorders, and in relatives of schizophrenic patients (Levy & Holzman, 1997). Abnormal functioning in this domain is associated with disrupted functioning and decreased metabolism in the frontal cortex (Ross, Thaker, Holcomb, Cascella, Medoff, & Tamminga, 1995), particularly the DLPC (Evdokimidis, Liakopoulous, Constantinides, & Papageorgiou, 1996), reflecting the diminished capacity of the frontal lobes to inhibit reflexive responses. With regard to executive functioning, several studies have concluded that there is no specific executive functioning deficit in schizophrenia (e.g., Goldberg, Saint-Cyr, & Weinberger, 1990; Scarone, Abbruzzesse, & Gambini, 1993) as measured by the Wisconsin Card Sorting Test (WCST). Other investigations have found the opposite pattern of results (Goldman-Rakic, 1996; Laurent et al., 2000), particularly with regard to the 'categories completed' index (Laurent et al., 2000). Examinations of working memory and attention, which will be focused on in depth here, have also pointed to dysfunction in the frontal lobes.

Attention

Given that attentional difficulties are a prominent neurocognitive deficit in schizophrenia, attention is a neurocognitive domain that has received particular focus in the literature as it relates to the disorder. Attention is a prefrontal function (Maier, Franke, Haine, Kopp, & Rist, 1992); the frontal lobes are associated with attention as the endpoint of an axis that includes the thalamus, reticular activating system (Gualtieri, 1995), and the anterior cingulate gyrus (Haznedar, Buchsbaum, Hazlett, Shihabuddin, New, & Siever, 2004). Emphasizing the connection between the frontal lobes and schizophrenia, both frontal lobe and schizophrenia patients are impaired on measures of sustained attention (Buchsbaum et al., 1990).

Myriad studies have documented the occurrence of impaired sustained attention in schizophrenia patients as compared to control participants (e.g., Braff, 1993; Cornblatt & Keilp, 1994; Mirsky, Yardley, Jones, & Walsh, 1995; Nuechterlein, 1991; Roitman et al., 1997). A low hit rate and a high rate of false alarms on various versions of the continuous performance task best characterizes the profile of the schizophrenia patients on measures of sustained attention (Michie et al., 2000). Such a deficit appears to be a stable trait marker rather than a state characteristic as it occurs independent of the expression of clinical symptoms, such as hallucinations or delusions (Cornblatt, Winters, & Erlenmeyer-Kimling, 1989; Michie et al., 2000) or the decline of other indices such as IQ (Weickert, Goldberg, Gold, Bigelow, Egan, & Weinberger, 2000). This deficit also appears independent of the chronicity or severity of symptoms (Orzack & Kornetsky, 1971). Neuroleptic treatment shows promise in ameliorating the attention deficit; a sample of neuroleptic-medicated schizophrenia patients performed equally as well as control participants in one study (Jones, Cardno, Sanders, Owen, & Williams, 2001), although these results could be related to the negative symptom profile of the sample. A meta-analysis (Nieuwenstein, Aleman, & de Haan, 2001) and an examination of patients with the deficit syndrome of schizophrenia (chararacterized by primary, chronic negative symptoms; Buchanan, Strauss, Breier, Kirkpatrick, & Carpenter, 1997) both showed that negative symptoms are associated with particularly pronounced sustained attention deficits.

Working memory

Another neurocognitive domain that has received considerable attention in the literature is working memory, which is defined as a system for temporarily maintaining and manipulating information during the performance of a range of cognitive tasks, including comprehension, learning, and reasoning (Baddeley, 1986). Considerable research has supported the idea that the working memory comprises three domains: the central executive, which is an attentional control system; the phonological loop, which holds auditory information via rehearsal; and the visuospatial sketchpad, which maintains and manipulates visuospatial images (Baddeley, 1986). These three areas provide a computational area for holding items of information 'online' as they are recalled, manipulated, and associated with ideas and incoming information (Goldman-Rakic & Selemon, 1997). Working memory is theorized to mediate performance on many neurocognitive tests if performance is dependent on information that is not immediately present in the environment at the time of response and/or if the information requires updating on a moment-to-moment basis (Goldman-Rakic, 1991), such as when registering and remembering feedback on the Wisconsin Card Sorting Test. In fact, working memory appears to mediate overall performance on this task (Gold, Carpenter, Randolph, Goldberg, & Weinberger, 1997).

Working memory appears to be mediated by the DLPC. Performance on tests sensitive to DLPC function is impaired in schizophrenia patients. For instance, deficits in verbal, visual, and spatial working memory are all correlated with volume loss in the DLPC (Goldman-Rakic & Selemon, 1997), and studies of nonhuman primates show that lesions in this area affect working memory performance on a variety of tasks, including oculomotor delayed response tasks (Goldman-Rakic, 1991). Similarly, in humans, neurocognitive (Baddeley, & Della Salla, 1998), lesion, and functional magnetic resonance imaging studies (Barch, Braver, Nystrom, Forman, Noll, & Cohen, 1997; Cohen, Perlstein, Braver, & Nystrom, 1997) have implicated the DLPC as well. In addition, positron emission tomography studies have shown that while healthy subjects demonstrate activation of the DLPC during the Wisconsin Card Sorting Test (Rezai, Andreasen, Alliger, & Cohen, 1990), frontal cerebral blood flow is reduced during the administration of the same task in schizophrenia patients (Goldberg et al., 1990).

A growing body of literature supports the hypothesis that the behavioral disruption observed in schizophrenia arises from deficits in the working memory (Goldman-Rakic, 1991). Negative symptoms are associated with working memory failures in the DLPC, and working memory dysfunction may be a fundamental deficit underlying the cognitive features of schizophrenia.

Goldman-Rakic and Selemon (1997) hold that "the disorganized thought process in schizophrenia patients that manifests itself in idiosyncratic content may be reducible to an impairment of neural mechanisms by which symbolic representations are both retrieved from the long-term memory and held in mind to guide behavior" (pp. 437–438). This assertion is supported by research that demonstrates that working memory impairments interact with interpersonal criticism to predict the emergence of psychotic thinking (Rosenfarb et al., 2000), showing that the behavior guidance properties of working memory are impaired in schizophrenia.

Given the impaired performance of schizophrenia patients on a range of working memory tasks, it is assumed that schizophrenia patients have functional and/or structural deficits in the DLPC. Working memory can be viewed as a particularly reliable endophenotypic marker; there is a significant and stable association between schizophrenia and working memory impairment independent of medication status or negative and positive symptoms, suggesting that such impairment is a trait rather than a state marker (Aleman & de Haan, 2000; Kurtz, Ragland, Bilker, Gur, & Gur, 2001).

Considerable evidence shows that individuals with schizophrenia have impaired working memory on a variety of tasks. Spatial working memory is one area in which schizophrenia patients show deficits. For example, Park and Holzman (1992) and Carter, Robertson, Nordahl, Chaderjian, Kraft, & O'Shara-Celaya (1996) determined that schizophrenia is associated with spatial working memory impairments. Another study (Park & Holzman, 1993) confirmed these results using similar methods. As with attention, however, this deficit may be partially ameliorated by neuroleptic medications. Atypical antipsychotic medications (e.g., risperidone, olanzapine) appear to improve spatial working memory to some degree after four to eight weeks of treatment (Flashman & Green, 2004; Harvey, Green, McGurk, & Meltzer, 2003).

Although deficits were found in spatial working memory, Park and Holzman (1992) did not find auditory working memory deficits in their sample. On the basis of these results, they concluded on the basis of these results that the working memory deficits of schizophrenia are domain-specific: that is, the deficits are specific to visuospatial processes rather than verbal or auditory ones. Other research has supported the view that these deficits are pervasive and not limited to one domain, however. Gold and colleagues (1997) found that schizophrenia patients exhibit impaired auditory working memory, utilizing a letter number sequencing task that required the storage, manipulation, and recall of a series of letters and numbers presented aurally. In a study examining each of the domains of working memory, Perry, Heaton, Potterat, Roebuck, Minassian, and Bratt (2001) provide more evidence that the working memory deficit in schizophrenia is pervasive: schizophrenia patients performed worse than a standardization sample on tests of auditory and visuospatial working memory. Moreover, in the schizophrenia group, performance on these measures was correlated, providing evidence for a pervasive deficit.

Language and verbal memory

Reduced activity in the DLPC is not the only area that appears to be significantly involved in the neurocognitive impairments of schizophrenia, particularly in language and verbal memory. The left temporal area, which interconnects with the DLPC (e.g., Cannon, 1996), is associated with verbal skills (e.g., Ragland et al., 2004), and schizophrenia patients exhibit abnormalities in both the left temporal area and in verbal domains.

It appears that working memory partially mediates performance on verbal learning and memory tests, but available data show that putative left temporal defects contribute to impaired performance on verbal learning and memory tests, independent of DLPC function. With regard to the establishment of abnormal functioning in the left temporal area, Lawrie and Abukmeil (1998) reviewed 40 papers that examined structural volumes in the brains of schizophrenia patients. Small percentages of volume reduction in the left temporal area were revealed by several studies, as were large increases in the lateral ventricles, which may contribute to temporal structural volume reduction. Although these reductions in left temporal volume are relatively small (i.e., 3.5%; Lawrie, Adams, Thornley, & Joy, 2000), they are consistent with small volumetric reductions found across brain regions (Lawrie et al., 2000). These changes appear to be neurodevelopmental in nature and associated with genetic transmission of the liability for schizophrenia; first- and second-degree relatives of schizophrenia patients also show temporal lobe reductions, although they are only significantly smaller in the right temporal lobe (Lawrie et al., 2002). It is important to note that while left temporal reductions are present, but not statistically significant in family members, null results may be due to greater variance in measurements in the left compared to the right lobe (Lawrie et al., 2002). Statistical significance notwithstanding, even small changes in temporal volume may affect cognition. Family members of schizophrenia patients demonstrate deficits relative to controls in verbal memory, and also exhibit subtle anomalies in verbal communication (Docherty & Gordinier, 1999). In addition, the family members included in the study were aged 16–25; this is relatively early in the high-risk stage, and further volume reductions may occur over time.

In what way are these volume reductions significant for the phenomenology of schizophrenia? Several investigations have revealed implications for symptom presentation, outcome, and neurocognitive functioning. For instance, left temporal volume reduction accounts for a portion of the variance (i.e., 27% of cumulative variance of left temporal, left hippocampal, and right ventricular volume) in poor outcome, as defined by length of hospitalization, symptom severity, employment and performance, and social contacts (Rossi, Bustini, Prosperini, Kalyvoka, Stratta, & Daneluzzo, 2000). It is important to note that these outcome indices, as measured by a single instrument, were combined into a summary score, and it is not clear what the contribution of left temporal volume is in relation to the individual indices.

Supporting these findings, however, semantic fluency, which arises from the left temporal lobe, is impaired in first-episode schizophrenia patients (Giovannetti, Goldstein, Schullery, Barr, & Bilder, 2003).

Temporal lobe abnormalities appear to be a predictor of risk for the development of the symptoms of schizophrenia. In neuroleptic-naïve first-episode patients, left temporal gray matter reduction precedes psychotic symptoms (Hietala et al., 2003), and is associated with longer duration of the episode (Hietala et al., 2003; Keshavan, Schooler, Sweeney, Haas, & Pettigrew, 1998). The contention that gray matter reduction precedes symptom presentation is further supported by data presented by Cannon and colleagues (2002), who determined that fetal hypoxia is strongly associated with temporal lobe volume reductions, and by other examinations of neuroleptic-naïve first-episode patients (Gur, Maany, Mozley, Swanson, Bilker, & Gur, 1998).

Despite evidence that temporal lobe volume reductions are associated with poor outcome (e.g., employment and social contacts; Rossi et al., 2000) and symptom presentation, one investigation (Gur et al., 1998) resulted in counter-intuitive findings: that is, the rate of temporal volume reduction actually predicted improvement in the occurrence of hallucinations and delusions in first-episode patients, and lower temporal volume was associated with improvement in flat affect and avolition in previously-treated patients, even when controlling for medication dose. As would be expected, these reductions were associated with less improvement in negative symptoms in the first-episode patients. It is noteworthy, however, that this study was the first to examine the association of volume change and clinical presentation, and methodological replications and/or refinements may produce results more consistent with expectations.

With regard to neurocognitive functioning, the left temporal lobe is generally associated with verbal functioning, including language fluency and verbal memory (e.g., Stone, Thermenos, Tarbox, Poldrack, & Seidman, 2005). Less temporal volume reduction is generally associated with less neuropsychological decline in several domains, including verbal functioning (Gur et al., 1998), with the exception of one surprising finding that better verbal functioning is associated with greater reduction in non-neuroleptic-naïve patients.

It appears that overactivation in this area, despite volume reductions, is associated with impairments in verbal functioning. For instance, left temporal hypermetabolism in schizophrenia patients is associated with poor verbal memory (Gur et al., 1997). More specifically, Ragland and colleagues (2004) found that overactivation of the left temporal lobe (particularly the medial region) is associated with impaired recognition. This was found in concert with evidence of underactivation of the DLPC. In contrast, while another study (Hofer et al., 2003) found intact verbal recognition in patients, verbal encoding appeared to be associated with less activation of the left lateral temporal area. A complementary study showed that relative overactivation, as compared to control participants, is observed during tasks of verbal fluency, whereas control participants display activation in the prefrontal cortex during these tasks (Yurgelun-Todd, Waternaux, Cohen, Gruber, English, & Renshaw, 1996).

Taken together, schizophrenia is associated with a wide range of metabolic, structural, and cognitive abnormalities. All appear to be associated, in some fashion, with symptom presentation and outcome. Establishment of the neurocognitive profile of schizophrenia and that of substance use will serve as a background for the primary goal of this chapter: to discern if there is a worse cognitive profile in schizophrenia patients with a co-occurring substance use disorder than in individuals with only one of the disorders.

Studies comparing dually diagnosed and nonsubstance-using schizophrenia patients

It has now been established that schizophrenia and substance use are both associated with a range of neurocognitive deficits. To briefly review, schizophrenia is associated with myriad cognitive impairments, which appear to arise largely from metabolic and structural abnormalities in the DLPC and left temporal lobe. Affected domains include sustained attention, working memory, verbal functioning, and executive functioning. As reviewed in prior chapters, substance use disorders are also associated with a variety of cognitive impairments, most strikingly in the domains of memory and executive functioning.

Given these findings, the question remains as to whether the combination of substance use and schizophrenia leads to further deleterious neurocognitive consequences. Are there additive effects? There is a paucity of research examining the issue of possible additive neurocognitive effects of substance use in schizophrenia. To date, fewer than twenty studies have been performed which have directly compared schizophrenia patients with and without a co-occurring substance use disorder. This section will consider each of those studies in order to contribute to the surprising conclusion that substance use largely does not appear to produce additional neurocognitive deficits above and beyond those found in schizophrenia.

With regard to theoretical expectations for these studies, Tracy and colleagues (1995) propose two models: the exacerbation model, which assumes that dually diagnosed patients will evince a neurocognitive profile similar to nonabusing patients but of a worse magnitude, and the interactive model, which proposes that the dually diagnosed will exhibit a neurocognitive profile that is unique to their cohort. In that these studies examined domains in which schizophrenia patients show extensively documented deficits and not other areas, they fall under the rubric of the exacerbation model. In the sections below, investigations that met with positive results will be considered first, and then investigations which concluded that substance abuse does not exacerbate the neurocognitive deficits of schizophrenia will be discussed.

Evidence for exacerbation of neurocognitive impairment in dual diagnosis

Several studies have determined that there is an incremental effect of substance use on neurocognitive functioning over and above that observed in schizophrenia alone. Each of these studies examined a group of patients who used only cocaine (Serper, Bergman, Copersino, Chou, Richarme, & Cancro, 2000a; Serper, Copersino, Richarme, Vadhan, Cancro, 2000b; Sevy, Kay, Opler, & Van Praag, 1990) or alcohol (Nazzaro, 1996). As emphasized in the discussion of methodological considerations in a later section, capturing a group that was homogenous with regard to substance of choice is a methodological strength that may have contributed to positive results.

In one study (Sevy et al., 1990), schizophrenia patients and patients with a history of cocaine dependence were evaluated on a variety of memory indices, including immediate and delayed recall, recognition, and effectiveness in conceptual encoding. Individuals with a history of cocaine use displayed impairments on indices of verbal memory, semantic encoding, and recall; surprisingly, these same patients performed better than did patients without a history of cocaine use on measures of attention. Although some patients did have a history of the use of other illicit substances, none were using them at the time of their study participation. The prior use of these other substances did not appear to have an effect on cognition; memory deficits were specific to cocaine use. That these patients were abstinent from cocaine may underscore the potentially enduring effects of the drug on the brain, particularly because when cocaine history was statistically controlled, other drugs of abuse appeared to have no effect on cognition.

Consistent with the above results, a study (Serper et al., 2000a) that compared current cocaine users and schizophrenia patients with or without a diagnosis of cocaine dependence found that cocaine-using schizophrenia patients performed worse than did cocaine users or nonusing patients on measures of verbal encoding, delayed recall, and recognition; in contrast, these patients did not show a deficit in semantic organization, as the patients with a history of cocaine use evidenced (Sevy et al., 1990). Performance of cocaine users and nonusing patients did not differ on any measure. On a more extensive battery (Serper et al., 2000b), schizophrenia patients who were recently abstinent from cocaine use showed a significant impairment in the retention of a list of words over a long delay, but did not differ from nonusing patients on measures of working memory and resistance to interference, sustained attention, or indices of executive functioning. Given that these patients were abstinent from cocaine at the time of testing, it may seem that these results align with those of Sevy and colleagues (1990), who found that cocaine-abstinent patients had enduring cognitive deficits beyond those of nonusing patients. However, these patients were only recently abstinent (i.e., within days of study participation), so it is unclear whether the effects of recent cocaine use could have contributed to these results.

The final study that supports Tracy et al.'s (1995) exacerbation model is an unpublished dissertation investigation performed by Nazzaro (1996), which also focused on a homogenous substance-using group: alcohol-dependent patients. Nazzaro hypothesized that those in the co-occurring group would have more severe neurocognitive deficits than those in the nonusing group, and that these differences would be less pronounced as time spent abstinent accumulated. These hypotheses were supported in one domain: individuals with schizophrenia and alcohol dependence performed more poorly than did schizophrenia patients on measures of visual memory. Executive function, attention, and verbal memory did not differ between the groups. Given this significant result, Nazzaro's hypothesis that increased abstinence would result in improvement of deficits was borne out: impairment improved with increased sobriety. These results are interesting and somewhat difficult to interpret in light of the other evidence presented here due to the fact that alcohol has a different deficit profile than do the other drugs of abuse (Tracy et al., 1995). Perhaps alcohol is unique in conferring acute neurocognitive deficit exacerbations in visual memory, although it is unclear why visual memory would show pronounced deficits while verbal memory is spared, given that chronic alcohol abuse can result in global memory deficits (i.e., in Korsakoff's syndrome).

Although these studies support the hypothesis that there is an exacerbation of neurocognitive deficits related to substance use, only four of the studies discussed in this paper that examined this issue met with positive results. The next section will review studies that found no additive effect.

Evidence to the contrary: There is no additive effect

The preponderance of evidence suggests that substance use does not contribute to a more impaired neurocognitive profile in schizophrenia patients. Even when patient groups are examined on the basis of the existence of cognitive impairment versus no cognitive impairments, rates of substance abuse do not differ between the impaired and nonimpaired groups in any of a multitude of cognitive domains (Holthausen et al., 2002). Indeed, some substance-abusing patients appear to perform better than their nonusing counterparts on some measures; although schizophrenia patients who abused marijuana had difficulty on a measure of resistance to interference, their performance exceeded that of nonusers on measures of verbal and visual memory. This section expands on these findings and summarizes studies which have determined that there is no exacerbation of the neurocognitive deficits of schizophrenia when there is co-occurring substance use.

Although it was not a direct focus of their study, Cleghorn, Kaplan, Szechtman, Szechtman, and Brown (1990) examined a subset of 38 schizophrenia patients who reported prior substance abuse, some of whom were being treated with neuroleptics. They performed as well as did controls on measures of motor functioning, planning, and memory. These patients were not compared with nonsubstance-abusing patients. These results are odd because schizophrenia patients generally perform worse than controls even if they do not have a prior history of substance use. One would expect that the addition of a substance use history would lead to significant results. However, one interesting feature did emerge from this study: patients with and without a history of substance use who were being treated with neuroleptics performed worse on the above measures than did controls and patients who were not on a neuroleptic regimen. Overall, it does not appear that substance use contributed to neurocognitive deficits in this study.

Cleghorn, Kaplan, Szechtman, Szechtman, Brown, and Franco (1991) performed the first study with a focus on examining the issue of neurocognitive profiles of dually diagnosed and nondually diagnosed schizophrenia patients. They examined medicated and nonmedicated first-episode schizophrenia patients with a 17-measure neurocognitive battery examining domains such as full-scale IQ, executive functioning, and psychomotor speed. In both the medicated and unmedicated groups, there were no significant differences between substance users and nonusers on any of the measures. It is important to note, however, that these were first-episode patients. It is possible that some patients were experiencing a relatively acute psychotic disorder (e.g., a brief psychotic episode) and not schizophrenia *per se*; this could contribute to negative results. This conjecture is supported by an investigation (Fitzgerald et al., 2004) which concluded that those with substance-induced first-episode psychosis evinced better neurocognitive performance in a comprehensive neurocognitive battery than did first-episode patients whose psychosis was related to schizophrenia (according to DSM-IV diagnostic criteria); thus, replication of this study with only patients who have a confirmed diagnosis of schizophrenia is warranted.

Symptom presentation was also examined in this study. Substance-using patients had significantly more positive symptoms than did nonusers. While the neurocognitive results in this study were negative, this finding has important implications for treatment. Whatever the etiological relation between substance use and an excess of positive symptoms, these data have value in describing the characteristics of substance-using schizophrenia patients, leading to a conclusion that positive symptoms may need to be addressed more aggressively in this group.

A 1996 investigation by Nixon, Hallford, and Tivis found similar results, albeit with a less extensive neurocognitive battery. They used a test of psychomotor functioning and a face-recognition task and discovered that nonsubstance using and dually diagnosed schizophrenia patients performed similarly on these measures. Notably, alcohol-dependent participants without schizophrenia did not perform significantly better than did the schizophrenia patients. Additionally, dually diagnosed patients had higher anxiety and depression scores than did nonusing patients.

Similar results were found in a study that examined social functioning, quality of life, and neurocognitive functioning in dually-diagnosed and nonabusing schizophrenia patients (Addington & Addington, 1997). As Nixon and colleagues (1996) discovered, substance use can have a deleterious effect in functional domains, defined in this study as overall quality of life (e.g., educational and occupational functioning, social support). However, substance-abusing participants performed just as well as nonabusing patients on measures of verbal fluency, attention, executive functioning, and different domains of memory. Pencer and Addington (2003) also found no association between cognitive functioning and substance use (in first-episode psychosis patients), although, like in the studies above, substance use was associated with functional factors (i.e., an increase in positive symptoms). This pattern of results contributes to a treatment heuristic: namely, that dually diagnosed patients would benefit from treatment of symptoms beyond typical schizophrenia symptoms, and that substance-using patients should not require different treatment strategies with regard to their neurocognitive functioning (i.e., more concrete instructions) from their nonusing counterparts.

In a similar study, an unpublished dissertation by Snyder (1998) examined archival neurocognitive battery data from a population of inpatients. The battery included measures of attention, memory, executive function, and visuospatial abilities. No significant differences were found on any of these measures. Of course, using archival data comes with its limitations. For example, standardized procedures might not have been used to confer a substance use or schizophrenia diagnosis, which could result in a misclassification of study participants. This is especially true in an inpatient unit in which chart review and site-specific brief interviews may be used to confer diagnoses, rather than a structured, standardized interview. Still, these results contribute to a pattern which reveals a lack of neurocognitive exacerbation in dually diagnosed patients.

Cooper, Liberman, Tucker, Nuechterlein, Tsuang, and Barnett (1999) employed strict sampling procedures and included only cocaine-using individuals. All participants were assessed on an inpatient unit. In contrast to studies of cocaine-using patients cited in the above section, however, this study did not find an exacerbation of cognitive symptoms. Both at admission and 18 days following admission, nonsubstance-using and substance-using groups did not differ on any of the neurocognitive measures. This study has two main strengths in comparison to other studies in this section: by focusing on cocaine users alone, these researchers avoided the possible confound of the different neurocognitive effects of different drugs. Second, they used structured and standardized clinical assessments, possibly preventing misdiagnoses and erroneous group assignment. This approach represents an improvement over the archival strategy of Snyder (1998). With regard to why these results differ from those of the studies that examined patients with a history of cocaine use, abstinence was not an inclusion criterion for this study. Thus, the acute effects of cocaine may have contributed to the results.

Psychomotor speed and executive functioning were the focus of Smelson, Davis, Di Pano, Johnson, Losonczy, and Ziedonis (2002), who also used a narrow sampling approach in their study. Their results, however, diverged from the pattern found by previous researchers. Surprisingly, cocaine-using patients actually performed *better* on most neurocognitive tests than did nonusing schizophrenia patients. That the subjects were recently abstinent from cocaine makes the results even more unexpected; one might expect significant psychomotor slowing in patients who were "crashing." Of course, this is the intuitive interpretation. It could also be that recently abstinent cocaine users experience a rebound of cognitive clarity after a period of recovery from cocaine use. It is unclear, however, why these recently abstinent patients performed well on these tests while the similarly abstinent patients in the study by Serper and colleagues (2000b) performed worse than did nonusing schizophrenia patients.

While differences were found between groups in another sample of cocaine-dependent patients (Smelson et al., 2003), impaired performance was not evidenced in the dually diagnosed group alone. Rather, while dual diagnosis patients performed worse than did nonabusing patients on a task of fine motor coordination and on one of immediate attention, the nonabusing patients performed worse on tests of psychomotor speed. No differences were found between groups on measures of executive functioning, verbal fluency, resistance to interference, working memory, and another task of immediate attention. Thus, there did not appear to be a global cognitive impairment in dual diagnosis patients as compared to nonabusing patients. Significant differences in motor coordination may have been related to a dopamine system doubly compromised by both the pathophysiology of schizophrenia and the effects of cocaine use (Smelson et al., 2003).

Despite some differences in results among studies using only cocaine-using schizophrenia patients as a population of interest, these studies underscore the necessity of parsing out homogenous groups of substance users while investigating possible additive effects of schizophrenia and substance abuse. These were the only studies to find significant differences of any sort between the two groups, even if in the unexpected direction. Based on this, it does not seem a stretch to conclude that future studies should use homogenous groups, as heterogeneity may lead to spurious negative results. The next section considers this and other reasons why the current body of literature does not overwhelmingly support the contention that substance use exacerbates the neurocognitive deficits of schizophrenia.

What factors might be associated with this general lack of exacerbation?

A multitude of factors could be responsible for the overall surprising lack of additive neurocognitive effects in patients with co-occurring substance use and schizophrenia. This section will speculate upon several of those reasons.

First, and perhaps most parsimoniously, there could have been underreporting of substance use in the group designated as nonsubstance abusing. For example, Cleghorn and colleagues (1991) noted that they did not give drug screen tests to the participants. This would naturally lead to the appearance of a lack of additive effects because the groups were not essentially different. In future studies, this could be controlled for by the use of urinalysis, although recent abstinence may lead to negative urine test results even if the individual is a frequent user. Moreover, neurocognitive deficits associated with substance abuse are partially reversible with abstinence (Meek, Clark, Solana, 1989). More ambitious (and well-funded) investigators may consider the use of hair toxicology analysis.

Following from the concept of drug-use status confirmation, many of the studies cited above did not control for the effects of dose and frequency of use on cognitive function. This is important in determining who is most likely to demonstrate neurocognitive deficits and in interpreting null findings; if many of the users were using low doses or used infrequently, the sample heterogeneity could contribute to a lack of demonstrated deficits. At least one study has determined that cognitive effects of cocaine only emerge after prolonged use of high doses (Bolla, Rothman, & Cadet, 1999).

Second, it is a well-known observation that schizophrenia is a highly heterogeneous syndrome. One attempt to classify possible subtypes of the disorder places individuals into groups with primarily negative or primarily positive symptoms (e.g., Crow, 1982). Some researchers postulate that the negative symptom group contains a syndrome subtype known as the deficit syndrome (Carpenter, Heinrichs, & Wagman, 1988), which comprises individuals with primary and enduring negative symptoms. The deficit syndrome group has been shown in a variety of investigations to have a different neurocognitive profile than those in the nondeficit syndrome group, including poorer performance on measures of executive functioning (Bryson, Whelahan, & Bell, 2001), eye tracking (Ross et al., 1997), and attention (Buchanan & Carpenter, 1994).

None of the studies cited here differentiated between deficit and nondeficit syndrome individuals. It is a possibility that neglecting to account for the presence of members of the subtype groups in these studies could have contributed to a veiling of the true state of nature. Deficit syndrome schizophrenia patients exhibit a less severe pattern of substance use than do nondeficit patients (Kirkpatrick et al., 1996) and have a lowered risk of polysubstance abuse (Kirkpatrick, Messias, & Tek, 2003), while thought disorganization, a positive symptom, is associated with an increased risk of alcohol and marijuana abuse (Kirkpatrick et al., 2003). It is possible that many of the individuals in the nonsubstance-using groups in these studies actually had the deficit form of the disorder. This presents a confound because the poorer neuropsychological profile of the deficit syndrome could have resulted in these patients not appearing different from those in the co-occurring groups, even if co-occurrence is actually associated with an exacerbation of neurocognitive symptoms. In addition, neuroleptic treatment can contribute to a worse (e.g., Cleghorn et al., 1990) or better (Flashman & Green, 2004) neurocognitive profile. Patients with different types of symptoms may be treated with different forms of antipsychotic medications, the effects of which could confound results.

Related to this, there appears to be a subgroup of individuals with schizophrenia who do not evidence cognitive deficits (Holthausen et al., 2002). Heavy inclusion of such individuals in the substance-using group could contribute to negative results.

Third, as discussed earlier, most of the substance-using groups in these studies misused a wide variety of substances. Perhaps using such heterogeneous groups is not prudent; although neurocognitive deficits have been found to be associated with a wide range of substances, some substances have specific aspects to their neurocognitive signature. As reviewed by Tracy and colleagues (1995), heroin is associated with unstructured problem-solving deficits, alcohol use is associated with abstraction, perceptual motor, and immediate memory problems, and marijuana is not believed to contribute to extensive neurocognitive deficits. Future studies, following the lead of Cooper, Liberman, Tucker, Nuechterlein, Tsuang, and Barnett (1999) and other researchers, who focused on cocaine use, should examine more homogeneous groups of substance-using patients. This is especially salient given that studies that found differences between illicit substance-abusing and non-abusing patients focused on cocaine alone. If this is not feasible, studies using groups with a heterogeneous substance-use profile may be able to control for this potential confound, if sample sizes are large enough, by statistically controlling for such heterogeneity.

Finally, in evaluating these studies as a whole, it is difficult to make cross-study comparisons. This prevents making definitive conclusions about the effects of substance use on neurocognitive functioning in schizophrenia. Each study evaluated different aspects of neurocognitive functioning, some several domains, others only two. This prevents one from identifying systematic patterns across the corpus of literature, at least at this early stage when there are very few studies examining this issue. Future efforts should seek to duplicate the results of earlier studies, using the same or similar measures.

Trait dimensions and shared pathophysiology: An interactive model of co-occurrence

Previous sections have noted that there are some similarities between the neurocognitive deficit profiles of substance use and schizophrenia. To date, few studies have compared the neurocognitive profiles of schizophrenia and substance use without co-occurrence; therefore, it is unclear if the severity of deficits seen in substance use is comparable with the severity of deficits found in schizophrenia. Collingwood and Harrell (1999) compared psychosis patients with substance abusers and found that the groups did not differ in terms of cognitive impairment, but this sample included patients with a range of psychotic disorders and not only schizophrenia, which could have impacted the results. Given the pervasive and severe deficit profile of schizophrenia, it is possible that schizophrenia provides for worse deficits than does substance use alone. There is a genetic–environmental reaction range (e.g., Gottesman & Shields, 1972) associated with a variety of characteristics; perhaps schizophrenia pushes individuals to their predetermined neurocognitive deficit limit. Thus, substance use would fail to create deficits above and beyond those associated with the effects of schizophrenia.

Keeping these pervasive preexisting deficits in mind, how can this pattern of negative results add to our understanding of dual diagnosis in schizophrenia? Previous theories of co-occurrence did not take into account neurocognitive findings. The following model builds on previous theory and incorporates neurocognitive data.

First, consider how the schizophrenic brain is characterized by diffuse and severe hypofrontality. As reviewed earlier, this is evident in imaging studies and tests of frontal functions such as executive functioning, working memory, and attention. Chambers, Krystal, and Self (2001) note that frontal deficits reduce inhibitory control, while dopamine and glutamate dysregulation in the nucleus accumbens could facilitate hyper-response to drugs. The extreme reinforcing effects of drug use and a lack of behavioral inhibition resulting from hypofrontality would combine to prompt the schizophrenic individual to continuously seek drugs. In this vein, substance use and schizophrenia arise from the same dysfunction, that is, a shared pathophysiology distinct from that seen in substance use. How do the data discussed here support this theory? If there is a preexisting pathophysiology that underlies the onset of both schizophrenia and substance use, neurocognitive deficits would likely not be exacerbated by substance use because, as discussed above, the disease process itself would result in reaching predetermined neurocognitive deficit limits. This could account for the pattern of negative results; in schizophrenia, it appears that neurocognitive deficits could be a precursor to substance use, not a result. An already damaged cognitive system may lead people to seek drugs, but the substances would not worsen the deficits of someone whose brain had already reached its limits.

This explains the largely negative results; it does not explain, however, why some individuals with schizophrenia become substance users while others do not. One might expect that a shared physiological vulnerability would lead inexorably to co-occurrence; what spares the non-users? To review, Blanchard and colleagues (2000) postulated that trait negative affectivity, impulsivity, and skills deficits are instrumental in a schizophrenia patient's choice to use drugs. Tying these theories together, trait impulsivity in schizophrenia may be tied to a lack of inhibition related to hypofrontality. While many schizophrenia patients may demonstrate such neurologically-based impulsivity, the behavioral outcomes of it may be modulated by individual difference factors such as trait negative affect, as well as coping and social skills.

The drug-using behavior of schizophrenia patients likely results from an interaction of a variety of factors. First, a physiologically-mediated tendency toward disinhibition and impulsivity can contribute to environmental stressors and to responses to those stressors that are not well planned and that may not be successful. Individual difference factors such as trait negative affectivity and social and problem-solving skills (which may also be frontally mediated) jointly determine one's response to those stressors. High trait negative affectivity and skills deficits can lead, as Blanchard and colleagues (2000) suggested, to using substances to cope with internal (negative affect) and external (environmental, social) stressors, while those with low negative affectivity and fewer skills deficits can identify and exercise other coping options. In those who use drugs to cope, the physiological vulnerabilities (e.g., dopamine dysregulation) that can lead to hyper-response to substances (Chambers et al., 2001) encourages further drug use. Thus, drug use in schizophrenia could arise from an interaction of neurological and individual difference factors, with neurocognitive dysfunction contributing to a cascade of environmental stressors, the coping response to which (drug use) is reinforced by enhanced physiological pleasure. Further neurocognitive dysfunction will not be demonstrated due to the extent of preexisting deficits. To date, nobody has examined the interaction of neurocognitive and individual difference factors with regard to substance use in schizophrenia; this remains a topic of study for future research. Prospective studies of substance users, close to the onset of use and following them to chronic use, could help to determine the relationship of cognitive, substance-related, and individual difference factors in the phenomenology and pathophysiology of schizophrenia.

Functional and treatment considerations

Although it generally does not appear that substance use contributes to a worsening of neurocognitive symptoms, dual diagnosis in schizophrenia remains a focus of concern. Whether or not test performance suffers with the addition of substance use, functional outcomes of the dually diagnosed may be worse than for those who do not use substances. As detailed earlier, findings have been conflicting with regard to whether substance use definitively results in worse functional outcomes (e.g., symptom presentation, treatment response, social and occupational functioning), but this issue has not been examined with regard to neurocognitive deficits. It has already been demonstrated that the neurocognitive deficits of schizophrenia without substance use are associated with dysfunction in work, social effectiveness, activities of daily living (Teichner, Hormer, & Harvey, 2001; Velligan, Bow-Thomas, Mahurin, Miller, & Halgunseth, 2000), social skills acquisition, and social problem-solving ability (Green, 1996). Given that users and nonusers do not differ in their neurocognitive profiles, it may be illuminating to examine if poorer neurocognitive functioning within the substance-using group is associated with worse functional outcomes. This would serve the dual purpose of describing the functional abilities of those with lower neurocognitive abilities within the substance-using group and perhaps provide a basis for which to interpret previous conflicting findings about functional outcomes in the dual diagnosis population. Maybe it is the degree of neurocognitive functioning within this group that influences functional outcomes, not substance use status alone.

The issue of neurocognitive functioning also has an impact on treatment considerations. In substance-using populations, better attentional capacity is associated with higher attainment of treatment objectives (Teichner et al., 2001), and better overall cognitive functioning is associated with greater readiness to change drug-using behaviors (Blume, Davis, & Schmaling, 1999), although executive functioning deficits alone are not associated with acquisition of complex change processes (Morgenstern & Bates, 1999). Cognitive functioning also has implications for relapse regardless of initial success; in one study (Gregson & Taylor, 1977), 87% of substance abuse patients designated as having low cognitive functioning relapsed compared to 37% in the higher functioning group. Success and relapse after completing treatment aside, individuals with cognitive impairment may not even complete treatment; although they did not differ from a nonimpaired group in terms of treatment objectives in one study (Teichner, Horner, Roitzsch, Herron, & Thevos, 2002), more impaired individuals dropped out of treatment.

How can knowledge of cognitive deficits help to formulate treatments for substance abuse in schizophrenia? Bellack and Gearon (1998) emphasize that given the pervasive cognitive deficits of schizophrenia patients, treatments must reduce demands on cognitive capacity, which makes behavioral skills-based treatments promising candidates for the treatment of the dually diagnosed. Knowledge of frontal deficits likely resulting in behavioral disinhibition points to the possibility of intervening at the level of such impulsivity. Such an intervention would likely be two-tiered: Training patients in distress-tolerance skills so that they will not immediately turn to drugs to cope with acute stressors may be helpful, while at the same time providing instruction in problem-solving skills so as to enhance the repertoire with which one can approach a problem, thereby encouraging patients to consider other coping options. Symptom considerations, such as an excess of positive symptoms (Cleghorn et al., 1991) and of depression and anxiety (Nixon et al., 1996), compared to nonusing patients, should not be ignored.

While the extent of co-occurring substance use and schizophrenia remains a vexing problem with regard to theories of co-occurrence, treatment, and possible increased resource consumption, it is heartening to discover that, at this time, neurocognitive deficits in the dually diagnosed generally do not appear to be exacerbated, methodological considerations notwithstanding. Time and additional research will be able to determine if this remains the case.

References

Addington, J., & Addington, D. (1997). Substance abuse and cognitive functioning in schizophrenia. *Journal of Psychiatry and Neuroscience, 22,* 99–104.

Addington, A., & Duchak, V. (1997). Reasons for substance use in schizophrenia. *Acta Psychiatrica Scandinavica, 96,* 329–333.

Aleman, A., & de Haan, E. (2000). Antipsychotics and working memory in schizophrenia. *Science, 289,* 56–57.

Andreasen, N., Rezai, K., & Alliger, R. (1992). Hypofrontality in neuroleptic-naïve patients and in patients with chronic schizophrenia: Assessment with xenon 133 single-photon emission computed tomography and the Tower of London. *Archives of General Psychiatry, 49,* 943–958.

Baddeley, A. (1986). *Working memory.* New York: Oxford University Press.

Baddeley, A., & Della Salla, S. (1998). Working memory and executive control. In A. Roberts & T. Robbins (Eds.), *The prefrontal cortex: Executive and cognitive functions* (pp. 9–21). London: Oxford University Press.

Barch, D., Braver, T., Nystrom, L., Forman, S., Noll, D., & Cohen, J. (1997). Dissociating working memory from task difficulty in human prefrontal cortex. *Neuropsychologia, 35,* 1373–1380.

Basso, M., Nasrallah, H., Olson, S., & Bornstein, R. (1998). Neuropsychological characteristics of negative, disorganized, and psychotic symptoms in schizophrenia. *Schizophrenia Research, 31,* 99–111.

Bellack, A., & Gearon, S. (1998). Substance abuse treatment for people with schizophrenia. *Addictive Behaviors, 23,* 749–766.

Blanchard, J., Brown, S., Horan, B., & Sherwood, A. (2000). Substance use disorders in schizophrenia: Review, integration, and a proposed model. *Clinical Psychology Review, 20,* 207–234.

Blanchard, J., & Neale, J. (1994). The neuropsychological signature of schizophrenia: Generalized or differential deficit? *American Journal of Psychiatry, 151,* 40–48.

Blume, A., Davis, M., & Schmaling, K. (1999). Neurocognitive dysfunction in dually-diagnosed patients: A potential roadblock to motivating behavior change. *Journal of Psychoactive Drugs, 31,* 111–115.

Bolla, K., Rothman, R., & Cadet, J. (1999). Dose-related neurobehavioral effects of chronic cocaine use. *Journal of Neuropsychiatry and Clinical Neurosciences, 11,* 361–369.

Braff, D. (1993). Information processing and attention dysfunctions in schizophrenia. *Schizophrenia Bulletin, 19,* 233–259.

Bryson, G., Whelahan, H., & Bell, M. (2001). Memory and executive function impairments in deficit syndrome schizophrenia. *Psychiatry Research, 102,* 29–37.

Buchanan, R., & Carpenter, W. (1994). Domains of psychopathology: An approach to the reduction of heterogeneity in schizophrenia. *Journal of Nervous and Mental Disease, 182,* 193–204.

Buchanan, R., Strauss, M., Breier, A, Kirkpatrick, B., & Carpenter, W. (1997). Attentional impairments in deficit and nondeficit forms of schizophrenia. *American Journal of Psychiatry, 154,* 363–370.

Buchsbaum, M., Neuchterlein, K., Haier, R., Wu, J., Sicotte, N., Hazlett, E., et al. (1990). Glucose metabolic rate in normals and schizophrenics during the continuous performance task assessed by positron emission tomography. *British Journal of Psychiatry, 156,* 216–227.

Bühler, B., Hambrecht, M., Löffler, W., van der Heiden, W., & Häfner, H. (2002). Precipitation and determination of the onset and course of schizophrenia by substance abuse: A retrospective and prospective study of 232 population-based first illness episodes. *Schizophrenia Research, 54*, 243–252.

Cannon, T. (1996). Abnormalities of brain function and structure in schizophrenia: Implications for aetiology in pathophysiology. *Annals of Medicine, 28*, 533–539.

Cannon, T., van Erp, T., Rosso, I., Huttunen, M., Lönnqvist, J., Pirkola, T., et al. (2002). Fetal hypoxia and structural brain abnormalities in schizophrenic patients, their siblings, and controls. *Archives of General Psychiatry, 15*, 35–41.

Carey, K., Carey, M., & Simons, J. (2003). Correlates of substance use disorder among psychiatric outpatients: Focus on cognition, social role functioning, and psychiatric status. *Journal of Nervous and Mental Disease, 191*, 300–308.

Carpenter, W., Heinrichs, D., & Wagman, A. (1988). Deficit and non-deficit forms of schizophrenia: The concept. *American Journal of Psychiatry, 145*, 578–583.

Carter, C., Robertson, L., Nordahl, T., Chaderjian, M., Kraft, L., & O'Shara-Celaya, L. (1996). Spatial working memory deficits and their relation to negative symptoms in unmedicated schizophrenia patients. *Biological Psychiatry, 40*, 930–932.

Chambers, A., Krystal, J., & Self, D. (2001). A neurobiological basis for substance abuse comorbidity in schizophrenia. *Biological Psychiatry, 50*, 71–83.

Cleghorn, J., Kaplan, R., Szechtman, B., Szechtman, R., & Brown, G. (1990). Neuroleptic drug effects on cognitive function in schizophrenia. *Schizophrenia Research, 3*, 211–219.

Cleghorn, J., Kaplan, R., Szechtman, B., Szechtman, R., Brown, G., & Franco, S. (1991). Substance abuse and schizophrenia: Effect on symptoms but not on cognitive function. *Journal of Clinical Psychiatry, 52*, 26–30.

Cohen, J., Perlstein, W., Braver, T., & Nystrom, L. (1997). Temporal dynamics of brain activation during a working memory task. *Nature, 386*, 604–608.

Collingwood, L., & Harrell, E. (1999). Performance of psychotic and substance abuse patients with or without head injury on the Halstead-Reitan battery. *Applied Neuropsychology, 6*, 88–95.

Cooper, L., Liberman, D., Tucker, D., Nuechterlein, K., Tsuang, J., & Barnett, H. (1999). Neurocognitive deficits in the dually diagnosed with schizophrenia and cocaine abuse. *Psychiatric Rehabilitation Skills, 3*, 231–245.

Cornblatt, B., & Keilp, J. (1994). Impaired attention, genetics, and the pathophysiology of schizophrenia. *Schizophrenia Bulletin, 20*, 31–46.

Cornblatt, B., Winters., L., & Erlenmeyer-Kimling, L. (1989). Attentional markers of schizophrenia: Evidence from the New York High-Risk Study. In S. Schulz & C. Tamminga (Eds.), *Schizophrenia: Scientific progress* (pp. 83–92). London: Oxford University Press.

Crow, T. (1982). Two syndromes in schizophrenia? *Trends in Neuroscience, 5*, 351–354.

Docherty, N., & Gordinier, S. (1999). Immediate memory, attention, and communication disturbances in schizophrenia and their relatives. *Psychological Medicine, 29*, 189–197.

Drake, R., Osher, F., & Wallach, M. (1991). Homelessness and dual diagnosis. *American Psychologist: Special Issue on Homelessness, 46*, 1149–1158.

D'Souza, D., Perry, E., MacDougall, L., Ammerman, Y., Cooper, T., Wu, Y., et al. (2004). The psychotomimetic effects of intravenous delta-9-tetrahydrocannabinol in healthy individuals: Implications for psychosis. *Neuropsychopharmacology, 29*, 1558–1572.

Evdokimidis, L., Liakopoulos, D., Constantinides, L., & Papageorgiou, C. (1996). Cortical potential with antisaccades. *Neurophysiology, 98,* 377–384.
Fitzgerald, D., Lucas, S., Redoblado, M., Winter, V., Brennan, J., Anderson, J., et al. (2004). Cognitive functioning in young people with first episode psychosis: relationship to diagnosis and clinical characteristics. *Australian and New Zealand Journal of Psychiatry, 38,* 501–510.
Flashman, L., & Green, M. (2004). Review of cognition and brain structure in schizophrenia: Profiles, longitudinal course, and effects of treatment. *Psychiatric Clinics of North America, 27,* 1–18.
Giovannetti, T., Goldstein, R., Schullery, M., Barr, W., & Bilder, R. (2003). Category fluency in first-episode schizophrenia. *Journal of the International Neuropsychological Society, 9,* 384–393.
Gold, J., Carpenter, C., Randolph, C., Goldberg, T., & Weinberger, R. (1997). Auditory working memory and Wisconsin Card Sorting Test performance in schizophrenia. *Archives of General Psychiatry, 54,* 159–165.
Goldberg, T., Saint-Cyr, J., & Weinberger, D. (1990). Assessment of procedural learning and problem solving in schizophrenic patients by Tower of Hanoi type tasks. *Journal of Neuropsychiatry and Clinical Neurosciences, 2,* 165–173.
Goldman-Rakic, P. (1991). Prefrontal cortical dysfunction in schizophrenia: The relevance of working memory. In B. Carroll (Ed.), *Psychopathology and the brain.* New York: Raven Press.
Goldman-Rakic, P. (1996). The functional parcellation of the dorsolateral prefrontal cortex and the heterogeneous facets of schizophrenia. In S. Matthysse, D. Levy, J. Kagan, & F. Benes (Eds.), *Psychopathology: The evolving science of mental disorders* (pp. 7–33). New York: Cambridge University Press.
Goldman-Rakic, P., & Selemon, L. (1997). Functional and anatomical aspects of prefrontal pathology in schizophrenia. *Schizophrenia Bulletin, 23,* 437–458.
Gottesman, I., & Shields, J. (1972). *Genetics and schizophrenia: A twin study vantage point.* Oxford, UK: Academic Press.
Green, M. (1996). What are the functional consequences of neurocognitive deficits in schizophrenia? *American Journal of Psychiatry, 153,* 321–330.
Gregson, R., & Taylor, G. (1977). Prediction of relapse in men alcoholics. *Journal of Alcohol Studies, 38,* 1749–1760.
Gruzelier, J., Seymour, K., Wilson, L., Jolley, A., & Hirsch, S. (1988). Impairments on neuropsychologic tests of temporohippocampal and frontohippocampal functions and word fluency in remitting schizophrenia and affective disorders. *Archives of General Psychiatry, 45,* 623–629.
Gualtieri, C. (1995). The contribution of frontal lobes to a theory of psychopathology. In J. Ratey (Ed.), *Neuropsychiatry of personality disorders* (pp. 149–171). Cambridge, MA: Blackwell Science.
Gur, R.C., Ragland, J., Mozley, L., Mozley, D., Smith, R., Alavi, A., et al. (1997). Lateralized changes in regional cerebral blood flow during performance of verbal and facial recognition tasks: Correlations with performance and "effort." *Brain and Cognition, 33,* 388–414.
Gur, R.E., Maany, V., Mozley, D., Swanson, C., Bilker, W., & Gur, R.C. (1998). Subcortical MRI volumes in neuroleptic-naïve and treated patients with schizophrenia. *American Journal of Psychiatry, 155,* 1711–1717.
Hambrecht, M., & Häfner, H. (2000). Cannabis, vulnerability, and the onset of

schizophrenia: An epidemiological perspective. *Australian and New Zealand Journal of Psychiatry, 34,* 468–475.

Harvey, P., Green, M., McGurk, S., & Meltzer, H. (2003). Changes in cognitive functioning with risperidone and olanzapine treatment: A large-scale, double-blind, randomized study. *Psychopharmacology, 169,* 404–411.

Haznedar, M., Buchsbaum, M., Hazlett, E., Shihabuddin, L., New, A., & Siever, L. (2004). Cingulate gyrus volume and metabolism in the schizophrenia spectrum. *Schizophrenia Research, 71,* 249–262.

Hietala, J., Cannon, T., van Erp, T., Syvälahti, E., Vilkman, H., Laasko, A., et al. (2003). Regional brain morphology and duration of illness in never-medicated first-episode schizophrenia patients. *Schizophrenia Research, 64,* 79–81.

Hofer, A., Weiss, E., Golazewski, S., Siedentopf, C., Brinkhoff, C., Kremser, C., et al. (2003). An fMRI study of episodic encoding and recognition of words in patients with schizophrenia in remission. *American Journal of Psychiatry, 160,* 911–918.

Hoff, A., Riordan, H, O'Donnell, D., Morris, L., & DeLisi, L. (1992). Anomalous lateral sulcus asymmetry and cognitive function in first-episode schizophrenia. *Schizophrenia Bulletin, 18,* 257–272.

Holthausen, E., Weirsma, D., Sitskoorn, M., Hijman, R., Dingemans, P., Schene, A., et al. (2002). Schizophrenic patients without neuropsychological deficits: Subgroup, disease severity, or cognitive compensation? *Psychiatry Research, 112,* 1–11.

Izenwasser, S. (2004). The role of the dopamine transporter in cocain abuse. *Neurotoxicology Research, 6,* 379–383.

Jackson, C., Fein, D., Essock, S., & Mueser, K. (2001). The effects of cognitive impairment and substance use on psychiatric hospitalizations. *Community Mental Health Journal, 37,* 303–312.

Jones, L., Cardno, A., Sanders, R., Owen, M., & Williams, J. (2001). Sustained and selective attention as measures of genetic liability to schizophrenia. *Schizophrenia Research, 48,* 263–272.

Kendler, K. (1985). A twin study of individuals with both schizophrenia and alcoholism. *British Journal of Psychiatry, 147,* 48–53.

Kendler, K. (1995). Genetic epidemiology in psychiatry: Taking both genes and environment seriously. *Archives of General Psychiatry, 52,* 895–899.

Keshavan, M. Schooler, N., Sweeney, J., Haas, G., & Pettegrew, J. (1998). Research and treatment strategies in first-episode psychosis: The Pittsburgh experience. *British Journal of Psychiatry, 172* (Suppl. 33), 60–65.

Kirkpatrick, B., Amador, X., Flaum, M., Yale, S., Gorman, J., Carpenter, W., et al. (1996). The deficit syndrome in the DSM-IV field trial: I. Alcohol and other drug abuse. *Schizophrenia Research, 20,* 69–77.

Kirkpatrick, B., Messias, M., & Tek, C. (2003). Substance abuse and the heterogeneity of schizophrenia. *Schizophrenia Research, 62,* 293–294.

Kovasznay, B., Bromet, E., Schwartz, J., & Ram, R. (1993). Substance abuse and onset of psychotic illness. *Hospital and Community Psychiatry, 44,* 567–571.

Kurtz, M., Ragland, J., Bilker, W., Gur, R., & Gur, R. (2001). Comparison of the continuous performance task with and without working memory demands in healthy controls and patients with schizophrenia. *Schizophrenia Research, 48,* 307–316.

Laurent, A., Biloa-Tang, M., Bougerol, T., Duly, D., Anchisi, A., Bosson, J., et al. (2000). Executive/attentional performance and measures of schizotypy in patients with schizophrenia and in their nonpsychotic first degree relatives. *Schizophrenia Research, 46*, 269–283.

Lawrie, S. & Abukmeil, S. (1998). Brain abnormality in schizophrenia: A systematic and quantitative review of volumetric magnetic resonance imaging studies. *British Journal of Psychiatry, 172*, 110–120.

Lawrie, S., Adams, C., Thornley, B., & Joy, C. (2000). Comprehensiveness of systematic review: Update. *British Journal of Psychiatry, 176*, 396–397.

Lawrie, S., Whalley, H., Abukmeil, S., Kestelman, J., Miller, P., Best, J., et al. (2002). Temporal lobe changes in people at high risk of schizophrenia with psychotic symptoms. *British Journal of Psychiatry, 181*, 138–143.

Levy, D., & Holzman, P. (1997). Eye tracking dysfunction and schizophrenia: An overview with special reference to the genetics of schizophrenia. *International Review of Psychiatry, 9*, 365–371.

Luo, X., Kranzler, H., Lappalainen, J., Charney, D., Zuo, L. Erdos, J., et al. (2004). CALCYON gene variation, schizophrenia, and cocaine dependence. *American Journal of Medical Genetics (Neuropsychiatry Genetics), 125*, 25–30.

Maier, W., Franke, P., Haine, C., Kopp, B., & Rist, F. (1992). Neuropsychological Indicators of the vulnerability to schizophrenia. *Progress in Neuropsychopharmacology and Biological Psychiatry, 16*, 703–715.

Meek, P., Clark, H., & Solana, V. (1989). Neurocognitive impairment: The unrecognized component of dual diagnosis in substance abuse treatment. *Journal of Psychoactive Drugs, 21*, 153–160.

Michie, P., Kent, A., Stienstra, R., Castine, Z., Johnston, J., Dedman, K., et al. (2000). Phenotypic markers as risk factors in schizophrenia: Neurocognitive functions *Australia and New Zealand Journal of Psychology, 34* (suppl.), 574–585.

Mirsky, A., Yardley, S., Jones, B., & Walsh, D. (1995). Analysis of the attention deficit in schizophrenia: A study of patients and their relatives in Ireland. *Journal of Psychiatric Research, 29*, 23–42.

Morgenstern, A., & Bates, M. (1999). Effects of executive function impairment on change processes and substance use outcomes in 12-step treatment. *Journal of Studies on Alcohol, 60*, 846–855.

Mueser, K., Yarnold, P., Levinson, D., & Singh, H. (1990). Prevalence of substance abuse in schizophrenia: Demographic and clinical correlates. *Schizophrenia Bulletin, 16*, 31–56.

Nazzaro, D. (1996). Neuropsychological differences between patients diagnosed with schizophrenia and comorbid schizophrenia and alcohol dependence. *Dissertation Abstracts International: Section B: The Sciences and Engineering, 63*, 2596.

Negrete, J. (2003). Clinical aspects of substance abuse in persons with schizophrenia. *Canadian Journal of Psychiatry, 48*, 14–20.

Nieuwenstein, M., Aleman, A., & de Haan, E. (2001). Relationship between symptom dimensions and neurocognitive functioning in schizophrenia: A meta-analysis of Wisconsin Card Sorting Test and continuous performance task studies. *Journal of Psychiatric Research, 35*, 119–125.

Nixon, S., Hallford, H., & Tivis, R. (1996). Neurocognitive function in alcoholic, schizophrenic, and dually diagnosed patients. *Psychiatry Research, 64*, 35–45.

Nuechterlein, K. (1991). Vigilance in schizophrenia and related disorders. In S. Steinhauer & J. Gruzelier (Eds.), *Neuropsychology, psychophysiology, and information processing, Handbook of schizophrenia, Volume 5* (pp. 397–433). New York: Elsevier Science.

Orzack, M., & Kornetsky, C. (1971). Environmental and familial predictors of attention behavior in chronic schizophrenics. *Journal of Psychiatric Research, 9*, 21–29.

Park, S., & Holzman, P. (1992). Schizophrenics show spatial working memory deficits. *Archives of General Psychiatry, 49*, 975–982.

Park, S., & Holzman, P. (1993). Association of working memory deficit and eye tracking dysfunction in schizophrenia. *Schizophrenia Research, 11*, 55–61.

Pencer, A., & Addington, J. (2003). Substance use and cognition in early psychosis. *Journal of Psychiatry and Neuroscience, 28*, 48–54.

Perlstein, W., Carter, C., Noll, D., & Cohen, J. (2001). Relation of prefrontal cortex dysfunction to working memory and symptoms in schizophrenia. *American Journal of Psychiatry, 158*, 1105–1113.

Perry, W., Heaton, R., Potterat, E., Roebuck, T., Minassian, A., & Bratt, D. (2001). Working memory in schizophrenia: Transient online storage vs. executive functioning. *Schizophrenia Bulletin, 27*, 157–176.

Potvin, S., Stip, E., & Roy, J-Y. (2003). Schizophrenia and addiction: An evaluation of the self-medication hypothesis. *Encephale, 29*, 193–203.

Ragland, J. D., Gur, R. C., Valdez, J., Turetsky, B., Elliot, M., Kohler, C., et al. (2004). Event-related fMRI of frontotemporal activity during word encoding and recognition in schizophrenia. *American Journal of Psychiatry, 161*, 1004–1015.

Randolph, C., Gold, J., Carpenter, C., Goldberg, T., & Weinberger, D. (1993). The neuropsychology of schizophrenia. In K. Heilman & Valenstein, E. (Eds.), *Clinical neuropsychology* (pp. 499–518). London: Oxford University Press.

Regier, D., Farmer, M., Rae, D., Locke, B., Keith, S., Judd, L., et al. (1990). Comorbidity of mental disorders with alcohol and other drug abuse: Results from the ECA study. *Journal of the American Medical Association, 264*, 2511–2518.

Rezai, K., Andreasen, N., Alliger, R., & Cohen, G. (1990). The neuropsychology of the prefrontal cortex. *Archives of Neurology, 50*, 636–642.

Roitman, S., Cornblatt, B., Bergman, A., Obuchowski, M., Mitropolan, V., Keefe, R., et al. (1997). Attentional functioning in schizotypal personality disorder. *American Journal of Psychiatry, 154*, 655–660.

Rosenfarb, I., Neuchterlein, K., Goldstein, M., & Subotnik, K. (2000). Neurocognitive vulnerability, interpersonal criticism, and the emergence of unusual thinking by schizophrenia patients during family transactions. *Archives of General Psychiatry, 57*, 1174–1179.

Ross, D., Thaker, G., Holcomb, H., Cascella, N., Medoff, D., & Tamminga, C. (1995). Abnormal smooth pursuit eye movements in schizophrenic patients are associated with cerebral glucose metabolism in oculomotor regions. *Psychiatry Research, 58*, 53–67.

Ross, D., Thaker, G., Buchanan, R., Kirkpatrick, B., Lahti, A., Medorff, D., et al. (1997). Eye tracking disorder in schizophrenia is characterized by specific ocular motor deficits and is associated with the deficit syndrome. *Biological Psychiatry, 42*, 781–796.

Rossi, A., Bustini, M., Prosperini, P., Kalyvoka, A., Stratta, P., & Daneluzzo, E. (2000). Neuromorphological abnormalities in schizophrenic patients with good and poor outcome. *European Archives of Psychiatry and Clinical Neuroscience, 250*, 73–75.

Rubino, T., Vigano, D., Massi, P., & Parolaro, D. (2001). The psychoactive ingredient of marijuana induces behavioural sensitization. *European Journal of Neuroscience, 14*, 884–886.

Scarone, S., Abbruzzesse, S., & Gambini, O. (1993). The Wisconsin Card Sorting Test discriminates schizophrenia patients and their siblings. *Schizophrenia Research, 10,* 103–107.

Serper, M., Alpert, M., Richardson, N., & Dickson, S. (1995). *American Journal of Psychiatry, 152,* 1464–1469.

Serper, M., Bergman, A., Copersino, M., Chou, J., Richarme, D., & Cancro, R. (2000a). Learning and memory impairment in cocaine-dependent and comorbid schizophrenic patients. *Psychiatry Research, 93,* 21–32.

Serper, M, Copersino, M., Richarme, D., Vadhan, N., & Cancro, R. (2000b). Neurocognitive functioning in recently abstinent, cocaine-abusing schizophrenic patients. *Journal of Substance Abuse, 11,* 205–213.

Sevy, S., Kay, S., Opler, L., & Van Praag, H. (1990). Significance of cocaine history in schizophrenia. *Journal of Nervous and Mental Disease, 178,* 642–648.

Shi, W., Pun, C., & Zhu, Y. (2004). Psychostimulants induce low-frequency oscillations in the firing activity of dopamine neurons. *Neuropsychopharmacology, 29,* 2160–2170.

Smelson, D., Davis, C., Di Pano, R., Johnson, V., Losonczy, M., & Ziedonis, D. (2002). Executive and motor skill functioning among cocaine-dependent schizophrenics and non-drug-abusing schizophrenics. *Journal of Nervous and Mental Disease, 190,* 200–202.

Smelson, D., Davis, C., Eisenstein, N., Engelhart, C., Williams, J., Losonczy, M., et al. (2003). Cognitive disparity in schizophrenics with and without cocaine dependency. *Journal of Substance Abuse Treatment, 24,* 75–79.

Smythies, J. (1997). Oxidative reactions and schizophrenia: A review-discussion. *Schizophrenia Research, 24,* 357–364.

Snyder, A. (1998). The neurocognitive functioning of patients with schizophrenia and a substance use disorder. *Dissertation Abstracts International: Section B: The Sciences & Engineering, 59,* 3075.

Soyka, M., Albus, M., Kathmann, N., & Finelli, A. (1993). Prevalence of alchol and drug abuse in schizophrenic inpatients. *European Archives of Psychiatry and Clinical Neuroscience, 242,* 362–372.

Stone, W., Thermenos, H., Tarbox, S., Poldrack, R., & Seidman, J. (2005). Medial temporal and prefrontal lobe activation during verbal encoding following glucose ingestion in schizophrenia: A pilot fMRI study. *Neurobiology of Learning and Memory, 83,* 54–64.

Tamminga, C., Thaker, G., & Buchanan, R. (1992). Limbic system abnormalities identified in schizophrenia using positron emission tomography with fluorodeoxyglucose and neocortical alterations with deficit syndrome. *Archives of General Psychiatry, 49,* 522–530.

Teichner, G., Horner, M., & Harvey, R. (2001). Neuropsychological predictors of the attainment of treatment objectives in substance abuse patients. *International Journal of Neuroscience, 106,* 253–263.

Teichner, G., Horner, M., Roitzsch, J., Herron, J., & Thevos, A. (2002). Substance abuse treatment outcomes for cognitively impaired and intact outpatients. *Addictive Behaviors, 27,* 751–763.

Tracy, J., Josiassen, R., & Bellack, A. (1995). Neuropsychology of dual diagnosis: Understanding the combined effects of schizophrenia and substance use disorders. *Clinical Psychology Review, 15,* 67–97.

Velligan, D., Bow-Thomas, C., Mahurin, R., Miller, A., & Halgunseth, L. (2000). Do specific neurocognitive deficits predict specific domains of community function in schizophrenia? *Journal of Nervous and Mental Disease, 188,* 518–524.

Weickert, T., Goldberg, T., Gold, J., Bigelow, L., Egan, M., & Weinberger, D. (2000). Cognitive impairments in patients with schizophrenia displaying preserved and compromised intellect. *Archives of General Psychiatry, 57,* 907–913.

Yurgelun-Todd, D., Waternaux, C., Cohen, B., Gruber, S., English, C., & Renshaw, P. (1996). Functional magnetic resonance imaging of schizophrenia patients and comparison subjects during word production. *American Journal of Psychiatry, 153,* 200–205.

Zubin, J., & Spring, S. (1977). Vulnerability: A new view of schizophrenia. *Journal of Abnormal Psychology, 86,* 103–126.

Part III

Future Directions

13 If only the hangover preceded intoxication: An integration of behavioral economic and neuropsychological approaches to impulsive choice

John R. Monterosso, Ari Kalechstein, and Xochitl Cordova

Why is it so difficult for addicted individuals to quit, even if they believe it is in their vital interest? On typically smaller scales, behavior that runs counter to recognized best interest is ubiquitous (e.g., overeating, credit card debt, overconsumption of passive entertainment, etc.); however, it is one of the fascinating aspects of addiction that the divergence between perceived best interest and actual behavior is extreme. As such, addiction provides a useful context in which to study the interplay between motivational conflict and the struggle for self-control.

The goal of this chapter is to review what behavioral economic theories and research can tell us about this topic, which we will refer to as "impulsive choice," and then to consider how neuropsychology might be integrated with the behavioral economic perspective. We begin with a brief introduction to behavioral economics, followed next by a summary of basic research on the "temporal discounting" model of impulsive choice, then we consider several behavioral economic theories of self-control, and finally we attempt to integrate neuropsychological literature with these behavioral economic models.

What is behavioral economics?

Because the reader of this book may not be familiar with behavioral economics, a brief introduction may be useful. "Behavioral economics" is something of a rebellious faction within the broader field of economics. Traditional economics has been perhaps the most successful of the social sciences (the only one deemed important enough for a Nobel Prize!), in part through extremely disciplined methodology. Paramount in this discipline is a set of modeling axioms. While the specifics of these axioms are beyond the scope of this chapter, the assumptions collectively characterize individuals as consistent "rational maximizers" of whatever goals they hold. To the extent that the reality of human behavior has been demonstrated to violate "rational maximization", the neoclassical economist's position is that the departure is not sufficiently significant to warrant a revision of economic assumptions (Friedman, 1953).

In opposition to the neoclassical economists, behavioral economists hold that economic analysis can be improved by revising the axioms away from complete rationality and toward "bounded rationality," a concept that was formulated by Herbert Simon (and for which he received a Nobel Prize in 1978). Simon railed against what he saw as the neoclassical notion that economic theories were "not falsified in any interesting or relevant sense when their empirical predictions of microphenomena are found to be grossly incompatible with the observed data." (1978). As the name implies, Simon's "bounded rationality" proposes significant constraints on the decision-maker that could be incorporated into economic models without, he believed, undermining their rigor.

In a related series of papers, Daniel Kahneman and Amos Tversky's work on Prospect Theory (Kahneman & Tversky, 1979) provided another major milestone for behavioral economics. Prospect Theory offers an empirically derived formulation of *subjective* utility and probability to substitute for the formulation of utility and probability that conforms to the economic axioms of rationality (psychologist Kahneman's 2002 co-receipt of the Nobel Prize in economics for this work was no doubt unsettling to the strict neoclassical economist!). In addition to their break from neoclassic theoretical convention, the collective works of Simon and Kahneman and Tversky brought a greater interest and reliance on laboratory experiments to the field of economics. As we will argue below, the thriving approach of behavioral economics has allowed modeling rigor to be applied to the analysis of impulsive choice.

Behavioral economics of impulsive choice

The challenge continually faced by individuals struggling with addiction is to forgo the relatively immediate reward or relief available from drugs, in the service of attaining the relatively delayed benefits of sobriety (e.g., financial, social, and health benefits). The difference in immediacy between the rewards of drug use versus sobriety is critical; no doubt, it would be easy to quit smoking if the enjoyable aspects of smoking a cigarette arrived 20 years after the puff, but each puff carried a risk of immediate health disaster. As Samuel Butler brilliantly put it, *"If the headache would only precede the intoxication, alcoholism would be a virtue."* Thus, the behavioral economic approach to addiction has focused primarily on the effect of delay on the valuation of expected outcomes. Pioneering work by George Ainslie as early as the 1970s showed that this effect was not a simple matter of computation (Ainslie, 1975, 1982); Ainslie's exploration of the "temporal discount function" and its implications is the starting place of this chapter.

The temporal discount function is a mathematical characterization of the relationship between the expected delay associated with a reinforcer and the motivational value of that reinforcer. The basic idea is that the further in time an expectancy is, the less power that expectancy has to motivate behavior. In animal experiments, temporal discount functions are assessed using behavioral choice methodologies. For example, in Mazur's "adjusting procedure" (1987), pigeons were forced to choose between two response keys: one that resulted in some (adjusted) amount of immediate grain, and the other that resulted in a (fixed) larger amount of grain, but only after a delay. If the pigeon exhibited a preference for the key associated with the "later-larger" (LL) reward, the amount of grain associated with the "smaller-sooner" (SS) reward was increased on the next block of trials. Conversely, if the pigeon preferred the SS reward, then the amount of grain associated with the SS reward was *decreased* on the next block of trials. In this way, the procedure arrived at "indifference-points" – the amount of immediate grain that was equally preferred to the fixed LL alternative. For example, through a testing session with a particular pigeon, the experimenter might discover that the "value" of 10 units of grain delayed by 3 seconds was equal to the value of 6 units of immediate grain – thus value is "discounted" by 40% in 3 seconds (assuming a linear relationship between amount and value for simplicity). By computing indifference points for a series of delays, the character of temporal discounting can be plotted on a graph, and a single "temporal discount function" can be calculated that (to varying degrees) fits empirically derived indifference point data.

Methodologies for assessing rate of discounting in humans

A variety of paradigms have been used to quantify steepness of temporal discounting in humans. Although human experiments on temporal discounting cannot reasonably achieve the control of context and sheer number of trials possible in experiments using samples of pigeons and rats, the logic that underlies human temporal discount experiments is the same as that underlying nonhuman experimentation. In human experiments, participants are asked to make a series of choices between LL and SS alternatives and, as in the animal experiments, the inferred indifference points over a range of delays allow the computation of a temporal discount function (Figure 13.1). In terms of the rewards used in such studies, points (Forzano & Logue, 1994), health outcomes (Chapman, 1996, 2000; Chapman, Brewer, Coups, Brownlee, Leventhal, & Leventhal, 2001; van der Pol & Cairns, 2001), hypothetical drug or alcohol (Bickel, Odum, & Madden, 1999; Madden, Bickel, & Jacobs, 1999; Madden, Petry, Badger, & Bickel, 1997; Petry, 2001), hypothetical money with context (e.g., "you just won some amount at a casino") (Bohm 1994; Chapman 1996; Chesson & Viscusi, 2000; Thaler 1981), hypothetical money without context (Ainslie & Haendel, 1983; Fuchs 1982; Madden et al., 1997), actual money (Ainslie & Haendel, 1983; Crean, de Wit, & Richards, 2000; Kirby & Herrnstein, 1995; Richards, Zhang, Mitchell, &

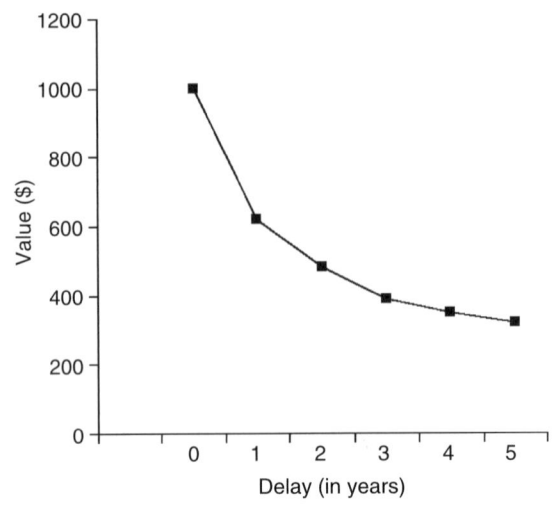

Figure 13.1 Value as a function of delay; based on Green et al., 1997. Each point indicates the average valuation of a hypothetical $1000 for a group of normal adults given a particular delay. For example, for the average subject, $1000 delayed by 3 years was valued as approximately equal to an immediate $400.

de Wit, 1999; Wallace, 1979), consumer goods (Kirby & Herrnstein, 1995), food (Forzano & Logue, 1994; Mischel & Grusec, 1967; Mischel, Grusec, & Masters, 1969), and juice (Logue, King, Chavarro, & Volpe, 1990) have all been used. Less frequently, choices among punishments have been used, including shocks (Cook & Barnes, 1964; Hare 1966; Mischel et al., 1969) and aversive noise (Navarick 1982). In terms of the procedures used, some studies have used choices among a fixed set of alternatives (Ainslie & Haendel, 1983; Kirby & Marakovic, 1996; Kirby, Petry, & Bickel, 1999; Monterosso, Ehrman, Napier, O'Brien, & Childress, 2001; van der Pol & Cairns, 2001), some have used a titration procedure with choice stimuli generated so as to narrow in on the subject's level of discounting (Crean et al., 2000; Kirby & Herrnstein, 1995; Madden et al., 1997; Richards et al., 1999), while other studies have required subjects to generate indifference amounts rather than to make choices (Cairns & van der Pol, 2000; Chapman, 1996).

Temporal discounting and "impulsivity"

There is some inconsistency with regard to the relationship between temporal discount rate and the term "impulsivity". Within behavioral economic research, the temporal discount rate is often treated as an operational index of an individual's or a group's level of impulsivity (Bickel et al., 1999; Bradshaw & Szabadi, 1992; Green, Myerson, & McFadden, 1997). That is to say, "impulsiveness" is operationalized as steep temporal discounting. Notice that this does not capture at least part of the everyday sense of the term "impulsive," which includes the evaluation of a behavior as having occurred suddenly and with minimal deliberation. Steep temporal discounting – a great willingness to trade value for immediacy – is no less "impulsive" in the behavioral economic sense if it occurs after long deliberation than if it occurs with no deliberation. This distinction will be particularly relevant when we consider the neurological lesion literature, which includes a lesion-syndrome that is associated with both undervaluation of delayed consequences and unusually *long* deliberation in decision-making.

Of course, in addition to its everyday use, the term "impulsivity" is also extensively used in the clinical and personality psychological literature. It has been convincingly argued that there are multiple constructs underlying the use of the term in these disciplines (Evenden, 1999) and so it is not surprising that putative measures of impulsivity are often only modestly intercorrelated (Corulla, 1987; Parker, Bagby, & Webster, 1993). Various taxonomies of impulsivity have been offered, such as functional and dysfunctional impulsivity (Dickman, 1990) and motoric, motivational, and cognitive impulsivity (Evenden, 1999; Patton, Stanford, & Barratt, 1995).

In contrast to the behavioral economic literature, "impulsivity" in these taxonomies is in part equated with "the tendency to deliberate less than most people of equal ability before taking action." (Dickman, 1990, p. 95). For clinical and personality researchers then, the relationship between impulsivity and delay discounting is an empirical question. Across a variety of disorders thought to relate to impulsivity (including substance abuse discussed below) and a variety of personality measures of impulsivity, modest associations have often been observed between impulsivity and steeper temporal discounting (Cherek, Moeller, Schnapp, & Dougherty, 1997; Crean et al., 2000; Kirby et al., 1999; Madden et al., 1997; Richards et al., 1999; Vuchinich & Simpson, 1998).

Application of temporal discounting assessment to addiction

The most expedient method for relating temporal discount rates to addiction is to compare the discount rates of addicted and nonaddicted populations. In particular, it has been hypothesized that addicted populations may discount more steeply with delay – that they may be more "temporally myopic" than nonaddicted populations (Ainslie, 1975; Bickel et al., 1999; Madden et al., 1997; Vuchinich & Tucker, 1988). Across a range of addicted populations, the evidence has been consistent with this hypothesis. Using hypothetical money, a heterogeneous group of substance-dependent subjects discounted more steeply than controls (Ainslie & Haendel, 1983); heavy social drinkers and problem drinkers both discounted delayed rewards more steeply than did light drinkers (Vuchinich & Simpson, 1998); smokers discounted delayed rewards more steeply than nonsmokers (Bickel et al., 1999; Cairns & van der Pol, 2000; Fuchs, 1982), and opioid-dependent patients discounted money more steeply than controls (Bretteville-Jensen, 1999; Madden et al., 1997, 1999).

Similar results were obtained using actual monetary rewards. Compared to controls, heroin-dependent subjects chose more immediate nickels over tokens exchangeable for dimes in 10 days (Wallace, 1979), regular smokers discounted money more steeply than did a population who had never smoked (Mitchel, 1999), and heroin-dependent subjects had steeper discount functions than demographically matched controls (Kirby et al., 1999). Furthermore, Odum, Madden, Badger, and Bickel (2000) found that heroin addicts who shared needles discounted money more steeply than heroin addicts who did not.

Impulse control in addiction: Precommitment and intrapersonal bargaining

Despite the studies cited above, human experimental data on temporal discounting should be interpreted with caution. As has been reviewed elsewhere (Ainslie & Monterosso, 2002; Loewenstein & Prelec, 1992; Roelofsma, 1996), the literature contains numerous anomalies (e.g., low correlations across domains, much greater variability among human than animal subjects, and preference for delay of some good outcomes and for immediacy of some bad outcomes). It is evident that individuals' tendency to make impulsive choices cannot be so readily distilled to a single number. At least part of complication, we argue, stems from self-control processes that affect the choices that people make in and out of the laboratory. While these self-control mechanisms emerge in part as a consequence of the way value is discounted with delay, they are processes distinct from temporal discounting (Ainslie, 1975, 1992, 2001). That is to say, self-control is not, on this account, merely a low level of temporal discounting. Rather self-control consists of mechanisms that change the operative contingencies at stake in a given decision, which are then subject to temporal discounting. We consider two categories of self-control mechanisms: precommitment and intertemporal bargaining. Later, we will consider possibilities with regard to the underlying neuropsychology of these mechanisms.

Precommitment

Up until now, we have glossed over the particular nature of the function relating delay to value (i.e., the temporal discount function). For reasons we will only characterize in general terms, the nature of the temporal discount function has been a key point of controversy between neoclassical economists and behavioral economists. Orderly "rational" behavior requires that, to whatever extent value is discounted with delay, it must be discounted by a fixed rate per unit of time (similar to the way bank accounts change with time). Neoclassical models of behavior have assumed this "exponential discounting" (so-called because it is represented by a function in which the delay parameter is an exponent) because it maintains rational stability of preference. Just as the larger of two equal-interest savings accounts will always remain larger, regardless of when the accounts were started and how much money they started with, so too does exponential discounting imply that the more valued of two rewards fixed in time remains the more valued, regardless of how far away in time the individual is from these rewards. This stability is referred to as "delay independence" because it allows that any fixed delay can be added to a set of rewards without changing their value relative to each other (Figure 13.2A).

However, laboratory and field assessments of temporal discount functions consistently show that, for both humans and nonhumans, value is not discounted by a fixed proportion per unit of time. Instead, value is inversely proportional to delay (for review see Green & Myerson, 1994). While the percent interest accrued by your money for a day of sitting in the bank is the same regardless of how long it has been there, the percent devaluation of reward when given the addition of a fixed delay varies as a function of total delay. The subjective difference between expecting an immediate $100 and $100 in 3 months is proportionately greater than the difference between expecting $100 in 12 months versus $100 in 15 months. Human and nonhuman temporal discounting data are generally reasonably well characterized by the simple nonexponential temporal discount function:

$$V = \frac{A}{1+KD} \quad (13.1)$$

where V denotes the value of the reinforcer given delay, A is amount in some arbitrary unit, D is the delay to the reinforcer, and the parameter "K" is set to

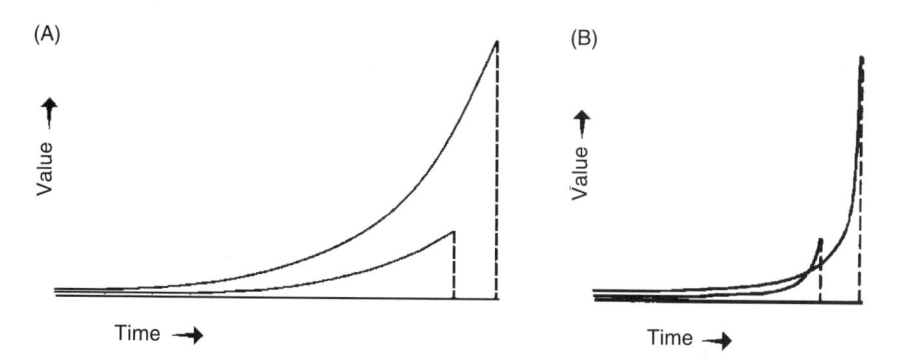

Figure 13.2 (A) Exponential discount curves from two rewards of different sizes available at different times. There is no delay at which the preference switches. (Reprinted with permission from Ainslie, 2001, p. 32.) (B) Hyperbolic discount curves from two rewards of different sizes available at different times. The smaller reward is more valued just in the period when its availability is relatively immediate.

the value that allows the function to most closely match observed data, with higher values indicating steeper temporal discounting (Mazur, 1987). This proportional, or "hyperbolic," discounting is important because, as a result, preference between a fixed pair of alternatives will predictably reverse as a result of the mere passage of time (delay dependence; Figure 13.2B). The implications of delay dependence are far-reaching, and will be discussed at length below. For now, suffice to say that proportional discounting has been looked to as a basis for understanding why immediately available rewards, such as cocaine, might be compelling even to an individual who believes she would be better in the long run if she abstained (Ainslie, 1975; Bickel et al., 1999; Kirby et al., 1999; Madden et al., 1999).

Because preference among a fixed set of alternatives can vary predictably as a function of the passage of time (*delay dependence*), it follows that in some cases one of the obstacles faced in trying to attain current preferences is the expected preference at some point in the future; thus, in the analysis of impulsive choice, and defenses against it, it may be more productive to model the individual as a series of successive selves in partial conflict, rather than as a single self moving through time (Ainslie, 1992; Monterosso, Ainslie, Toppi-Mullen, & Gautt, 2002). Consider a smoker trying to quit, and imagine she currently is not craving a cigarette, perhaps because she has just smoked a cigarette. If she is serious about quitting, she may currently have a clear preference for abstaining in the future, but an equally clear expectation that her own future self poses a threat to this current preference. She may thus be expected to behave strategically toward the competitive interests of her future self – that is, to try to *precommit* to her current interests.

The most direct method of precommitment is to arrange for some external control or influence, as illustrated in the story of Ulysses and the Sirens. Prior to hearing the Siren's voices, Ulysses held a preference for hearing them and living to tell about it. He also knew that if he heard the singing, his future self would hold a fatal preference to direct his ship toward the sound and crash against the rocks. To block this anticipated preference reversal, he tied himself to the mast (and directed his shipmates to wear earplugs) in order to secure his current preference.

While truly binding precommitment is often not possible, partial precommitments are often possible, in which the current self increases the likelihood of attaining its preference by altering the contingencies that future selves will face. For instance, if an alcoholic checks into a detoxification facility far away from the available drug or takes Antabuse, then the alcoholic is partially precommitting in accordance with current preferences by making it more costly or less pleasurable to resume drug use. Less extreme precommitments might include asking friends for assistance in order to remain abstinent or even declaring in public that you have quit drug use. Someone who has told all her friends she has quit smoking certainly has not eliminated the possibility of smoking, but she has altered the contingencies in favor of her current preference by adding the cost of embarrassment associated with smoking to the contingencies that future selves will face. Reputation may thus be a major vehicle of commitment (Becker, 1960).

Interestingly, precommitment by external manipulation has been demonstrated even in pigeons (Ainslie, 1974; Green & Rachlin, 1996), though only in a situation where the commitment method was highly salient. Precommitment itself does not require great cognitive sophistication: it follows mechanistically from hyperbolic discounting. The LL reward discounted for its associated delay is simply greater at the time of precommitment than is the discounted SS reward (to the right of the intersection of the curves in Figure 13.2B).

In his theoretical analysis of precommitment, Ainslie (1992, 2001) classifies the above types of precommitments as "extrapsychic" to contrast from precommiting tactics that occur internally ("intrapsychic"). Organisms' responses to stimuli depend on their attention to those stimuli, and on their own emotional state. Control of attention can be used to guard against preference reversal; for example, someone struggling to maintain fidelity to a spouse may not allow herself to notice the flirtations of an attractive other. Attending to such information may foreseeably lead to the likelihood of creating preferences in opposition to current preferences. Attentional control can occur as either deliberate avoidance of information or an avoidance that is itself not acknowledged. The latter case is the repression that Freud at one time held to be the cornerstone of all defensive processes (Freud, 1956). The repressive individual avoids unwanted thoughts, feelings, or behaviors by not attending to the psychically loaded information.

Emotions such as fear, jealousy, and arousal can, to a point, be vicious circles. After the emotion is underway, there is a lower threshold for further emotional activity of the same kind, until some satiation point is reached (Skinner, 1953, pp. 235–236, 239–240). If a person expects an emotion to make a currently unpreferred reward dominant, he may commit himself not to choose the reward through early inhibition of that emotion. There have been some experimental demonstrations of emotional control. For instance, Walter Mischel and colleagues found that while children below around 6 years were poor at self-control, many older children were often able to resist the temptation of an immediately available marshmallow in favor of a more preferred reward. Those that succeeded in avoiding the impulsive preference reversal often used emotional control in the form of thinking about the immediately available marshmallow in a "cool" way, or by imagining it to be undesirable (Mischel & Mischel, 1983; Mischel & Moore, 1980).

Beyond precommitment

Tactics that commit choice in advance are sometimes evident in addicts' efforts to avoid temptation. However, precommitment behaviors are probably not what people ordinarily have in mind when they refer to willpower or self-control; precommitments are more like strategies deployed when people lack confidence in their willpower. We sometimes do not need to bind ourselves by some physical device, contract, or even reputation to keep our intentions steady. It is certainly good advice for an addict to avoid the haunts where her substance is readily available, but most people who have given up a bad habit do not depend on keeping temptation at a distance or out of sight and/or attention. People who have given up smoking, for instance, often say that they "just did it" one day (Premack, 1970). They are said to have used *willpower*. If they relapse, they are more apt to attribute it to an exceptional circumstance – the pressure of an exam, depression over a failed relationship – than to the imminent availability of a cigarette. Rationalization, not proximity, is the most notorious threat to willpower.

Intertemporal bargaining and "the universal" of willpower

Writers since antiquity have related willpower to choosing according to principle: that is, choosing in categories containing a number of expectable choices rather than just the choice at hand. Aristotle said that impulsive choice (*"akrasia"*) was the result of choosing according to "particulars" instead of "universals" (Aristotle, 1984: *Nicomachean Ethics* 1147a, pp. 24–28); Kant said that the highest kind of decision-making involved making all choices as if they defined universal rules (the "categorical imperative"; Kant, 1793/1960, pp. 15–49); the Victorian psychologist Sully said that "will" consists of uniting "particular actions ... under a common rule" so that "they are viewed as members of a class of actions subserving one comprehensive end" (Sully, 1884, p. 663). The fundamental insight is that you increase your self-control by choosing according to category rather than on a case-by-case basis (e.g. a preference for being a nonsmoker, even if you prefer this particular cigarette).

"Intertemporal bargaining" (Ainslie, 1975, 1992, 2001) provides an account of how individuals unite "particular actions ... under a common rule" (Sully, 1884). The flavor of this model can be conveyed by what philosophers call a "thought experiment." Consider a smoker who is preparing to initiate abstinence, but currently craves a cigarette. Suppose an angel whispers in her ear that it is a forgone conclusion that she is destined to smoke a pack a day from tomorrow on. Given this certainty, she would, we think, have no incentive to turn down the desired cigarette – it would seem pointless. What if the destiny revealed by the angel was instead that she was never to smoke again from tomorrow on? Here, too, there seems to be little incentive left to turn down the cigarette – it would be harmless. Fixing future smoking choices in either direction evidently makes smoking the dominant current choice. Only if future smoking is in doubt does a current abstention seem worth the effort. But why should fixing future smoking behavior make a difference to the choice at hand? In normal circumstances, there is no necessary connection between current and future choices anyway. One literally makes one choice at a time. However, self-control evidently is in some important way related to the conception that more than "just one" episode is in the balance with a given choice.

While the above example may provide some *prima facie* evidence that perceiving a connection between current choices and future choices is relevant to self-control, it also raises questions. In particular, why does the bundling of future choices together with a current single choice diminish impulsivity, and what mechanism underlies spontaneous bundling? With regard to the first question, less steep temporal discounting when future choices are bundled with current choices is predicted by the hyperbolic temporal discount function. While value declines dramatically when a relatively small delay is added to an immediate reward, the effect of adding a similar additional delay to a reward that is already much delayed is very small: $100 now may be far better than $100 in 3 months, but what is the difference between $100 in 6 years and the same in 6 years and 3 months? The relatively flat discounting of rewards when delay is already large implies a potential for great increases in value if a series of expected future rewards are added together – and there is good evidence that the discounted values of series of rewards are additive (Mazur, 1997). Unlike exponential curves, hyperbolic curves level off with longer delays. As such, the added value from a series of alternative rewards, if bundled together, will favor the LL rewards increasingly as the series lengthens (Figure 13.3).

Experiments with both human and rodent subjects confirm a greater

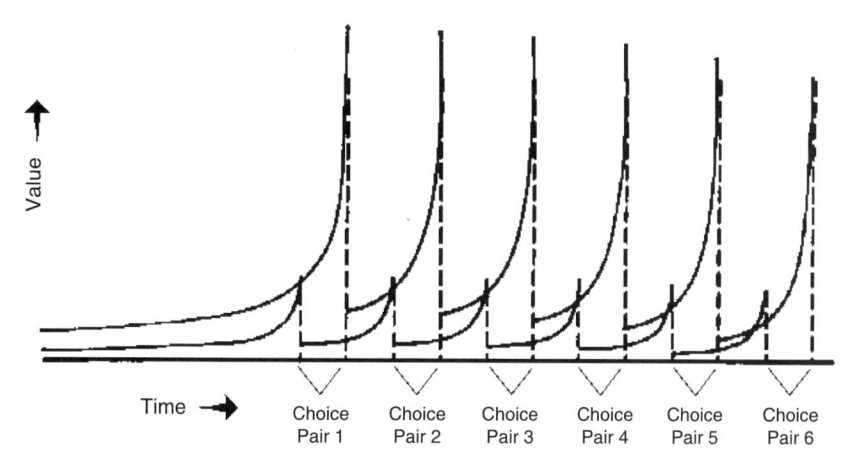

Figure 13.3 Summed hyperbolic curves from a series of larger–later rewards and a series of smaller–sooner alternatives (vertical dashed lines). Each curve depicts the summed discounted values of all future (more to the right) rewards in the series. Thus the curves of choice pair 1 are the sum of curves 1–6, and the curves of choice pair 2 are the sum of 2–6, etc. As the series gets longer and the summed curves peak higher above the current rewards, the initial period of temporary preference (the period in which the smaller–sooner curve is higher than its larger–later alternative) shrinks to zero. (Figure modified from Ainslie, 2001, p. 83).

tolerance for delay with bundled rewards. Kirby and Guastello (2001) gave college students choices between smaller and earlier rewards (SS) and larger but more delayed alternatives (LL), both with money and food. In one condition, the choice was made five times, each time separated by a week. In another condition, the choice was made between the two alternatives up front and for all five weeks at once. As predicted from the summation of hyperbolically discounted rewards, preference for the LL alternative was increased in the condition in which a series of choices was bundled together. Indeed, when Kirby and Guastello merely suggested to student subjects that the subjects' current choices might serve as predictions of their future choices, preference for LL alternatives increased, although not as much as when the experimenters bundled the choices directly (Kirby & Guastello, 2001).

In a recent study, the same phenomenon of decreased impulsive choice with bundling was demonstrated in rats (Ainslie & Monterosso, 2003). Eight rats were run through two conditions of a procedure designed to determine how much immediate sugar water was equal in value to a delayed standard reward of 150 ml after a 3 second interval. In one condition of the procedure, choices were made on a trial-by-trial basis while in another condition every choice determined the reward that would be delivered for three consecutive trials. As predicted by hyperbolic discounting, preference for the LL alternative was greater for all subjects in the bundled condition.

Of course, unlike the case of the rats described above, self-control requires the individual to spontaneously bundle future choices with current choices. What mechanism underlies spontaneous bundling? An astute person is aware that preferences are volatile. The best way to predict behavior in the face of a future temptation is to see what occurs with a similar temptation in the present. Consider a smoker whose preference for cigarettes is roughly described by Figure 13.2B. That is, while she prefers smoking in the immediate future, she also prefers nonsmoking in the more distant future. If she is deciding today on a plan for her entire smoking future, the dominant option is to choose to smoke in the near future, but plan to abstain thereafter. To make concrete, consider the near future "January," and thereafter "February" onwards. So our smoker decides she will smoke in January and not smoke from February onwards. But what happens in February? Without bundling, in February she will simply change her mind, since now the dominant plan in terms of discounted payoffs is to smoke in February and quit from March onwards. But of course, the same reversal left unchecked would occur when March becomes the present.

By April she may see the pattern of unrealized plans. She may notice her preference to stop smoking in May looks just like last month's preference to stop smoking in April and, ultimately, the plan may lose credibility. She may think something like "If I break last month's plan to not smoke in April, I am going to do the same next month with my current plan to not smoke in May." The credibility of attaining abstinence from May and beyond may thus depend upon not smoking in April. If, for simplicity, we consider her credibility to herself to be all or none, then our smoker who sees her situation in this way is left with the *de facto* options of smoking from the present onwards versus not smoking from the present onwards. If the lifetime of not smoking is preferred when given such a conception, the product is a "personal rule" (Ainslie, 1992, 2001) such as "I cannot smoke any cigarettes." The expectation of smoking future is therein tied to one's own adherence, or, more accurately, one's own perceptions of her adherence to her rule in the present.

The current choice may thus function as a test case. An individual thereby looks principled, but what literally happens is that her successive selves are engaged in a situation similar to a repeated prisoner's dilemma, which they come to solve in the same way as tacit interpersonal bargainers. Each expects future selves to perceive the current choice as a precedent for cooperation or defection, and this expectation adds to those incentives that depend on that choice alone (see Ainslie & Monterosso, 2002). In this regard, repeated prisoners' dilemma between individuals has been used to model phenomena related to impulse control (Monterosso et al., 2002).

In principle, personal rules make it possible for a person never to prefer small early alternatives at the expense of the series of larger later ones. She may successfully keep temptations nearby without succumbing to them; however, although she may always prefer a series of LL rewards to the SS one at hand, she must even more strongly prefer to have both. The danger is no longer one of the poorer reward coming so close that she will suddenly choose it, but of her finding a credible distinction between this choice and the other members of the series that form the greater part of her expected outcome. Proximity is still a contributor to her temptation, of course, but the deciding factor is no longer whether a prior commitment is too weak but whether a tentative loophole currently looks to her like she could get away with it. The person will not experience this situation as the exotic voyage past some Siren or other, but as a simultaneous struggle between two ways of conceiving a choice. Her rules have enabled her to live in close proximity to her temptations, but while she is there the struggle will be continuous rather than episodic. Lapses will occur through loopholes, variously clever and inept, rather than through a global shift of preference in favor of the forbidden activity. A person is apt to express preference for the course of action required by her rule even as she is evading it, as Sjoberg and Johnson (1978) found in their study of smoking lapses.

Neuropsychology of impulsive choice

In the previous discussion, we have implied a specific relationship between temporal discounting and self-control. Temporal discounting refers to devaluation as a function of delay. Self-control is not the absence of this, but rather specific processes that the organism (in some cases probably only humans) engages in which enable the attainment of LL rewards that would otherwise be lost to temporary preference reversal. In our discussion of the relevant neuropsychological literature, we follow this same scheme; we begin with neuropsychological literature that appears to relate directly to the motivational influence of expected delayed consequences (i.e., temporal discounting). From there we turn to the reviewed mechanisms of self-control, and consider how individual differences in neuropsychological functioning might relate to individual differences in the capacity for engaging in these mechanisms.

Neuropsychology of temporal discounting: Focus on the ventromedial prefrontal cortex

Over the last decade, and especially over the last five years, researchers have sought to clarify the degree to which ventromedial prefrontal cortex (VMPFC) mediates the valuation of delayed rewards. The VMPFC sector includes both the gyrus rectus and the mesial half of the orbital gyri, as well as the inferior half of the medial prefrontal surface, from its most caudal aspect to its most rostral in the frontal pole. Mesial sectors of areas 10 and 11, areas 12, 13, and 25, and subgenual sectors of areas 24 and 32 of Brodmann are included in this sector (Damasio, 1995). Interest in the relationship with VMPFC function and motivation for delayed rewards has grown out of Antonio Damasio and Antoine Bechara's work with VMPFC lesion patients. Patients with lesions in the VMPFC do not typically present with impaired performance on standard neuropsychological measures of frontal lobe functioning. However, "real-life" impairments in decision-making and social behavior have been well documented in these individuals (Bechara, Damasio, Damasio, & Anderson, 1994, Bechara, Damasio, Damasio, & Lee, 1999, Bechara, Tranel, & Damasio, 2000; Mavaddat, Kirkpatrick, Rogers, & Sahakian, 2000; Rogers et al., 1999a; Tranel, Bechara, & Damasio, 2000). Damasio describes the prototypical VMPFC lesion patient as being:

> controlled largely by immediate prospects and indeed appear insensitive to the future. This suggests that [they] suffer from a profound exaggeration of what may be a normal basic tendency, to go for the now rather than bank on the future . . . We might describe the predicament of these patients as a "myopia for the future" . . .
>
> (Damasio, Tranel, & Damasio, 1991, p. 217)

Damasio and colleagues suggest that the functional basis of the deficits observed in VMPFC patients is a failure to achieve a visceral reaction ("somatic marker") in response to "thoughts" about rewarding or punishing events that are not currently present in the immediate environment (Bechara et al., 1999). This is consistent with the anatomy of the VMPFC, which has dense interconnections with limbic structures known to govern emotional responses (Derryberry & Tucker, 1992). VMPFC patients may thus lack the requisite substrates for turning abstract knowledge of future consequences into emotional/limbic responses. Consistent with this hypothesis, VMPFC patients show blunted physiological responses to pictures depicting emotionally laden scenes (Damasio, Grabowski, Frank, Galaburda, & Damasio, 1994).

It is worth pointing out that while the behavioral syndrome seen in VMPFC lesion patients may be related to "impulsivity" in the behavioral economic sense of steep temporal discounting, their behavior is quite divergent from "impulsivity" in the sense used by personality and clinical researchers. Far from being impetuous decision-makers, VMPFC lesion patients show a propensity to be indecisive about even trivial decisions (Damasio gives the example of a VMPFC lesion patient who could not decide which of two routes to take on the drive home from his visit to the laboratory). Similarly, impulsivity is sometimes associated with an inability to sustain attention (Dickman, 1993); VMPFC patients, by contrast, have trouble *breaking* attention. Damasio writes, "When the job called for interrupting an activity and turning to another, [a VMPFC lesion patient] might persist nonetheless, seemingly losing sight of his main goal." (Damasio et al., 1991, p. 36).

Iowa and Cambridge Gambling Tasks

Despite their functional impairment, VMPFC patients perform normally on most neuropsychological test batteries (Damasio et al., 1994). Because traditional neuropsychological tests, particularly measures of executive function, are relatively insensitive to the functional impairments displayed by VMPFC patients, Damasio's group set out to devise a neuropsychological test sensitive to VMPFC-related deficits. They developed the "Iowa Gambling Task" (Bechara, et al., 1994; Bechara, Damasio, Tranel, & Anderson, 1998; Bechara, Damasio, Tranel, & Damasio, 1997; Bechara, Tranel, Damasio, & Damasio, 1996; Bechara et al., 1999), which requires participants to repeatedly choose cards from four decks (sometimes using computerized decks). The decks vary in terms of expected payoff and expected penalty. The payoffs are designed so that decks with larger immediate gains also have much larger intermittent penalties ("bad decks"), while decks with smaller immediate gains also have sufficiently smaller intermittent penalties such that they are "good decks." Although this scheme does not literally pit short-term interests against long-term interests (the expected value of any number of bad deck choices is negative and the expected value of any number of good deck choices is positive), participants may conceive of the payoffs of bad decks as individually more attractive, while viewing good decks as, as one research participant from Monterosso et al. (2001) put it, the "slow and steady best option" in the long-run. VMPFC patients tend to choose many more cards from "bad decks" than controls.

In some studies using the task, skin conductance response (SCR) levels were recorded while the task was being performed. While the SCRs of VMPFC patients are normal in *response* to the rewards and penalties they receive, they are severely blunted during the *anticipation* of those rewards relative to controls (Bechara et al., 1997). Tranel, Bechara, and Denburg (2002) observed a similar blunting of anticipatory SCR in unilateral VMPFC lesion with damage in the right but not left hemisphere.

In the Iowa Gambling Task, participants are not directly shown the payoff structure of the task. While this uncertainty may enhance the face validity of the task (real life uncertainties rarely come with exact probabilities attached), the lack of specified contingencies makes the functional interpretation of poor performance on the Gambling Task ambiguous. For example, an individual may choose from inferior decks either because he is failing to take long-range interests into account or because he is *unaware* of the actual contingencies. In part motivated by this concern, Rogers and colleagues designed another task to be sensitive to VMPFC functioning, in which contingencies were made explicit. In their "Cambridge Gambling Task," participants are asked to make gambles among choices in which odds explicitly favor one of the available options. While the outcomes of individual trials may be uncertain, performance is optimized if participants choose the option with better odds on every trial. Compared to controls, VMPFC patients (but not patients with damage to the dorsolateral prefrontal cortex) deliberate longer on their choices, and choose the lower probability option on significantly more trials (Rogers et al., 1999b).

Iowa and Cambridge Gambling Tasks in drug-abusing populations

The performances of substance-abusing populations and controls have been compared on both the Iowa Gambling Task and the Cambridge Gambling Task. In a comparison of 30 polysubstance abusers and 24 drug-naive controls, drug abusers made significantly more high-reward/higher-punishment choices than did controls on the Iowa Gambling Task (Grant, Contoreggi, & London, 2000). Based on this pattern of results, the authors conjectured that the "... bias towards immediate rewards despite even more substantial long-term adverse consequences, reflects dysfunction of the [VMPFC]." (Grant, Contoreggi, & London, 1997, p. 1943). A similar deficit in performance on the Iowa Gambling Task has been reported among alcohol and stimulant abusers (Bechara, Dolan, Denburg, Hindes, Anderson, & Nathan, 2001), opiate-dependent tobacco smokers (Rotheram-Fuller, Shoptaw, Berman, & London, 2004), and marijuana users (Whitlow et al., 2004).

Rogers et al. (1999a) compared performance on the Cambridge Gambling Task of chronic amphetamine users, chronic opioid users, and control subjects. Similar to VMPFC patients, chronic amphetamine abusers deliberated longer and chose unfavorable gambles on significantly more rounds than controls. Chronic opiate users also differed from control subjects in terms of deliberation time, but not in terms of the choices they made (Rogers et al., 1999a).

While the poor performance of drug-abusing populations on the Iowa and Cambridge Gambling Tasks is consistent with the idea that these populations have poor VMPFC functioning, it certainly should not be taken as conclusive on this point. First, the relationship between the task and life behavior is not well established, as convergent validity data are still rather limited. Moreover, the tasks are complex, and so the sources of variability in performance may vary greatly. Bechara and colleagues have reported poor performance on amygdala-lesion populations similar in magnitude to that observed in VMPFC lesion populations (Bechara et al., 1999). And furthermore, some (less striking) deficits are observed in patients with more posterior frontal lesions (Bechara et al., 1998). Thus while VMPFC impairment appears to be sufficient to disrupt performance on the tasks, it does not appear to be necessary.

Although the deficits on the Iowa Gambling Task are theorized to possibly reflect "inability to assess future consequences" (Grant et al., 2000, p. 1185), it is not clear whether variability in performance on the task, as well as on the Cambridge Gambling Task, is well correlated with temporal discount rate measurements. To our knowledge, the only data correlating performance on the measures were collected among a small group ($n=32$) of cocaine-dependent individuals (Monterosso et al., 2001). A modest, significant correlation was observed between bad deck choices on the Iowa Gambling Task and steeper temporal discounting ($r=.36$), while reaction time but not choices on the Cambridge Gambling Task was similarly modestly correlated with temporal discounting ($r=.33$). It is noteworthy that performances on the Iowa and Cambridge Gambling tasks were not significantly correlated with each other in that small sample of cocaine-dependent participants.

Caveats regarding the role of the VMPFC

Mapping the VMPFC as the substrate of motivation for delayed consequences is assailable on a number of grounds. First, the region is large and, as suggested by the multitude of Brodman areas included, it is heterogeneous in terms of cytotechtonic make-up. Doubtlessly the VMPFC is functionally heterogeneous. At the same time, more sophisticated analyses taking a systems approach to the topic of motivation look at the role of the VMPFC in conjunction with other regions, especially, though not exclusively, in the striatum. For example, Wagar and Thagard's (2004) model of cognitive-affective processing hypothesizes that the VMPFC provides cognitive information about contingencies, while the amygdala provides emotional information, and both of these inputs are critically integrated in the nucleus accumbens. The critical role posited for the nucleus accumbens is particularly interesting in light of data indicating that lesion of that region in rats (and not two of its primary cortical afferents, the anterior cingulate cortex and medial prefrontal cortex) results in greater preference for SS rewards in a delay-discounting procedure (Cardinal, Pennicott, Sugathapala, Robbins, & Everitt, 2001). Furthermore, a study of human subjects making intertemporal choices while undergoing functional magnetic resonance imaging (fMRI) recently reported that VMPFC activation was observed in the presence of an "immediate alternative" in the choice pair, and not when both alternatives in the pair were delayed (McClure, Laibson, Loewenstein, & Cohen, 2004). However, the rewards used in that study were a gift certificate for Amazon.com, so it is arguable that these rewards were not literally immediate (Ainslie & Monterosso, 2004). The same study observed activation in the lateral prefrontal cortex and the parietal cortex in association with intertemporal decision-making more generally. Interestingly, using cell recording, Paul Glimcher and colleagues have observed single cells in the parietal cortex of monkeys that fire in correspondence to the value of expected reward (see Glimcher, 2003, chapter 10). So while the VMPFC appears to play an important role in the motivation for delayed expectancies, it may be a far from simple one.

Neuropsychology of self-control

The behavioral economic mechanisms of self-control described above – precommitment and intertemporal bargaining – reflect complex management of behaviors. With the exception of precommitment in situations where a precommitting alternative is made highly salient, they probably are exclusively human phenomena. We know of no existing work that explicitly relates these mechanisms to underlying cognitive capacities, as conceived by neuropsychology, and we think there is important potential for such an attempt. We offer some hypotheses, as well as consider some existing data that may be relevant. In particular, we conjecture that the executive functions of working memory, response inhibition, and (more speculatively) episodic memory each may be related to the application of mechanisms of self-control.

Working memory is taxed in self-control

Working memory is a limited-capacity system, responsible for the maintenance and manipulation information within attention that contributes to a wide range of cognitive operations (Baddeley, 1996a, 1996b; Ragland et al., 2002). The cognitive processing hypothesized to underlie choice bundling requires attentional shifting between several types of information (i.e., the value of the immediate temptation, the value of future abstinence, past episodes that bear on the current situation, and estimates of future likely behavior given either choice in the present setting). Given these computational demands, it is plausible that variability in working memory capacity is a determinant of variability in effective choice bundling.

Although not directly tested, there is evidence that supports this hypothesis. Finn and colleagues have argued that working memory plays a critical role in substance abuse decisions by facilitating "the shifting of influence on decisions from high-salient stimuli to less salient stimuli" (Finn & Hall, 2004, p. 578). With respect to the present context, the reward of drug for a dependent individual is sure to be the most salient contingency at least some of the time, and so the weighing of alternate considerations is apt to tax working memory.

One way to establish the involvement of working memory in a behavioral process is through the use of a secondary extrinsic memory load in a dual-task paradigm (e.g., Ashcraft & Kirk, 2001; Baddeley, 1996b). On this approach, if the additional tax on working memory undermines performance of the primary task, it can be inferred that the primary task has some reliance on working memory. Hinson, Jameson, and Whitney (2003) used this approach to assess whether working memory was taxed in an intertemporal choice task much like the ones described above using hypothetical and real monetary rewards. As predicted by the authors and by the idea that self-control taxes working memory, the dual-task manipulation increased the steepness by which value was discounted with delay.

Ward and Mann (2000) observed a possibly related finding using a more ecologically valid paradigm. Their experiment measured the spontaneous consumption of milkshake while a group of restrained eaters and a group of unrestrained eaters were under either high or low cognitive load. In the high-cognitive load condition, participants tried to remember a series of art slides – a task that greatly relies on active rehearsal thus taxing working memory. Among unrestrained eaters, consumption was reduced in the high-cognitive load condition, perhaps because the task distracted attention away from the provided food. However, for restrained eaters, the opposite pattern was observed; this group consumed *more* milkshake under the greater cognitive load. It is possible that this effect was mediated by the disrupting effect of working memory load of the active intertemporal bargaining processes necessary to continually restrain eating.

In the domain of substance abuse, Finn and Hall (2004) recently observed that among individuals high in social deviance (a group for whom negative consequences may be of relatively low salience) lower working-memory capacity, as assessed by a digit span task, predicted more alcohol-related problems. It may be the case that among this group the limitations on working-memory capacity resulted in a diminished tendency to deploy choice-bundling processes that weigh against problem drinking behavior.

Response inhibition may facilitate intertemporal bargaining and intrapsychic precommitment

Consider a smoker who would like to quit smoking and who is offered a cigarette. There is direct and rapid consideration supporting motivation to smoke – the individual need only access the association between the stimulus and the positive feelings associated with it (CS-US). In contrast, bundling effects that might weigh against taking the cigarette are slower, and less direct. Even if they are deployed, the requisite processing for choice bundling is likely to produce expectancies that might oppose smoking hundreds of milliseconds subsequent to the CS-US link favoring smoking. Given this latency, these mechanisms may depend on a more basic effective mechanism of "response inhibition," which we define as "the intentional prevention of a behavior that is underway or that is otherwise automatically evoked (i.e., "pre-potent") (Monterosso, Aron, Cordova, Xu, & London, 2005). Response inhibition capacity is assessed with tasks such as the Stop-Signal Task (Logan, Schachar, & Tannock, 1997), which measures how long it takes an individual to abort a simple motor response already underway.

Response inhibition may play a more direct role in intrapsychic methods of precommitment, especially attentional control. If attending to a particular stimulus is identified as creating a risk of preference reversal, adept response inhibition may be critical in keeping attentional control from the stimulus (or thought), or at least keeping it from lingering there for enough time to cause the reversal. Response inhibition may thus be critical for intrapsychic precommitment and intertemporal bargaining because suppression of rapid, conditioned responses favoring the SS temptation may allow time for slower mechanisms favoring self-control to guide behavior (Jentsch & Taylor, 1999). Consistent with this conjecture, substance abusers with comorbid attention deficit hyperactivity disorder (ADHD) – a population marked by impairment of inhibitory control (Nigg, 2001) – have poorer treatment outcomes than matched substance-dependent individuals without ADHD (Biederman, Wilens, Mick, Faraone, & Spencer, 1998; Carroll & Rounsaville, 1993; Whitmore, Mikulich, Thompson, Riggs, Aarons, & Crowley, 1997).

Episodic memory and self-control

Episodic memory refers to a neurocognitive system that enables human beings to remember past personal events. As conceived by Tulving (2002), episodic memory is tantamount to the individual "traveling back in time" and reexperiencing events. Interestingly, amnesia that is specific to such episodic memory is associated not just with an inability to mentally travel back in time, but with an inability to project oneself into the future as well. For example, a patient known as K.C., after a motorcycle injury, suffered both an "utter inability to remember any events, circumstances or situations from his own life" (Tulving, 2002, p. 14) as well as an inability to project himself in the future. Tulving stated, "Thus, when asked, he cannot tell the questioner what he is going to do later on that day, or the day after, or at any time in the rest of his life."(p. 14).

It is likely that for such an individual the mechanisms of self-control would be profoundly limited. In situations that are highly repetitive in which a salient precommitting option is available (as with Ainslie's pigeons, 1974), an absence of episodic memory should not be a barrier to self-control. However, a lack of episodic memory might preclude precommitment in situations that contain some measure of novelty, since precommitment there would require drawing on projection of oneself in the future and episodic memory of situations conceived as similar, both to identify the risk of preference reversal (e.g., "that is just what I was thinking yesterday and then last night I binged") and the precommitting solution (e.g., "If I break-up with my boyfriend who smokes crack, I think I can stay away from it"). It is possible that even within the normal range of variation of episodic memory, better episodic memory may be associated with more effective deployment of precommitment.

With the increased subtlety of the intertemporal reasoning deployed in choice bundling, the demands on episodic memory are even greater. Recall that in domains where self-control is required, the most attractive option given hyperbolic discounting is always "binge-today, diet tomorrow." Here, self-control resides first in the conception that this is not a credible alternative. Again, episodic memory of past plans may provide the starting point (e.g., that is what I said yesterday), but, in this case, whether or not the individual binges is hypothesized to rest on an implicit equation that includes the individual's estimate of how likely it is that her future self will diet if she binges today (a probability of zero at the limit, but certainly not zero always) versus the likelihood that her future self will diet if she diets today (a probability of one at the limit, but in domains of struggle probably much lower typically). The difference between the second probability and the first must be sufficiently large to outweigh the opportunity cost of forgoing the reward of the immediate binge. Furthermore, as discussed above, the real threat in domains where bundling is evident is rationalization. If there is something unique about a current temptation (e.g., it is my birthday, or I had a particularly bad day today), perhaps it is possible that a binge today will not portend future binging. After all, it is not my birthday tomorrow. This approach is a gamble – if tomorrow's self remembers the episode not as a true special case, but rather as a failure to abide by her diet, the estimated probability that her future self will diet tomorrow if she diets today may drop enough to undermine resolve altogether. To be sure, the individual always exists as a momentary self, but the bargaining process underlying sophisticated self-control resides in a subtle recursive inferential process between episodic memory of past selves and projected future selves. For the individual with weak episodic memory, and thus only dim representations of each, the force of the immediate temptation may be unlikely to be offset.

Final comment

In the past decade, an emergent literature has utilized the concepts of behavioral economics to explain why substance-dependent individuals are unable to maintain abstinence or quit, even when the consequences of substance misuse are clear to them. The resulting framework extends well beyond simple temporal discount rate assessment to mechanisms of self-control available to cognitively sophisticated organisms. Behavioral economics does not integrate cognition into explanation of temporal discounting. We speculate that:

(1) Variability in deployment of self-control mechanisms is related to real-world problems, including substance abuse and dependence.
(2) Individual differences in neuropsychological functioning (perhaps working memory, response inhibition and episodic memory) mediate individual differences in the capacity to deploy self-control mechanisms.

By integrating the behavioral economics and neurocognition, a more comprehensive understanding of addiction and recovery may be achieved.

Acknowledgment

This work was supported by NIH Grant K01 DA0051-01A1.

References

Ainslie, G. (1974). Impulse control in pigeons. *Journal of the Experimental Analysis of Behavior, 21,* 485–489.
Ainslie, G. (1975). Specious reward: a behavioral theory of impulsiveness and impulse control. *Psychological Bulletin, 82,* 463–496.
Ainslie, G. (1982). A behavioral economic approach to the defense mechanisms: Freud's energy theory revisited. *Social Science Information, 21,* 735–779.
Ainslie, G. (1992). *Picoeconomics: The strategic interaction of successive motivational states within the person.* New York: Cambridge University Press.
Ainslie, G. (2001). *Breakdown of will.* New York: Cambridge University Press.
Ainslie, G., & Haendel, V. (1983). The motives of the will. In K. A. Druley. E. Gottheil, T. E. Skoloda, & H. M. Waxman (Eds.), *Etiologic aspects of alcohol and drug abuse* (pp. 119–140). Springfield, IL: Charles C. Thomas.
Ainslie, G., & Monterosso, J. (2002). Hyperbolic discounting lets empathy be a motivated process. In N. Heather & R. E. Vuchinich (Eds.), *Choice, behavioral economics and addiction* (pp. 35–62). New York: Elsevier Science.
Ainslie, G., & Monterosso, J. (2003). Building blocks of self-control: increased tolerance for delay with bundled rewards. *Journal of the Experimental Analysis of Behavior, 79,* 37–48.
Aristotle (1984). *The complete works of aristotle* (ed. by J. Barnes). Princeton: Princeton University Press.
Ashcraft, M. H., & Kirk, E. P. (2001). The relationships among working memory, math anxiety, and performance. *Journal of Experimental Psychology: General, 130,* 224–237.
Baddeley, A. (1996a). Exploring the Central Executive. *Quarterly Journal of Experimental Psychology, 49A,* 5–28.
Baddeley, A. (1996b). The fractionation of working memory. *Proceedings of the National Academy of Science, 93,* 13468–13472.
Bechara, A., Damasio, A. R., Damasio, H., & Anderson, S. W. (1994). Insensitivity to future consequences following damage to human prefrontal cortex. *Cognition, 50,* 7–15.

Bechara, A., Damasio, H., Damasio, A. R., & Lee, G. P. (1999). Different contributions of the human amygdala and ventromedial prefrontal cortex to decision-making. *Journal of Neuroscience, 19*, 5473–5481.

Bechara, A., Damasio, H., Tranel, D., & Anderson, S. W. (1998). Dissociation of working memory from decision making within the human prefrontal cortex. *Journal of Neuroscience, 18*, 428–437.

Bechara, A., Damasio, H., Tranel, D., & Damasio, A. R. (1997). Deciding advantageously before knowing the advantageous strategy. *Science, 275*, 1293–1955.

Bechara, A., Dolan, S., Denburg, N., Hindes, A., Anderson, S. W., & Nathan, P. E. (2001). Decision-making deficits, linked to a dysfunctional ventromedial prefrontal cortex, revealed in alcohol and stimulant abusers. *Neuropsychologia, 39*, 376–389.

Bechara, A., Tranel, D., & Damasio, H. (2000). Characterization of the decision-making deficit of patients with ventromedial prefrontal cortex lesions. *Brain, 123*, 2189–2202.

Bechara, A., Tranel, D., Damasio, H., & Damasio, A. R. (1996). Failure to respond autonomically to anticipated future outcomes following damage to prefrontal cortex. *Cerebral Cortex, 6*, 215–225.

Becker, H. S. (1960). Notes on the concept of commitment. *American Journal of Sociology, 66*, 32–40.

Bickel, W. K., Odum, A. L., & Madden, G. J. (1999). Impulsivity and cigarette smoking: Delay discounting in current, never, and ex-smokers. *Psychopharmacology, 146*, 447–454.

Biederman, J., Wilens, T., Mick, E., Faraone, S., & Spencer, T. (1998). Does attention-deficit hyperactivity disorder impact the developmental course of drug and alcohol abuse and dependence? *Biological Psychiatry, 44*, 269–273.

Bohm, P. (1994). Time preference and preference reversal among experienced subjects: the effects of real payments. *Economic Journal, 104*, 1370–1378.

Bradshaw, C. M., & Szabadi, E. (1992). Choice between delayed reinforcers in a discrete-trials schedule: The effect of deprivation level. *Quarterly Journal of Experimental Psychology. B, Comparative and Physiological Psychology, 44B*, 1–16.

Bretteville-Jensen, A. L. (1999). Addiction and discounting. *Journal of Health Economics, 18*, 393–407.

Cairns, J., & van der Pol, M. (2000). Valuing future private and social benefits: The discounted utility model versus hyperbolic discounting models. *Journal of Economic Psychology, 21*, 191–205.

Cardinal, R., Pennicott, D., Sugathapala, L., Robbins, T., & Everitt, B. (2001). Impulsive choice induced in rats by lesions of the nucleus accumbens core. *Science, 292*, 2499–2501.

Carroll, K. M., & Rounsaville, B. J. (1993). History and significance and childhood attention deficit disorder in treatment-seeking cocaine abusers. *Comprehensive Psychiatry, 34*, 75–82.

Chapman, G. B. (1996). Temporal discounting and utility for health and money. *Journal of Experimental Psychology: Learning, Memory, and Cognition, 22*, 771–791.

Chapman, G. B. (2000). Preferences for improving and declining sequences of health outcomes. *Journal of Behavioral Decision Making, 13*, 203–218.

Chapman, G. B., Brewer, N. T., Coups, E. J., Brownlee, S., Leventhal, H., & Levanthal, E. A. (2001). Value for the future and preventive health behavior. *Journal of Experimental Psychology: Applied, 7*, 235–250.

Cherek, D. R., Moeller, F. G., Schnapp, W., & Dougherty, D. M. (1997). Studies of violent and nonviolent male parolees: I. Laboratory and psychometric measurements of aggression. *Biological Psychiatry, 41*, 514–522.

Chesson, H., & Viscusi, W. K. (2000). The heterogeneity of time–risk tradeoffs. *Journal of Behavioral Decision Making, 13*, 251–258.

Cook, J. O., & Barnes, L. W., Jr. (1964). Choice of delay of inevitable shock. *Journal of Abnormal and Social Psychology, 68*, 669–672.

Corulla, W. J. (1987). A psychometric investigation of the Eysenck Personality Questionnaire (Revised) and its relationship to the I.7 Impulsiveness Questionnaire. *Personality and Individual Differences, 8*, 651–658.

Crean, J. P., de Wit, H., & Richards, J. B. (2000). Reward discounting as a measure of impulsive behavior in a psychiatric outpatient population. *Experimental and Clinical Psychopharmacology, 8*, 155–162.

Damasio, A. R., Tranel, D., & Damasio, H. C. (1991). Somatic markers and the guidance of behavior: Theory and preliminary testing. In H. S. Levin, H. M. Eisenberg and A. L. Benton (Eds.), *Frontal lobe function and dysfunction* (pp. 217–229). New York: Oxford University Press.

Damasio, H. (1995). *Human brain anatomy in computerized images.* New York: Oxford University Press.

Damasio, H., Grabowski, T., Frank, R., Galaburda, A. M., & Damasio, A. R. (1994). The return of Phineas Gage: clues about the brain from the skull of a famous patient. *Science, 264*, 1102–1105.

Derryberry, D., & Tucker, D. M. (1992). Neural mechanisms of emotion. *Journal of Consulting and Clinical Psychology, 60*, 329–338.

Dickman, S. J. (1990). Functional and dysfunctional impulsivity: Personality and cognitive correlates. *Journal of Personality and Social Psychology, 58*, 95–102.

Dickman, S. J. (1993). Impulsivity and information processing. In W. G. McCown & J. L. Johnson (Eds.), *The impulsive client: Theory, research, and treatment* (pp. 151–184). Washington, DC: American Psychological Association.

Evenden, J. (1999). Varieties of impulsivity. *Psychopharmacology. Special Impulsivity, 146*, 348–361.

Finn, P. R., & Hall, J. (2004). Cognitive ability and risk for alcoholism: Short-term memory capacity and intelligence moderate personality risk for alcohol problems. *Journal of Abnormal Psychology, 113*, 569–581.

Forzano, L. B., & Logue, A. W. (1994). Self-control in adult humans: Comparison of qualitatively different reinforcers. *Learning and Motivation, 25*, 65–82.

Freud, S. (1956). On the history of the psychoanalytic movement. *The standard edition of the complete works of Sigmund Freud.* London: Hogarth.

Friedman, M. (1953). *Essays in positive economics.* Chicago: University of Chicago Press.

Fuchs, V. R. (1982). Time preferences and health: An exploratory study. *Economic Aspects of Health.* Chicago, IL: University of Chicago Press.

Glimcher, P. W., & Rustichini, A. (2004). Neuroeconomics: The consilience of brain and decision. *Science, 306*, 447–452.

Grant, S., Contoreggi, C., & London, E. (1997). Drug abusers show impaired performance on a test of orbitofrontal function. *Society for Neuroscience, 23*, 1943.

Grant, S., Contoreggi, C., & London, E. D. (2000). Drug abusers show impaired performance in a laboratory test of decision making. *Neuropsychologia, 38*, 1180–1187.

Green, L., & Myerson, J. (1994). Temporal discounting and preference reversals in choice between delayed outcomes. *Psychonomic Bulletin and Review, 1*, 383–389.

Green, L., Myerson, J., & McFadden, E. (1997). Rate of temporal discounting decreases with amount of reward. *Memory and Cognition, 25*, 715–723.

Green, L., & Rachlin, H. (1996). Commitment using punishment. *Journal of the Experimental Analysis of Behavior, 65*, 593–601.

Hare, R. D. (1966). Preference for delay of shock as a function of its intensity and probability: Psychopathy and choice of immediate versus delayed punishment. *Psychonomic Science, 5*, 393–394.

Hinson, J. M., Jameson, T. L., & Whitney, P. (2003). Impulsive decision making and working memory. *Journal of Experimental Psychology: Learning, Memory, and Cognition, 29*, 298–306.

Jentsch, J. D., & Taylor, J. R. (1999). Impulsivity resulting from frontostriatal dysfunction in drug abuse: Implications for the control of behavior by reward-related stimuli. *Psychopharmacology. Special Impulsivity, 146*, 373–390.

Kahneman, D., & Tversky, A. (1979). Prospect theory: an analysis of decisions under risk. *Econometrica, 47*, 313–327.

Kant, I. (1793/1960). *Religion within the limits of reason alone.* New York: Harper & Row.

Kirby, K. N., & Guastello, B. (2001). Making choices in anticipation of similar future choices can increase self-control. *Journal of Experimental Psychology: Applied, 7*, 154–164.

Kirby, K. N., & Herrnstein, R. J. (1995). Preference reversals due to myopic discounting of delayed reward. *Psychological Science, 6*, 83–89.

Kirby, K. N., & Marakovic, N. N. (1996). Delay-discounting probabilistic rewards: Rates decrease as amounts increase. *Psychonomic Bulletin and Review, 3*, 100–104.

Kirby, K. N., Petry, N. M., & Bickel, W. K. (1999). Heroin addicts have higher discount rates for delayed rewards than non-drug-using controls. *Journal of Experimental Psychology: General, 128*, 78–87.

Loewenstein, G., & Prelec, D. (1992). Anomalies in intertemporal choice: Evidence and an interpretation. *Quarterly Journal of Economics* (*May*), 573–577.

Logan, G. D., Schachar, R., & Tannock, R. (1997) Impulsivity and inhibitory control. *Psychological Science, 8*, 60–64.

Logue, A. W., King, G. R., Chavarro, A., & Volpe, J. S. (1990). Matching and maximizing in a self-control paradigm using human subjects. *Learning and Motivation, 21*, 340–368.

Madden, G. J., Bickel, W. K., & Jacobs, E. A. (1999). Discounting of delayed rewards in opioid-dependent outpatients: Exponential or hyperbolic discounting functions? *Experimental and Clinical Psychopharmacology, 7*, 284–293.

Madden, G. J., Petry, N. M., Badger, G. J., & Bickel, W. K. (1997). Impulsive and self-control choices in opioid-dependent patients and non-drug-using control participants: drug and monetary rewards. *Experimental and Clinical Psychopharmacology, 5*, 256–262.

Mavaddat, N., Kirkpatrick, P. J., Rogers, R. D., & Sahakian, B. J. (2000). Deficits in decision-making in patients with aneurysms of the anterior communicating artery. *Brain, 123*, 2109–2117.

Mazur, J. (1987). An adjusting procedure for studying delayed reinforcement. In M. Commons, J. Mazur, J. Nevin, & H. Rachlin (Eds.), *The effect of delay and of intervening events on reinforcement value* (pp. 55–73). Hillsdale, NJ: Lawrence Erlbaum Associates.

Mazur, J. E. (1997). Choice, delay, probability, and conditioned reinforcement. *Animal Learning and Behavior, 25*, 131–147.

Mischel, H., & Mischel, W. (1983). The development of children's knowledge of self-control strategies. *Child Development, 54*, 603–619.

Mischel, W., & Grusec, J. (1967). Waiting for rewards and punishments: Effects of time and probability on choice. *Journal of Personality and Social Psychology, 5*, 24–31.

Mischel, W., Grusec, J., & Masters, J. C. (1969). Effects of expected delay time on the subjective value of rewards and punishments. *Journal of Personality and Social Psychology, 11*, 363–373.

Mischel, W., & Moore, B. (1980). The role of ideation in voluntary delay for symbolically-presented rewards. *Cognitive Therapy and Research, 4*, 211–221.

Mitchel, S. (1999). Measures of impulsivity in cigarette smokers and non-smokers. *Psychopharmacology, 146*, 455–464.

Monterosso, J., & Ainslie, G. (1999). Beyond discounting: possible experimental models of impulse control. *Psychopharmacology, 146*, 339–347.

Monterosso, J., Ainslie, G., Toppi-Mullen, P., & Gault, B. (2002). The fragility of cooperation: A false feedback study of a sequential iterated prisoner's dilemma. *Journal of Economic Psychology, 23*, 437–448.

Monterosso, J., Aron, A., Cordova, X., Xu, J., & London, E. (2005). Deficits in response inhibition associated with chronic methamphetamine abuse. *Drug and Alcohol Dependence, 79*, 273–277.

Monterosso, J., Ehrman, R., Napier, K. L., O'Brien, C. P., & Childress, A. R. (2001). Three decision-making tasks in cocaine-dependent patients: Do they measure the same construct? *Addiction, 96*, 1825–1837.

Navarick, D. (1982). Negative reinforcement and choice in humans. *Learning and Motivation, 13*, 361–377.

Nigg, J. T. (2001). Is ADHD a disinhibitory disorder? *Psychological Bulletin, 127*, 571–598.

Odum, A. L., Madden, G. J., Badger, G. J., & Bickel, W. K. (2000). Needle sharing in opioid-dependent outpatients: Psychological processes underlying risk. *Drug and Alcohol Dependence, 60*, 259–266.

Parker, J. D., Bagby, R. M., & Webster, C. D. (1993). Domains of the impulsivity construct: A factor analytic investigation. *Personality and Individual Differences, 15*, 267–274.

Patton, J. H., Stanford, M. S., & Barratt, E. S. (1995). Factor structure of the Barratt Impulsiveness Scale. *Journal of Clinical Psychology, 51*, 768–774.

Petry, N. M. (2001). Substance abuse, pathological gambling, and impulsiveness. *Drug and Alcohol Dependence, 63*, 29–38.

Premack, D. (1970). Mechanisms of self-control. In W. I. Hunt (Ed.), *Learning mechanisms and smoking* (pp. 107–125). Chicago: Aldine Publishing Company.

Ragland, J. D., Turetsky, B. I., Gur, R. C., Gunning-Dixon, F., Turner, T., Schroeder, L., et al. (2002). Working memory for complex figures: an fMRI comparison of letter and fractal n-back tasks. *Neuropsychology, 16*, 370–379.

Richards, J. B., Zhang, L., Mitchell, S. H., & de Wit, H. (1999). Delay or probability discounting in a model of impulsive behavior: Effect of alcohol. *Journal of the Experimental Analysis of Behavior, 71*, 121–143.

Roelofsma, P. H. M. P. (1996). Modelling intertemporal choices: An anomaly approach. *Acta Psychologica, 93*, 5–22.

Rogers, R. D., Everitt, B. J., Baldacchino, A., Blackshaw, A. J., Swainson, R., Wynne, K., et al. (1999a). Dissociable deficits in the decision-making cognition of chronic amphetamine abusers, opiate abusers, patients with focal damage to prefrontal cortex, and tryptophan-depleted normal volunteers: evidence for monoaminergic mechanisms. *Neuropsychopharmacology, 20*, 322–339.

Rogers, R. D., Owen, A. M., Middleton, H. C., Williams, E. J., Pickard, J. D., Sahakian, B. J. et al. (1999b). Choosing between small, likely rewards and large, unlikely rewards activates inferior and orbital prefrontal cortex. *Journal of Neuroscience, 19*, 9029–9038.

Rotheram-Fuller, E., Shoptaw, S., Berman, S. M., & London, E. (2004). Impaired performance in a test of decision-making by opiate-dependent tobacco smokers. *Drug and Alcohol Dependence, 73*, 79–86.

Simon, H. (1978). *The sciences of the artificial.* Karl Taylor Compton Lectures. Cambridge: MIT Press.

Sjoberg, L., & Johnson, T. (1978). Trying to give up smoking: A study of volitional breakdowns. *Addictive Behaviors, 3*, 149–164.

Skinner, B. F. (1953). *Science and human behavior.* New York: Macmillan.

Sully, J. (1884). *Outlines of psychology.* New York: Appleton.

Thaler, R. (1981). Some empirical evidence on dynamic inconsistency. *Economic Letters, 8*, 201–207.

Tranel, D., Bechara, A., & Denburg, N. (2002). Assymmetric funtional roles of right and left ventromedial prefrontal cortices in social conduct, decision-making, and emotional processing. *Cortex, 38*, 589–612.

Tranel, D., Bechara, A., & Damasio, A. R. (2000). Decision making and the somatic marker hypothesis. In M. S. Gazzaniga (Ed.), *The new cognitive neurosciences* (2nd ed., pp. 192–214). Cambridge: MIT Press.

Tulving, E. (2002). Episodic memory. *Annual. Review of Psychology, 53*, 1–25.

van der Pol, M., & Cairns, J. (2001). Estimating time preferences for health using discrete choice experiments. *Social Science and Medicine, 52*, 1459–1470.

Vuchinich, R. E., & Simpson, C. A. (1998). Hyperbolic temporal discounting in social drinkers and problem drinkers. *Experimental and Clinical Psychopharmacology, 6*, 292–305.

Vuchinich, R. E., & Tucker, J. A. (1988). Contributions from behavioral theories of choice to an analysis of alcohol abuse. *Journal of Abnormal Psychology, 97*, 181–195.

Wagar, B., & Thagard, P. (2004) Spiking Phineas Gage: A neurocomputational theory of cognitive-affective integration in decision making. *Psychological Review, 111*, 67–79.

Wallace, C. (1979). The effects of delayed rewards, social pressure, and frustration on the response of opiate addicts. *NIDA Monograph Series, 25*, 6–25.

Ward, A., & Mann, T. (2000). Don't mind if I do: Disinhibited eating under cognitive load. *Journal of Personality and Social Psychology, 78*, 753–763.

Whitlow, C. T., Liguori, A., Livengood, L. B., Hart, S. L., Mussat-Whitlow, B. J., Lamborn, C. M., et al. (2004). Long-term heavy marijuana users make costly decisions on a gambling task. *Drug and Alcohol Dependence, 76*, 107–111.

Whitmore, E. A., Mikulich, S. K., Thompson, L. L., Riggs, P. D., Aarons, G. A., & Crowley, T. J. (1997). Influences on adolescent substance dependence: conduct disorder, depression, attention deficit hyperactivity disorder, and gender. *Drug and Alcohol Dependence, 47*, 87–97.

14 The influence of environmental context on the effects of drugs of abuse

Jason M. Uslaner, Hans S. Crombag, and Terry E. Robinson

Drug addiction is not for everyone. The vast majority of individuals who experiment with potentially addictive drugs do not become addicted. Even for the drugs with the greatest addictive potential, such as tobacco and heroin, less than one-third of the individuals who try these drugs go on to become compulsive users or addicts (Anthony, Warner, & Kessler, 1994; Wagner & Anthony, 2002). This fact does not minimize the seriousness of substance abuse and addiction; for the unfortunate minority, substance dependence is an extremely unpleasant state. What this fact does make clear, however, is that the psychological and physiological effects of drugs differ greatly between individuals (Deroche-Gamonet, Belin, & Piazza, 2004; Robinson, 2004). Why do some who experiment with drugs become addicts, while others can use drugs casually without any signs of addiction?

Undoubtedly, this is one of the most important questions facing drug addiction research. While the influence of genetic variables is well documented, heritability (h^2) only accounts for a portion of the variance, with large between-drug and between-study differences: h^2 ranges from 0 to ~0.8 (Bierut et al., 1998; Pedersen, 1981; Tsuang et al. 1998; van den Bree, Johnson, Neale, & Pickens, 1998). Clearly, factors other than the primary pharmacological actions of the drug or the genetic makeup of the individual are important in determining drug effects.

One variable that has been generally overlooked by researchers examining the effects of drugs of abuse is the *environmental context* in which drugs are taken. Drug users do not generally self-administer drugs of abuse in laboratories or hospitals; however, one may form the wrong impression that they do while perusing the methods sections of most journal articles dedicated to the analysis of drug effects. In the world outside the experimental setting, addictive drugs are taken in a wide variety of environmental contexts, which can differ in terms of their physical attributes, the cultural norms, and the societal expectations surrounding the use and effects of a particular drug.

Given this discrepancy, it is reasonable to ask why most investigations aimed at elucidating the effects of drugs of abuse are conducted in laboratories or hospitals, where the rich context normally surrounding drug administration has been stripped away. Of course, experimental researchers offer a number of reasonable explanations for designing studies in this manner. For example, the controlled environment provided by a laboratory or hospital minimizes the likelihood that confounds will affect the study results. In contrast, naturalistic studies, in which drug users are examined in the environment in which they usually self-administer drug, are often confounded by uncontrollable variables. Moreover, the effects of drugs have long been assumed to result chiefly from their primary pharmacological actions. Drug effects are generally considered in terms of ligand–receptor interactions, and according to common thought these should not differ as a function of the environmental context in which drug administration takes place.

Contrary to this long-standing belief, accumulating evidence has shown that the effects produced by drugs of abuse vary dramatically as a function of the environmental context in which drugs are administered (Falk & Feingold, 1987). These findings have been documented across various types of study methodologies, including fieldwork, quasi-experimental studies, and experimental research in which the environment surrounding drug administration is systematically manipulated by the experimenter. These studies show that the subjective, cognitive, behavioral, physiological, and neurobiological effects of drugs are influenced by the environment in which they are administered. In other words, *all* of the major types of drug effects are influenced by the context surrounding drug administration.

Despite the evidence that environmental context influences the entire spectrum of drug effects, these findings have not been integrated into studies examining the neuropsychological consequences of drugs of abuse in humans nor in research aimed at developing pharmacotherapy for drug addiction. In this chapter we will describe some of the best characterized and most pronounced environmental influences on drug effects, highlight the implications of these findings, and suggest future studies in which these implications can be further explored. The chapter will begin by considering the results of some nonexperimental findings suggesting that environmental factors influence drug effects. Then, we will review the results of well-controlled experimental studies with human subjects, in which the environment of drug administration has been systematically manipulated in order to evaluate the effect of such manipulations on drug effects. Finally, we will examine the results of some preclinical work, which suggests that the environment of drug administration can have a profound influence on the neurobiological effects of drugs of abuse.

Nonexperimental studies

Cross-cultural examinations

Accounts suggesting that drug effects are influenced by the context in which drugs are taken originate from cross-cultural descriptions of the behavioral and subjective effects of drugs. These accounts provide a useful starting point for considering the influence of context because cross-cultural differences are much greater than the contextual variation one can create in a controlled laboratory setting.

Alcohol is a drug with a long history of use and wide geographic distribution, and therefore there is a large body of research documenting the influence of culture on the effects of alcohol (for reviews see MacAndrew & Edgerton, 1969; Marshall, 1979). This literature reveals that a simple dose–effect analysis, without consideration for contextual variables, does not adequately account for the behavioral and subjective changes produced by this drug.

For example, when not intoxicated, the Abipore people of Paraguay are described as very calm and quiet, "Nothing licentious, indecent, or uncourteous, is discoverable in their actions. In their daily meetings, all is quiet and orderly. Confused vociferations, quarrels or sharp words have no place there." (Dobrizhoffer, 1822, Vol. 3, p. 136, as cited in MacAndrew & Edgerton, 1969). During a drinking party, however, their behavior is strikingly different, "Disputes are frequent among them concerning preeminence in valour, which produce confused clamours, fighting ... and is sometimes carried on for many hours with much vociferation of the combatants, and no less effusion of blood" (Dobrizhoffer, 1822, Vol. 2, pp. 436–437, as cited in MacAndrew & Edgerton, 1969).

Despite these observations, it would be erroneous to conclude that alcohol promotes disinhibition or aggression. Indeed, in other communities with very different cultural norms and expectations regarding drug effects, alcohol induces behavior that contrast vividly with those observed among the Abipores. For example, the people of Ifaluk Island, part of the Carolines, display very different behavioral responses to alcohol, "Some of the men drink glass after glass in the course of an evening. A slightly bleary look about the eyes, and a tendency to be jovial or sentimentally friendly, were the only effects we noticed" (Burrows, 1957, p. 44, as cited in MacAndrew & Edgerton, 1969). Thus, it appears that alcohol can produce opposite effects, ranging from disinhibition and aggression to slight bleariness and joviality, depending on the environmental context in which it is consumed.

Of course, one does not have to travel to Paraguay or the Caroline Islands to realize the extent to which context can modulate the behavioral effects of alcohol. One can merely go to a local sports bar during a football match and observe a group of fans who have drunk a bit too much and compare their behavior to a young couple who drink a bit too much on a first date. The differences will be just as apparent.

Reports indicating that drug effects vary across cultures are not limited to alcohol. For example, the hallucinogenic effects of peyote and LSD are likewise dependent on the sociocultural context in which these drugs are taken (Aberle & Moore, 1991; Blum, 1964; Wallace, 1959), as are the subjective effects of THC (Du Toit, 1977; Falk & Feingold, 1987; Rubin & Comitas, 1975).

When the environmental context of the drug user changes

Although the cross-cultural studies described above are intriguing, it is difficult to determine whether the environmental context is directly modifying the effects of the drug being consumed. Other factors may be responsible, such as the degree to which one's culture affects developmental processes or genetic differences across cultures, which in turn may influence a drug's effects. In some cases, however, this ambiguity is minimized. Specifically, there are cases when the culture surrounding the drug user suddenly changes. If environmental context directly modulates the effects of drugs, then one would predict that such an abrupt shift in context would also result in an alteration in drug effects.

The best-known case describing a sudden change in the environment of a group of drug users is that of the numerous Vietnam soldiers who had used heroin while abroad, and then were brought back home to the United States when their tours of duty were completed. In this case, the majority of heroin-abusing soldiers stopped using heroin upon returning to the USA (Robins, Davis, & Goodwin, 1974; Robins, Helzer, & Davis, 1975). These included the heaviest users in Vietnam, who had "reported daily narcotic use for at least one month, or . . . had experienced a period of physical dependence or withdrawal . . ." (O'Brien, Nace, Mintz, Meyers, & Ream, 1980, p. 335).

Of even greater relevance to the current discussion are the approximately 32–50% of the Vietnam veterans who were heavy narcotic users while in Vietnam *and continued* to use heroin after returning to the United States (O'Brien et al., 1980; Robins, 1993; Robins et al., 1974). Astonishingly, despite lapsing when they came back to America, these individuals were unlikely to become readdicted to heroin. Only 6–12% of those who used narcotics upon return showed the behavioral symptoms that accompany addiction or experienced any physical withdrawals once stopping, and only 14% sought any treatment for their problem (O'Brien et al., 1980; Robins et al., 1975). These rates are far lower than would be expected based on the results of studies examining rates of heroin relapse in which the subjects did not experience such a dramatic change in the environmental context of drug administration in which the relapse rate ranges from ~55% to 71% (Gossop, Green, Phillips, & Bradley, 1989; Gossop, Stewart, Browne, & Marsden, 2002; Hser, Anglin, & Powers, 1993). Thus, for these soldiers, the change in environmental setting apparently altered the addictive consequences of heroin exposure.

Other reports also indicate that the reinforcing effects of narcotic analgesics, such as heroin, can be dramatically influenced by the environment in which they are administered. For example, despite being given high doses of these drugs to alleviate pain while in the hospital, relatively few patients experience serious withdrawal effects or craving for these drugs upon being released (Lindesmith, 1947; Zinberg, 1974, 1984).

The idea that a change in context can dramatically alter the psychological and behavioral effects of drugs of abuse is further supported by data concerning the number of psychedelic-induced visits to the Massachusetts Mental Health Center and New York City's Bellevue hospital during the mid- and late 1960s (Zinberg, 1984). When psychedelic drug usage first gained popularity in the New England states in the mid-1960s, approximately one-third of all admissions to these psychiatric hospitals resulted from the ingestion of psychedelics. However, by the late 1960s, the rate had dropped dramatically. Importantly, the reason for this sudden drop in hospital admissions was not due to a sudden decrease in psychedelic consumption. Instead, the primary factor appeared to be a lessening in users' anxiety levels prior to drug administration, resulting from a greater knowledge concerning the effects of psychedelics, as these drugs had received increases in popularity, publicity, and user-to-user communication about their effects (Zinberg, 1984). A similar phenomenon has been reported concerning marijuana-induced anxiety attacks in the 1920s (Becker, 1967). Thus, changes in expectancies resulting from environmental influences can dramatically modulate a drug's effects (see below for further discussion concerning the influence of expectancies).

It is worth mentioning here an account of an entirely opposite phenomenon, in which the drug being used by a group of individuals suddenly changed, while the context of drug administration and expectancies of the users stayed the same. In the mid-1960s, heroin supplies in St. Louis had run dry, and long-time heroin addicts began injecting the only white powder available, methamphetamine. Although methamphetamine is normally considered to have very different physiological and psychoactive effects than heroin, the users experienced the same sort of psychological and behavioral effects that they had while using heroin previously (Jackson, 1978). As the author of this account writes, "The addicts maintained the heroin subculture on a methamphetamine metabolism" (p. 269).

Experimental studies: humans

The above reports suggest that the context of drug administration can dramatically influence the effects of addictive drugs, but these accounts cannot be considered definitive for several reasons. First, there are no placebo controls in these studies, so one cannot conclude whether environmental context is actually modulating the effects produced by drug, or simply producing or influencing a placebo effect. In addition, since there is no control over drug intake, the average dose administered by the particular group of individuals being described may vary substantially, preventing direct comparisons between groups. Finally, contextual variables were not directly manipulated and differ widely from case to case, so it is difficult to determine which environmental variables are critical in modulating the behavioral and subjective effects of drugs.

The shortcomings of naturalistic studies have been addressed by experimental studies in which the experimenters have systematically manipulated the environmental context surrounding drug administration. In the following sections we discuss some of the environmental influences on drug effects that have been discovered by performing controlled experiments with human subjects.

Expectancies

The environmental context of drug administration can influence the drug effects that are expected by the drug user. As put by Howard Becker, "*expectancies* of these (drug) effects ... are *themselves* a function of the social organization of knowledge in different social settings or subcultures" (Becker, 1967). In other words, the expectancies that an individual has are determined by the context of drug administration. Expectancies may be influenced by societal beliefs and practices, communication between drug users, or the individual's experience with the drug in a particular environmental context.

In the laboratory expectancies can be manipulated in many ways, such as varying the description given by the researcher to a test subject concerning the effects of a drug to be ingested, or by altering the context of drug administration, thereby indirectly influencing the expectancies of the user. Using these procedures, it has been found that expectancies influence the behavioral, subjective, and physiological effects produced by a variety of psychoactive drugs.

Much of the experimental research on expectancies has used alcohol, because it is so widely consumed and most people have had the opportunity to form expectancies about its effects. For example, expectations concerning alcohol-induced euphoria and disinhibition are greater when consumption takes place in an on-campus bar, as compared to inside the laboratory (Wall, McKee, & Hinson, 2000). Importantly, these pre-drink expectancies modulate alcohol-induced euphoria and disinhibition (Wall, Thrussell, & Lalonde, 2003), as well as total alcohol consumption when subjects are allowed to consume it *ad libitum* (Lindman, 1982). Furthermore, when receiving alcohol and expecting alcohol, as opposed to when expecting a nonalcoholic beverage, individuals report greater alcohol-induced pleasurable effects (Laberg, 1986; Marlatt & Rohsenow, 1980), self-administer greater amounts of alcohol (Laberg & Loberg, 1989), report greater anxiolytic effects (de Boer, Schippers, Schippers, & van der Staak, 1993), and show decreased motor steadiness (Laberg & Loberg, 1989). Interestingly, much of the influence of expectancies on the effects of alcohol is overcome when very high doses of alcohol are consumed, indicating that expectancies shift the dose–effect curve for these effects (Martin, Earleywine, Finn, & Young, 1990; Martin & Sayette, 1993; O'Boyle, Binns, & Sumner, 1994). Of additional interest, there have been findings suggesting that the effect of expectancies on alcohol-induced sensorimotor impairment and reinforcement is greater in alcohol-dependent individuals, as compared to moderate drinkers (Laberg & Loberg, 1989).

Expectancies also modulate the effects of other drugs of abuse, including the subjective effects produced by caffeine (Griffiths & Woodson, 1988; Stern, Chait, & Johanson, 1989), THC (Cami, Guerra, Ugena, Segura, & de la Torre, 1991; Kirk, Doty, & de Wit, 1998; Stark-Adamec, Adamec, & Pihl, 1981), nicotine (Hughes, Pickens, Spring, & Keenan, 1985), and amphetamine (Mitchell, Laurent, & de Wit, 1996). In addition, the behavioral and physiological effects of psychostimulant drugs are influenced by expectancies. For example, the sensorimotor effects of amphetamine (Lyerly, Ross, Krugman, & Clyde, 1964) and the cardiovascular effects produced by cocaine (Muntaner, Cascella, Kumor, Nagoshi, Herning, & Jaffe, 1989) are enhanced when subjects are expecting to receive the drug, as compared to when subjects are expecting placebo.

The influence of the group

In experimental studies, individuals typically receive drugs in isolation, yet most drug use in the natural environment occurs at social gatherings or in the company of other individuals also administering drug. Several naturalistic observations have underlined the importance of this discrepancy by showing that the amount of drug consumption is increased when others are also consuming drugs, as compared to when consumption occurs in isolation (Cutler & Storm, 1975; Harford, Feinhandler, O'Leary, & Dorman, 1983; Sommer, 1965). Indeed, recent experimental studies indicate that the number of other drug users in the environment of drug administration can have a dramatic influence on the effects produced by drugs of abuse.

For example, alcohol- and THC-induced euphoria are enhanced when other subjects in the environment are also consuming these drugs, as compared to when consumption occurs alone (Doty & de Wit, 1995; Jones, 1971; Lindman, 1982; Pliner & Cappell, 1974; Sher, 1985, Del Porto & Masur, 1984). Furthermore, subjective ratings of THC-induced "conceptual disorganization", "introspective behavior", and "emotionality" are significantly enhanced when THC is consumed in a group (Del Porto & Masur, 1984). In addition, alcohol is self-administered to a greater extent and is enjoyed more when consumed in a group (Doty & de Wit, 1995; Pliner & Cappell, 1974).

There are a variety of ways in which group size may modulate the effects of drugs of abuse. Some evidence indicates that the presence of others influences the expectancies of drug effects since, as previously noted, most drug consumption occurs in groups. Indeed, when alcohol consumption occurs in a group, expectancies concerning the effects of alcohol are enhanced and the expectancies have a greater influence on the subjective effects (Sher, 1985). Social modeling also appears to contribute to the effect of group size. For example, when individuals drink alcohol with others, they consume similar quantities as the members in their group (Caudill & Marlatt, 1975; Collins, Parks, & Marlatt, 1985; DeRicco, 1978; Garlington & Dericco, 1977). This factor also influences the subjective and behavioral effects of THC (Becker,

1953) and hallucinogenic drugs (Becker, 1967). Finally, there is evidence that drugs of abuse, such as amphetamine and alcohol, directly increase socialization, and socialization is itself pleasurable (Griffiths, Stitzer, Corker, Bigelow, & Liebson, 1977; Higgins, Hughes, & Bickel, 1989; Higgins & Stitzer, 1988; Stitzer, Griffiths, Bigelow, & Liebson, 1981).

Studies have also shown that the social setting in which drug is administered can influence the physiological effects of drugs of abuse. Thus, the ability of amphetamine to elevate body temperature and heart rate is increased when the drug is administered in the presence of others (de Wit, Clark, & Brauer, 1997). In contrast, some physiological effects of drugs, such as alcohol-induced dizziness and sleepiness, are actually decreased when consumption occurs in a group setting (Lindman, 1982; Pliner & Cappell, 1974), indicating that not all effects of drugs of abuse are influenced in the same direction by social setting.

A drug for the task at hand

Thus far, we have considered the influence of contextual variables that are passively experienced. One is not normally active in determining the expectancies of the drug in their environment or the number of people surrounding him/her. However, individuals do interact with the environmental situation in which they find themselves. In this section we discuss how drug effects may be altered by the specific task or behavior that the individual is engaged in at the time of drug consumption, and by the feedback from the environment following completion of a particular task.

Various studies demonstrate that the behavioral and cognitive effects of psychoactive drugs vary as a function of task requirements. For example, although amphetamine is thought to promote impulsivity, this behavioral effect is critically dependent on the task in which the individual is engaged. Fillmore, Rush, and Marczinski (2003) presented subjects with a first cue signaling the likelihood that a second cue would signal that the individual was to engage in a response (go) or to inhibit a response (no-go) (the first cue would predict, with 80% accuracy, the second cue). When the initial cue correctly predicted response inhibition, amphetamine did not promote impulsive responding. Only when presented with the cue predicting response execution did amphetamine promote impulsivity. Thus, amphetamine's effects on impulsivity were entirely task-dependent, varying as a function of the environmental stimulus (the cue) presented. Similar effects have been observed with alcohol-induced impulsivity (Marczinski & Fillmore, 2003).

The reinforcing effects of drugs of abuse have also been shown to be dependent on task requirements. For example, Silverman, Kirby, and Griffiths (1994) showed that, after individuals had familiarized themselves with the effects of three different-colored capsules (amphetamine, the benzodiazepine triazolam, or placebo) and two different tasks (requiring either vigilance or relaxation), subjects chose to administer amphetamine over either placebo or triazolam when engaged in the task requiring vigilance. On the other hand, subjects self-administered triazolam over amphetamine or placebo when engaged in the relaxation task (Silverman, Kirby, & Griffiths, 1994). Similar findings have been reported with cocaine and caffeine (Jones, Garrett, & Griffiths, 2001; Silverman, Mumford, & Griffiths, 1994). These findings suggest that stimulants are more reinforcing when the individual is active, but central nervous system depressants have greater reinforcing effects when the individual is relaxed.

Feedback from the environment during or following completion of a task can also modulate the behavioral and cognitive effects of psychoactive drugs. Thus, on a go/no-go task similar to the one described above, the ability of alcohol to increase impulsivity is attenuated by reinforcing subjects for correctly inhibiting responses (Fillmore & Vogel-Sprott, 2000). Feedback from the environment has also been shown to modulate alcohol-induced disruption of sensorimotor skills (Sdao-Jarvie & Vogel-Sprott, 1991; Vogel-Sprott, Kartechner, & McConnell, 1989; Zack & Vogel-Sprott, 1997).

Feedback from the environment further influences the reinforcing effects of drugs of abuse. For example, whereas subjects generally choose to self-administer placebo over diazepam [i.e. diazepam is avoided (de Wit, Uhlenhuth, & Johanson, 1985; Johanson & Uhlenhuth, 1980)], forced diazepam administration coupled with monetary reinforcement for performing a computer task enhances the reinforcing properties of diazepam, such that subjects subsequently self-administer diazepam when given the choice [i.e. it has become reinforcing (Alessi, Roll, Reilly, & Johanson, 2002)]. Similar findings have been reported for the benzodiazepine alprazolam, as well as for amphetamine (Comer, Haney, Foltin, & Fischman, 1996; Haney, Comer, Foltin, & Fischman, 1997). It is interesting to speculate that other environmental variables acting as positive reinforcers, such as the social interactions generally accompanying drug use, could enhance the reinforcing effects of drugs of abuse in a similar fashion (Wikler, 1971). Indeed, affiliation with drug-using peers is a powerful predictor of drug use and dependence (see Chilcoat & Anthony in Dishion, Patterson, & Reid, 1988; Higgins & Katz, 1998).

Environmental context modulates the neurobiological effects of drugs of abuse

In contrast to the relatively large amount of data on the influence of environmental context on the behavioral and subjective effects of drugs of abuse, much less is known about the influence of the environment on the *neurobiological* effects of drugs. However, given that context modulates the behavioral, cognitive, subjective, and reinforcing effects of drugs of abuse, and assuming that the neurobiological effects of drugs determine these psychological effects, then it follows that the environmental context must also influence the neurobiological effects of drugs. This section is dedicated to

The effect of ambient temperatures on the neurotoxic effects of MDMA and other amphetamine-like compounds

Most laboratories maintain a temperature that is optimal for the health of the animal subjects, but drug users do not always take drugs in contexts with such optimal temperatures. This is especially true for the amphetamine-like compound 3,4-methylenedioxymethamphetamine (MDMA), or Ecstasy, which has become especially popular at all-night rave parties that typically become increasingly warm and humid. As reports of MDMA-induced fatalities at raves increased in number during the 1990s (Chadwick, Curry, Linsley, Freemont, & Doran, 1991; Randall, 1992), it became apparent that high ambient temperatures may influence the effects of MDMA. Indeed, there had been a few scattered reports in the scientific literature indicating this possibility with other amphetamine-like compounds (Chance, 1946; Swinyard, Clark, Miyahara, & Wold, 1961).

Recently, there have been many studies examining the influence of ambient temperature on the toxic effects produced by MDMA, as well as other amphetamine-like compounds. For example, the ability of MDMA, methamphetamine, and d-methylenedioxyamphetamine (MDA) to induce depletion of striatal dopamine-containing terminals (Miller & O'Callaghan, 1994) and striatal, cortical, and hippocampal serotoninergic terminals (Malberg & Seiden, 1998; Miller & O'Callaghan, 1995) is dramatically influenced by the temperature of the room in which these drugs are given, with higher temperatures resulting in greater drug-induced toxicity. Astonishingly, the neurotoxic effects produced by these drugs can be dramatically enhanced by increasing the room temperature by just a few degrees centigrade. In contrast, testing animals in even moderately cooler room temperatures can almost completely protect them from the neurotoxic effects of these drugs (Miller & O'Callaghan, 1994, 1995; Xie, McCann, Kim, Yuan, & Ricaurte, 2000).

The neural mechanisms involved in associative tolerance to morphine-induced analgesia

It is well documented that repeated treatment with narcotic analgesics can produce tolerance to their analgesic effects, and that this effect can be critically dependent on the context of drug administration. For example, when repeatedly treated in the same environmental context, tolerance to the analgesic effects of a morphine challenge is expressed when drug is given in the same environment as pretreatment (drug-paired environment), but not when the drug challenge occurs in a different unpaired environment (Adams, Yeh, Woods, & Mitchell, 1969; Kayan, Woods, & Mitchell, 1969; Siegel, 1975,

1977). This difference in tolerance does not appear to be simply quantitative. For example, there is evidence that animals fail to show savings, or an enhanced development of tolerance as a result of prior experience with morphine, when treatment is moved to the unpaired environment (Siegel, 1975).

This form of associative tolerance was traditionally thought to be the result of a conditioned compensatory response opposite to the drug effect [i.e. hyperalgesia (Siegel, 1975)], but this idea has recently been questioned. For example, there is evidence suggesting that morphine itself produces an unconditioned hyperalgesic response that is initially masked by morphine's analgesic effects, but is eventually observed when morphine's analgesic effects wear off (Blasig, Herz, Reinhold, & Zieglgansberger, 1973; Kim, Fields, & Barbaro, 1990; Larcher, Laulin, Celerier, Le Moal, & Simonnet, 1998) or when naloxone is co-administered with morphine (Kayan, Woods, & Mitchell, 1971; Kim et al., 1990; Tilson, Rech, & Stolman, 1973). Thus, it is now believed that the hyperalgesic response is the unconditioned response (UR), which after repeated pairing with an environment [ultimately becoming a conditioned stimulus (CS)], is evoked as a conditioned response (CR) when the animal is brought to the paired environment (Bespalov, Zvartau, & Beardsley, 2001). Thus, associative tolerance to morphine's analgesic effects may result from a CR that is qualitatively similar to, rather than opposite, an effect produced by opioids (Bespalov et al., 2001; McNally & Westbrook, 1998).

Regardless of the nature of the CR, the neural mechanisms underlying associative tolerance to morphine's analgesic effects are just beginning to be explored. In an elegant study, Mitchell, Basbaum, and Fields (2000) showed that neuronal activity in the basolateral and/or lateral amygdala is important for associative tolerance. Thus, Fos-like immunoreactivity, an index of neuronal activity, is increased in the basolateral and lateral amygdala following a morphine challenge in the paired environment, but not when given in the unpaired environment nor when given to animals expressing nonassociative morphine tolerance (induced by implanting a pellet that slowly releases morphine). Furthermore, the expression of associative tolerance seems to be dependent on the actions of cholecystokinin (CCK) on the CCK-2 receptor in the amygdala. Thus, the expression of associative tolerance, but not nonassociative tolerance, is blocked by infusing a CCK-2 receptor antagonist into the lateral portion of the amygdala. In contrast, associative tolerance is neither disrupted by administration of a CCK-1 receptor antagonist into the amygdala, nor by infusing a CCK-2 antagonist into brain regions outside the amygdala.

Additional studies indicate that different mechanisms at the spinal cord may also distinguish associative tolerance from nonassociative tolerance. For example, it has been reported that intrathecal infusion of a neurotensin receptor partial agonist blocks associative tolerance without influencing nonassociative tolerance (Grisel, Watkins, & Maier, 1996). In contrast, infusion of the NMDA receptor antagonist MK-801 has been found to block nonassociative tolerance without affecting the associative component (Trujillo & Akil, 1994; but see McNally & Westbrook (1998)). These findings are especially intriguing, as they indicate that the neural mechanisms underlying associative and nonassociative tolerance are qualitatively different. Thus, the behavior and brain systems engaged by morphine when it is given in the same environment as the animal has received it in the past are very different than when morphine is given in a different context.

The neurobiological effects of amphetamine, cocaine, and morphine differ as a function of environmental novelty

It is well established that intermittent injections of amphetamine, cocaine, and morphine produce psychomotor sensitization, or an increase in the psychomotor-activating effects produced by a given dose of drug. It is now also clear that the environmental context of drug administration can dramatically modulate the development and expression of sensitization (Anagnostaras & Robinson, 1996; Beck, Chow, & Cooper, 1986; Ellinwood & Kilbey, 1975; Hirabayashi & Alam, 1981). For example, the induction of psychomotor sensitization is enhanced when these drugs are given immediately after the animal is placed into an unfamiliar and distinct (i.e. novel) environment, as compared to when these drugs are administered to animals in their home cage (Badiani, Anagnostaras, & Robinson, 1995; Badiani, Browman, & Robinson, 1995; Badiani, Oates, & Robinson, 2000; Crombag, Badiani, & Robinson, 1996). With certain doses of these drugs, treatment in the novel environment produces robust behavioral sensitization, but treatment at home fails to produce sensitization. Furthermore, the expression of sensitization is enhanced when animals receive a drug challenge in the environment in which they received pretreatment, as compared to when they receive the challenge in a different context (Anagnostaras & Robinson, 1996; Hinson & Poulos, 1981; Post, Lockfeld, Squillace, & Contel, 1981). These findings are particularly interesting in light of evidence indicating that behavioral sensitization is relevant to drug addiction (see Robinson & Berridge, 1993, for discussion).

Recently, our laboratory has attempted to characterize the ability of environmental context to modulate the neurobiological effects of amphetamine, cocaine, and morphine. Using the immediate early gene, c-*fos*, as a marker of neuronal activity, we have shown that amphetamine-, cocaine-, and morphine-induced c-*fos* mRNA expression can be dramatically influenced by environmental novelty. Thus, these drugs induce significantly greater levels of c-*fos* expression in the caudate-putamen, nucleus accumbens, and several regions of the cortex when they are given in a novel environment, as compared to when they are given to animals in their home cage (Badiani, Oates, Day, Watson, Akil, & Robinson, 1998; Ferguson, Thomas, & Robinson, 2004; Ostrander et al., 2003; Uslaner, Badiani, Day, Watson, Akil, & Robinson, 2001a).

As gene induction is a first step in synaptic plasticity, we recently examined whether environmental context also influences the ability of these drugs to produce morphological changes in neuronal processes. Indeed, we have shown that cocaine administered in a novel environment promotes greater increases in dendritic spine density in the nucleus accumbens and caudate-putamen, as compared to when drug is given at home (Li, Acerbo, & Robinson, 2004).

In addition, we have demonstrated that the neuronal circuitry engaged by these drugs differs according to the context of drug treatment (Badiani, Oates, Day, Watson, Akil, & Robinson, 1999; Ferguson et al., 2004; Uslaner et al., 2001a). When amphetamine, cocaine, or morphine is given to animals in their home cage, they induce c-*fos* expression almost exclusively in substance P/dynorphin mRNA positive cells (SP+ cells) in the caudate-putamen. These SP+ cells project directly to more caudal structures, such as the substantia nigra, via the so-called "direct pathway" (Albin, Young, & Penney, 1989). When given to animals in a novel environment, amphetamine, cocaine, and morphine induce c-*fos* in the SP+ cells, and in addition they induce significant levels of c-*fos* expression in cells in the caudate-putamen that are positive for enkephalin mRNA (ENK+). These ENK+ cells project to more caudal structures, such as the substantia nigra, via the so-called "indirect pathway", which synapses in the globus pallidus and subthalamic nucleus *en route* to more caudal structures (Albin et al., 1989). Importantly, this difference in the ability to engage ENK+ cells does not merely represent a shift in the dose–response curve. Even very high doses of these drugs given at home fail to induce c-*fos* in very many ENK+ cells (Uslaner, Norton, Watson, Akil, & Robinson, 2003).

Further supporting the idea that environmental novelty modulates the circuitry engaged by these drugs, amphetamine- and cocaine-induced c-*fos* expression in the subthalamic nucleus is enhanced when these drugs are given in a novel environment, as compared to when they are given at home (Uslaner et al., 2001b; Uslaner et al., 2003). As noted above, the subthalamic nucleus is part of the indirect pathway that is influenced by ENK+ cells.

Finally, we have also shown that the context of drug administration modulates the neurotransmitter systems that underlie the neurobiological effects of amphetamine. For example, the ability of dopamine and glutamate antagonists to attenuate amphetamine-induced c-*fos* expression differs as a function of environmental novelty (Ferguson, Norton, Watson, Akil, & Robinson, 2003).

Taken together, this series of studies shows that the context of drug administration regulates the ability of amphetamine, cocaine, and morphine to induce gene transcription in brain areas thought to be critical for the reinforcing and cognitive effects of these drugs, modulates the neural circuitry and neurotransmitter systems engaged by these drugs, and influences the ability of drugs of abuse to produce persistent neuroplastic adaptations that may mediate drug addiction. Some of these differences are not merely quantitative, but are qualitative differences in drug effects that are dependent upon the context in which the drug is administered.

Conclusion, implications, and future directions

The evidence presented in this chapter clearly indicates that the environmental context in which drugs are experienced modulates many of their effects. The behavioral and psychological effects of drugs of abuse vary as a function of culture, the physical properties of the environment, expectancies, social contexts, tasks in which the individual is engaged, and feedback from the environment. In addition, the neurobiological effects of drugs of abuse are also influenced to a great extent by the context of drug administration. These findings have considerable implications for future studies aimed at elucidating the effects of psychoactive drugs, as well as for discovering treatments for drug addiction.

Whereas the overarching goal of drug addiction research is to understand the effects of drugs of abuse in the environment in which they are typically administered, there are some obvious constraints to this endeavor when conducting experimental studies. Indeed, simply by observing the drug user, the experimenter alters the environment in some way. Of course, this hindrance is relatively minor in comparison to the problems that arise for studies designed to examine the *neurobiological* effects of drugs, in which devices such as neuroimaging machines are needed. Nevertheless, the studies mentioned in this chapter emphasize how important it is that the environment surrounding drug administration in experimental studies remains *as similar as possible* to that in which the drug user normally consumes drugs.

Recent efforts to do so have been fruitful. For example, several laboratories have designed bars or pubs that more closely resemble the environment in which most individuals consume alcohol (see above). These studies have demonstrated that the effects of alcohol consumption in these "on-campus bars" are quite different than those observed when consumption occurs in the standard laboratory setting. Furthermore, several laboratories interested in imaging the neurobiological correlates underlying drug addiction have begun using drug-related cues, or had subjects imagine drug-related experiences, in an attempt to recreate the environment in which drug use normally occurs. These studies have been successful at identifying brain regions involved in cue-induced craving (Childress, Mozley, McElgin, Fitzgerald, Reivich, & O'Brien, 1999; Sell, Morris, Bearn, Frackowiak, Friston, & Dolan, 1999; Volkow et al., 1999). For example, regions of the limbic system, such as the amygdala, as well as several cortical areas are active when individuals are presented with drug-related cues or are imagining drug-related environments. Unfortunately, no study to date has examined the effects of these contextual variables on *drug-induced* neuronal activity in humans. Such studies are critical for understanding the neurobiological consequences of drugs of abuse as they occur in the user's typical environment of drug administration.

Furthermore, by elucidating the effects of drugs as they occur in the user's drug-taking environment, the goal of developing treatments for drug addiction will be greatly facilitated. Preclinical studies have demonstrated that the neural circuitry engaged by drugs of abuse markedly differs as a function of the environmental context in which the drug is administered. Thus, it seems likely that the pharmacological treatments that are necessary to antagonize the effects of drugs of abuse may be quite different for the user in his/her drug-taking environment, as compared to the laboratory or hospital. No study that we know of has directly assessed this possibility. Moreover, while the effects of drugs of abuse have been shown to vary as a function of environmental context, the effects of drugs that could be used for pharmacotherapeutic purposes may likewise differ according to the context in which they are given. Very little attention has been paid to this possibility, but if it were the case, it would have quite important consequences for identifying pharmacological treatments for drug addiction (or for any psychological disorder, for that matter).

Although control is necessary for conducting experimental studies, it is not impossible to maintain control while providing an environment that closely resembles that in which drug users normally take drugs. The challenge of designing creative experiments can and should be met to produce data with greater external validity. We must shift our emphasis from a purely pharmacology-centered approach, to an approach that emphasizes pharmacology/nonpharmacology interactions.

References

Aberle, D. F., & Moore, H. C. (1991). *The Peyote religion among the Navaho* (2nd ed.). Norman: University of Oklahoma Press.

Adams, W. J., Yeh, S. Y., Woods, L. A., & Mitchell, C. L. (1969). Drug–test interaction as a factor in the development of tolerance to the analgesic effect of morphine. *Journal of Pharmacology and Experimental Therapeutics, 168,* 251–257.

Albin, R. L., Young, A. B., & Penney, J. B. (1989). The functional anatomy of basal ganglia disorders. *Trends in Neuroscience, 12,* 366–375.

Alessi, S. M., Roll, J. M., Reilly, M. P., & Johanson, C. E. (2002). Establishment of a diazepam preference in human volunteers following a differential-conditioning history of placebo versus diazepam choice. *Experimental and Clinical Psychopharmacology, 10,* 77–83, 101–103.

Anagnostaras, S. G., & Robinson, T. E. (1996). Sensitization to the psychomotor stimulating effects of amphetamine: modulation by associative learning. *Behavioral Neuroscience, 110,* 1397–1414.

Anthony, J. C., Warner, L. A., & Kessler, R. C. (1994). Comparative epidemiology of dependence on tobacco, alcohol, controlled substances, and inhalants: basic findings from the national comorbidity survey. *Experimental and Clinical Psychopharmacology, 2,* 244–268.

Badiani, A., Anagnostaras, S. G., & Robinson, T. E. (1995). The development of sensitization to the psychomotor stimulant effects of amphetamine is enhanced in a novel environment. *Psychopharmacology (Berlin), 117,* 443–452.

Badiani, A., Browman, K. E., & Robinson, T. E. (1995). Influence of novel versus home environments on sensitization to the psychomotor stimulant effects of cocaine and amphetamine. *Brain Research, 674*, 291–298.

Badiani, A., Oates, M. M., Day, H. E., Watson, S. J., Akil, H., & Robinson, T. E. (1998). Amphetamine-induced behavior, dopamine release, and c-*fos* mRNA expression: modulation by environmental novelty. *Journal of Neuroscience, 18*, 10579–10593.

Badiani, A., Oates, M. M., Day, H. E., Watson, S. J., Akil, H., & Robinson, T. E. (1999). Environmental modulation of amphetamine-induced c-*fos* expression in D1 versus D2 striatal neurons. *Behavioral Brain Research, 103*, 203–209.

Badiani, A., Oates, M. M., & Robinson, T. E. (2000). Modulation of morphine sensitization in the rat by contextual stimuli. *Psychopharmacology (Berlin), 151*, 273–282.

Beck, C. H., Chow, H. L., & Cooper, S. J. (1986). Initial environment influences amphetamine-induced stereotypy: subsequently environment change has little effect. *Behavioral and Neural Biology, 46*, 383–397.

Becker, H. S. (1953). Becoming a marihuana user. *American Journal of Sociology, 59*, 235–242.

Becker, H. S. (1967). History, culture and subjective experience: an exploration of the social bases of drug-induced experiences. *Journal of Health and Social Behavior, 8*, 163–176.

Bespalov, A. Y., Zvartau, E. E., & Beardsley, P. M. (2001). Opioid–NMDA receptor interactions may clarify conditioned (associative) components of opioid analgesic tolerance. *Neuroscience and Biobehavior Review, 25*, 343–353.

Bierut, L. J., Dinwiddie, S. H., Begleiter, H., Crowe, R. R., Hesselbrock, V., Nurnberger, J. I., et al. (1998). Familial transmission of substance dependence: alcohol, marijuana, cocaine, and habitual smoking. *Archives of General Psychiatry, 55*, 982–988.

Blasig, J., Herz, A., Reinhold, K., & Zieglgansberger, S. (1973). Development of physical dependence on morphine in respect to time and dosage and quantification of the precipitated withdrawal syndrome in rats. *Psychopharmacologia, 33*, 19–38.

Blum, R. H. (1964). *Utopiates; the use & users of LSD 25*. New York: Atherton Press.

Cami, J., Guerra, D., Ugena, B., Segura, J., & de la Torre, R. (1991). Effect of subject expectancy on the THC intoxication and disposition from smoked hashish cigarettes. *Pharmacology, Biochemistry and Behavior, 40*, 115–119.

Caudill, B. D., & Marlatt, G. A. (1975). Modeling influences in social drinking: an experimental analogue. *Journal of Consulting and Clinical Psychology, 43*, 405–415.

Chadwick, I. S., Curry, P. D., Linsley, A., Freemont, A. J., & Doran, B. (1991). Ecstasy, 3-4 methylenedioxymethamphetamine (MDMA), a fatality associated with coagulopathy and hyperthermia. *Journal of the Royal Society of Medicine, 84*, 371.

Chance, M. R. A. (1946). Aggregation as a factor influencing the toxicity of sympathomimetic amines in mice. *Journal of Pharmacology and Experimental Therapeutics, 87*, 214–249.

Childress, A. R., Mozley, P. D., McElgin, W., Fitzgerald, J., Reivich, M., & O'Brien, C. P. (1999). Limbic activation during cue-induced cocaine craving. *American Journal of Psychiatry, 156*, 11–18.

Collins, R. L., Parks, G. A., & Marlatt, G. A. (1985). Social determinants of alcohol consumption: the effects of social interaction and model status on the self-administration of alcohol. *Journal of Consulting and Clinical Psychology, 53*, 189–200.

Comer, S. D., Haney, M., Foltin, R. W., & Fischman, M. W. (1996). Amphetamine self-administration by humans: modulation by contingencies associated with task performance. *Psychopharmacology (Berlin)*, *127*, 39–46.

Crombag, H. S., Badiani, A., & Robinson, T. E. (1996). Signalled versus unsignalled intravenous amphetamine: large differences in the acute psychomotor response and sensitization. *Brain Research*, *722*, 227–231.

Cutler, R. E., & Storm, T. (1975). Observational study of alcohol consumption in natural settings. The Vancouver beer parlor. *Journal of Studies on Alcohol*, *36*, 1173–1183.

De Boer, M. C., Schippers, G. M., & van der Staak, C. P. (1993). Alcohol and social anxiety in women and men: pharmacological and expectancy effects. *Addictive Behavior*, *18*, 117–126.

De Wit, H., Clark, M., & Brauer, L. H. (1997). Effects of d-amphetamine in grouped versus isolated humans. *Pharmacology, Biochemistry and Behavior*, *57*, 333–340.

De Wit, H., Uhlenhuth, E. H., & Johanson, C. E. (1985). Drug preference in normal volunteers: effects of age and time of day. *Psychopharmacology (Berlin)*, *87*, 186–193.

Del Porto, J. A., & Masur, J. (1984). The effects of alcohol, THC and diazepam in two different social settings. A study with human volunteers. *Research Communications in Psychology, Psychiatry and Behavior*, *9*, 201–212.

DeRicco, D. A. (1978). Effects of peer majority on drinking rate. *Addictive Behavior*, *3*, 29–34.

Deroche-Gamonet V., Belin D., & Piazza P. V. (2004) Evidence for addiction-like behavior in the rat. *Science*, *305*, 1014–1017.

Dishion, T. J., Patterson, G. R., & Reid, J. R. (1988). Parent and peer factors associated with drug sampling in early adolescence: implications for treatment. *NIDA Research Monograph*, *77*, 69–93.

Doty, P., & de Wit, H. (1995). Effect of setting on the reinforcing and subjective effects of ethanol in social drinkers. *Psychopharmacology (Berlin)*, *118*, 19–27.

Du Toit, B. M. (1977). *Drugs, rituals and altered states of consciousness*. Rotterdam: A. A. Balkema.

Ellinwood, E. H., Jr., & Kilbey, M. M. (1975). Amphetamine stereotypy: the influence of environmental factors and prepotent behavioral patterns on its topography and development. *Biological Psychiatry*, *10*, 3–16.

Falk, J. L., & Feingold, D. A. (1987). Environmental and cultural factors in the behavioral actions of drugs, In H. Y. Meltzer (Ed.), *Psychopharmacology: the third generation of progress* (pp. 1503–1510). New York: Raven Press.

Ferguson, S. M., Norton, C. S., Watson, S. J., Akil, H., & Robinson, T. E. (2003). Amphetamine-evoked c-*fos* mRNA expression in the caudate-putamen: the effects of DA and NMDA receptor antagonists vary as a function of neuronal phenotype and environmental context. *Journal of Neurochemistry*, *86*, 33–44.

Ferguson, S. M., Thomas, M. J., & Robinson, T. E. (2004). Morphine-induced c-fos mRNA expression in striatofugal circuits: modulation by dose, environmental context and drug history. *Neuropsychopharmacology*, *29*, 1664–1774.

Fillmore, M. T., Rush, C. R., & Marczinski, C. A. (2003). Effects of *d*-amphetamine on behavioral control in stimulant abusers: the role of prepotent response tendencies. *Drug and Alcohol Dependence*, *71*, 143–152.

Fillmore, M. T., & Vogel-Sprott, M. (2000). Response inhibition under alcohol: effects of cognitive and motivational conflict. *Journal of Studies on Alcohol*, *61*, 239–246.

Garlington, W. K., & Dericco, D. A. (1977). The effect of modelling on drinking rate. *Journal of Applied Behavior Analysis, 10*, 207–211.

Gossop, M., Green, L., Phillips, G., & Bradley, B. (1989). Lapse, relapse and survival among opiate addicts after treatment. A prospective follow-up study. *British Journal of Psychiatry, 154*, 348–353.

Gossop, M., Stewart, D., Browne, N., & Marsden, J. (2002). Factors associated with abstinence, lapse or relapse to heroin use after residential treatment: protective effect of coping responses. *Addiction, 97*, 1259–1267.

Griffiths, R. R., Stitzer, M., Corker, K., Bigelow, G., & Liebson, I. (1977). Drug-produced changes in human social behavior: facilitation by d-amphetamine. *Pharmacology, Biochemistry and Behavior, 7*, 365–372.

Griffiths, R. R., & Woodson, P. P. (1988). Reinforcing effects of caffeine in humans. *Journal of Pharmacology and Experimental Therapeutics, 246*, 21–29.

Grisel, J. E., Watkins, L. R., & Maier, S. F. (1996). Associative and non-associative mechanisms of morphine analgesic tolerance are neurochemically distinct in the rat spinal cord. *Psychopharmacology (Berlin), 128*, 248–255.

Haney, M., Comer, S. D., Foltin, R. W., & Fischman, M. W. (1997). Behavioral contingencies modulate alprazolam self-administration by humans. *Behavioral Pharmacology, 8*, 82–90.

Harford, T. C., Feinhandler, S. J., O'Leary, J., & Dorman, N. (1983). Drinking in bars: an observational study of companion status and drinking behavior. *International Journal of Addiction, 18*, 937–950.

Higgins, S. T., Hughes, J. R., & Bickel, W. K. (1989). Effects of d-amphetamine on choice of social versus monetary reinforcement: a discrete-trial test. *Pharmacology, Biochemistry and Behavior, 34*, 297–301.

Higgins, S. T., & Katz, J. L. (1998). *Cocaine abuse: behavior, pharmacology, and clinical applications*. San Diego, CA: Academic Press.

Higgins, S. T., & Stitzer, M. L. (1988). Effects of alcohol on speaking in isolated humans. *Psychopharmacology (Berlin), 95*, 189–194.

Hinson, R. E., & Poulos, C. X. (1981). Sensitization to the behavioral effects of cocaine: modification by Pavlovian conditioning. *Pharmacology, Biochemistry and Behavior, 15*, 559–562.

Hirabayashi, M., & Alam, M. R. (1981). Enhancing effect of methamphetamine on ambulatory activity produced by repeated administration in mice. *Pharmacology, Biochemistry and Behavior, 15*, 925–932.

Hser, Y. I., Anglin, D., & Powers, K. (1993). A 24-year follow-up of California narcotics addicts. *Archives of General Psychiatry, 50*, 577–584.

Hughes, J. R., Pickens, R. W., Spring, W., & Keenan, R. M. (1985). Instructions control whether nicotine will serve as a reinforcer. *Journal of Pharmacology and Experimental Therapeutics, 235*, 106–112.

Jackson, B. (1978). Deviance as success: the double inversion of stigmatized roles. In B. A. Babcock (Ed.), *The reversible world: Symbolic inversion in art and society* (pp. 258–271). Ithica: Cornell University Press.

Johanson, C. E., & Uhlenhuth, E. H. (1980). Drug preference and mood in humans: diazepam. *Psychopharmacology (Berlin), 71*, 269–273.

Jones, H. E., Garrett, B. E., & Griffiths, R. R. (2001). Reinforcing effects of oral cocaine: contextual determinants. *Psychopharmacology (Berlin), 154*, 143–152.

Jones, R. T. (1971). Marihuana-induced "high": influence of expectation, setting and previous drug experience. *Pharmacology Review, 23*, 359–369.

Kayan, S., Woods, L. A., & Mitchell, C. L. (1969). Experience as a factor in the development of tolerance to the analgesic effect of morphine. *European Journal of Pharmacology, 6*, 333–339.

Kayan, S., Woods, L. A., & Mitchell, C. L. (1971). Morphine-induced hyperalgesia in rats tested on the hot plate. *Journal of Pharmacology and Experimental Therapeutics, 177*, 509–513.

Kim, D. H., Fields, H. L., & Barbaro, N. M. (1990). Morphine analgesia and acute physical dependence: rapid onset of two opposing, dose-related processes. *Brain Research, 516*, 37–40.

Kirk, J. M., Doty, P., & de Wit, H. (1998). Effects of expectancies on subjective responses to oral delta9-tetrahydrocannabinol. *Pharmacology, Biochemistry and Behavior, 59*, 287–293.

Laberg, J. C. (1986). Alcohol and expectancy: subjective, psychophysiological and behavioral responses to alcohol stimuli in severely, moderately and non-dependent drinkers. *British Journal of Addiction, 81*, 797–808.

Laberg, J. C., & Loberg, T. (1989). Expectancy and tolerance: a study of acute alcohol intoxication using the balanced placebo design. *Journal of Studies on Alcohol, 50*, 448–455.

Larcher, A., Laulin, J. P., Celerier, E., Le Moal, M., & Simonnet, G. (1998). Acute tolerance associated with a single opiate administration: involvement of *N*-methyl-D-aspartate-dependent pain facilitatory systems. *Neuroscience, 84*, 583–589.

Li, Y., Acerbo, M. J. & Robinson, T. E. (2004). The induction of behavioural sensitzation is associated with cocaine-induced structural plasticity in the core (but not shell) of the nucleus accumbens. *European Journal of Neuroscience, 20*, 1647–1654.

Lindesmith, A. R. (1947). *Opiate addiction*. Bloomington, IN: Principia Press.

Lindman, R. (1982). Social and solitary drinking: effects on consumption and mood in male social drinkers. *Physiology and Behavior, 28*, 1093–1095.

Lyerly, S. B., Ross, S., Krugman, A. D., & Clyde, D. J. (1964). Drugs and placebos: The effects of instructions upon performance and mood under amphetamine sulphate and chloral hydrate. *Journal of Abnormal Psychology, 68*, 321–327.

MacAndrew, C., & Edgerton, R. B. (1969). *Drunken comportment: a social explanation*. New York: Aldine Publishing.

Malberg, J. E., & Seiden, L. S. (1998). Small changes in ambient temperature cause large changes in 3,4-methylenedioxymethamphetamine (MDMA)-induced serotonin neurotoxicity and core body temperature in the rat. *Journal of Neuroscience, 18*, 5086–5094.

Marczinski, C. A., & Fillmore, M. T. (2003). Preresponse cues reduce the impairing effects of alcohol on the execution and suppression of responses. *Experimental and Clinical Psychopharmacology, 11*, 110–117.

Marlatt, G. A., & Rohsenow, D. J. (1980). Cognitive processes in alcohol use: Expectancy and the balanced placebo design. In N. K. Mello (Ed.), *Substance abuse: Behavioral and biological research* (pp. 159–199). Greenwich: JA1 Press.

Marshall, M. (1979). *Beliefs, behaviors, & alcoholic beverages: a cross-cultural survey*. Ann Arbor: University of Michigan Press.

Martin, C. S., Earleywine, M., Finn, P. R., & Young, R. D. (1990). Some boundary conditions for effective use of alcohol placebos. *Journal of Studies on Alcohol, 51*, 500–505.

Martin, C. S., & Sayette, M. A. (1993). Experimental design in alcohol administration research: limitations and alternatives in the manipulation of dosage-set. *Journal of Studies on Alcohol, 54,* 750–761.

McNally, G. P., & Westbrook, R. F. (1998). Effects of systemic, intracerebral, or intrathecal administration of an N-methyl-D-aspartate receptor antagonist on associative morphine analgesic tolerance and hyperalgesia in rats. *Behavioral Neuroscience, 112,* 966–978.

Miller, D. B., & O'Callaghan, J. P. (1994). Environment-, drug- and stress-induced alterations in body temperature affect the neurotoxicity of substituted amphetamines in the C57BL/6J mouse. *Journal of Pharmacology and Experimental Therapeutics, 270,* 752–760.

Miller, D. B., & O'Callaghan, J. P. (1995). The role of temperature, stress, and other factors in the neurotoxicity of the substituted amphetamines 3,4-methylenedioxymethamphetamine and fenfluramine. *Molecular Neurobiology, 11,* 177–192.

Mitchell, J. M., Basbaum, A. I., & Fields, H. L. (2000). A locus and mechanism of action for associative morphine tolerance. *Nature Neuroscience, 3,* 47–53.

Mitchell, S. H., Laurent, C. L., & de Wit, H. (1996). Interaction of expectancy and the pharmacological effects of d-amphetamine: subjective effects and self-administration. *Psychopharmacology (Berlin), 125,* 371–378.

Muntaner, C., Cascella, N. G., Kumor, K. M., Nagoshi, C., Herning, R., & Jaffe, J. (1989). Placebo responses to cocaine administration in humans: effects of prior administrations and verbal instructions. *Psychopharmacology (Berlin), 99,* 282–286.

O'Boyle, D. J., Binns, A. S., & Sumner, J. J. (1994). On the efficacy of alcohol placebos in inducing feelings of intoxication. *Psychopharmacology (Berlin), 115,* 229–236.

O'Brien, C. P., Nace, E. P., Mintz, J., Meyers, A. L., & Ream, N. (1980). Follow-up of Vietman veterans. I. Relapse to drug use after Vietnam service. *Drug and Alcohol Dependence, 5,* 333–340.

Ostrander, M. M., Badiani, A., Day, H. E., Norton, C. S., Watson, S. J., Akil, H., et al. (2003). Environmental context and drug history modulate amphetamine-induced c-fos mRNA expression in the basal ganglia, central extended amygdala, and associated limbic forebrain. *Neuroscience, 120,* 551–571.

Pedersen, N., (1981). Twin similarity for usage of common drugs. *Progress in Clinical and Biological Research, 69C,* 53–59.

Pliner, P., & Cappell, H. (1974). Modification of affective consequences of alcohol: a comparison of social and solitary drinking. *Journal of Abnormal Psychology, 83,* 418–425.

Post, R. M., Lockfeld, A., Squillace, K. M., & Contel, N. R. (1981). Drug–environment interaction: context dependency of cocaine-induced behavioral sensitization. *Life Sciences, 28,* 755–760.

Randall, T. (1992). Ecstasy-fueled "rave" parties become dances of death for English youths. *Journal of the American Medical Association, 268,* 1505–1506.

Robins, L. N. (1993). The sixth Thomas James Okey Memorial Lecture. Vietnam veterans' rapid recovery from heroin addiction: a fluke or normal expectation? *Addiction, 88,* 1041–1054.

Robins, L. N., Davis, D. H., & Goodwin, D. W. (1974). Drug use by U.S. Army enlisted men in Vietnam: a follow-up on their return home. *American Journal of Epidemiology, 99,* 235–249.

Robins, L. N., Helzer, J. E., & Davis, D. H. (1975). Narcotic use in southeast Asia and afterward. An interview study of 898 Vietnam returnees. *Archives of General Psychiatry, 32*, 955–961.

Robinson, T. E. (2004). Neuroscience. Addicted rats. *Science, 305*, 951–953.

Robinson, T. E., & Berridge, K. C. (1993). The neural basis of drug craving: an incentive-sensitization theory of addiction. *Brain Research Reviews, 18*, 247–291.

Rubin, V. D., & Comitas, L. (1975). *Ganja in Jamaica: a medical anthropological study of chronic marihuana use.* The Hague: Mouton.

Sdao-Jarvie, K., & Vogel-Sprott, M. (1991). Response expectancies affect the acquisition and display of behavioral tolerance to alcohol. *Alcohol, 8*, 491–498.

Sell, L. A., Morris, J., Bearn, J., Frackowiak, R. S., Friston, K. J., & Dolan, R. J. (1999). Activation of reward circuitry in human opiate addicts. *European Journal of Neuroscience, 11*, 1042–1048.

Sher, K. J. (1985). Subjective effects of alcohol: the influence of setting and individual differences in alcohol expectancies. *Journal of Studies on Alcohol, 46*, 137–146.

Siegel, S. (1975). Evidence from rats that morphine tolerance is a learned response. *Journal of Comparative and Physiological Psychology, 89*, 498–506.

Siegel, S. (1977). Morphine tolerance acquisition as an associative process. *Journal of Experimental Psychology and Animal Behavior Processes, 3*, 1–13.

Silverman, K., Kirby, K. C., & Griffiths, R. R. (1994). Modulation of drug reinforcement by behavioral requirements following drug ingestion. *Psychopharmacology (Berlin), 114*, 243–247.

Silverman, K., Mumford, G. K., & Griffiths, R. R. (1994). Enhancing caffeine reinforcement by behavioral requirements following drug ingestion. *Psychopharmacology (Berlin), 114*, 424–432.

Sommer, R. (1965). The isolated drinker in the Edmonton beer parlor. *Quarterly Journal of Studies on Alcohol, 26*, 95–110.

Stark-Adamec, C., Adamec, R. E., & Pihl, R. O. (1981). The subjective marijuana experience: great expectations. *International Journal of Addiction, 16*, 1169–1181.

Stern, K. N., Chait, L. D., & Johanson, C. E. (1989). Reinforcing and subjective effects of caffeine in normal human volunteers. *Psychopharmacology (Berlin), 98*, 81–88.

Stitzer, M. L., Griffiths, R. R., Bigelow, G. E., & Liebson, I. (1981). Human social conversation: effects of ethanol, secobarbital and chlorpromazine. *Pharmacology, Biochemistry and Behavior, 14*, 353–360.

Swinyard, E. A., Clark, L. D., Miyahara, J. T., & Wold, H. H. (1961). Studies on the mechanism of amphetamine toxicity in aggregated mice. *Journal of Pharmacology and Experimental Therapeutics, 256*, 506–512.

Tilson, H. A., Rech, R. H., & Stolman, S. (1973). Hyperalgesia during withdrawal as a means of measuring the degree of dependence in morphine dependent rats. *Psychopharmacologia, 28*, 287–300.

Trujillo, K. A., & Akil, H. (1994). Inhibition of opiate tolerance by non-competitive N-methyl-D-aspartate receptor antagonists. *Brain Research, 633*, 178–188.

Tsuang, M. T., Lyons, M. J., Meyer, J. M., Doyle, T., Eisen, S. A., Goldber, J., et al. (1998). Co-occurrence of abuse of different drugs in men: the role of drug-specific and shared vulnerabilities. *Archives of General Psychiatry, 55*, 967–972.

Uslaner, J., Badiani, A., Day, H. E., Watson, S. J., Akil, H., & Robinson, T. E. (2001a). Environmental context modulates the ability of cocaine and amphetamine to induce c-*fos* mRNA expression in the neocortex, caudate nucleus, and nucleus accumbens. *Brain Research, 920*, 106–116.

Uslaner, J., Badiani, A., Norton, C. S., Day, H. E., Watson, S. J., Akil, H., et al. (2001b). Amphetamine and cocaine induce different patterns of c-*fos* mRNA expression in the striatum and subthalamic nucleus depending on environmental context. *European Journal of Neuroscience, 13*, 1977–1983.

Uslaner, J. M., Norton, C. S., Watson, S. J., Akil, H., & Robinson, T. E. (2003). Amphetamine-induced c-fos mRNA expression in the caudate-putamen and subthalamic nucleus: interactions between dose, environment, and neuronal phenotype. *Journal of Neurochemistry, 85*, 105–114.

Van den Bree, M. B. M., Johnson, E. O., Neale, M. C., & Pickens, R. W. (1998). Genetic and environmental influences on drug use and abuse/dependence in male and female twins. *Drug and Alcohol Dependence, 52*, 231–241.

Vogel-Sprott, M., Kartechner, W., & McConnell, D. (1989). Consequences of behavior influence the effect of alcohol. *Journal of Substance Abuse, 1*, 369–379.

Volkow, N. D., Wang, G. J., Fowler, J. S., Hitzemann, R., Angrist, B., Gatley, S. J., et al. (1999). Association of methylphenidate-induced craving with changes in right striato-orbitofrontal metabolism in cocaine abusers: implications in addiction. *American Journal of Psychiatry, 156*, 19–26.

Wagner, F. A., & Anthony, J. C. (2002). From first drug use to drug dependence: developmental periods of risk for dependence upon marijuana, cocaine, and alcohol. *Neuropsychopharmacology, 26*, 479–488.

Wall, A. M., McKee, S. A., & Hinson, R. E. (2000). Assessing variation in alcohol outcome expectancies across environmental context: an examination of the situational-specificity hypothesis. *Psychology of Addictive Behavior, 14*, 367–375.

Wall, A. M., Thrussell, C., & Lalonde, R. N. (2003). Do alcohol expectancies become intoxicated outcomes? A test of social-learning theory in a naturalistic bar setting. *Addictive Behavior, 28*, 1271–1283.

Wallace, A. F. (1959). Cultural determinants of response to hallucinatory experience. *Archives of General Psychiatry, 1*, 58–69.

Wikler, A. (1971). Present status of the concept of drug dependence. *Psychological Medicine, 1*, 377–380.

Xie, T., McCann, U. D., Kim, S., Yuan, J., & Ricaurte, G. A. (2000). Effect of temperature on dopamine transporter function and intracellular accumulation of methamphetamine: implications for methamphetamine-induced dopaminergic neurotoxicity. *Journal of Neuroscience, 20*, 7838–7845.

Zack, M., & Vogel-Sprott, M. (1997). Drunk or sober? Learned conformity to a behavioral standard. *Journal of Studies on Alcohol, 58*, 495–501.

Zinberg, N. E. (1974). The search for rational approaches to heroin use. In P. G. Bourne (Ed.), *Addiction* (pp. 149–174). New York: Academic Press.

Zinberg, N. E. (1984). *Drug, set, and setting: the basis for controlled intoxicant use.* New Haven: Yale University Press.

Author index

Aarons, G. A. 425
Abbruzzesse, S. 381
Abdollah, S. 60
Abdulla, F. A. 238
Aberle, D. F. 437
Abood, M. E. 143
Abukmeil, S. 384
Abu-Shaar, M. 143
Acerbo, M. J. 447
Aceto, M. D. 238
Acker, C. F. 328
Adachi, Y. 327
Adamec, R. E. 441
Adams, C. 384
Adams, K. M. 47, 56, 298–299, 300, 303, 356
Adams, R. D. 328
Adams, W. J. 444
Adamse, M. 119
Addington, A. 378
Addington, D. 390
Addington, J. 390
Adelson, M. 305
Adem, A. 238
Adinoff, B. 124, 125
Adkins, L. M. 334
Adler, L. 79, 83
Adler, L. E. 244
Adler, S. 352
Agartz, I. 60, 334
Aggleton, J. P. 58
Agmo, A. 78
Aharonovich, E. 128, 221
Ahlgren, P. 56
Ahmed, I. 46, 47, 55, 56, 57, 62
Ainslie, G. 408, 409, 410, 411, 412, 414, 415, 416, 418, 419, 424, 425
Akil, H. 263, 446, 447
Alam, M. R. 446
Albin, R. L. 447
Albus, M. 375
Aldrich, M. R. 140
Aleman, A. 381, 383
Aleman, V. 264
Alessi, S. M. 443

Allard, J. 338
Allen, D. 82, 83, 98
Allgulander, C. 96
Alliger, R. 380, 382
Alpérovitch, A. 323, 326, 338
Alpert, M. 378
Altschul, D. 54
Alvarez, J. F. 306
Amara, S. G. 111–112
Amaral, D. G. 58
Amass, L. 121, 266
Amen, D. G. 359
Ames, D. 334, 337
Ames, N. 350
Anagnostaras, S. G. 446
Anderson, D. C. 121
Anderson, G. M. 177
Anderson, H. 10
Anderson, R. 10
Anderson, S. W. 124, 125, 273, 274, 420, 421, 422
Andersson, K. 233
Andreasen, N. 380, 382
Andreski, P. 227
Andrews, B. T. 118
Andrews, C. 116
Anggard, E. 215
Anglin, D. 438
Anglin, M. 207
Angrist, B. 79, 83, 215
Angst, J. 361
Angunawela, I. 334
Annon, J. 207
Anthony, J. C. 435, 443
Anttila, T. 326
Aoki, J. 241
Apfelbaum, J. L. 306
Appel, P. W. 276
Araki, M. 334
Aranko, K. 79, 80
Araujo, D. M. 245–246
Arcand, L. 50
Ardila, A. 119, 120, 122, 129, 364
Arevalo, C., de 157

Argyrakis, A. 96
Aristotle 416
Armstrong, M. A. 333
Arnall, C. 229
Arneric, S. P. 239
Arnett, M. 274
Aron, A. 426
Aronen, H. J. 47, 60
Aronson, M. J. 292, 294, 295, 296
Arora, P. K. 354
Arria, A. M. 327
Arsura, E. L. 209
Artero, S. 338
Ashby, F. G. 229
Ashcraft, M. H. 425
Ashton, H. 79, 80, 81, 82, 86
Assaad, J. M. 58
Aston-Jones, G. 264
Atkinson, R. M. 329, 330, 335
Attaway, C. M. 240
Aubert, I. 245–246
Auerbach, J. G. 85
Augsburger, M. 302, 305
Aulakh, C. S. 180
Avants, S. K. 300
Avenevoli, S. 228
Avila, A. H. 352
Avrith, D. B. 116
Aycicegi, A. 234
Ayd, F. J. 100
Ayre, F. 279, 298, 300
Azrin, R. L. 119, 127, 128

Babst, D. V. 302
Bach, P. B. 304
Bachman, J. G. 7, 10, 12, 16, 20, 24, 26, 28, 31, 35, 36, 143
Backman, L. 235
Badcock, R. 79, 82
Baddeley, A. 382, 424, 425
Badger, G. J. 127, 128, 274, 288, 412
Badiani, A. 446, 447
Bagary, M. 96
Bagasra, O. 358
Bagby, G. J. 358
Bagby, R. M. 411
Baggott, M. J. 181
Bailey, L. 82
Baker, K. G. 57, 58
Baker, P. J. 228
Bakhit, C. 179
Bakos, N. 157
Baldinger, B. 230
Baldwin, G. C. 352
Balfour, H. H. 353
Balster, R. L. 178
Baltazar, P. L. 83
Balter, B. B. 75
Balter, M. B. 75, 79, 86
Bannerman, D. M. 59

Bannon, A. W. 239
Baram, D. A. 158
Barbaro, N. M. 445
Barberger-Gateau, P. 332, 336
Barbone, F. 97, 99
Barch, D. 382
Barker, A. 334
Barker, M. J. 75, 86, 87, 88, 89, 91, 93, 338
Barker, W. 331
Barnes, L. W. 410
Barnett, H. 390, 393
Barnett, M. J. 339
Baron, J. A. 246
Barr, W. 385
Barratt, E. S. 411
Barrett-Connor, C. 326
Barrett-Connor, E. 235, 236
Barry, D. 44
Bartzokis, G. 121, 352
Basbaum, A. I. 445
Basil, M. D. 236
Basile, A. S. 182
Basile, M. 184
Basso, A. M. 362
Basso, M. 380
Basso, M. R. 350, 351, 363
Bateman, C. 158
Bates, M. 396
Bates, M. E. 44
Bates, T. C. 230, 233
Batkai, S. 144
Batra, A. 47
Battaglia, G. 174
Battig, K. 228, 230, 232
Bauer, L. O. 122, 127, 128
Bauman, M. D. 58
Bautista, A. P. 357
Baxter, L. R. J. 116
Bayer, B. M. 352
Baylis, L. L. 116
Beal, J. E. 159
Beale K. S. 240
Beardsley, P. M. 178, 445
Bearn, J. 287, 302, 448
Beauchamp, N. J. 242
Beauvais, J. 128
Bechara, A. 121, 124, 125, 273, 274, 420, 421, 422, 423
Beck, A. T. 212
Beck, C. H. 446
Beck, J. 171, 196
Becker, H. S. 415, 439, 440, 441–442
Beckwith, B. E. 51, 228, 233
Becona, E. 227
Beecher, H. K. 292
Beekman, A. T. 227
Beevers, G. 235
Begaud, B. 338–339
Begleiter, H. 50, 51
Behl, C. 144

Behm, F. M. 239
Beiser, A. 333
Belanger, A. J. 335
Belanger, H. 236
Belin, D. 435
Bell, C. M. 97
Bell, D. S. 215
Bell, M. 392
Bell, N. 229, 230, 231, 232, 233
Bell, S. L. 229, 231
Bellack, A. 376, 377, 386, 388, 393, 396
Belleville, R. E. 288
Belman, A. L. 350
Benavides, J. 182
Bengochea, O. 60
Benkelfat, C. 58, 116
Bennett, D. A. 330
Bennett, R. C. 302
Benowitz, N. L. 232, 239
Benson, D. F. 120
Beresford, T. 324
Beresford, T. P. 83
Berger, J. R. 364
Bergman, A. 387
Bergman, H. 95
Bergman, J. 112
Berkman, L. 338
Berkman, L. F. 235
Berman, J. 351–352
Berman, J. S. 158
Berman, S. M. 273, 274, 300, 422
Bernas, M. J. 358
Bernik, M. A. 92, 95
Berridge, K. C. 446
Berthold, T. 189
Bespalov, A. Y. 445
Best, D. 305
Best, P. J. 61
Better, W. E. 118, 267
Beylich, K.-M. 302
Bhattachary, S. 192, 193, 194, 195
Bickel, W. K. 127, 128, 274, 287, 288, 305, 409, 410, 411, 412, 414, 442
Biederman, J. 425
Biegon, A. 113, 143, 144
Bienias, J. L. 330
Bierut, L. J. 45, 435
Bigelow, G. E. 287, 288, 289, 291, 292, 293, 294, 304, 305, 442
Bigelow, L. 381
Bilder, R. 385
Bilecen, D. 54
Bilgic, B. 328, 334
Bilker, W. 383, 385
Bilsky, E. J. 177
Binns, A. S. 440
Birch, B. R. P. 79
Birch, R. 158
Bird, M. 178
Birkett, D. J. 76

Birks, J. 334, 337
Bisogno, T. 143
Bixler, E. O. 84
Bjork, J. M. 53
Blair, R. J. 58
Blanchard, J. 376, 377, 378, 379, 380, 394, 395
Blaney, T. 304
Blasig, J. 445
Bleiberg, J. 119
Bleich, A. 305
Blessing, W. W. 180
Blin, O. 59
Block, R. I. 119, 120, 129, 152, 153, 155, 359
Blomberg, R. D. 302
Blomstrand, C. 264
Bloom, F. E. 78
Bloome, B. 158
Blum, R. H. 437
Blume, A. 396
Bo, P. 56
Boardman, A. 239
Boberg, M. 235
Boccellari, A. A. 300
Bochner, F. 295
Bodner, G. 305
Bogunovic, O. J. 100
Bohm, P. 409
Bohn, P. B. 83
Boileau, I. 58
Boivin, J. 99, 100
Boivin, J. F. 337
Bolla, K. I. 113, 116, 117, 119, 120, 121, 126, 127, 129, 153, 156, 352, 392
Bolton, J. 287, 302
Bonci, A. 46
Bond, G. E. 326
Bondi, M. W. 364
Bonita, R. 335
Bonner, T. I. 143
Bontempi, B. 244
Bonthius, D. J. 54, 60
Boone, K. B. 349, 350
Booth, M. 139
Boreham, J. 237
Borgis, K. J. 332
Borg, S. 95, 96, 294
Borgs, P. 358
Bormann, J. 78
Bornstein, R. A. 349, 350, 351, 354, 356, 357, 358, 359, 360, 363, 380
Borsutzky, S. 328
Bortolotto, Z. A. 265
Bosch-Morell, F. 60
Bosman, M. 229, 230
Bourin, M. 84
Boutcher, S. H. 228, 232
Bow-Thomas, C. 395
Bowden, S. C. 44
Bowirrat, A. 45, 55
Bowyer, J. F. 180, 185

Boysen, G. 333
Bradley, B. 294, 438
Bradshaw, C. M. 410
Brady, C. M. 158
Brady, J. V. 178
Brady, K. T. 119, 120, 227
Braestrup, C. 78
Braff, D. 381
Braida, D. 264
Bramlage, A. 53
Brammer, M. 266
Bramness, J. G. 99–100
Brand, M. 328
Brandt, K. M. 53
Bratt, D. 383
Brauer, L. H. 442
Braun, D. W. 158
Braun, G. 177
Braun, U. 177
Braus, D. F. 188
Braver, T. 382
Breeder, A. 171
Breier, A. 79, 82, 83, 382
Breiter, H. C. 58, 59, 118
Breivogel, C. S. 143
Bremner, K. E. 96
Brennan, E. 159
Breslau, N. 227
Brewer, N. T. 409
Bricolo, R. 183
Brien, J. F. 60
Brioni, J. D. 239
Britt, R. H. 86
Britton, K. T. 362
Broderick, J. P. 117
Brodkin, J. D. 180
Brody, A. L. 242
Broening, H. W. 180
Brokate, B. 328
Bromet, E. 375
Brooks, B. P. 174
Brooner, R. K. 305
Brouhard, B. 360
Brower, K. 357
Brown, B. S. 305
Brown, G. 388, 389, 396, 392, 393
Brown, G. G. 47, 56
Brown, H. 75, 79
Brown, K. 156
Brown, R. A. 227
Brown, R. R. 296
Brown, R. W. 240
Brown, S. 376, 377, 378, 379, 394, 395
Brown, S. A. 47, 56
Browndyke, J. N. 352
Browne, N. 438
Brownlee, S. 409
Brownstein, M. J. 143
Bruce, I. 325
Brunk, S. F. 158

Bryan, G. 196
Bryant, K. J. 127
Bryceland, J. 178
Bryson, G. 392
Buccafusco, J. J. 240, 244
Buchanan, R. 380, 382, 392
Buchert, R. 186
Buchner, D. M. 302
Bucholz, K. K. 45
Buchsbaum, M. 381
Buck, A. 189
Buckner, R. L. 51
Budd, R. D., K. 302
Budney, A. J. 127, 128, 146
Buffet-Jerrott, S. E. 337
Bühler, B. 378
Bunney, B. S. 264
Bunzow, J. R. 112, 175
Buono, D. 353
Burger, C. 152
Burke, C. 207
Burr, G. 56
Burton, M. J. 116
Buschke, H. 333
Bush, G. 116
Bushman, B. J. 52
Busquets, X. 265
Bustini, M. 384, 385
Busto, U. 96
Butelman, E. R. 238
Butler, S. 408
Butters, M. A. 329, 330
Butters, N. 44, 56, 61, 328, 334
Buzzi, R. 232

Cadet, J.-L. 113, 118, 119, 120, 121, 127, 129, 153, 156, 267, 352, 392
Caggiula, A. R. 230
Cahill, L. 229
Cairns, J. 409, 410, 411
Calhoun, V. D. 54
Callaway, C. W. 175, 177
Callaway, E. 232
Camargo, E. E. 352
Cami, J. 275, 287, 288, 292, 293, 299, 441
Campbell, A. M. 359
Campbell, K. 50
Cancela, L. M. 362
Cancro, R. 387, 391
Canfield, D. R. 112
Cannon, T. 380, 384, 385
Canter, A. 158
Cantillon, M. 331
Cantos, E. L. 56
Canu, W. 245
Capitanio, J. P. 58
Cappell, H. 441, 442
Carboni, E. 182
Cardenas, V. A. 46, 56, 352
Cardinal, R. N. 59, 423

Cardno, A. 381
Cardon, L. R. 237
Carey, C. 154, 155
Carey, K. 376
Carey, M. 376
Carlen, P. L. 329
Carlin, A. S. 155, 298–299, 300, 303
Carmelli, D. 234, 235, 237, 241, 242
Carpenter, C. 380, 382, 383
Carpenter, W. 382, 392
Carrigan, M. H. 119, 120
Carroll, K. M. 127, 425
Carter, C. 182, 380, 383
Carter, J. D. 192, 193, 194, 195
Cary, M. S. 329, 330
Cascella, N. 381
Cascella, N. G. 441
Cascio, M. G. 143
Casellas, P. 182
Castner, S. A. 208
Catafau, A. M. 56, 327
Catlin, M. C. 60
Caudill, B. D. 441
Cavalheiro, E. A. 265
Cecyre, D. 245–246
Celerier, E. 445
Cerhan, J. R. 234, 237
Cervilla, J. A. 234, 237
Cestaro, V. L. 56
Chaderjian, M. 383
Chadwick, I. S. 444
Chadwick, O. 10
Chaisson, R. E. 354
Chait, L. D. 441
Chambers, A. 394, 395
Chambers, J. H. 82, 83, 98
Chan, S. F. 298, 299
Chance, M. B. 239
Chance, M. R. A. 444
Chang, A. E. 158
Chang, L. 187, 210, 215, 218, 350
Changeux, J. P. 240
Chao, C. C. 353
Chapman, G. B. 409, 410
Charuvastra, C. 304
Chatham, L. R. 305
Chatwal, J. P. 359
Chavarro, A. 410
Chen, M. 335, 336
Chen, W. T. 235
Chen, Y. 75, 80, 81, 83, 86, 95, 98, 100, 117
Cheng, R. 227
Cherek, D. R. 411
Cherner, M. 361
Cherpitel, C. J. 98
Chessick, R. D. 288
Chesson, H. 409
Cheung, E. H. 47, 56
Chew, M. L. 339
Chilcoat, H. D. 227, 443

Childers, S. R. 143
Childress, A. 121, 123, 125
Childress, A. R. 410, 421, 423, 448
Chirurgi, V. A. 349
Chiu, N. Y. 152
Cho, A. K. 177
Choi, M. 306
Choi, S. J. 121
Chokshi, S. K. 119
Chorlian, D. B. 50
Chou, J. 387
Chouinard, G. 78
Chow, H. L. 446
Christensen, L. Q. 302
Christian, J. C. 234, 235, 237
Chui, H. C. 332, 335, 337
Chutuape, M. A. 305
Cimbura, G. 302
Ciraulo, D. A. 79, 86
Civelli, O. 112
Clark, H. 392
Clark, H. W. 119
Clark, L. D. 444
Clark, M. 442
Clark, W. C. 158
Clarkson, J. E. 99
Clayton, T. 334, 337
Cleghorn, J. 388, 389, 396, 392, 393
Clemens, P. 246
Cleveland, M. F. 236
Clifford, S. T. 50
Clyde, D. J. 441
Co, C. 184
Coakley, D. 325
Coalson, D. W. 292
Cochrane, K. J. 292, 294, 295, 296
Coenen, A. 82–83
Coffey, B. J. 84
Coffey, D. 246
Coffey, S. F. 119, 120
Cohen, A. J. 294
Cohen, B. 386
Cohen, G. 382
Cohen, J. 87, 380, 382
Cohen, L. 122
Cohen, L. S. 85
Cohen, R. S. 188
Colado, M. I. 180
Colditz, G. A. 333
Coleman, R. E. 151, 239, 359
Coleman, V. 75, 76, 79, 85
Coles, M. G. 53
Collado-Morente, L. 60
Collier, A. C. 349
Collingwood, L. 393–394
Collins, A. C. 238
Collins, E. D. 287
Collins, G. H. 328
Collins, M. 92
Collins, R. L. 441

Colliver, J. D. 22, 140
Collomp, K. 77, 85
Colombo, J. A. 182
Colrain, I. M. 233
Colsher, P. L. 323
Comer, S. D. 287, 443
Comitas, L. 437
Commenges, D. 331
Commins, D. L. 182
Commissaris, R. L. 176
Compton, D. M. 240
Compton, W. M. 22, 140
Concha, M. 1992; 354, 355, 357, 363
Cone, E. J. 288, 292
Conley, F. K. 86
Conners, C. K. 245
Connolly, J. F. 83
Conrath, C. L. 246
Constantinides, L. 381
Contel, N. R. 446
Contoreggi, C. 121, 422, 423
Cook, C. C. 334
Cook, I. A. 210
Cook, J. O. 410
Cook, M. R. 228, 229, 232, 237
Cook, R. T. 357
Cooper, H. M. 52
Cooper, J. R. 78, 304
Cooper, L. 390, 393
Cooper, S. J. 446
Copeland, J. R. 329
Copersino, M. L. 277, 298, 387, 391
Corballis, P. 230
Cord, B. J. 179
Cordova, X. 426
Corker, K. 442
Cornblatt, B. 381
Corne, L. 337, 339
Cornish, J. W. 123
Correia, C. J. 289
Corrigall, W. A. 238
Corulla, W. J. 411
Coups, E. J. 409
Courchesne, E. 50
Court, J. A. 238
Couture, A. 328
Cowan, R. L. 187
Cowen, P. J. 117
Cox, J. L. 325
Craig, D. 230, 231, 232
Craig, R. J. 304
Crean, J. P. 409, 410, 411
Crews, D. J. 228, 232
Crippa, J. A. 152
Cristiani, S. A. 359, 360
Croft, R. J. 155, 192, 193, 194, 195
Crombag, H. S. 446
Cronin, C. 158
Crow, T. 392
Crowe, S. F. 75, 79, 86, 87, 88, 89, 91, 93, 338

Crowley, T. J. 227, 425
Crunican, M. A. 294, 295, 296
Cummings, J. L. 56, 326, 328, 329, 333
Cunningham, V. J. 97
Curran, H. V. 79, 82, 83, 95, 98, 183, 272, 287, 302, 305
Curry, P. D. 444
Cushman, P. 294
Cutler, R. E. 441
Cutter, H. S. 294, 295, 296
Czuczwar, S. J. 265

Dackis, C. A. 122
D'Agostino, R. B. 326, 333, 335
Dahlgren, L. A. 244
Daingerfield, M. 289, 304
Dam, M. 327
Damasio, A. R. 124, 125, 273, 274, 420, 421, 422, 423
Damasio, H. C. 121, 124, 125, 273, 274, 420, 421, 422, 423
Daneluzzo, E. 384, 385
Dani, J. A. 238, 246
Daniel, D. G. 96
Daniels, B. A. 79, 82
Danielsen, U. T. 56
Dannals, R. F. 186
Danos, P. 266, 353
Dansky, B. S. 119, 120
Daras, M. 118
Darke, S. 215, 272, 273, 300, 305
Dartigues, J. F. 331
Darwin, W. D. 288, 292
Datta, H. 264
Daugherty, J. R. 302
Daumann, J. 188, 190, 191, 192, 194
Daunais, J. B. 113
D'Aunno, T. 304
Davanipour, Z. 235
Davidson, M. C. 231, 240
Davies, A. G. 46
Davies, M. F. 77, 78
Davies, S. N. 144
Davis, C. 391
Davis, D. H. 438
Davis, F. C. 229
Davis, G. C. 227
Davis, J. W. 245
Davis, L. J. 329, 323, 337
Davis, M. 58, 396
Davis, P. E. 276, 277, 293, 298
Dawe, G. S. 238
Dawson, D. A. 340
Dawud-Noursi, S. 207
Day, H. E. 446, 447
Day, R. O. 239
Dazzi, L. 359
Deacon, R. M. J. 59
Dealberto, M. J. 338
Deary, I. J. 234, 234, 324, 339

DeBiasi, M. 246
De Blas, A. L. 78
De Boer, M. C. 440
Debski, T. D. 231
DeCarli, C. 241, 242
De Castro, S. 355
Decker, M. D. 302
Decker, M. W. 239
De Costa, B. R. 143
Deeg, D. J. 227
Degenhardt, L. 147, 148
Degrado, T. R. 152
De Haan, E. 381, 383
Deif, A. 155
Delafuente, J. C. 352
De la Torre, R. 441
Delaveau, P. 59
De Leon, J. 227
DeLisi, L. 380
Dellaportas, C. 86
Della Salla, S. 382
Del Pesce, M. 354, 355, 363
Del Porto, J. A. 441
Del Rio, M. C. 306
Denburg, N. 422
Deng, J. 235
Den Heeten, G. J. 186
Denihan, A. 325
Depatie, L. 244
De Petrocellis, L. 143
DeRicco, D. A. 441
Deroche-Gamonet, V. 435
Derryberry, D. 420
Desmond, J. E. 47, 48
De Souza, E. B. 174, 181, 182, 183
Des Rosiers, M. H. 114
DeVane, C. L. 352
Devane, W. A. 143
De Visser S. J. 98
De Vlugt, Y. 53
De Wit, H. 153, 292, 409–410, 411, 441, 442, 443
Dhuna, A. 121
Di, S. V. 120, 128, 129
Diaz, F. J. 227
Di Carlo, G. 157
Dick, D. M. 45, 46
Dickman, S. J. 411, 421
Dickson, D. W. 350
Dickson, S. 378
Diehr, P. 242
Dierker, L. C. 228
Dietze, P. 289, 305
Di Franco, M. J. 354
Difranza, J. R. 237
Di Furia, L. 183
Diksic, M. 54
Dillon, W. P. 46
DiMaio, V. J. 302
Di Marzo, V. 143

Dingle, G. A. 358
Dinn, W. M. 234
Dinnis, A. K. 229
Di Pano, R. 391
Di Sclafani, V. 46
Dishion, T. J. 443
Dittert, S. 277
Djousse, L. 333
Dlugosch, G. 294
Dlugos, C. A. 57
Docherty, J. R. 180
Docherty, N. 384
Dolan, R. J. 58, 60, 448
Dolan, S. 422
Dole, V. P. 263, 294, 304
Doll, R. 99
Domino, E. F. 243
Donaldson, D. I. 51
Donny, E. C. 239
Doran, B. 444
Dore, C. J. 86
Dorman, N. 441
Doty, P. 441
Dougherty, D. M. 53, 411
Doyle, T. 45
Drachman, D. 330, 331
Dragunow, M. 143
Drake, A. I. 364
Drake, R. 375
Drummer, O. H. 100
D'Souza, D. 377
Duara, R. 331
Duchak, V. 378
Ducimetiere, P. 326
Due, D. L. 240
Dufouil, C. 323, 326, 338
Dufour, M. 325
Dunne, M. P. 228, 232, 233
Dunphy, S. C. 83
Duran, S. D. 210
Durlak, J. A. 87
Durvasula, R. S. 352, 353, 363
Du Tertre, A. C. 84
Du Toit, B. M. 437
Dworkin, S. I. 116, 184
Dyer, K. R. 295
Dysarz, F. A. 143

Eap, C. B. 304
Earleywine, M. 140, 440
Easton, C. 127, 128
Eaton-Williams, P. 228
Eaves, L. 227
Ebmeier, K. P. 183, 186
Eckardt, M. 83
Edelmann, R. J. 293
Edelstein, S. L. 235, 236, 326
Edenberg, H. 45
Eder, H. 277, 278, 281, 300
Edgerton, R. B. 437

Edwards, J. A. 228, 230
Egan, M. 381
Ehrenreich, H. 155
Ehrman, R. 121, 123, 410, 421, 423
Eisen, S. A. 45
Eisenman, A. J. 289, 304
Eklund, C. 294
El, S. A. 155
El-Bassel, N. 305
Eldreth, D. A. 121, 153, 156
Elias, M. F. 326
Elias, P. K. 326
Eling, P. 82–83, 328
Ellinwood, E. H. J. 83, 446
Ellis, R. J. 46
Ellison, R. C. 333
Elrod, K. 240
Elton, M. 53
Elwood, P. C. 234, 235, 237
Emre, M. 328, 334
Ende, G. 188
Endo, K. 241
Engelbrektson, K. 95
Engelhart, C. 119
English, C. 386
Enoka, R. M. 229
Epstein, L. H. 230, 231
Erbaugh, J. 212
Erkinjuntti, T. 332, 335, 337
Erlenmeyer-Kimling, L. 381
Ernst, M. 230, 232, 234, 238, 241, 242, 361
Ernst, T. 187, 210, 350
Erwin, W. J. 119, 120, 129
Eslinger, P. J. 237
Espinosa, J. 331
Essex, M. 354
Essock, S. 375
Esteban, B. 180
Estes, S. L. 230, 242
Estruch, R. 56
Etco, N. L. 58
Etienne, M. A. 242
Evans, D. 330
Evans, M. 359
Evdokimidis, L. 381
Evenden, J. 411
Everitt, B. 423
Everitt, B. J. 59
Evert, D. L. 56, 61, 62
Ezekiel, F. 46

Faber, E. S. 58
Fadayel, G. M. 176
Faett, D. G. 327
Fage, D. 182
Fagerstrom, K. O. 239, 246
Fahey, M. A. 112
Fales, H. M. 78
Falk, J. L. 436, 437
Fann, W. E. 334

Fant, R. V. 288
Fantegrossi, W. E. 172, 173, 175, 176, 177, 178, 180, 181, 185
Faraone, S. 425
Farfel, G. M. 180
Farkas, L. 79
Farmer, M. E. 53
Farquhar-Smith, W. P. 157
Farre, M. 287, 288, 292, 293
Fass, R. J. 349, 350, 354, 357
Fastbom, J. 338
Faull, R. L. M. 143
Faure, P. 240
Fawzy, R. K. 155
Fein, D. 375
Fein, G. 46, 120, 128, 129
Feingold, D. A. 436, 437
Feinhandler, S. J. 441
Feldman, R. S. 360
Felong, A. M. 57
Ferguson, D. A. 50
Ferguson, S. M. 446, 447
Feria-Velasco, A. 264
Ferini Strambi, L. 83
Fertig, J. 230
Feskens, E. J. M. 237, 326
Fichtner, H. 328
Fields, F. R. 296
Fields, H. L. 445
Fife-Schaw, C. 230
File, S. E. 83, 229
Fillmore, M. T. 442, 443
Finch, E. 305
Finelli, A. 375
Finkbeiner, T. 272, 300
Finlayson, R. E. 329, 323, 337
Finn, P. R. 53, 424, 425, 440
Finnigan, F. 305
Fiore, M. C. 325
Fiorentine, R. 207
Fischer, G. 277, 278, 281, 300
Fischer, H. S. 173
Fischer, M. E. 241
Fischermann, T. 188, 191
Fischman, M. W. 116, 178, 208, 212, 287, 288, 352, 443
Fischman, V. S. 215
Fisher, J. 100
Fitzgerald, D. 389
Fitzgerald, J. 448
Fitzpatrick, A. L. 331, 334
Flanary, H. G. 288
Flashman, L. 383, 393
Fleishaker, J. C. 82, 83, 98
Fleming, S. E. 230
Fleming, T. 155
Flemming, D. 292
Fleshner, M. 229
Foerg, F. E. 127, 128
Foley, D. J. 235, 237

Author index   465

Folks, D. G. 76
Folli, D. 291
Folstein, M. F. 330, 331
Foltin, R. W. 212, 288, 443
Ford, J. M. 51
Forman, S. 382
Fornai, F. 182
Forno, L. S. 208
Foroud, T. 45, 46
Forsell, Y. 338
Forster, A. 96
Forza, G. 183
Forzano, L. B. 409, 410
Foster, D. J. 295
Fought, R. L. 302
Foulds, J. 229, 230, 231, 232, 233
Fountain, D. 3
Fournier, L. 53
Fowler, J. S. 54, 56
Fox, A. M. 152
Frackowiak, R. S. 448
Franceschi, D. 54
Francis, H. 354
Franco, S. 389, 396, 392
Frank, K. 289, 304
Frank, L. R. 47, 56
Frank, R. 421
Franke, P. 381
Franken, I. H. 353
Franklin, T. R. 121, 352
Fraser, H. F. 288, 289, 292, 293
Fratiglioni, L. 331, 336
Freedman, R. 244
Freeman, D. H. 335, 337
Freemont, A. J. 444
Freier, D. O. 354
Freire-Garabal, M. 362
Freud, S. 415
Freund, T. F. 143, 144, 157
Fride, E. 143, 157, 354
Fried, P. 156, 157
Friedman, D. P. 113
Friedman, G. D. 333
Friedman, H. 353, 354, 360
Friedman, M. 408
Friedrich, P. 78
Frisoni, G. B. 336
Friston, K. J. 448
Friswell, J. 59
Frith, C. D. 58
Frowein, H. W. 50
Fuchs, B. A. 354
Fuchs, V. R. 411
Fuh, J. L. 235
Fujishima, Y. 327
Fujitani, N. 210
Fujiwara, E. 328
Fujiwara, M. 243
Fukuda, H. 241
Fukui, S. 361

Fuller, R. K. 325
Fuller, R. W. 178
Fullerton, J. R. 296
Funderburk, F. R. 120, 127
Fuseler, J. 357
Fuster, J. M. 56

Gaiefsky, M. 350
Galaburda, A. M. 421
Galambos, R. 50
Galanis, D. J. 235, 237
Gale, A. 228, 230
Galiegue, S. 143, 182
Gallagher, D. W. 77
Galve-Roperh, I. 144
Galynker, I. I. 267
Gambini, O. 381
Gamma, A. 176, 189
Gansler, D. A. 46, 47, 55, 56, 57, 62, 328
Ganzini, L. 330, 335
Garavan, H. 127
Garcia-Estrada, J. 264
Garcia-Sevilla, J. A. 265
Garlington, W. K. 441
Garman, R. H. 265
Garnham, N. J. 192, 193, 194
Garrett, B. E. 443
Garriott, J. C. 302
Garvey, M. J. 83
Garzone, P. D. 82, 83, 98
Gaskell, R. K. 329
Gastpar, M. 272, 300
Gault, B. 414, 419
Gauthier, S. 245–246, 337
Gawin, F. H. 119, 122
Gearon, S. 396
Gebo, K. A. 354
Gee, K. W. 182
Gekker, G. 353
Gelkopf, M. 305
Geller, A. M. 81, 98
Gentry, M. V. 228
Georgiou, G. 47, 56
Gerkovich, M. M. 228, 229, 232, 237
Gerra, G. 267, 294, 300
Gershon, S. 215
Gerth, C. W. 148
Geschwind, N. 121
Gescuk, B. 47
Geyer, M. A. 175, 176, 177
Ghatan, P. H. 54, 241, 242
Ghia, J. 158
Ghoneim, M. M. 82, 83, 98, 119, 120, 129,
    155, 212
Giardini, A. 56
Gibb, J. W. 178, 179, 183
Gibson, M. A. 60
Giedd, J. N. 352
Giesbrecht, N. 98
Gilbert, D. G. 230, 242

Gill, J. S. 333
Gill, T. M. 240
Gilman, S. 47, 56
Gilmore-Thomas, K. K. 304
Gioino, G. 362
Giordani, B. 246
Giovannetti, T. 385
Givens, B. 240
Gjerde, H. 302
Glabus, M. F. 183, 186
Glantz, M. D. 22, 140
Glass, M. 143, 144
Glassman, R. 100
Glennon, R. A. 172, 173, 176
Gleser, G. C. 296
Glimcher, P. 424
Glue, P. 97
Goa, C. 335, 336
Goate, A. 45
Goeders, N. E. 113
Goeters, S. 229, 232
Gold, G. 332
Gold, J. 380, 381, 382, 383
Gold, L. H. 177
Gold, M. L. 294
Gold, M. S. 122
Goldberg, E. 56
Goldberg, J. 45
Goldberg, S. R. 112, 145–146, 292
Goldberg, T. 380, 381, 382, 383
Goldberger, B. A. 288, 292
Golding, J. G. 79, 86
Goldman, P. S. 208
Goldman-Rakic, P. S. 208, 380, 381, 382, 383
Goldmann, H. 46
Goldstein, A. 277, 300, 303
Goldstein, M. 380, 383
Goldstein, R. 385
Goldstein, R. Z. 115
Golombok, S. 92, 94, 95, 96
Gomberg, E. 324
Gong, Z. H. 238
Gonzalez, B. 351–352
Gonzalez, G. 48, 263
Gonzalez, R. 154, 155
Gonzalez-Pinto, A. 227
Gonzalo, L. M. 60
Goodall, E. M. 117
Goodwin, D. W. 51, 438
Gordinier, S. 384
Gordon, A. M. 99
Gordon, N. 302
Gordon, N. B. 276, 281
Gorelick, P. B. 325
Gorell, J. M. 245
Gorenstein, C. 83, 92, 95
Gori, E. 264
Gorissen, M. 82–83, 98
Gorny, G. 264
Gorter, R. 159

Gossop, M. 294, 305, 438
Gottesman, I. 377, 394
Gottschalk, C. 128, 352
Gottschalk, L. A. 296
Gould, K. L. 352
Gourevitch, M. N. 353
Gouzoulis-Mayfrank, E. 155, 188, 191
Govitrapong, P. 354
Grabowecky, M. F. 50
Grabowski, J. 305
Grabowski, T. 421
Graeber, M. B. 182
Graham, C. 228, 229, 232, 237
Gralla, R. J. 158
Grammer, G. G. 328, 334
Granados, R. 180
Grandinetti, A. 245
Grandy, D. K. 112
Granon, S. 240
Grant, B. F. 22, 140
Grant, I. 45, 150, 154, 155, 159, 298–299, 300, 303, 349, 350, 364
Grant, S. 121, 125, 422, 423
Grant, S. A. 49
Grant, T. M. 288, 292
Graupner, L. 233, 234
Gravenstein, J. S. 292
Graves, A. B. 235, 236, 331, 336
Gray, F. 156, 157
Gray, J. A. 59, 230, 233, 231, 238, 244
Gray, R. 238
Gray, S. L. 337
Green, A. R. 180
Green, B. 145
Green, J. E. 356, 357, 358, 363
Green, L. 410, 413, 415, 438
Green, M. 215, 383, 393, 395
Green, M. F. 221
Greenwald, M. K. 293
Greenwood, K. M. 338
Greenwood, K. M. 75, 86, 87, 88, 89, 91, 93
Greer, G. R. 196
Gregg, J. 158
Gregson, R. 396
Greiner, L. H. 332
Greiner, P. A. 332
Greist, J. H. 81, 82, 84
Grenden, J. 357
Grevert, P. 277, 300, 303
Griesar, W. S. 230, 231
Griffin, G. 143
Griffin, M. R. 302
Griffith, J. D. 174
Griffiths, R. R. 86, 178, 305, 441, 442, 443
Grillon, C. 50
Gritz, E. R. 276
Grob, C. S. 187
Grobe, J. E. 230
Gronbaek, M. 333
Gross, K. 272, 287, 281, 290

Gross, S. D. 238
Grotenhermen, F. 141
Grottick, A. J. 240
Grow, R. W. 45
Grubb, M. 59
Gruber, A. J. 155
Gruber, S. 386
Gruber, S. A. 153
Grunberg, N., E. 235
Grundy, R. I. 144
Grusec, J. 410
Gruzelier, J. 380
Gruzelier, J. G. H. 155
Gualtieri, C. 381
Guastello, B. 418
Gudelsky, G. A. 176, 180
Gudex, C. 81, 82, 85
Gudjonsson, G. H. 95
Guerra, D. 275, 299, 441
Guerrera, M. P. 237
Guimon, J. 265
Gunnarsdottir, E. D. 122
Gunne, L. M. 215
Gunthner, A. 47
Gur, R. 383
Gur, R. C. 385
Gur, R. E. 385
Gurling, H. 266, 300
Gurpegui, M. 227
Gurvit, H. 328, 334
Gustafsen, S. 228, 232
Guthrie, S. 243
Gutstein, H. B. 263
Guy, G. 139
Guy, T. D. 230
Guzman, M. 144
Gylfadottir, G. 244

Haan, M. N. 236
Haas, G. 385
Haavik, C. O. 171, 195
Haber, R. 45
Habraken, J. B. 186
Hack, S. 233
Hader, S. 355
Haefely, W. E. 77
Haendel, V. 409, 410, 411
Haertzen, C. A. 288, 292, 293
Häfner, H. 376, 377–378, 379
Hagenah, J. M. 246
Haine, C. 381
Hakan, R. 238
Hakkinen, S. 305
Hale, C. R. 228
Halgren, E. 50, 51, 52, 53
Halgunseth, L. 395
Hall, C. B. 333
Hall, J. 424, 425
Hall, M. 244
Hall, W. 140, 147, 148, 215

Hall, W. G. 240, 305
Haller, J. 157
Hallford, H. 390, 396, 389
Halliday, G. M. 56, 57, 58, 60
Halliday, R. 232
Hallstrom, C. 86
Hambrecht, M. 376, 377–378, 379
Hamid, S. 238
Hamil, W. L. 155
Hammersley, R. 305
Hampson, A. J. 144
Hanagasi, H. A. 328, 334
Handelsman, L. 292, 294, 295, 296, 305
Hando, J. 215
Haney, M. 443
Hanggi, D. 54
Hanlon, J. 338
Hannerz, J. 359
Hans, S. L. 85
Hanson, G. R. 178, 179, 183
Hanson, K. L. 192, 193, 194, 195
Harding, A. J. 56, 57, 58, 60
Hardman, H. F. 171, 195
Hardy, D. J. 210
Hare, R. D. 410
Harford, T. C. 441
Harper, C. G. 45, 46, 56, 57, 58
Harrell, E. 393–394
Harris, C. L. 234
Harris, G. C. 264
Harris, G. J. 46, 47, 55, 56, 57, 62, 352
Harris, H. W. 264
Harris, J. 305
Harris, L. 158
Harris, L. S. 178
Harris, T. B. 235, 237
Hart, R. 128
Hartley, L. R. 228, 232, 233
Hartman, D. E. 352, 356, 358, 364
Harvey, J. A. 178
Harvey, P. 383
Harvey, R. 395, 396
Harwood, D. 331
Harwood, H. J. 3
Haselhorst, R. 54
Hasenfratz, M. 228, 230, 232
Hasin, D. 128, 221
Hatsukami, D. K. 244
Hatzidimitriou, G. 179
Hauger, R. 362
Haughton, V. M. 241
Haut, J. S. 51
Hauw, J-J. 332
Hawkins, K. A. 300
Hawkins, R. A. 265
Hawley, C. J. 86
Hawthorne, J. W. 305
Hayward, R. 305
Hazlett, E. 381
Haznedar, M. 381

He, H. 235
He, S. Y. 210
Heard, J. E. 229
Heath, A. 45
Heath, A. C. 227
Heath, C. 237
Heaton, R. K. 119, 127, 128, 349, 350, 357, 365, 383
Hebert, L. E. 330
Hebert, R. 333
Hege, S. G. 83
Heilman, K. M. 243
Heinrichs, D. 392
Heishman, S. J. 228, 229, 230, 231, 232, 234, 237, 238, 246, 292, 294
Hell, D. 176
Hellenbrand, W. 245
Heller, W. 242
Helligers, C. A. M. 83
Helzer, L. N. 438
Hemby, S. E. 184
Hemmelgarn, B. 99, 100, 337
Hendrie, H. 329
Hendriks, V. M. 353
Henn, F. A. 188
Hennekens, C. H. 333
Henningfield, J. E. 227, 228, 229, 230, 231, 232, 233, 237, 288, 292
Henriksen, L. 56
Hepner, I. J. 264
Herbert, L. E. 237
Herbert, M. 230
Herkenham, M. 143, 157
Hermann, H. 144
Hernandez-Tristan, R. 157
Herning, R. I. 118, 231, 267, 441
Herranz, R. 56
Herrera, B. 239
Herrera, C. 230, 234
Herrera, D. G. 60
Herrnstein, R. J. 409, 410
Herron, J. 396
Herzig, K. 232
Herz, A. 445
Hesselbrock, V. M. 122
Hietala, J. 385
Higa, M. 235
Higgins, G. A. 240
Higgins, S. T. 117, 127, 128, 288, 442, 443
Hildebrandt, H. 328
Hill, E. 357
Hill, H. E. 288
Hill, R. D. 235
Hill, S. Y. 47, 266, 279, 298, 300
Hillebrand, J. 305
Hillyard, S. A. 50, 51
Hiltunen, A. J. 294, 295
Hindes, A. 422
Hindmarch, I. 99, 230, 231, 232, 233, 306
Hindmarsh, T. 359

Hines, S. E. 53
Hinkin, C. H. 364
Hinrichs, J. V. 82, 83, 98
Hinson, J. M. 425
Hinson, R. E. 440, 446
Hirabayashi, M. 446
Hirai, S. 361
Hiramatsu, M. 177
Hiripi, E. 227
Hirsch, S. 380
Hitzemann, R. J. 56
Ho, A. 113
Ho, C. H. 209
Hoeldtke, R. D. 293
Hofer, A. 385
Hoff, A. 380
Hoff, A. L. 119, 122
Hoffer, L. D. 244
Hoffer, M. 227
Hoffman, A. J. 174
Hoffman, S. J. 228, 229, 232, 237
Hogan, D. B. 325, 339
Hohmann, A. G. 157
Holcomb, H. 381
Holcomb, P. J. 51
Holicky, B. A. 288, 292
Hollander, E. 122
Hollister, L. E. 86
Holman, B. L. 118
Holroyd, C. B. 53
Holthausen, E. 388, 393
Holzman, P. 380, 383
Homewood, J. 264
Hommer, D. W. 47, 60, 79, 82, 83
Hong, R. 210
Honkanen, R. 302
Hooks, N. T. 292, 293
Horak, M. 277
Horan, B. 376, 377, 378, 379, 394, 395
Horn, J. L. 239
Hornak, J. 116
Horner, M. 395, 396
Horschitz, S. 186
Horvath, T. B. 50
Hoth, A. 339
Houlihan, M. E. 230
House, H. 158
Howe, M. N. 234
Howlett, A. C. 143
Hser, Y. I. 438
Huang, A. 99, 100, 337
Huang, D. B. 305
Huang, S. M. 143
Huang, W. 331
Hubbell, C. L. 177
Hubner, C. B. 178
Huddleston, J. 288
Hudson, J. I. 155
Huestis, M. A. 155
Huettel, S. A. 240

Hughes, J. R. 227, 244, 441, 442
Hui, Y. Z. 177
Hummerich, R. 186
Humpel, C. 173
Humphreys, D. F. 152
Hunter, D. J. 354
Hurd, Y. L. 112
Hurt, R. D. 329, 323, 337
Hutner, N. 47

Iga, J. 334
Iguchi, M. Y. 305
Ikonomidou-Turski, C. 265
Ilinsky, I. A. 57
Ilivitsky, V. 229, 230
Infante, M. 245
Ingram, M. V. 328, 334
Ingvar, D. H. 114
Ingvar, M. 54
Insel, T. R. 83, 181
Ireland, S. J. 119
Irvine, E. E. 229
Irwin, M. 362
Isaacs, J. P. 292
Isbell, H. 289, 304
Isen, A. M. 229
Isensee, B. 227
Ishikawa, A. 246
Ishimoto, Y. 334
Isner, J. M. 119
Iversen, L. L. 139, 144, 151, 154, 358
Iwasa, M. 327
Iyo, M. 219, 220, 361
Izenwasser, S. 184
Izzo, A. A. 157

Jääskeläinen, I. P. 50
Jackson, B. 439
Jackson, C. 375
Jackson, M. 75, 86, 87, 88, 89, 91, 93, 329, 338
Jackson, W. J. 240
Jacob, P. 239
Jacob, R. G. 231
Jacob, T. 45
Jacobs, E. A. 409, 412, 414
Jacobs, H. 246
Jacobsen, L. K. 184, 189, 352
Jacobson, R. R. 92, 328
Jaffe, J. 441
Jaffe, J. H. 288
Jagust, W. J. 236, 349
Jain, A. K. 158
Jajich, C. L. 335, 337
James, D. 156
James, G. H. 51
James, M. 233
Jameson, T. L. 425
Janal, M. N. 158
Jankovic, J. 364
Janosky, J. 265

Janson, V. E. 239
Jarrard, L. E. 238
Jarusuraisin, N. 214
Jarvis, M. J. 231, 234, 237
Jasinski, D. R. 174, 227, 292, 293, 295
Jay Frye G. D. 240
Jefferson, J. W. 81
Jeffery, P. J. 352
Jeffike, M. A. 58
Jeffnigan, T. L. 56
Jenner, F. A. 96
Jensen, M. K. 227
Jentsch, J. D. 359, 425
Jernigan, T. L. 334, 355
Jerrells, T. R. 357
Jittiwutikan, J. 214
Joe, G. W. 305
Joels, S. 234, 237
Johannesson, T. 244
Johanson, C. E. 116, 441, 443
Johns, A. 147, 148
Johnsen-Soriano, S. 60
Johnson, A. E. 238
Johnson, B. A. 117
Johnson, C. C. 245
Johnson, E. O. 227, 435
Johnson, M. 178, 179, 183
Johnson, M. P. 177
Johnson, M. R. 143
Johnson, R. E. 288
Johnson, S. E. 112
Johnson, T. 419
Johnson, V. 391
Johnson-Greene, D. 47, 56
Johnston, L. D. 7, 10, 12, 16, 20, 24, 26, 28, 31, 35, 36, 143
Johnstone, E. C. 183, 186
Jollant, F. 80
Jolles, J. 234, 235, 237
Jolley, A. 380
Jones, B. 381
Jones, B. E. 288, 289, 293
Jones, C. 274, 299, 300
Jones, G. M. 230, 233, 231, 244
Jones, H. E. 443
Jones, L. 381
Jones, M. 192, 193, 194
Jones, R. T. 181, 441
Jones, T. 97
Jonsson, J. E. 244
Jonsson, L. E. 215
Jonsson, S. 359
Jordan, B. 350
Joseph, H. 304
Josiassen, R. 376, 377, 386, 388, 393
Joy, C. 384
Joyce, E. M. 83, 123
Juan, D. 335, 336
Judd, B. W. 333, 335, 337
Judd, L. L. 53, 150, 298–299, 300, 303

Juge, O. 96
Junck, L. 47
June, H. L. 287, 292, 293
June, L. 231, 232, 233
Jungreis, C. A. 242
Justice, J. B. 112

Kaboli, P. J. 339
Kagerer, S. 277
Kahn, A. 47, 56
Kahn, D. A. 361
Kahn, H. J. 246
Kahneman, D. 408
Kaiser, A. H. 357
Kaito, M. 327
Kajdacsy-Balla, A. 358
Kajimura, N. 96
Kalbe, E. 328
Kalechstein, A. D. 207, 210, 215, 217, 219, 221
Kales, A. 84
Kalia, M. 181
Kalmijn, S. 234, 235, 237, 326
Kalyvoka, A. 384, 385
Kameyama, M. 243
Kameyama, T. 177
Kaminski, B. J. 178
Kanayama, G. 153
Kanazawa, I. 228, 233
Kandel, D. B. 227
Kandel, E. R. 78
Kaneta, H. 327
Kang, C. 230, 234
Kanitz, R. D. 332
Kannel, W. B. 335
Kano, M. 144
Kanof, P. D. 292, 294, 295, 296
Kant, I. 416
Kao, C. H. 361
Kaplan, E. 121
Kaplan, R. 388, 389, 396, 392, 393
Kaplan, S. 239
Karch, S. B. 209
Karlix, J. L. 352
Kartechner, W. 443
Kaslow, R. A. 358
Kassel, J. D. 228, 230, 246
Kathmann, N. 375
Kato, A. 327
Katona, I. 143
Katz, J. L. 86, 98, 443
Katz, M. J. 333
Katzman, R. L. 329, 330, 331
Kaufman, M. J. 58, 117, 266
Kavanagh, D. 145
Kawachi, I. 337
Kay, S. 387
Kayan, S. 444, 445
Kaye, F. J. 230
Ke, V. 334
Keenan, R. M. 441

Kehne, J. H. 176, 181
Kehr, J. 112
Keilp, J. 381
Keith, S. J. 53
Kellar, K. J. 238
Kelleher, L. M. 156
Kellogg, S. H. 238
Kelly, D. 291
Kelly, T. H. 212
Keltner, N. L. 76
Kelton, M. C. 246
Kempen, G. I. 227
Kendler, K. S. 227, 377
Kenny, G. N. 49
Kerich, M. J. 60
Kerman, I. A. 143
Kerr, J. S. 230, 231, 232, 233, 306
Kerr, S. A. 51
Keshavan, M. 385
Kessels, R. P. 328
Kessler, J. 328
Kessler, R. 227
Kessler, R. C. 435
Khandat, A. 245
Khuri, E. T. 304
Kilander, L. 235, 237
Kilbey, M. M. 446
Kim, D. H. 445
Kim, H. 46
Kim, K. Y. 334
Kim, P. 240
Kim, S. 444
Kim, S. W. 116
Kindermann, S. S. 47, 56
King, D. E. 118
King, G. R. 410
King, K. 119, 122
King, M. B. 86
Kingstone, A. 51
Kirby, K. C. 442, 443
Kirby, K. N. 274, 409, 410, 411, 412, 414, 418
Kirby, M. 325
Kirk, E. P. 425
Kirk, J. M. 441
Kirkby, K. C. 79, 82
Kirkley, S. M. 328
Kirkpatrick, B. 382, 391, 392
Kirkpatrick, P. J. 420
Kish, S. J. 181, 183, 184, 265
Kishida, S. 209
Kitani, M. 241, 335, 337
Kiuchi, Y. 80
Kjelstrup, K. G. 59, 60
Klar, H. M. 329
Klatsky, A. L. 333
Kleber, H. D. 122, 274, 294, 299, 300
Kleckham, J. 287, 302
Klein, R. M. 231
Klein, R. S. 353
Klein, T. W. 353, 354, 360

Kleinrok, Z. 265
Klett, C. J. 294, 304
Klono., D. C. 118
Kloos, A. 245
Klopp, J. 50, 52, 53
Klose, U. 334
Klosterkotter, J. 148
Kluin, K. J. 47
Kluwig, J. 272, 300
Knight, K. 96
Knight, R. T. 50
Knoller, N. 159
Knopick, C. 233
Knott, V. J. 229, 230, 231
Kobayashi, S. 241, 335, 337
Kobayashi, T. 80
Koelega, H. S. 49
Koeppe, R. A. 47, 243
Koepsell, T. D. 302
Kofke, W. A. 265
Koide, H. 241
Kolb, B. 264
Koob, G. F. 177, 362
Kopell, B. S. 50, 212
Kopp, B. 381
Korbo, L. 60
Korin, H. 279
Kornetsky, C. 178, 381
Kornetsky, C. H. 288
Kornhuber, J. 60
Kornreich, C. 293
Korttila, K. 80, 83, 98
Kos, J. 232
Kosten, T. R. 118, 122, 124, 128, 352
Kotchabhakdi, N. 354
Kovacs, E. J. 357
Kovasznay, B. 375
Koves, T. R. 184
Kovner, R. 354, 355, 363
Krabbendam, L. 328
Kraft, L. 383
Krajewski, K. 352
Kramer, J. C. 215
Krauss, B. 272, 287, 281, 290
Krebs, S. J. 228, 233
Kreek, M. J. 113, 238, 305, 352
Kress, Y. 350
Krieg, J. C. 95
Kril, J. J. 56, 57, 58, 60
Kringelbach, M. L. 116
Kritz-Silverstein, D. 235, 236, 326
Kroft, C. L. 47
Kroll, P. 357
Kromhout, D. 237, 326
Kronfol, Z. 357
Krugman, A. D. 441
Kruse, W. H. 100
Krystal, J. 394, 395
Krystal, J. H. 48, 189, 266, 267
Ksir, C. 238

Kudoh, A. 337
Kuehnle, J. C. 293
Kuhar, M. J. 111–112
Kuhn, C. 351–352
Kukull, W. A. 329, 330
Kuller, L. 236
Kuller, L. H. 331, 334
Kulsakdinun, C. 174
Kultas-Ilinsky, K. 57
Kumar, V. 331
Kumari, V. 241, 232
Kumor, K. M. 441
Kundurovic, Z. 334
Kunos, G. 144, 157
Kure, K. 350
Kurth, C. 60
Kurtz, M. 383
Kuslansky, G. 333
Kutas, M. 51
Kuyt, F. 239

Laakso, M. P. 47, 60
LaBar, K. S. 58
Laberg, J. C. 440
Lader, M. H. 75, 80, 82, 83, 86, 92, 94, 95, 96, 98
Lagnaoui, R. 323, 338–339
La Harpe, R. 265
Lai, R. 334, 337
Lalonde, R. N. 440
Lamas, X. 287, 288, 292, 293
Lamb, R. J. 112, 178
Lancaster, F. E. 47
Landers, D. M. 228, 232
Landi, F. 337
Lane, B. 54
Lane, S. B. 264
Lange, N. 58
Langendorf, F. G. 121, 122
Langrod, J. 304
Lantos, J. 304
Larcher, A. 445
Larrieu, S. 332, 336
Larson, E. B. 329, 330
LaRue, A. 237
Lasagna, L. 292
Lassen, N. A. 114
Latowsky, M. 295
Lau, M. A. 53
Laulin, J. P. 445
Launer, L. J. 234, 235, 237, 325, 326, 336
Laurent, A. 381
Laurent, C. L. 441
Lavenex, P. 58
LaVigne, G. 155
Lawlor, B. 325
Lawrence, N. S. 230, 241
Lawrie, S. 384
Lawson, C. W. 97
Leamon, M. 360

Leavitt, S. B. 304
Leccese, A. P. 127
Ledent, C. 157
Ledesert, B. 244
LeDoux, J. E. 59
Lee, G. P. 420, 421, 423
Lee, M. B. 58
Lee, S.-C. 333
Lee, T. M. 298, 299
Leenders, K. L. 361
Lees, A. 192, 193, 194
Lefkowitz, D. 242
Lehmann, P. 305
Le Houezec, J. 232
Leibovici, D. 244
Leifert, K. 272, 300
Lemay, S. 246
Lemeshow, S. 331
Lemmens, G. M. 266
Le Moal, M. 445
Lenne, M. G. 289, 305
Leonard, S. 244
Leonido-Yee, M. 210
Leshner, Alan I. 147
Letenneur, L. 331, 332, 336
Leuchter, A. F. 210
Levanthal, E. A. 409
Leveille, S. G. 302
Levin, E. D. 230, 232, 239, 240, 243, 244, 245
Levin, H. S. 349
Levin, J. M. 58, 115
Levine, A. J. 364
Levine, S. R. 118
Levinson, D. 375
Levy, D. 380
Levy, M. L. 214
Levy, R. 230, 233, 231, 244
Lewczuk, P. 60
Leweke, F. M. 148
Lewinsohn, P. M. 227
Lewis, R. F. 46, 47, 55, 56, 57, 62
Leyton, M. 58
Lezak, M. D. 120
Li, J. 235, 335, 336
Li, M. 239
Li, M. D. 227
Li, T. K. 45
Li, Y. 447
Liakopoulos, D. 381
Liang, B. 357–358
Liao, D. 236, 241
Liao, J. 227
Liberman, D. 390, 393
Lichter, D. G. 56
Lichtor, J. L. 292
Liddiard, H. 276, 277, 298
Liddle, P. F. 97
Lieb, R. 227
Liebson, I. A. 287, 287, 288, 289, 291, 292, 293, 294, 304, 305, 442

Liechti, M. E. 176
Lim, K. O. 46–47, 48, 54, 56, 57, 121, 334
Lin, K. N. 235
Lindesmith, A. R. 438
Lindman, R. 440, 441, 442
Lindsay, J. 210, 333
Ling, W. 210, 294, 304
Linnoila, M. 53, 305
Linsley, A. 444
Lipton, R. B. 333
Lischner, H. W. 358
Lishman, W. W. 328
Lithell, H. 235, 237
Littlefield, D. C. 215
Liu, H. C. 235
Liu, X. 121
Livermore, G. 3
Lloyd, D. H. 174
Lloyd, G. K. 244
Løberg, T. 44, 48, 326, 440
Locke, B. Z. 53
Lockfeld, A. 446
Lodemann, E. 272, 300
Loeber, R. T. 150, 151, 152
Loewenstein, G. 412, 424
Löffler, W. 378
Logan, B. K. 99
Logan, G. D. 425
Logan, J. 51
Logue, A. W. 409, 410
Lolait, S. J. 143
Lombardo, T. W. 230
Lomeña, F. J. 56
London, E. D. 113, 115, 118, 121, 219, 230, 232, 234, 238, 266, 273, 274, 300, 352, 422, 423, 426
Longstreth, W. T. 241, 242, 331, 334
Looi, J. C. 333
Lopez, A. D. 237
Lopez De Armentia, M. 58
Losonczy, M. 391
Lovestone, S. 234, 237
Lowe, J. V. 152
Lu, L. 113
Lubomski, M. 119, 122
Lucas, D. M. 302
Lucas, G. M. 354, 355
Lucas, L. R. 361
Luchsinger, J. A. 331, 332
Luciana, M. 192, 193, 194, 195
Lucki, I. 75, 81, 92, 95, 98
Luebbers, S. 192, 193, 194, 195
Lundqvist, T. 359
Lunell, E. 239
Luo, X. 378
Lutz, B. 144
Lyden, P. D. 209
Lyerly, S. B. 441
Lyman, W. D. 350
Lyndon, R. W. 86

Lynn, A. B. 143
Lynskey, M. 147, 148
Lyons, D. 113
Lyons, M. J. 45, 157
Lyvers, M. 291, 292, 300

Ma, J. Z. 227
Maany, V. 385
Maas, L. C. 54, 125
McAllister, S. D. 144
MacAndrew, C. 437
McArthur, J. C. 350, 357
Mcavay, G. J. 338
McBay, A. J. 302
McCanlies, N. 294
McCann, U. D. 179, 181, 186, 210, 444
McCardle, K. 192, 193, 194, 195
McCarthy, G. 58
McCaul, M. E. 292
McClernon, F. J. 242
McCloskey, L. W. 302
McConnell, D. 443
McDaid, J. 180
McDonald, J. 153
McDonald, S. 272, 273, 300
MacDonald, D. 228, 232, 233
MacDonald, S. 98
McDougle, M. 293
McElgin, W. 448
McEvoy, J. 244
McFadden, E. 410
McGaugh, J. L. 229
McGinty, V. 54
McGue, M. 45
McGurk, S. 233, 383
McGurn, B. 324, 339
McGwinn, G. 100
McHugh, S. B. 59
McInerney, S. C. 58
Mackay, A. J. 155
MacKay, S. 46
McKee, S. A. 440
McKernan, J. F. 158
McKhann, G. 330, 331
McKnelley, W. 291
MacLean, C. J. 227
McLellan, A. T. 123, 305
Macleod, J. 147, 148, 149
McMahon, F. G. 158
McMaster, S. E. 178
McMillan, D. E. 304
McMillan, T. M. 276, 277, 298
McNally, G. P. 445, 446
McNamee, H. B. 293
McNaughton, N. 59
McNeal, M. A. 330
McSorley, K. 229, 230, 231, 232, 233
Madden, G. J. 274, 409, 410, 411, 412, 414
Madden, J. A. 119
Maddux, J. F. 302

Madhusoodanan, S. 100
Madras, B. K. 112
Maeda, Y. 177
Maeir, S. 85
Maejima, T. 144
Maglione, M. M 207
Maguire, R. P. 361
Mahoney, C. 229, 230
Mahurin, R. 395
Maibach, E. W. 236
Maier, W. 381
Majoie, C. B. 186
Makela, P. 158
Makriyannis, A. 159
Malberg, J. E. 180, 186, 444
Maldonado, R. 145, 146, 157
Malizia, A. L. 77, 78, 97
Mallon, K. F. 349
Malouf, R. 334, 337
Maltzman, I. 50, 51, 52, 53
Mancuso, G. 229, 230, 231, 232, 240
Mangan, G. L. 230, 233
Mann, A. 234, 237
Mann, K. 47, 334
Mann, T. 425
Mannheimer, D. I. 75, 79, 86
Manolio, T. A. 236, 242
Manschreck, T. C. 119
Mansky, P. A. 293
Mantsch, J. R. 113
Marakovic, N. N. 410
March, J. 245
Marcourakis, T. 95
Marcus, J. 85
Marczinski, C. A. 442
Marder, K. 351
Margolin, A. 300
Marinkovic, K. 50, 51, 52, 53
Markesbery, W. R. 332
Markowitsch, H. J. 328
Marks, I. M. 81
Marks, M. J. 238
Marks, S. 118
Marlatt, G. A. 440, 441
Marlink, R. 354
Marois, R. 50
Marona-Lewicka, D. 177
Marrocco, R. T. 231, 240, 242
Marsden, J. 305
Marsden, J. 438
Marsh, D. M. 53
Marshall, J. 246
Marshall, M. 437
Marsicano, G. 144
Martin, B. 187
Martin, B. R. 143, 238
Martin, C. D. 230, 234
Martin, C. S. 440
Martin, D. J. 349, 350
Martin, E. M. 349

Martin, M. 157
Martin, P. R. 57
Martin, W. R. 288, 292, 293, 295
Mash, D. C. 184
Mason, A. P. 302
Mason, W. A. 58
Masover, B. 277, 300, 303
Massi, P. 377
Masters, J. C. 410
Masur, J. 441
Mathalon, D. H. 46–47, 51, 54, 56, 57, 334
Mathew, R. J. 151, 152, 356, 359
Mathieu-Kia, A. M. 113, 238
Mathys, K. 361
Matoba, R. 210
Matochik, J. A. 121, 153
Matsuda, L. A. 143
Matsumura, K. 327
Matsuyama, E. 210
Matthew, R. J. 96
Matthews, D. B. 61
Mattila, M. J. 79, 80, 83, 98, 305
Mattioni, T. A. 118
Mattson, M. P. 187
Mattson, S. N. 60
Matz, B. 230
Maudsley, S. 187
Mauldin-Jourdain, M. L. 58
Mavaddat, N. 420
Maxwell, J. C. 11, 36
Maxwell, S. 304
Mayer, K. 354
Mayer-Oakes, S. A. 325, 339
Mayeux, R. 331, 332
Maylor, E. A. 51
Mazas, C. A. 53
Mazur, J. 409, 414, 417
Mazzola-Pomietto, P. 180
Meader, K. J. 324, 339
Mechoulam, R. 143, 144, 159
Medoff, D. 381
Meek, P. 392
Meek, P. S. 119
Meisch, R. A. 305
Meketon, M. J. 292
Melamed, J. I. 119
Melega, W. P. 208
Melen, M. 229, 230, 231, 232, 240
Melgaard, B. 56
Meliska, C. J. 228, 230
Mellinger, G. D. 75, 79, 86
Mello, N. K. 47, 112
Meltzer, H. 383
Meltzer, H. Y. 180, 233
Melvin, L. S. 143
Mena, I. 124
Mencl, W. E. 189
Mendelson, J. 212
Mendelson, J. H. 47, 58, 121, 266
Mendez, M. F. 326, 328, 329

Menelaou, A. 295
Menzaghi, F. 244
Meray, R. 240
Merikangas, K. R. 228
Messias, M. 392
Mesulam, M.-M. 61
Mets, T. 337, 339
Mewaldt, S. P. 82, 83, 98, 212
Meyer, J. M. 45
Meyer, J. S. 333, 335, 337
Meyer, R. E. 272, 287, 281, 290, 293
Meyerhoff, D. J. 46, 56, 352, 357
Meyers, A. L. 438
Meyerson, B. 238
Micallef-Roll, J. 59
Michie, P. 381
Michie, P. T. 152
Mick, E. 425
Miguel, R. de 157
Mikhael, M. A. 266, 279, 298, 300
Mikulich, S. A. 227
Mikulich, S. K. 425
Mikuriya, T. H. 140
Millar, K. 49
Miller, A. 395
Miller, B. L. 56, 241, 242
Miller, D. B. 179, 180, 181, 444
Miller, E. 350
Miller, F. B. 304
Miller, G. A. 242
Miller, M. W. 60
Miller, N. S. 80, 95
Miller, R. A. 79
Millman, R. 171
Mills, A. T. D. 155
Millsaps, C. 119
Milne, G. M. 143
Minassian, A. 383
Minicuci, N. 183
Mintz, J. 438
Mintzer, M. Z. 83, 96, 273, 274, 277, 289, 298, 355
Mirin, S. M. 293
Mirsattari, S. M. 364
Mirsky, A. 381
Mirza, N. R. 240
Mischel, H. 415
Mischel, W. 410, 415
Mitchel, S. 412
Mitchell, C. L. 444, 445
Mitchell, J. E. 244
Mitchell, J. M. 445
Mitchell, S. H. 409–410, 411, 441
Mittenberg, W. 119, 129
Mittleman, M. A. 331, 334
Miyahara, J. T. 444
Miyasato, K. 227
Miyatake, T. 246
Mock, J. 212
Moeller, F. G. 53, 190–191, 411

Moeller-Hartmann, W. 188, 191
Mohns, L. 154
Mohs, R. C. 212
Mokler, D. J. 176
Molchan, S. E. 83
Molina, V. A. 362
Molitor, T. W. 353
Molliver, M. E. 179, 180
Molloy, B. B. 178
Momenan, R. 47, 60
Monroy, F. 210
Monteiro, M. G. 51
Monterosso, J. R. 121, 215, 217, 410, 412, 414, 418, 419, 421, 423, 424, 426
Montgomery, I. M. 79, 82
Moodley, P. 92, 94, 96
Moore, B. 415
Moore, H. C. 437
Moore, R. D. 354, 355
Moore, T. 159
Moosmann, B. 144
Mora, F. 116
Moran, S. 294, 295, 296
Morel, D. 96
Morens, D. M. 245
Morgan, C. A. 352
Morgan, M. J. 119, 181, 183
Morgenstern, A. 396
Mori, M. 209, 219
Mørland, J. 99–100, 302
Morris, J. S. 58
Morris, J. 448
Morris, L. 380
Morse, R. M. 329, 323, 337
Mortel, K. F. 333, 335, 337
Mortimer, J. A. 235, 236, 332
Moselhy, H. F. 47, 56
Moser, E. I. 59, 60
Moser, M. B. 59, 60
Moskowitz, H. 276
Moss, H. B. 327
Motta, S. 129
Mozley, D. 385
Mozley, P. D. 448
Mueser, K. 375
Mukamal, K. J. 331, 334
Mullan, B. A. 57
Mullani, N. 352
Mullen, F. M. 196
Muller, C. 233
Mulsant, B. H. 339
Mulvihill, L. E. 53
Mumford, G. K. 443
Munjack, D. J. 83
Munro, C. A. 329, 330
Munro, S. 143
Muntaner, C. 441
Murakami, A. 293
Muriach, M. 60
Murison, R. 59, 60

Murphy, D. L. 83, 180
Murphy, F. C. 231
Murphy, H. B. M. 119
Murray, S. 119, 122
Musa, M. N. 82
Museo, E. 240
Muto, J. J. 302
Myerson, J. 410, 413

Näätänen, R. 50
Nabeshima, T. 177
Nace, E. P. 438
Nader, M. A. 113
Naegele, T. 334
Nagel, B. J. 61
Nagoshi, C. T. 49, 53, 441
Nahas, G. G. 158
Nair, B. S. 360
Nair, M. 357
Nair, N. P. V. 79, 83
Nakagawa, Y. 327
Nakamura, H. 243
Nakayama, Y. 243
Namba, H. 361
Napier, K. L. 121, 410, 421, 423
Naranjo, C. 173
Nardin, R. 121, 266
Nash, J. F. 176, 180
Nasrallah, H. A. 349, 350, 354, 357, 380
Natarajan, L. 155
Nath, A. 364
Nathan, P. E. 422
Navarick, D. 410
Navia, B. 350
Nayeem, N. 77
Naylor, H. 232
Nazzaro, D. 387, 388
Neale, J. 380
Neale, M. C. 227, 435
Negrete, J. 375
Negrete, J. C. 119
Negus, S. S. 112
Nelson, J. 78
Nelson, J. A. 350
Nencini, P. 181
Ness, J. 339
Ness, R. 292, 294, 295, 296
Nestler, E. J. 264
Nestoros, J. N. 79, 83
Neuchterlein, K. 380, 383
Neutel, C. I. 100
New, A. 381
Newhouse, P. A. 228, 229, 244, 246
Newman, S. 302
Newton, C. 353, 354, 360
Newton, T. F. 210, 212, 214, 215, 217, 218, 219, 221
Ni, L. 243
Niaura, R. 52
Nichols, D. E. 173, 174, 177, 180

Nichols, M. B. 174
Nicolás, J. M. 56
Nielsen, B. B. 357
Nielsen, L. M. 302
Nielsen, S. L. 302
Nieuwenstein, M. 381
Nigg, J. T. 425
Nilsson, B. 114
Nilsson, L. 235
Nimmerrichter, A. 57
Nixon, S. 390, 396, 389
Nobel, K. 100
Noll, D. 380, 382
Nomoto, Y. 243
Nordahl, T. 383
Nordahl, T. E. 210, 360
Nordberg, A. 238, 239
Norton, C. S. 447
Noteboom, J. T. 229
Nottet, H. S. 353
Novelly, R. A. 274, 299, 300
Noyes, R. 158
Nuechterlein, K. 381, 390, 393
Nunes, E. 128, 221
Nunez, M. J. 362
Nunez-Iglesias, M. J. 362
Nur, K. 210
Nurminen, N. 58, 59
Nutt, D. J. 76, 77, 78, 97
Nutt, J. G. 174
Nyberg, L. 235
Nyman, H. 235, 237
Nystrom, L. 382
Nyswander, M. E. 263, 304

Oates, M. M. 446, 447
Obana, W. G. 118
Obara, H. 327
Obergriesser, T. 188
O'Boyle, D. J. 440
O'Brien, C. P. 121, 123, 410, 421, 423, 438, 448
Obrocki, J. 189
O'Callaghan, J. P. 179, 180, 181, 444
O'Carroll, R. 327
O'Carroll, R. E. 183, 186
O'Connor, S. 122
O'Doherty, J. 58, 116
O'Donnell, D. 380
O'Donnell, V. M. 334
Odum, A. L. 409, 410, 411, 412, 414
Oei, T. P. 358
Offen, S. 59
Ogata, H. 80
Ohman, A. 58
Ohman, B. 238
Ohmori, T. 334
Ohnishi, T. 120
Ohno-Shosaku, T. 144
Ohta, K. 209
Okamoto, K. 209
Oken, B. S. 230, 231
Oldman, D. 117
O'Leary, D. S. 151, 359
O'Leary, J. 441
Olesen, J. 242
Olmstead, R. E. 239
Olson, S. 380
O'Malley, P. M. 7, 10, 12, 16, 20, 24, 26, 28, 31, 35, 36, 143
O'Malley, S. S. 50, 119, 120, 127, 128
O'Neill, J. 56, 352
Onishi, S. 210
Opgenoorth, E. 277, 278, 281, 300
Opler, L. 387
Oquendo, M. A. 80
Ordorica, P. I. 235, 236, 237
Orgogozu, J. M. 331
Orgozo, J. M. 331
Ornstein, T. J. 280
Orr, L. E. 158
Ortner, R. 277, 278, 281, 300
Orzack, M. 381
Oscar-Berman, M. 44, 45, 46, 47, 55, 56, 57, 61, 62, 328
O'Shara-Celaya, L. 383
O'Shea, E. 180
Osher, F. 375
Oslin, D. 329, 330
Ostfeld, A. M. 335, 337
Ostrander, M. 446
Ott, A. 336
Owen, M. 381

Pacher, P. 144, 157
Pacifici, R. 360
Page R. D. 236
Palva, E. 80, 83, 98
Pandey, G. 80
Panikashvili, D. 144
Pantoni, L. 335, 337
Papageorgiou, C. 381
Papke, R. A. 241
Pappas, N. R. 54
Para, M. F. 349, 350, 354, 357
Parasuraman, R. 50
Paredes, R. G. 78
Paris, P. 304
Park, C. H. 182
Park, S. 233, 383
Parker, J. D. 411
Parkinson, J. A. 59
Parks, G. A. 441
Parks, R. W. 244
Parmentier, M. 157
Parolaro, D. 377
Parrott, A. C. 171, 175, 183, 192, 193, 194, 229, 230, 231, 232
Parsons, O. A. 44, 45, 47
Partington, J. E. 296
Pascani, K. 56

Pascual-Leone, A. 121
Patat, A. 99
Patel, T. 184
Paterniti, S. 323, 338
Paterson, D. 238, 239
Paterson, D. L. 365
Patterson, G. R. 443
Patterson, J. F. 79, 83
Pattie, A. 234, 339
Patton, J. H. 411
Paty, I. 99
Pau, C. W. 298, 299
Paulson, O. B. 56, 242
Paulus, M. P. 210, 215, 218, 220, 221
Pauly, J. R. 238
Paus, T. 116
Payeur, R. 84
Payte, J. E. 304
Pearlson, G. D. 115, 118, 352
Pearson, J. 265
Pedersen, A. E. 357
Pedersen, N. 435
Pedersen, N. P. 180
Peeke, H. S. 233
Peeke, S. C. 233
Pellett, O. L. 233
Pencer, A. 390
Penkower, L. 358
Penney, J. B. 447
Pennicott, D. 423
Pennings, E. J. 127
Penninx, B. W. 227
Pentney, R. J. 57
Perera, K. M. 96
Perez, J. A. 209
Perez-Stable, E. J. 239
Perkins, K. A. 228, 229, 230, 231, 233
Perlstein, W. 380, 382
Perrettand, D. I. 58
Perrochet, B. 207
Perry, W. 383
Pertwee, R. G. 143, 144
Pescor, F. T. 288
Peselow, E. 79, 83
Peternell, A. 277, 278, 281, 300
Peterson, D. 334
Peterson, E. L. 227, 245
Peterson, J. B. 49, 52, 53
Peterson, P. K. 353
Peterson, R. C. 228, 229, 232, 237, 326, 327
Petitto, J. 354
Peto, R. 237
Petrakis, I. L. 48
Petros, T. V. 51, 228, 233
Petrovitch, H. 235, 336
Petry, N. M. 274, 288, 355, 409, 410, 411, 412, 414
Pettegrew, J. 385
Pettigrew, L. C. 364
Pettit, H. O. 112

Petty, C. S. 302
Petursson, H. 75, 95, 96
Pezawas, L. M. 266, 300, 353
Pfeffer, A. Z. 296
Pfefferbaum, A. 46–47, 48, 50, 51, 54, 56, 57, 60, 334
Phan, V. 61
Phillips, B. K. 328, 334
Phillips, G. 438
Phillips, G. T. 294
Phillips, S. C. 57
Piazza, P. V. 435
Pickens, R. W. 435, 441
Pickering, A. 92
Pickworth, W. B. 231, 288
Pidoplichko, V. I. 246
Pierce, D. R. 60
Pierce-Shimomura, J. T. 46
Pihl, R. O. 49, 52, 53, 58, 441
Pikkarainen, M. 58, 59
Pilatus, U. 188, 191
Pillai, A. K. 83
Pillai, R. 360
Pillay, S. S. 153
Pinard, G. 99, 100, 337
Pineda, J. A. 230, 234
Piomelli, D. 143, 144, 159
Pirola, R. 83
Pitkänen, A. 58, 59
Pitts, W. M. 334
Pletscher, A. 178
Pliner, P. 441, 442
Poland, R. E. 187
Poldrack, R. 385
Polich, J. 50
Poling, A. 178
Pollack, B. G. 339
Pollack, H. A. 304
Pollack, M. H. 75, 83, 84
Pomara, N. 121
Pomerantz, R. J. 358
Pomerleau, C. S. 229, 230, 232
Pomerleau, O. F. 229, 230, 232, 246
Pompeia, S. 92, 95
Pope, H. G. 149–150, 153, 154, 155
Porjesz, B. 50, 51
Porrino, L. J. 113
Poser, S. 96
Poser, W. 96
Post, B. 233
Post, R. M., R. 446
Postma, A. 328
Potter, A. 228
Potter, M. 305
Potterat, E. 383
Potvin, S. 378
Poulos, C. X. 446
Poulsen, H. A. 140
Powell, J. E. 296
Powell, J. H. 192, 193, 194, 195

Powell, T. 96
Power, C. 364
Power, J. 58
Power, K. G. 94
Powers, K. 438
Powers, R. H. 119
Prelec, D. 412
Premack, D. 416
Preston, K. L. 267, 287, 288, 289, 291, 292, 293, 305
Preusser, D. F. 302
Price, B. B. 294, 295, 296
Price, D. 330, 331
Price, I. R. 234
Price, L. J. 120, 128, 129
Price, R. 350
Prince, M. 234, 237
Pritchard, W. S. 230
Prohovnik, I. 361
Prosperini, P. 384, 385
Provost, S. C. 231, 232
Pubill, D. 182
Pugh, K. R. 189
Puissant, V. I. 182
Pukay-Martin, N. D. 359, 360
Pulley, L. 100
Pulman, J. R. 79, 83
Pulvirenti, L. 362
Pun, C. 377

Qiu, C. 331
Quarton, G. C. 212
Quenzer, L. F. 360
Quinn, D. I. 239
Quirion, R. 243, 245–246
Quirt, K. 229, 230

Rabbitt, P. M. 51
Rachlin, H. 415
Radcliffe, K. A. 238
Radic, A. 325
Radtke, R. 242
Radu, E. W. 54
Rae, D. S. 53
Raft, D. 158
Ragan, P. 47
Ragland, J. D. 383, 384, 385, 424
Raichle, M. E. 114
Rajan, A. S. 238
Ram, R. 375
Ramirez, G. 358
Randall, T. 444
Randolph, C. 380, 382, 383
Randolph, W. F. 196
Rao, V. S. 331
Rashbaum, W. K. 350
Rassnick, S. 178
Ratti, M. T. 56
Rauch, S. L. 58
Rawlings, R. R. 47, 60

Rawlins, J. N. P. 59
Ray, W. A. 302
Razani, J. 349, 350
Razdan, R. K. 143
Ream, N. 438
Rech, R. H. 176, 445
Redman, J. R. 289, 305
Reed, D. 245
Reed, R. 150
Reed, T. 234, 235, 237, 241, 242
Reed, T. E. 49
Reeves, A. 246
Reger, M. 349, 350
Regier, D. 375
Regier, D. A. 53
Rehncrona, S. 114
Reid, J. R. 443
Reid, L. D. 177
Reilly, M. P. 443
Reinhold, K. 445
Reinsel, R. A. 96
Reiter, S. R. 83
Reith, M. E. 111
Reivich, M. 448
Reneman, L. 186, 187, 188
Renner, J. 231, 232, 233
Rennick, P. M. 298–299, 300, 303
Renshaw, P. 386
Renvoize, E. B. 329
Repo, E. 47, 60
Reulbach, U. 60
Revell, A. 230, 232
Reyes, R. B. 279, 298, 300
Reynolds, J. N. 60
Rezai, K. 380, 382
Rezvani, A. H. 240
Rhee, G. S. 177
Ricaurte, G. A. 179, 180, 181, 185, 196, 208, 444
Rice, J. P. 45
Rice, K. C. 172, 173
Rice, R. R. 350
Richards, J. B. 153, 409–410, 411
Richards, M. 234, 237
Richards, S. M. 99
Richardson, M. P. 60
Richardson, N. 378
Richarme, D. 387, 391
Richfield, E. K. 143
Richter, R. W. 265
Rickels, K. 75, 81, 92, 95, 98
Ridderinkhof, K. R. 53
Riddle, W. R. 57
Riedel, G. 144
Riggs, P. D. 227, 425
Riley, E. P. 60
Riley, K. P. 332
Rio, D. 47
Riordan, H. 380
Rioux, G. F. 83

Rippeth, J. D. 361, 362, 363
Risberg, J. 54, 152, 359
Risbrough, V. B. 244
Rissanen, A. M. 159
Rist, F. 381
Ritchie, C. W. 334, 337
Ritchie, K. 244, 338
Ritz, M. C. 112
Rivier, L. 302, 305
Robbins, S. J. 123
Robbins, T. 423
Robbins, T. W. 59, 123, 229
Roberts, G. 229
Robertson, L. 383
Robertson, L. C. 349
Robins, L. N. 438
Robinson, C. D. 276
Robinson, J. E. 127, 128
Robinson, J. H. 230
Robinson, S. F. 238
Robinson, T. E. 264, 435, 446, 447
Robitaille, Y. 245–246
Robles, E. 304
Robson, P. 158
Robson, P. J. 139
Rochford, J. 155
Rockwood, K. 333
Rodgers, J. 155
Rodrigo, E. K. 86
Rodriguez, L. A. 53
Rodriguez Holguin, S. 50
Roebuck, T. 383
Roebuck, T. M. 60
Roelofsma, P. H. M. P. 412
Rogers, R. D. 215, 217, 280, 420, 422
Rogers, R. L. 333, 335, 337
Rogish, M. 235, 236, 237
Rogowska, J. 153
Rohrbaugh, J. W. 50
Rohrer, M. S. 288
Rohsenow, D. J. 440
Roitman, S. 381
Roitzsch, J. 396
Rolfe, T. 156
Roll, J. M. 443
Rollings, J. 92
Rolls, E. T. 59, 116
Romach, M. 86
Roman, G. C. 241, 333, 335, 337
Romanelli, L. 238
Ron, M. 96
Rönnbäck, L. 264
Roque, C. T. 56
Roscher, D. 96
Rose, J. E. 238, 239, 240, 242, 243, 244
Rose, J. S. 267, 300, 353
Rose, M. E. 265
Rosecrans, J. A. 176
Roseman, J. M. 100
Rosen, B. R. 58, 59

Rosenbaum, J. F. 83, 85
Rosenbaum, M. 171, 196
Rosenberg, D. E. 288, 289, 293
Rosenberger, P. H. 349, 351, 354, 355, 357
Rosenbloom, M. J. 47, 48, 54, 56, 57, 334
Rosenfarb, I. 380, 383
Rosenheck, R. 48
Rosenthal, R. 87
Ross, C. A. 352
Ross, D. 381, 392
Ross, G. W. 245, 336
Ross, J. 215
Ross, M. H. 58
Ross, S. 441
Ross, T. J. 230, 241
Rosselli, M. 119, 120, 122, 129, 364
Rossi, A. 384, 385
Rossner, S. 159
Roth, B. L. 180, 293
Roth, M. D. 352
Roth, R. H. 78, 359
Roth, W. T. 50, 212
Rothenberg, S. 272, 287, 281, 290, 294, 295, 296
Rotheram-Fuller, E. 273, 274, 300, 422
Rothfleisch, J. 49, 52
Rothlind, J. C. 356, 358
Rothman, R. 392
Rothman, R. B. 119, 120, 129, 175
Rothrock, J. F. 209
Rotrosen, J. P. 121
Rounsaville, B. J. 127, 274, 299, 300, 425
Rourke, S. B. 44, 48, 326
Roush, B. W. 178
Rouveix, B. 354
Rowan-Szal, G. A. 305
Rowell, P. P. 239
Roy, A. 119, 351–352
Roy, C. W. 114
Roy, J.-Y. 378
Roy-Byrne, P. P. 76, 77, 81, 82
Rubenstein, R. 209
Rubin, D. C. 240
Rubin, V. D. 437
Rubino, T. 377
Rubinstein, A. 350
Rubinstein, K. J. 292, 295, 296
Ruble, D. C. 296
Rudnick, G. 174, 175
Rugg, M. D. 51
Ruitenberg, A. 332, 333
Rumbold, G. R. 289, 305
Runge, K. 328
Rush, C. R. 442
Russell, J. D. 86
Russell, M. A. 229, 230, 231, 232, 233
Russell, S. 51
Rusted, J. M. 228, 233, 234
Rustembegovic, A. 334
Ruttenber, A. J. 184

Ryan, J. 158
Rybicki, B. A. 245

Sabate, E. 355
Sabol, K. E. 175, 180
Saccone, N. L. 45
Sachdev, P. S. 333
Sachdeva, K. 209
Sackeim, H. A. 361
Sadzot, B. 176
Sah, P. 58
Saha, N. 264
Sahakian, B. J. 123, 230, 233, 231, 244, 420
Sahin, H. A. 328, 334
Saint-Cyr, J. 381, 382
Sairenchi, T. 335
Sakol, M. S. 94
Sakurai, Y. 228, 233
Sala, M. 264
Salam, S. A. 83
Salamero, M. 56
Salgado-Pineda, P. 59
Salinsky, J. V. 86
Sallan, S. E. 158
Salo, R. 217, 360
Salzman, C. 100
Sanberg, P. R. 245
Sanchez, C. 144
Sanchez, V. 175
Sanchez-Ramos, J. R. 118
Sanders, R. 381
Sanders-Bush, E. 178
Sandler, A. 230, 234
Sangameswaran, L. 78
Sannerud, C. A. 178
Santana, S. 119
Sapcanin, A. 334
Sargent, T. 173
Saria, A. 173
Sarid-Segal, O. 79, 86
Sarter, M. 240
Sastry, B. V. 239
Sathananthan, G. 215
Sato, S. 327
Saunders, M. 181
Saur, M. R. 176
Savage, V. R. 264
Saveanu, R. V. 356, 357, 358, 363
Savolainen, L. 47, 60
Saxton, J. 329, 330
Sayette, M. A. 440
Scabini, D. 50
Scaramucci, A. 333
Scarone, S. 381
Scatton, B. 182
Schachar, R. 425
Schatz, D. S. 173
Schatz, I. 210
Scheen, A. J. 159
Scheffel, U. 186

Scheffers, M. K. 53
Schellenberg, G. D. 234, 235, 237
Schendan, H. E. 46
Scherr, P. A. 330
Schieve, J. F. 114–115
Schifano, F. 183
Schilling, R. F. 305
Schindler, S. D. 277, 278, 281, 300
Schinka, J. A. 235, 236, 237
Schippers, G. M. 440
Schiwy, W. 82
Schleifer, L. 153
Schloss, P. 186
Schmahmann, J. D. 57, 58
Schmaling, K. 396
Schmauss, C. 95
Schmidt, C. J. 175, 176, 181
Schmidt, V. 305
Schnapp, W. 411
Schneider, B. 119
Schneider, N. G. 239
Schnieden, H. 246
Schnohr, P. 333
Schoenbaum, E. E. 353
Schofield, P. R. 77
Schooff, K. 298–299, 300, 303
Schooler, N. 385
Schottenfeld, S. 272, 287, 281, 290
Schramke, C. 330
Schroger, E. 50
Schroth, G. 47, 334
Schuckit, M. A. 51, 220
Schuh, K. J. 287, 292, 293
Schulenberg, J. E. 7, 12, 16, 20, 24, 26, 28, 31, 35, 36, 14
Schullery, M. 385
Schultz, L. R. 227
Schuster, C. R. 178, 196, 208, 292
Schut, R. 353
Schwartz, J. 375
Schwarz, M. 265
Schweinsburg, A. D. 61
Schweitzer, C. 354
Schweizer, E. 81, 84
Scott, D. 54
Scott, H. F. 113
Sdao-Jarvie, K. 443
Sears, E. 54
Seeger, U. 57
Seeley, J. R. 227
Seeman, T. 338
Seevers, M. H. 171, 195
Segu, L. 184
Segura, J. 441
Seiden, L. S. 175, 178, 180, 181, 186, 196, 208, 444
Seidman, J. 385
Seifritz, E. 54
Seitz, D. 57
Sekine, Y. 219, 220, 360

Selby, M. J. 119, 127, 128
Selemon, L. 380, 382, 383
Self, D. 394, 395
Sellers, E. M. 96
Sell, L. A. 266, 448
Selmeci, G. 111
Selnes, O. A. 351
Semple, D. M. 183, 186
Seppala, T. 79, 80, 83, 98
Sergejew, A. A. 156
Serper, M. 378, 387, 391
Serventi, K. L. 47, 48
Seto, T. 210
Sevy, S. 387
Sexton, J. E. 231
Seymour, K. 380
Shah, A. 327
Shaham, Y. 113
Shaper, A. G. 337
Sharkansky, E. J. 53
Sharma, P. L. 264
Shea, S. 331, 332
Shear, P. K. 47, 56, 57, 334
Sheikh, J. I. 100
Shemanski, L. 236
Shepard, J. D. 113
Sher, K. J. 441
Shergold, K. 233
Sherrington, C. S. 114
Sherwood, A. 376, 377, 378, 379, 394, 395
Sherwood, N. 228, 229, 230, 231, 232, 233, 240, 306
Shi, W. 377
Shi, W. X. 264
Shields, J. 377, 394
Shiffman, S. 230
Shih, R. 54
Shihabuddin, L. 381
Shim, I. 240
Shimizu, H. 80
Shimohama, S. 243
Shinderman, M. S. 304
Shine, P. 96
Shinton, R. 235
Shirtcliff, E. A. 242
Shohami, E. 144, 157
Shoptaw, S. 273, 274, 300, 422
Shorr, R. I. 302, 339
Shrotriya, R. C. 80, 83, 98
Shuer, L. S. 86
Shulgin, A. T. 171, 173, 174, 177, 196
Shytle, R. D. 245
Sibley, D. 357
Siddiqui, M. 331, 332
Sidney, S. 333
Sieberer, M. 246
Siebert, D. J. 293
Siegal, D. 209
Siegel, S. 184, 444, 445
Sieghart, W. 77

Siesjo, B. K. 114
Siever, L. 381
Silbershatz, H. 326
Silva, D. 245
Silver, A. A. 245
Silverman, K. 442, 443
Simmons, A. 266
Simon, B. B. 239
Simonnet, G. 445
Simonov, P. V. 61
Simons, J. 376
Simpson, C. A. 411
Simpson, D. D. 305
Simpson, H. M. 302
Simpson, R. J. 86
Sims, J. 272, 273, 300
Sims, R. V. 100
Singh, A. 228, 245
Singh, G. 239
Singh, H. 375
Singleton, E. G. 229, 231
Sinha, R. 50
Sinz, E. H. 265
Sirocco, K. 82, 83, 98
Siscovick, D. S. 331, 334
Sjoberg, L. 419
Skegg, D. C. G. 99
Skilling, T. A. 53
Skinhoj, E. 242
Skinner, A. 230, 234
Skinner, B. F. 415
Skinner, J. S. 228, 232
Sklair-Tavron, L. 264
Skolnick, P. 354
Skoog, I. 332, 335
Skudlarski, P. 189
Skurtveit, S. 99–100
Slater, M. D. 236
Slikker, W. 177, 180
Sloan, J. W. 295
Sloan, M. A. 118
Slukvin, I. 357
Smelson, D. A. 119, 391
Smirne, S. 83
Smith, D. M. 329
Smith, G. 158
Smith, G. M. 292
Smith, H. R. 113
Smith, J. E. 116, 184
Smith, M. E. 51
Smith, N. T. 146
Smith, R. C. 245
Smith, S. S. 325
Smyth, C. 287, 302
Smythies, J. 377
Snaedal, J. 244
Snel, J. 53
Snell, J. D. 178
Snoddy, H. D. 178
Snowden, D. A. 332

Snyder, A. 390
Snyder, F. R. 229, 230, 231, 232
Soares, J. J. 58
Sodesaki, K. 210
Soeiro, R. 350
Sofic, E. 334
Soininen, H. 47, 60
Sokoloff, P. 112
Solana, V. 392
Solana, V. L. 119
Sole, A. 275, 299
Solowij, N. 150, 151, 152, 154, 155
Sommer, R. 441
Somogyi, A. A. 295
Song, A. W. 58
Soragna, D. 56
Sorensen, D. J. 349
Sorensen, H. 56
Sorensen, J. L. 294
Sosa, L. 357
Soyka, M. 277, 375
Spaan, M. 53
Spanos, L. J. 177
Spealman, R. D. 112
Speck, O. 210
Specka, M. 272, 300
Specter, S. 360
Speizer, F. E. 333
Spencer, T. 425
Sphire, R. D. 292
Spies, C. D. 357
Spiga, R. 305
Spilich, G. J. 231, 232, 233
Sprague, J. E. 177
Spring, S. 379
Spring, W. 441
Spurgeon, L. 230, 232, 234, 238
Squillace, K. M. 446
Squires, R. F. 78, 79
Srisurapanont, M. 214
Srivastava, B. I. 360
Srivastava, M. D. 360
Stadian, E. 330, 331
Staley, J. K. 184, 235
Stam, C. J. 353
Stamper, E. 207
Stampfer, M. J. 333
Stancliff, S. 304
Staner, L. 99
Stanford, M. S. 411
Stapleton, J. 229, 230, 231, 232, 233
Stapleton, J. M. 50
Stark-Adamec, C. 441
Starr, J. M. 234, 324, 339
Starzl, T. E. 327
Stastny, D. 305
Steele, N. 158
Steffenach, H. A. 59, 60
Stein, D. J. 122
Stein, E. A. 230, 240, 241, 243

Stein, M. B. 227
Steinberg, J. L. 53
Steinhauer, S. R. 47
Steinhoff, B. J. 60
Steinmetz, J. E. 53
Stelson, F. 246
Stephens, B. G. 209
Stephenson, D. T. 182
Stephenson, J. D. 238
Stern, K. N. 441
Stewart, D. 438
Stewart, S. A. 86
Stewart, S. H. 83, 337
Stiller, R. L. 230, 231, 265
Stinson, F. S. 22, 140
Stip, E. 378
Stitzer, M. L. 273, 274, 277, 287, 292, 293, 294, 298, 304, 305, 355, 442
Stolar, M. 228
Stolerman, I. P. 240
Stoller, K. B. 287, 288
Stolman, S. 445
Stone, D. 178, 179, 183
Stone, W. 385
Stone-Elander, S. 54
Storm, T. 441
Stough, C. 156, 192, 193, 194, 195, 230
Strain, E. C. 287, 288, 289, 291, 293, 304
Strang, J. 266, 287, 300, 302, 305
Strange, B. A. 60
Strategos, S. 209
Stratta, P. 384, 385
Strauss, L. 196
Strauss, M. 382
Streeter, C. 46, 47, 55, 56, 57, 62
Streit, W. J. 182
Streufert, S. 83
Strickland, T. L. 120, 352
Strumwasser, S. 120, 129, 364
Struwe, M. 159
Stunkard, A. 155
Stuss, D. T. 120
Su, K. H. 305
Subotnik, K. 380, 383
Sugathapala, L. 423
Sugiura, T. 143
Suissa, S. 99, 100, 337
Sullivan, C. K. 176
Sullivan, E. V. 11, 46–47, 48, 54, 55, 56, 57, 60, 62, 334, 355, 356
Sullivan, P. F. 227
Sully, J. 416
Sulser, F. 178
Sumner, J. J. 440
Sunderland, T. 83
Sutherland, G. J. 140
Sutter, T. W. 232
Suttitum, T. 354
Sutton, S. R. 229
Suzuki, K. 327

Svoboda, M. 56, 60
Swan, G. E. 227, 234, 235, 237, 241, 242
Swanson, C. 385
Sweeney, J. 385
Swerdlow, N. R. 362
Swettenham, J. 229, 230, 231, 232, 233
Swift, W. 140, 305
Swinyard, E. A. 444
Symonds, C. 158
Szabadi, E. 410
Szabo, G. 357
Szabo, Z. 186
Szechtman, R. 388, 389, 396, 392, 393
Szirmay, M. 157

Takahira, Y. 337
Takase, H. 337
Takeda, K. 327
Takeuchi, J. 80
Talland, G. A. 212
Tallman, J. 77
Tamminga, C. 380, 381
Tanaka, A. 243
Tancredi, O. 83
Tanda, G. 145–146
Tang, M. X. 331, 332
Taniguchi, T. 243
Tanizaki, Y. 241
Tannock, R. 425
Tansella, C. Z. 92
Tant, S. R. 152
Tao-Cheng, J. H. 184
Tapert, S. F. 47, 56, 61, 220
Tapia-Arizmendi, G. 264
Tarbox, S. 385
Tarter, R. E. 327
Tashkin, D. P. 352
Tata, P. R. 92
Tate, K. 156, 267
Tattersall, M. 86
Tawakina, T. 333
Taylor, A. J. 264
Taylor, D. 296
Taylor, G. 396
Taylor, J. R. 425
Taylor, M. D. 234
Taylor, R. C. 228, 229, 231, 232
Taylor, V. L. 175
Teichner, G. 395, 396
Tek, C. 392
Tennant, A. 234
Teo, R. K. 50
Teoh, S. K. 121, 266
terBrugge, K. 96
Terry, A. V. 244
Teuscher, F. 229, 232
Thagard, P. 423
Thaker, G. 380, 381
Thaler, R. 409
Thapar, P. 306

Thermenos, H. 385
Thevos, A. 396
Thiele, G. M. 357
Thiele, T. R. 46
Thomas, D. M. 182
Thomas, K. L. 143
Thomas, M. J. 446, 447
Thomas, R. E. 99
Thomasius, R. 192, 193, 194, 195
Thompson, A. K. 288, 289, 293
Thompson, L. L. 425
Thompson, N. 234, 237
Thompson, P. M. 210, 215
Thompson, W. 306
Thompson, W. K. 292
Thompson, W. O. 288
Thomson, A. D. 334
Thomson, J. L. 359
Thornley, B. 384
Thron, A. 188, 191
Thrussell, C. 440
Thulin, S. O. 152, 359
Thun, M. 237
Tiihonen, J. 97
Tilson, H. A. 445
Timm, C. 328
Tinklenberg, J. R. 212
Tinuper, P. 78
Tirelli, E. 229, 230, 231, 232, 240
Tivis, R. 390, 396, 389
Tobena, A. 275, 299
Tolbert, R. 196
Tollefson, G. D. 83
Tolliver, T. 180
Tolou-Shams, M. 46, 120, 128, 129
Tom, W. C. 265
Tonnesen, H. 357
Toppi-Mullen, P. 414, 419
Torry, D. 240
Toru, M. 80
Tosteson, T. 354
Touchon, J. 244
Tracy, J. 376, 377, 386, 388, 393
Tranel, D. 273, 420, 421, 422
Trier, M. 294
Triggs, T. J. 289, 305
Tringali, R. 327
Trites, R. 215
True, W. 45
Truelsen, T. 333
Trujillo, K. A. 446
Trupin, E. W. 155
Trzepacz, P. T. 327
Tsuang, J. 390, 393
Tsuang, M. T. 45, 435
Tsunematsu, T. 335, 337
Tsushima, Y. 241
Tuchman, A. J. 118
Tuck, R. R. 329
Tucker, D. 390, 393

Tucker, D. M. 242, 420
Tucker, J. A. 411
Tulving, E. 425
Tune, L. E. 339
Tumeh, S. S. 119, 124, 127
Tunving, K. 152, 359
Turchan, J. 362
Turchi, J. 240
Turcotte, N. 53
Turk, D. 230
Turken, A. U. 229
Turkington, T. G. 151, 152, 359
Turnbull, J. E. 305
Turner, M. D. 240
Turski, L. 265
Turski, W. A. 265
Tuvnes, F. A. 59, 60
Tversky, A. 408
Tyas, S. L. 336
Tyson, L. B. 158
Tzanis, E. 288
Tzourio, C. 245

Ueno, Y. 243
Ugena, B. 441
Uhl, G. R. 45
Uhlenhuth, E. H. 75, 79, 86, 443
Ullrich, T. 172, 173
Umbricht, A. 267
Uneklabh, T. 354
Ungerstedt, U. 112
Unützer, J. 95
Upadhyaya, H. P. 227
Uslaner, J. M. 446, 447

Vadhan, N. 387, 391
Valverde, O. 157
Van Asselen, M. 328
Van Boxtel, M. P. 234, 235, 237
Van de Kamp, J. L. 238
Van den Abell, T. 243
Van den Bree, M. B. M. 435
Van den Brink, W. 353
Van der Heiden, W. 378
Vanderploeg, R. D. 235, 236, 237
Van der Pol, M. 409, 410, 411
Van der Staak, C. P. 440
Van der Stelt, M. 144
Van Duijn, C. M. 336
Van Eijk, J. T. 227
Van Gaal, L. F. 159
Van Gool, C. H. 227
Van Gorp, W. G. 120, 221, 349
Van Heeringen, C. 80
VanHoven, M. K. 46
Van Laar, M. 99
Van Luijtelaar, G. 82–83
Van Praag, H. 387
Van Sickle, M. D. 157
Van Thiel, D. H. 327

Vantol, H. H. M. 112
Varma, V. K. 155
Varner, J. L. 50
Vaurio, O. 47, 60
Veldhuijzen, D. S. 97, 98, 100
Velligan, D. 395
Ventayol, P. 265
Verbaten, M. 99
Verdoux, H. 338–339
Verghese, J. 333
Verhaeghe, W. 337, 339
Verkes, R. J. 192, 193, 194, 195
Verrico, C. D. 359
Verschuren, M. W. 234, 235, 237
Verster, J. C. 97, 98, 99, 100
Veselis, R. A. 96
Vgontzas, A. N. 84
Victor, M. 57, 328
Vieregge, A. 246
Vieregge, P. 246
Vigano, D. 377
Viitanen, M. 336
Vikander, B. 95, 96
Villemagne, V. 208, 360
Vinciguerra, V. 159
Virkkunen, M. 53
Viscusi, W. K. 409
Vogel-Sprott, M. 53, 443
Volkerts, E. R. 97, 98, 99, 100
Volkow, N. D. 54, 56, 112, 115, 118, 119, 120, 122, 123, 124, 127, 152, 210, 211, 215, 217, 218, 352, 356, 448
Vollenweider, F. X. 176, 181, 189, 361
Volpe, J. S. 410
Von Felsinger, J. M. 292
Von Heijne, G. 54
Vuchinich, R. E. 411

Wade, D. T. 158
Wadsworth, M. J. 234, 237
Wagar, B. 423
Waggie, K. 354
Wagman, A. 392
Wagner, A. K. 337
Wagner, E. F. 227
Wagner, E. H. 302
Wagner, F. A. 435
Walker, D. J. 292
Walker, M. 337
Wall, A. 238
Wall, A. M. 440
Wall, S. C. 174, 175
Wallace, A. F. 437
Wallace, C. 410, 412
Wallace, E. A. 118
Wallace, R. B. 323
Wallach, M. 375
Wallin, A. 335, 337
Walls, C. 76, 98, 99
Walsh, D. 381

Walsh, J. M. 306
Walsh, S. L. 266, 287, 288, 292, 293
Walsh, T. 228
Walzer, C. 265
Wang, G. J. 54, 56, 218
Wang, G. Y. 357–358, 361
Wang, H. X. 336
Wang, J. Y. 335, 336
Wang, L. 58
Wang, P. N. 235
Wang, S. J. 235, 361
Wang, Y. 184, 235
Wanigaratne, S. 287, 302
Wannamethee, S. G. 337
Warburton, D. M. 228, 229, 230, 231, 232, 233, 234, 240, 244
Warburton, L. A. 300
Ward, A. 425
Ward, A. S. 212
Ward, C. H. 212
Ward, M. 82
Warkentin, S. 152, 359
Warner, A. 302
Warner, L. A. 435
Warner, M. R. 176
Warren, R. A. 302
Watanabe, A. 327
Waterman, B. 45
Waternaux, C. 386
Waters, A. J. 229
Waters, J. P. 140
Watkinson, B. 156, 157
Watson, R. R. 357–358, 360
Watson, S. J. 446, 447
Waugh, M. 359
Way, D. L. 358
Webber, M. P. 353
Weber, D. A. 118, 119, 127
Webster, C. D. 411
Wegerer, V. 60
Weickert, T. 381
Weidenheim, W. M. 350
Weidle, P. J. 355
Weinberger, D. 380, 381, 382, 383
Weiner, M. W. 46
Weingartner, H. J. 79, 82, 83
Weinstein, A. 125
Weiss, R. D. 47
Welch, K. M. 118
Welch, L. W. 57
Welch, R. 291
Wellman, M. C. 354, 355, 363
Wells, C. E. 329
Wells, S. 98
Welser, R. 230, 242
Welsh, R. 349, 350
Wendt, P. E. 54
Wesnes, K. 192, 193, 194, 228, 229, 230, 231, 232, 233
Wesson, D. R. 304

West, J. R. 54, 60
West, R. J. 231, 233
Westbrook, R. F. 445, 446
Wester, A. J. 328
Westman, E. C. 239
Wetterling, T. 332
Wetzel, S. 54
Wewers, M. E. 235
Whalen, P. J. 58
Whalley, L. J. 234, 324, 339
Wharton, M. 227
Wheeler, M. E. 51
Whelahan, H. 392
Whelan, K. T. 244
Whincup, P. H. 337
Whitacre, C. C. 349, 350, 354, 357
White, A. M. 61
White, H. K. 243, 244
White, J. M. 295
White, L. 245
White, L. R. 235, 237
White, P. M. 51
Whitehouse, P. J. 246
Whiteman, M. C. 234
Whiteman, M. 324, 339
Whitlow, C. T. 153, 422
Whitmore, E. A. 227, 425
Whitney, P. 425
Whittle, B. A. 139
Wicker, B. 59
Wickes, W. 272, 273, 300
Wide, R. J. 127
Widmann, U. 57
Wiethe, K. E. 152
Wig, N. N. 155
Wijetunga, M. 210
Wikkelso, C. 264
Wikler, A. 288, 443
Wilcock, G. 334
Wilens, T. 425
Wilens, T. E. 245
Wiley, C. A. 350
Wilk, S. 215
Wilker, A. 289, 304
Wilkinson, B. J. 245
Wilkinson, D. A. 355
Willcott, M. R. 57
Willett, W. C. 333
Willette, R. E. 306
Williams, J. 381
Williams, J. T. 246
Williams, M. J. 359
Williams, P. 86
Williams, R. 351–352
Williams, S. C. 266
Williams, T. R. 302
Williams, W. 47
Williamson, P. A. 242
Wilson, A. L. 244
Wilson, G. T. 52

Wilson, J. M. 184, 209
Wilson, J. R. 49, 53
Wilson, K. M. 265
Wilson, L. 380
Wilson, M. A. 180
Wilson, S. 97
Wilson, W. 244
Wilson, W. H. 83, 96, 151, 152, 356, 359
Wilson, W. P. 114–115
Winblad, B. 331, 336, 338
Winder, G. 230, 231
Winders, S. 235
Wing, L. L. 175
Winger, G. 86, 98, 172, 173, 178
Winsauer, P. J. 181
Winslow, J. T. 181
Winston, J. S. 58
Winters., L. 381
Wirsen-Meurling, A. 54
Wise, R. A. 52, 240
Wiser, A. 244
Witt, M. D. 350
Wittchen, H. U. 227
Witte, C. L. 358
Witte, E. A. 231, 240
Witte, M. H. 358
Wittling, W. 242
Wodak, A. 239
Wold, H. H. 444
Wolf, M. E. 302
Wolf, P. A. 241, 242, 326, 333, 335
Wolff, F. A. 127
Wolfson, T. 155
Wolkin, A. 121
Wong, A. 56, 60
Wong, C. T. 54
Wong, J. K. 302
Wonnacott, A. 238
Wood, P. L. 182
Woods, B. T. 47, 121, 266
Woods, J. H. 86, 98, 172, 173, 178
Woods, L. A. 444, 445
Woods, S. W. 300
Woodson, P. P. 232, 441
Woodward, K. G. 209
Woodward, R. 231, 232
Woolverton, W. L. 181, 208
Wuethrich, B. 47
Wyler, R. 240

Xie, T. 444
Xu, J. 426
Xu, Y. 243

Yague, A. G. 60
Yakazawa, T. 337
Yakehiro, M. 238
Yakimo, M. 291, 292, 300
Yamaguchi, S. 241, 335, 337
Yamamoto, B. K. 176, 177

Yamashita, K. 241, 335, 337
Yan, F. 293
Yanagisawa, M. 361
Yao, J. K. 327
Yardley, S. 381
Yarnold, P. 375
Yeh, S. H. 361
Yeh, S. Y. 444
Yen, D. J. 209
Yeomans, M. 171
Yetkin, F. Z. 241
Yeung, N. 53
Yim, G. K. 174
Ylinen, A. 58, 59
Yoritaka, A. 209
Yoshitake, T. 333
Young, A. B. 447
Young, A. C. 143
Young, C. W. 158
Young, R. 145, 176
Young, R. D. 440
Yuan, J. 179, 181, 444
Yuferov, V. 113
Yui, N. 361
Yule, W. 10
Yunger, L. M. 178
Yurgelun-Todd, D. A. 150, 151, 152, 153, 155, 386

Zack, M. 443
Zacny, J. P. 290, 292, 306
Zajdel, D. P. 230, 231
Zald, D. H. 116
Zandstra, S. M. 75
Zaragoza, J. G. 292
Zeidenberg, P. 158
Zekry, D. 332
Zelazo, P. D. 49, 52
Zelen, M. 158
Zernig, G. 173
Zhang, L. 353, 409–410, 411
Zhang, M. 235
Zhang, X. 238
Zhang, Z. 8, 14, 18, 25
Zhou, D. H. 335, 336
Zhou, F. C. 184
Zhou, H. 235
Zhou, Q. Y. 112
Zhu, Y. 377
Ziedonis, D. 391
Ziegler, J. A. 302
Ziegler, O. 159
Zieglgansberger, S. 445
Zinberg, N. E. 158, 438, 439
Zipursky, R. B. 54
Zubieta, J. K. 243
Zubin, J. 379
Zubovic, E. A. 50
Zumwalt, R. E. 302
Zvartau, E. E. 445

Subject index

Abstinent opioid abusers 276–277
Acute effects: alcohol 43–44; cocaine 117; dependent opioid abusers 281–288; marijuana 150–152; nicotine 228–231; nondependent opioid abusers 288–289
ADAM (Arrestee Drug Abuse Monitoring Program) 2–3, 8, 12, 13, 17, 22, 25
ADC (apparent diffusion coefficients) 188
ADHD (attention-deficit hyperactivity disorder) 129, 227, 230, 245, 246, 247, 426
Age/Aging: alcoholism and 46–47, 325–335; benzodiazepine use and neurocognitive disorders 337–339; smoking and 234–235; substance use and neuropsychological disorders 323–348
AIDS (acquired immune deficiency syndrome), 159, 349, 350, 352, 353, 354, 355, 360, 363, 358,
Alcohol 3–8, 37, 43–73, 323, 355–358; combination of cocaine and 127–128; comparison of opioid pharmacotherapies with 306; epidemiology of use in older adults 324; interaction studies of opioid pharmacotherapies with 305
Alzheimer's disease 243–244, 324, 325, 326, 327, 329, 330–332, 333, 334, 336, 338, 339; *see also* VaD
American Psychiatric Association 80, 81, 82, 83, 84, 85–86, 95, 98, 326; *see also* DSM-IV
amphetamine 280, 360–362, 446–447; *see also* MDMA; Methamphetamine
Animal models 77–80, 177–178, 208, 238–240, 263–265
ARCI (Addiction Research Center Inventory) 292, 293, 294
ARD (alcohol-related dementia) 326, 328–330, 334, 335, 339
Attentional networks 49–51
Attention/concentration 189, 193, 381–382

Behavioral economics 407–433
Bellevue hospital (New York City) 439
Benzodiazepines 28, 28–29, 37, 75–110, 337–339; epidemiology of use in older adults 325; interaction studies of opioid pharmacotherapies with 305
Binge and heavy drinking 37
Binswanger's disease 332
BMP (buprenorphine maintenance patients) 274, 277–278, 281, 302, 304, 305
Brain structures 55–62; *see also* CNS
Brodmann areas 420

Cambridge Gambling Task 422–423
Canada 325
Cannabis 157–159; *see also* Marijuana
CANTAB (Cambridge neuropsychological test automated battery) 280
Category test 298, 301
CCK (cholecystokinin) 445
Cerebrovascular effects: acute 117; residual 118–119
CEWG (Community Epidemiology Work Group) 3, 14, 15, 19, 23, 25, 28, 29, 31, 33–34, 35, 36
Chronic effects 234, 289–290
Cigarettes, *see* Nicotine
CNS (central nervous system) 77, 143, 144
Cocaine 12–15, 111–138, 351–353, 446–447
COGA (Collaborative Studies on Genetics of Alcoholism) 45
Cognition 211–218, 228–238
Cognitive effects: benzodiazepines 82–83; intoxication 48–55; nicotine 228–238; residual 86–95, 119–121
Cognitive functioning 326–327
Cognitive performance 267
Collaborative Neuropsychological Study of Polydrug Users 298
CPT (Continuous Performance Task) 189, 230, 243–245
CR (conditioned response) 445
Crack cocaine 1, 10, 12, 13, 14, 15, 19, 27, 31, 37, 111, 118, 427
Craving 123
Cross-cultural examinations 436–437
CS (conditioned stimulus) 425, 445

488 *Subject index*

CT (computerized tomography) scans 47, 95, 96, 266, 300–301

DAWN (Drug Abuse Warning Network) 16, 24, 32, 33; ED (emergency department) 2, 8, 11, 12–13, 22, 26, 28–29, 30, 31, 35, 36; ME (medical examiners) 2, 8, 13, 17, 22, 25, 27, 29
Dementia 243–244; *see also* Alzheimer's; ARD; VaD
Department of Health and Human Services (US) 228, 323, 324
DLPC (dorsolateral prefrontal cortex) 380, 381, 382, 383, 384, 385, 386
DOM (2, 5-dimethoxy-4-methylamphetamine) 176
Driving 97–100
Drug abusers 128, 129, 267, 298–299, 303, 364; dependent opioid, acute effects 281–288; Iowa and Cambridge Gambling Tasks in populations 422–423; neurobehavioral dysfunction 363; nonopioid, opioid abusers versus 279–280, 281, 290, 300; treatment relapse in 123
DSM-IV *(Diagnostic and Statistical Manual of Mental Disorders)* 22, 43, 111, 117, 145, 147, 214, 325, 328, 329, 330, 331, 332, 389
DSST (Digit Symbol Substitution Test) 273, 276, 287, 288–289, 291

Ecstasy, *see* MDMA
Electrophysiological studies 210–211
Emotional effects 95
Emotional functioning 122, 194–195
Environmental context 435–456
Epidemiological Catchment Area study 375
Epidemiology 1–39, 301–302, 324, 325; *see also* CEWG
Episodic memory 191
ERPs (event-related potentials) 49–51
EURODEM meta-analysis 331, 336
Executive function findings 231–233
Executive system functioning 194
Ex-smokers versus current smokers 236–237

FDA (US Food and Drug Administration) 325
fMRI (functional magnetic resonance imaging) 43, 47, 53, 54–55, 59, 114, 115, 118, 125, 126–127, 129, 149, 150, 153, 189–190, 191, 218, 220, 221, 230, 240–241, 242–243, 266, 301, 356, 380, 423–424
France 338

GABA (gamma-aminobutyric acid) 77–80, 82, 97, 144, 179, 338, 356
GAD (glutamate decarboxylase) 179
GBH (gamma hydroxybutyrate) 34–35
Gender: alcoholism and 47–48; smoking and 235–236

Genetics 45–46
Go/No-Go task 301
Gray matter 187

Halstead-Reitan Neuropsychological Battery 279, 296, 298–299
Hepatic encephalopathy 326, 327, 339
Heroin 23–25, 438
HIV infection 300, 305; neurobehavioral consequences of substance abuse and 349–375

Impulsive choice 407–433
Inhalants 9–11, 37
International Council on Alcohol, Drugs and Traffic Safety 306
Intertemporal bargaining 416–419, 425–426
Intoxication 80–85, 211–215, 267; effects of 48–55, 292–293, 304; mental health symptoms associated with 144–145
Iowa Gambling Task 124, 125, 421–423
Iowa Test of Achievement 120
IQ (Intelligence Quotient) 280, 296, 389

Ketamine 35–36

Laterality changes 242
Learning and memory findings 233–234
LL ("later-larger") reward 409, 415, 417, 418, 419
LSD (lysergic acid diethylamide) 10, 29–30, 34, 37, 142, 176, 196, 293, 437

Maddox Wing test 287, 291–292
Marijuana 20–23, 37, 139–170, 358–360
Massachusetts Mental Health Center 439
Mayo Clinic 326
MBD (Marchiafava-Bignami disease) 326
MCI (mild cognitive impairment) 326–327
MDMA (3, 4-methylenedioxymethamphetamine) 32–34, 171–206, 362; effect of ambient temperatures on neurotoxic effects of 444
Memory 233–234; nonverbal learning and 193; verbal, language and 384–386; *see also* Episodic memory; Working memory
Mental health symptoms/conditions 144–145, 147–149; alcohol and 48
Metabolic effects 118
Metabolic function 124–126
Methadone 25, 26–27, 263, 264, 265, 266, 267, 278, 288, 289, 292, 305, 354; high-dose 304; *see also* MMP
Methamphetamine 1, 15–20, 37, 178–179, 207–226
Mexico 293
Mini-Mental State Exam 326, 330
MMP (methadone maintenance patients) 272, 273, 274, 277, 279, 281, 290, 301, 355; daily dose 287, 300, 302; discontinuation 294–295; performance 280, 291, 293

Mood 194–195, 292–296, 300, 303
Morphine-induced analgesia 444–446
Motor/psychomotor speed 194
MRI (magnetic resonance imaging) 96, 114, 117, 359; *see also* fMRI; MRS
MRS (magnetic resonance spectroscopy) 187, 188
MTF (Monitoring the Future Survey) 1–2, 3, 9, 10, 12, 15–16, 20, 24, 26, 28, 31, 32–33, 35, 36

NART (Nelson Adult Reading Test) 275
National Institute of Justice 3, 31
Native religious users 293
Neurocognitive effects 117
Neuroimaging 210–211; *see also* CT; fMRI; PET; SPECT
NFLIS (National Forensic Laboratory Information System) 3, 14, 19, 23, 25, 28, 29, 30, 31, 32, 33, 35, 36
NIAAA (National Institute on Alcohol Abuse and Alcoholism) 45
Nicotine 227–262, 323
NIDA (National Institute on Drug Abuse) 1, 3, 10, 15, 23, 31, 147
NINCDS-ADRDA (Neurological and Communicative Disorders and Stroke and the Alzheimer's Disease and Related Disorders Association Joint Task Force) 330–331
NINDS-AIREN (National Institute of Neurological Disorders and Stroke and the Association Internationale pour la Recherche et l'Enseignement en Neurosciences) 332
NMDA ((N-methyl d-aspartate) 334, 445–446
NSDUH (National Survey on Drug Use and Health) 2, 7, 10, 12, 16, 20, 21, 24, 26, 28, 30, 31, 32, 33, 35, 36, 147, 324

Objective Opiate Withdrawal Scale 296
Opiates 25–28, 37, 353–355
Opioids 263–319

Parkinson's disease 209, 214, 245–246, 247, 329, 336
Pathophysiology 76–80, 300, 351; benzodiazepines 76–80; methamphetamine 280–211; opioids 263–267; schizophrenia 391, 393–395
PCAG (pentobarbital-chlorpromazinealcohol group) 292
PCP (phencyclidine) 30–32
Personality disorders 122
PET (positron emission tomography) 47, 53, 54–55, 96, 97, 114, 115, 118, 121, 124–125, 126, 129, 149, 150, 185, 186, 189, 240–241, 242–243, 265–266, 267, 327, 356
Physical health 48
Physiological changes 241–243

Polypharmacy 324, 339
POMS (Profile of Mood States) 292, 295, 296
Postmortems 46, 57, 76, 80, 113, 184, 185, 208–210, 265
Precommitment 412–415, 425–426
Psychedelic drugs 171, 173, 174, 439
Psychological effects 83–85
Psychomotor effects and impulsivity 52–54
Psychomotor findings 231
Psychomotor performance 267

QEEG (quantitative electroencephalography) 218

Race 236
Raven's Progressive Matrices 279
Relapse 123, 220
Residual effects: alcohol 43–44; benzodiazepines 85–95; marijuana 152–157; methamphetamine 215–220; opioid abusers in remission 280, 296–299, 300
Risk factors 299–300, 304, 324, 325

SAMHSA (Substance Abuse and Mental Health Services Administration) 2, 8, 10, 11, 12, 13, 16, 17, 22, 24, 25, 26, 27, 28, 29, 30, 31, 33, 35, 36, 227, 324–325
Schizophrenia 244–245; neurocognitive consequences of substance use in 375–404
SCR (skin conductance response) 421–422
Sedatives 28–29, 37
Self-control 407, 412, 415, 416–417, 418, 419, 420, 424–427
Semantic networks 51
Serotonin receptors 172, 174–177, 186–187, 188; *see also* SERT; SSRIs
SERT (serotonin reuptake transporter) 184, 186
Shipley-Hartford Scale 296
Smoking 324–325; *see also* Nicotine
SPECT (single photon emission computed tomography) 97, 114, 115, 122, 124, 126, 149, 150, 183, 184, 186, 187, 188–189, 208, 266, 267, 300, 327, 356
Speed, *see* Methamphetamine
SS ("smaller-sooner") reward 409, 415, 418, 419, 423, 426
SSRIs (serotonin selective reuptake inhibitors) 175–176
Subjective Opiate Withdrawal Scale 295, 296
Sweden 338

TEDS (Treatment Episode Data Set) 2, 8, 11, 12, 13, 16–17, 29, 30, 33, 35, 36
Temporal discounting 408–412
THC (delta-9 tetrahydrocannabinol) 139–141, 144, 145, 146, 150, 151, 153, 158, 161, 358–359, 437, 441
Tranquilizers 28–29, 37

UR (unconditioned response) 445
US (unconditioned stimulus) 425

VaD (vascular dementia) 324, 325, 326, 329, 330, 332–333, 336, 337, 339
VCI (vascular cognitive impairment) 332–333, 335
Vietnam 438
VMPFC (ventromedial prefrontal cortex) 420–424

WCST (Wisconsin Card Sorting Task) 194, 273, 275, 280, 291, 300, 381, 382
Weak Opiate Withdrawal Scale 295, 296
Wechsler Adult Intelligence Scale 298
White matter changes 241
WHO (World Health Organization) 85, 196, 207, 306, 332
Willpower 416–419
Withdrawal 88, 89, 92–95, 145–146; abrupt 101; effects of 294–295; intoxication and 76, 80–85, 211–215, 267; physiological and psychological 122–123
WKS (Wernicke-Korsakoff's syndrome), 326, 328, 334 339
Working memory 189–191, 382–383, 424–425